SUFFERING SAINTS

Jansenists and *Convulsionnaires* in France, 1640–1799

In Memoriam

To

Ronald S. Love

research partner, fellow traveler,
and friend

SUFFERING SAINTS

Jansenists and *Convulsionnaires* in France, 1640–1799

BRIAN E. STRAYER

sussex
ACADEMIC
PRESS
Brighton • Portland • Toronto

2 4 6 8 10 9 7 5 3 1

First published 2008 in Great Britain by
SUSSEX ACADEMIC PRESS
PO Box 139
Eastbourne BN24 9BP

Distributed in North America by
SUSSEX ACADEMIC PRESS
ISBS Publisher Services
920 NE 58th Ave #300, Portland, OR 97213, USA

British Library Cataloguing in Publication Data
A CIP catalogue record for this book is available from the British Library.

Library of Congress Cataloging-in-Publication Data
Strayer, Brian Eugene.
Suffering saints : Jansensists and Convulsionnaires in France, 1640–1799 / Brian Strayer.
p. cm.
Includes bibliographical references (p.) and index.
ISBN 978–1–84519–245–7 (h/c : alk. paper)
1. Jansenists—France. 2. Convulsionaries—France. 3. France—Church history—17th century. 4. France—Church history—18th century.
I. Title.

BX4723.S77 2008
282′.4409032—dc22

2007037714

Typeset and designed by SAP, Brighton & Eastbourne.

This book is printed on acid-free paper.

Contents

Graphs, Tables and Illustrations

Graphs and tables are between pages 192–205; illustrations, pages 112–117.

Graphs

Tables

Illustrations

Preface

Mention the Jansenists in front of a class of undergraduates and you are likely to get blank stares in return. Introduce the subject as an icebreaker at your next party and responses may vary from "Who were they?" to "Oh, yes, I've heard about them, but don't know much about them." Yet in the seventeenth and eighteenth centuries, the Jansenists, with their ascetic lifestyles and peculiar Augustinian twist on dogma, elicited the ire of both the Roman Catholic Church and the French state. Half a dozen papal bulls, dozens of royal *lettres de cachet*, scores of parlementary *arrêts* and *remonstrances*, and hundreds of sermons, pamphlets, and books attacked their beliefs between 1640 and 1799.

Although Jansenism (and its bizarre offshoot Convulsionism) enjoyed center-stage attention in France and across Europe for a century and a half, few historical surveys of this broad movement are available to the non-French reader today. J. D. Crichton's *Saints or Sinners?* (1996) focused only on seventeenth-century Jansenism, while William Doyle's *Jansenism* (2000) covered nearly three centuries in barely 100 pages. Alexander Sedgwick's *Travails of Conscience* (1998) dealt almost exclusively with the Arnauld family's role within the movement, while Dale Van Kley's *Religious Origins of the French Revolution* (1996) covered Calvinism, Jansenism, and other religious groups from the sixteenth to the end of the eighteenth century. These books, while thoroughly researched and well written, leave some questions unanswered.

Suffering Saints seeks to answer many of those questions, especially for readers unfamiliar with the persons, places, and events in the history of French Jansenism. Based on years of research in hundreds of primary and secondary sources from major archives and libraries in Paris and the United States, this comprehensive study of Jansenism and Convulsionism places the movement in the context of French political, social, economic, religious, and intellectual developments in the *ancien régime*. Students with a limited knowledge of Jansenism, its founders and their beliefs, will benefit from reading chapters 1 and 2, which provide biographical sketches of the key individuals (in chronological order) and briefly analyzes their major writings and their impact on the movement. Readers with a special interest in feminist history will find in chapters 3 and 4 a compelling narrative of the Port-Royal nuns' half-century struggle against Church and state to maintain their constitutional rights. College professors teaching classes in Old Regime France or focusing on religious controversies and the growth of toleration in Early Modern Europe will find in chapters 5 and 6 a description of the movement's internal conflicts and struggles against government and ecclesiastical persecution from 1713 to 1789. Even specialists in the field of Jansenist studies will find much that is new in this book. Chapters 1, 3, 4 and 9 contain updated historiographic sections that demonstrate what a minefield of controversial interpretations the historian of Jansenism must traverse. Chapters 6 and 8 offer innovative statistical analyses (based on the police archives at the Bibliothèque de l'Arsenal in Paris) of the differences in treatment that Jansenists and *convulsionnaires* at the Bastille received under Louis XIV and Louis XV.

Scholars unfamiliar with the Jansenist underground newspaper, the *Nouvelles Ecclésiastiques*, will gain fresh insights from the analyses of its contents found in chapters 5 through 8.

Finally, if a picture is worth a thousand words, this book presents twelve hitherto unpublished black and white sketches of life at Port-Royal des Champs, the controversial Jansenist convent southwest of Paris demolished by Louis XIV in 1709. I am especially grateful to M. Jean-Hugues Carbonnier, general secretary of the Société de l'histoire du protestantisme français, for granting permission to Sussex Academic Press to publish these rare prints taken from Manuscript 124 in the Collection Sainte-Beuve at the Bibliothèque de l'histoire du protestantisme français.

Historical surveys, by their very nature, emphasize breadth over depth. Although *Suffering Saints* attempts to discuss the key individuals, ideas, and events of the Jansenist movement in Paris and the Ile-de-France from 1640 to 1799, it would require more than one volume to adequately cover the topic of Jansenism in France and across Europe. Moreover, this book, as a companion volume to my *Huguenots and Camisards as Aliens in France, 1589–1789* (2001), focuses primarily on the theme of church–state conflicts and the slow growth of religious toleration in France. Those interested in further reading on this and related topics should consult the extensive bibliography found at the end of the book.

Acknowledgments

John Donne's famous line, "No man is an island, entire of itself," certainly applies to writing a book. From the shaping of ideas discussed in these pages to the preparation of final copy, I have enjoyed the encouragement and support of many individuals and institutions whose assistance I am happy to acknowledge.

It was at a conference of the Western Society for French History at Rosario Resort on Orcas Island, Washington, in 1992 that Professor Albert Hamscher of Kansas State University planted the seed for this book. He suggested that my life-long interest in religious liberty, my conservative religious education, and my familiarity with social control issues in *ancien régime* France made a perfect combination for writing a critical study of dissident religious groups such as the Huguenots, Camisards, Jansenists, and *Convulsionnaires*. Six years of research and writing (1994—1999) led to the publication of my book *Huguenots and Camisards as Aliens in France, 1598–1789: The Struggle for Religious Toleration* (Edwin Mellen Press, 2001). *Suffering Saints*, which focuses on the rise, persecution, and demise of Jansenism and convulsionism in France from 1640 to 1799, is the companion volume.

During the time devoted to research and writing, I have received generous financial support from the Office of Scholarly Research at Andrews University, Berrien Springs, MI, and from a Walter C. Utt research grant from Pacific Union College in Angwin, CA. Andrews' grants of more than $20,000 enabled me to spend several summers in Paris in 1995, 1997, 2000, 2003, and 2005, while the Utt grant of $30,000 paid for a teaching assistant and gave me a year-long sabbatical. During 2000–2001, I completed most of the research and writing for three subsequently published books: *Huguenots and Camisards as Aliens in France* (Edwin Mellen Press, 2001), *The Bellicose Dove: Claude Brousson and Protestant Resistance to Louis XIV, 1647–1698* (Sussex Academic Press, 2003), and *Suffering Saints* (Sussex Academic Press, 2008).

In the United States, I am most grateful for the help of Sandra White, Office of Interlibrary Loans at the James White Library of Andrews University, for helping me quickly obtain rare and recently published sources. In France, I wish to thank the dozens of staff members in the *Salle de Travaille*, *Manuscrits*, and *Périodiques* at the old Bibliothèque Nationale (rue de Richelieu) and at the Bibliothèque de l'Arsenal (Bastille Collection) for their absolutely indispensable services in obtaining rare manuscripts and printed materials. The young women at the Bibliothèque de l'Histoire du Protestantisme Français (Paris) brought me rare Jansenist and *convulsionnaire* sources from the Fonds Sainte-Beuve collection with cheerfulness and speed worthy of the Calvinist work ethic. They have also gone the extra mile in providing illustrations for this book.

As with my book *Lettres de cachet and Social Control in the Ancien Régime, 1659–1789* (Peter Lang Publishing, 1992), Dr. Jerry Thayer, Professor of Research and Statistical Methodology at Andrews University, helped me generate meaningful graphs and tables on the Jansenists and *convulsionnaires* detained at the Bastille from 1659 to 1789, a major statistical contribution of this book. I am indebted to Deborah Everhart, editor at Andrews University Press, for assisting me with the index and solving several computer glitches along the way.

Professor Ellen Weaver-Laporte, who volunteered to read an earlier draft of this manuscript, provided invaluable insights and timely criticism in several areas, particularly on the topics of monasticism, the Cistercian roots of Port-Royal, and Augustinian ideas within Jansenism. I have benefited enormously from her suggestions, and any lack of clarity on my part should not be laid at her doorstep.

Finally, I am grateful for the enthusiasm, cooperation, and expertise of Anthony Grahame, Editorial Director, and his staff at Sussex Academic Press, and for their patience and skill in transforming my efforts into this monograph. I hope that it will shed new light on the discussion concerning the meaning of religious pluralism, persecution, toleration, and liberty in *ancien régime* France.

BRIAN E. STRAYER
Andrews University
September 5, 2007

Introduction
Jansenism in France

To help readers understand the complexity of this religious controversy, *Suffering Saints* highlights twelve major themes which, like golden threads, can be traced through the fabric that comprised the Jansenist movement. These themes include suffering, saintliness, the search for truth, Gallicanism (as well as Richerism and conciliarism), church–state conflicts, contradictions and paradoxes, internal diversity, political thought and action, human interest stories, passive resistance, the impact of papal bulls, and the slow growth of toleration in France.

1. Suffering

Jansenists, true to their Benedictine roots and Cistercian heritage, adopted ascetic lifestyles, praised self-denial in others, expressed courage amidst persecution, found comfort in hard labor and severe penance, and (in the case of the *convulsionnaires*), deliberately tortured one another at religious gatherings. In a petition to Louis XIV in 1668, Antoine Arnauld (their chief spokesman) declared that Christians should defend the truth "by suffering; not by shedding others' blood, but by giving their own."[1] He encouraged the nuns at Port-Royal, a Jansenist convent in Paris, to view all their afflictions as "holocausts of [God's] love" to sanctify them and, in the end, to prepare them for crowns of glory.[2]

Like Antony, Cassian, Augustine, Pachomius, Basil, and scores of other hermits and cenobites during the previous millennium who served as their models, Jansenists embraced the ascetic lifestyles they imposed on themselves and others. Following the guidelines laid down by St. Augustine (397 AD), St. Jerome and John Cassian (420s AD), and in the famous sixth century *Rule* of St. Benedict, they adopted the practices of asceticism, including fasting, poverty, chastity, veiling, severe penance, long prayers, and minute self-examination.[3] When the abbess Angélique Arnauld reformed the convent of Port-Royal, for example, she imposed on the sisters a rigid regimen of prayer, liturgical services, poverty, simplicity, silence, solitude, and discipline. Their scorn for worldly comforts and pessimistic view of human nature, however, predisposed Jansenists to oppose not only sinful pleasures, but also much of the cultural progress of the age (Baroque art, music, dance, literature, and theatre) as spiritually worthless.

Asceticism combined with pious opposition to Church and state policies often brought persecution, but Jansenists, like the first century martyrs they imagined themselves to be, welcomed their sufferings. In scores of letters, Angélique Arnauld encouraged her friends to be happy amidst pain, find glory in affliction, seek hope in injustice, and suffer as faithful witnesses for the truth.[4]

By the end of the eighteenth century, however, the *convulsionnaires* had taken the theme of suffering to bizarre extremes. During the 1720s and 1730s, their outdoor public seances in Paris' Saint-Médard Cemetery often featured babbling in unknown tongues, writhing in convulsions, and alleged healing miracles. But after police repression drove them underground, their *secours* (secret meetings in homes) grew progressively more brutal as attendees beat, pierced, cut, burned, and crucified willing participants. By that time, suffering in defense of the truth had become sadomasochism for its own sake.

2. Saintliness

Although most Roman Catholic Church officials considered Jansenists at best schismatic and at worst, heretical, Jansenists saw themselves as "true Catholics" who followed the teachings of the fourth century Church Father St. Augustine. To them, Augustinianism—with its emphasis on man's original sin, God's efficacious grace, weak human willpower, and the necessity for strict morality—had been the essence of Catholicism for 1300 years. Jansenists considered Augustinianism the touchstone of orthodoxy, whereas their opponents the Jesuits considered Catholic dogma (shaped by history and incorporating the Council of Trent's theological innovations) as their orthodoxy. While the Jesuits espoused an optimistic view of human beings with free will, Jansenists held a pessimistic concept of sinful humans lacking free will.

Consequently, the best way to counteract one's sinful nature and prepare for God's saving grace was by walking "the narrow road of asceticism," the only true path for a saint. As described above, this life of self-denial included severe fasts, long prayers, solitude, self-examination, silence, and infrequent participation in Communion. But it also embraced other practices not adopted by mainstream Catholics: Mass in the vernacular, a strong emphasis on scripture, and, by the eighteenth century, a focus on the cross (rather than the sacred heart of Jesus). In their pursuit of saintliness, the Jansenist nuns at Port-Royal des Champs southwest of Paris adopted the triple solitude of Cistercians. First, by dwelling within walled enclosures, they separated themselves from the world; second, by living in tiny rooms, they isolated themselves from one another; third, by taking the vow of silence, they denied their selfish human nature.

To keep their souls pure, Jansenists, like religious ascetics of centuries past, contemplated death and dying. "Meditating on death," Pasquier Quesnel wrote in *Christian Instructions* (1671), "has always been seen by the Saints of the Old and New Testaments as the most certain preservative against sin."[5] Nuns and monks, having taken the three-fold vow of poverty, chastity, and obedience, became "dead" to the world and to themselves. In addition, dwelling on Christ's passion and crucifixion made one more willing to deny self. Thinking about death during bouts of sickness and pain kept one humble and prepared the soul for eternal life; illness itself became a "state of penance" to be borne willingly after the example of the suffering Christ. Jansenists welcomed suffering as a sanctifying, double grace that readied one for a "good death," the death of a saint in defense of the truth.[6]

3. Truth

Verité (truth) was the key word in Jansenist writings, for they saw themselves as defenders of certain doctrines (such as efficacious grace) neglected by the Catholic Church. They believed that truth, which comes from God, must be vigorously defended. Although at times suppressed, it would in the end triumph over falsehood if strong, independent-minded proponents (the "Friends of the Truth" as they called themselves) defended it. This search for truth inspired Jansenist educators to establish the *Petites Ecoles* ("little schools") to teach both girls and boys how to find "God's truth" and combat "Jesuit errors."

Their letters and books demonstrate just how much Jansenists hated error and slander. Angélique Arnauld told a friend that "it is necessary to repulse with force and vigor that which is said with such insolence against the truth . . . Forceful [arguments] that confuse the enemies of God and the Church are not unchristian."[7] Truth had the power to enlighten the ignorant and vanquish enemies, whose number by the eighteenth century included popes, kings, government ministers, bishops, the Jesuits, and the philosophes.

Indeed, truth was even worth dying for if necessary. In their ongoing battle with popes and kings over the Formulary (an oath required by various papal bulls that condemned Cornelius Jansen's book *Augustinus*), Jansenists put conscience above submission. Refusing to sign that "cowardly covenant with death," Blaise Pascal's sister Jacqueline, a nun at Port-Royal in 1661, exclaimed that "it is [time] for us to die for the truth."[8]

The spiritually sadistic *convulsionnaires* in the eighteenth century, with their penchant for martyrdom, were eager to die for the truth. Their apocalyptic focus on end-time events galvanized them to prepare the way for the return of Elijah by shedding their own blood. White-robed baptismal candidates were routinely asked: "Are you willing to die for the truth?" The correct response was: "To the degree that God gives me the grace to do it, such are [my] sentiments."[9]

4. Gallicanism, Richerism, Conciliarism

If theological truth was worth dying for, so too were certain political truths such as Gallicanism, Richerism, and conciliarism. Unlike the Jesuits, whose fourth vow of implicit obedience to the pope made them avid ultramontanists, the Jansenists never accepted the infallibility of popes and denied papal power over kings and bishops. Instead, they espoused a triple Gallicanism: episcopal (bishops to preserve their authority *vis-à-vis* popes and kings); royal (kings to be independent of popes); and parliamentary (Parlement to be free from the domination of Rome). Fearing a Jesuit conspiracy and papal domination, they boldly defended Gallican liberties—a position that attracted many merchants, lawyers, judges, and *parlementaires* to their ranks.

These liberties were encapsulated in the famous four "Gallican Articles" drafted by the General Assembly of the Clergy in 1681. These Articles state that in temporal matters French kings have absolute sovereignty; that in spiritual matters the pope's authority is subject to general church councils; that traditions and customs limit papal authority in France; and that papal decisions require the consent of the Gallican Church to be effective. Over the next century, adherence to these Articles often pitted Gallicans, Jansenists, Richerists, and *parlementaires* against the papacy, the monarchy, and the Jesuits in numerous debates over papal bulls condemning Jansenism.

"Richerism" took its name from Edmond Richer, dean of the Faculty of Theology at the Sorbonne, whose powerful *Book of Ecclesiastical and Political History* (1611) advanced several ideas that shaped church–state relations for the next two centuries. In his book, Richer asserts that French kings, sovereign by divine right, are independent of other authorities, including popes. In the Gallican Church, the exercise of power rests with the "body of pastors" (bishops, archbishops, cardinals) in general councils (the only infallible Church authority). Bishops, he states, should be elected by the clergy, gathered together in synods, and confirmed by the king and the people.[10]

Although separate in the seventeenth century, Richerism and Jansenism fused in the eighteenth century *parlementaire* resistance to Louis XIV and Louis XV—and Gallicanism was the glue that bonded them together. "Ecclesiastical democracy" reappeared in Pasquier Quesnel's works exalting the authority of the lower clergy, in the debates over the Bull *Unigenitus* (1713), in priests' demands in the 1770s for greater representation on diocesan panels, and in the National Assembly's discussion of the Civil Constitution of the Clergy in 1790.

Conciliarism—the appeal to Church councils rather than to the pope's authority—went hand in glove with Richerism and Gallicanism. Jansenist spokesmen like Antoine Arnauld and Pasquier Quesnel advocated conciliarism in their writings as an antidote to papal infallibility and the Formulary on the one hand and to the perceived arbitrariness of a divine right monarch on the other. Perhaps, Arnauld suggested in *Considerations on Matters in the Church* (1681), Church and state should operate in separate but complementary spheres.[11]

5. Church–state Conflicts

In real life, however, this proved impossible because in France, Church and state had been intertwined for 1200 years. Consequently, the Jansenists' outspoken defense of conciliarism, Gallicanism, and Richerism frequently embroiled them in controversies with both religious and political authorities.

Jansenists crossed swords with popes on several battlefields. In the political realm, they opposed those who advocated papal infallibility (not officially defined until the nineteenth century) and exalted the authority of Church councils. In theology, they emphasized the doctrines of St. Augustine (Augustinianism) more than the teachings of St. Thomas Aquinas (Thomism). As noted in section eleven below, they vociferously opposed the Formulary and the six papal bulls (from 1643 to 1713) that condemned the works of Jansen and Quesnel.

As Richerists, they clashed with several archbishops of Paris (Péréfixe, Harlay de Champvallon, and Noailles) over enforced signing of the Formulary, the distinction between *droit* (right) and *fait* (fact), and the orthodoxy of the two Port-Royal convents. Jansenist bishops demanded that their judicial authority be respected by Parlement and the Church hierarchy; they disagreed with Parlement's placing recalcitrant bishops on trial, a frequent practice during the 1730s and 1750s "refusal of sacraments" controversy.

Jansenists considered Jesuits enemies for several reasons. Theologically, they disagreed with their Molinist position on sufficient grace and free will. Philosophically, they opposed their lax morality and casuistry. Politically, they distrusted their tolerance for contrary dogmas and their love of hierarchical authority. Economically, they despised their imposing tributes on other religious groups in Catholic countries. Jansenist diatribes for 150 years labeled the Jesuits hypocrites, liars, persecutors, plotters, and murderers.

Jansenists occasionally found themselves at odds with the Gallican Church's highest administrative body, the General Assembly of the Clergy. Established in 1561, this Assembly of 30 to 60 bishops and other clergy met every five or ten years in Paris to vote on the *don gratuit* (cash gift) to the king, to lobby for Church reforms, and to find ways of combating heresy in the realm. Over time, its authority encompassed all spiritual and temporal matters relating to the French Church, including such matters as finances, censorship, ecclesiastical appointments, the Regale, the *vingtième,* and Jansenism. In their battle against Jansenism, the bishops saw Parlement as the "redoubtable enemy," especially during the eighteenth century.[12]

In addition, the administrative clergy in the Assembly often crossed swords with the Church's teaching clergy at the Sorbonne, the theological department within the University of Paris. Although the theology faculty saw themselves as the final judges in theological disputes, the Assembly frequently asserted its right to intervene and overrule if necessary the Sorbonne's decisions. In 1659, suspecting that the Office of the Holy Sacrament (supported by members of the Arnauld family close to the Sorbonne) had "a Jansenist spirit" about it, Archbishop François de Harlay, president of the Assembly, condemned the Office and asked Alexander VII to have the Inquisition examine it further. Then in 1682–83, another battle ensued when the Sorbonne opposed the Assembly's registration of the Four Gallican Articles and its continued efforts to rein in the faculties' authority in doctrinal matters. Further clashes occurred when the Assembly attempted to coerce the faculty into signing the Formulary and other oaths of orthodoxy.[13]

Staunchly Gallican, pro-Richerist, and anti-Jesuit, the theology faculty at the Sorbonne resented efforts by Louis XIV, the chancellor, and bishops to control their decisions regarding Jansenism. The Sorbonne registered the Bulls *Cum occasione* (1653) and *Ad sacram* (1656) only after years of debate stirred up by its pro-Jesuit dean Nicolas Cornet. Despite bullying by Louis XIV and Louis XV, its theologians refused to be silent in the "Case of Conscience" (1700) and refusal of sacraments (1750s) debates.

Louis XIV saw Jansenists as a cabal against Church and government authority, heretics and rebels whose "republicanism" clashed with his love of hierarchical authority. He and his successor Louis XV (unsuccessfully) marshaled popes, bishops, the Sorbonne, and Parlement to crush the movement with papal bulls, bishops' mandates, and *lettres de cachet* (royal arrest warrants). In response, Jansenists wrote books, filed lawsuits, signed petitions, and published a successful underground newspaper (the *Ecclesiastical News*).

The monarchy's repeated attempts to use Parlement to condemn Jansenism failed largely because many of its members sympathized with the movement and fought to protect their jurisdictional rights. Only when Louis XIV personally appeared at *lits de justice* did Parlement register the papal bulls of 1653 and 1657. But their opposition to the 1713 Bull and to the refusal of sacraments in the 1730s and 1750s opened a rift between the monarchy and the magistrates and helped cause the French Revolution.

6. Contradictions and Paradoxes

Being human, Jansenists evinced contradictions and paradoxes from time to time. Saint-Cyran confessed that he had a "celestial temperament" composed of "fire and ice, which makes me sometimes self-contradictory."[14] If one side of his temperament was cordial, happy, and kind, the other side tended toward austerity and melancholy, making him a somber man with a joyous heart, brilliant but excitable, stern yet affectionate. Although an inflexible defender of doctrinal truth, he could be calculating and devious in his political dealings with Cardinal Richelieu.

Blaise Pascal's *Provincial Letters* (1656), arguably the strongest defense of Jansenism in the seventeenth century, nonetheless engendered a mixed response from his Jansenist friends. Pierre Nicole considered the *Letters* a "just defense of truth" and Antoine Arnauld bragged that they had altered public opinion and "changed . . . the face of Jesuit affairs." But Antoine Singlin and Angélique Arnauld felt that their satirical tone and argumentative style did not constitute a model of Christian charity or piety.[15]

Likewise Jansenists' temporary liaison with Cardinal de Retz during the Fronde (1648–1653) represented a significant departure from their creed of rejecting the world. Their association with the controversial cardinal at a time when Retz opposed many of the king's ecclesiastical policies led Louis XIV and Cardinal Mazarin to consider them *frondeurs* (rebels); this damaged their public image for generations.

Consequently, Louis XIV considered the Jansenist nuns of Port-Royal de Paris and Port-Royal des Champs a "nest of heretics," despite the fact that they took vows of poverty, chastity, obedience, and stability like other Cistercian nuns. In other ways, however, they did not conform to monastic norms. For example, neither the nuns nor their students were compelled to attend Mass unless they felt worthy to take the sacraments. Their colleagues the *messieurs*, a group of pious hermits who lived at the hilltop farm called The Grange, took no monastic vows. In an era that considered manual labor socially discreditable if not shameful, they grew fruit and vegetables and milked cows while reading their Bibles and translating theological works.

7. Internal Diversity

Many of the paradoxes within Jansenism arose because of the tremendous spectrum of diversity within its ranks. The movement included liberals like Robert Arnauld d'Andilly and the Bishop of Comminges who sympathized with Jansenism but made accommodations to secular society because they hoped to advance within it, and therefore never adopted an ascetic ideology of their own. It embraced moderates like Antoine Arnauld and Pierre Nicole who sought a balance between compliance to authority and a demand for justice. In their struggle for goodness and truth, they created for themselves a more restricted sphere within the world. It also encompassed ascetics like Saint-Cyran, Martin de Barcos, Antoine Singlin, and Angélique Arnauld who lived lives of self-denial either at home or at Port-Royal and rejected everything they considered worldly. It absorbed extremists like Jacqueline Pascal and Guillaume Le Roy who made no concession to Church or state authority and who proclaimed goodness and right in an evil world they expected to persecute them.

Finally, in the eighteenth century, the rise of the fanatical *convulsionnaires* split the Jansenist movement into several antagonistic factions, including Figurists (who imitated the moments of Christ's passion), Visionaries (who had spiritual dreams), and Thaumaturges (who focused on healing miracles). As their seances became more violent and bizarre after the 1730s, groups took the names of their founders (as "Augustinians," "Margouillistes," "Vaillantistes," and "Ottinistes"). Finally, the introduction of the *grands secours* (crucifixions) further split the movement into "Secouristes" (who favored such sado-masochistic practices) and "Anti-Secouristes" (who opposed them).

Moreover, throughout the movement's history, divisions appeared in response to specific incidents or issues. Regarding the Formulary, Saint-Cyran felt one could sign it even if he did not believe that the five condemned propositions were found in Jansen's writings. Pierre Nicole sought a compromise measure based on the right/fact distinction. Antoine Arnauld, who argued that conscience and Christian sincerity prevented one from signing, advocated "respectful silence" instead. Jacqueline Pascal and the Port-Royal nuns, however, refused any compromise measures and initiated a program of civil disobedience described in section ten below.

8. Political Thought and Action

Although Jansenists professed to despise the world, they often found themselves drawn into secular debates and controversies because, in a divine right monarchy, many of their theological positions had social, economic, and political ramifications. As early as 1634, Cornelius Jansen, in his controversial *Mars Gallicus*, attacked Richelieu's diplomatic aims in Flanders and urged Louis XIII to sever his alliances with the Protestant Germans, Swedes, and Turks. Jansen debated what constituted a "just war" and suggested that when a king made military alliances against Catholic states, his subjects had no obligation to obey him. *Mars Gallicus* unleashed a hurricane of controversy among the *politiques* and *dévots* in France and across Europe.

As mentioned in section five, Jansenists' involvement with Cardinal de Retz during the Fronde further tainted their reputation as *frondeurs* espousing a "mentality of opposition" to Louis XIV and Mazarin. When the pro-Jansenist *duc* de Luynes rebelled, the king blamed Jansenism as the root cause, and when many Paris ecclesiastics supported Retz in his on-going battle with Mazarin, Louis held Port-Royal responsible. Several of the convent's most avid supporters—the *princesse* de Guémenée, the *duchesse* de Chevreuse, the *comte* de Chavigny, the *duc* de Liancourt—had close ties with actual *frondeurs*. In 1649 and 1652 Robert Arnauld d'Andilly, Antoine Arnauld's brother, wrote pamphlets attacking Mazarin and the Queen Mother for financial mismanagement, poor appointments to political offices, and failures in the war with Spain.

During the 1670s and 1680s, controversies over the Regale, the Formulary, and the Four Gallican Articles helped shape the politics of Port-Royal as Jansenists sought ways to balance Gallican liberties with papal power so that conciliarism could check ultramontanism in France. While Antoine Arnauld defended the pope and condemned Louis XIV for "usurping" regalian rights (taking Church property for profit), he also exalted the authority of Church councils as checks on papal power.[16]

The *convulsionnaires*, with their anti-social behavior and politically subversive ideas, upset this delicate balancing act between Church and state authority. While they never openly attacked Louis XV or Church officials, their religious, political, and social ideals subverted many of the cherished values of the *ancien régime*: order, hierarchy, corporate privilege. Their fraternal, egalitarian society and democratic, congregational polity constituted a serious indictment of the established order in both Church and state. Their claims of miraculous healing challenged the king's exclusive power to heal ("the king's touch"); likewise, their secret seances challenged the Church's right to control all religious activity. One *secouriste's* prayer, calling Louis XV an "errant and fugitive criminal," expressed the hope that "the Lord will undermine what you have built . . . and crush your house . . . that superb palace which for such a long time has been the seat of injustice and iniquity."[17]

Finally, although neither the Jansenists nor the *convulsionnaires* led the campaign to overthrow Chancellor Maupeau in 1770, they did participate in it, joining with old enemies (including the philosophes) who understood that the chancellor's reform program would undermine Parlement's authority. Led by the *abbé* Claude Mey and *parlementaire* Louis-Adrien Le Paige, these "Jansenist patriots" published 80 pamphlets comparing the "despotism" of Maupeou and past popes and contrasting Henri IV (the patriot-king) and Louis XV (the despot-king). They urged all true patriots to unite in checking the arbitrary power of Maupeou.[18]

9. Human Interest Stories

For 150 years, the rise, development, and decline of Jansenism in France unfolded amidst a human drama that witnessed pathos, humor, anguish, ecstasy, controversy, joy, brutality, and generosity. By means of human-interest stories, this book portrays the Jansenists as real people, not cardboard saints; they experienced love, happiness, and awe as well as sorrow, pain, and loss.

There is slapstick comedy in 1619 when Angélique d'Estrées, the dissolute abbess of Maubuisson, physically wrestles with Angélique Arnauld, the young abbess of Port-Royal, and temporarily prevents her from reforming Maubuisson by throwing her through the gate of the convent. There is bawdy humor when Luzancy Arnauld d'Andilly, a solitaire living at Port-Royal des Champs in 1645, has sex with his wife several times a night yet begs God for forgiveness for indulging his carnal appetite the next morning. There is wit when Cardinal de Retz in 1664 visits Versailles after twelve years in exile and responds to Louis XIV's observation that "your hair has grown whiter" by saying, "Sire, one grows whiter quickly when one has the misfortune of being in disgrace with Your Majesty."[19] There is delightful impertinence when, after listening to Archbishop of Paris Péréfixe's biased report on Port-Royal's "Little Schools," one ten-year-old pupil quips, "I admire the profoundness of God's judgments for having given us a prelate as ignorant as you are!"[20]

On the other hand, one senses the Port-Royal sisters' awe when in 1656, Blaise Pascal's niece Marguerite Périer, suffering excruciating pain from a cancerous ulcer near her left eye, is healed immediately at the touch of a thorn allegedly from Christ's crown of thorns on the cross. One feels the drama in 1668 when Robert Arnauld d'Andilly ushers his aging Uncle Antoine Arnauld into Louis XIV's throne room at Versailles. There, on his knees, Arnauld thanks the king "for the greatest happiness that has ever come to me" and praises him for bringing about the famous "Peace of the Church."[21] And in 1713, when Clement XI's Bull *Unigenitus* condemned 101 propositions in Pasquier Quesnel's book *Moral Reflections on the New Testament*, one can feel Quesnel's anguish as he reads it to three friends with tears streaming down his face—and then spends four hours in prayer.

Following the contorted history of the *convulsionnaire* movement is like watching the ever-changing acts in a vaudeville show. We see the pious ascetic Deacon Pâris in 1727 beating and starving himself into an early grave at St.-Médard Cemetery in Paris. Almost immediately, his tomb becomes a Mecca for pilgrims seeking miraculous healing, but the situation quickly degenerates as shouting, dancing, babbling, prophesying, and convulsions occur. The police move in, close down the cemetery, and begin jailing Jansenists. One is *Père* Creigny, the pistol-packing priest accused of convulsionism, sexual improprieties, and bilking his followers of 14,000 *livres* (and many pounds of chocolate); in 1735 Louis XV imprisons him at the chateau of Vincennes. Persecution forces the *convulsionnaires* underground and, as chapters 7 and 8 describe, they soon begin exhibiting behavior almost too bizarre to be believed.

10. Passive Resistance

Centuries before Henry David Thoreau, Mahatma Gandhi, and Martin Luther King, Jr. popularized methods of civil disobedience, the Jansenists pioneered both the theory and practice for resisting divine right authority in Church and state. As early as 1657, Antoine Arnauld defined two kinds of submission: positive (taking an oath to obey an ordinance) and negative (promising not to obstruct an ordinance). He stated that since Christians could not sin against their consciences and act contrary to truth, negative submission was acceptable when legitimate authorities tried to coerce one's conscience. Such "non-resistance," he said, "conserves the good order of States."[22]

For over a century, Jansenists used this argument to resist papal efforts to force them to sign the Formulary and to block royal attempts at coercing bishops and *parlementaires* into enforcing papal bulls in France. During the seventeenth century, a cohesive group of Port-Royal supporters used letters, speeches, books, petitions, and lawsuits to block government and Church actions against the convent. This pious propaganda upheld the values of truth, justice, liberty, charity, and grace, and opposed "blind obedience" to authority as harmful to one's conscience.

Although Angélique Arnauld had told her friends in 1653 to "Pray, weep, groan: your tears will do more than your writings,"[23] increasing government harassment after 1656 soon made her an advocate of passive resistance. Using Catholic canon law and patristic misogynistic attitudes to their advantage, Arnauld and her Port-Royal nuns argued that as women, they were "weaker vessels" forbidden to study Latin and canon law or engage in theological debates. Therefore, in their ignorance, they should not be required to sign a Formulary whose issues they could not understand; instead, Church officials should accept their "respectful silence" as a token of their submission.

Port-Royal's abbesses used this "theology of weakness" (what Daniella Kostroun calls "the feminist paradox")[24] to effectively defy what they considered the illegitimate use of authority by Louis XIV, the pope, and the archbishop of Paris when they tried to force them to sign the Formulary "against God's will." Thus, they blended defiance and acquiescent suffering into a balancing act of passive opposition. Putting their consciences above conformity, they walked a fine line between martyrdom and rebellion. By taking this stand—and being willing to die for it—the nuns shaped the theological, legal, rhetorical, and gender-based argument for resistance earlier advanced by Antoine Arnauld.

Adopting a tone of wounded innocence, naivete, and deep earnestness, these clever nuns used reams of paper and barrels of ink in their own defense. Seeing every exercise of Church or state authority against them—no matter how small—as "persecution," they wrote hundreds of protest letters. Manipulating elections, forcing signatures on the Formulary, transferring nuns, selling convent property, refusing them the sacraments, imprisoning their lawyer—all were unjust "afflictions" they could not endure. Although Archbishop Péréfixe denounced them as "pure as angels and proud as Lucifer," their campaign of passive resistance delayed the closing of Port-Royal des Champs for half a century.

11. Impact of Papal Bulls

But the nuns were not the only ones working like the devil for the Lord. With the best of intentions, three popes between 1643 and 1713 issued six bulls that had the effect of poisoning church–state relations in France and Europe for a century and a half.

Although Urban VIII's *In eminenti* (1643) did not specifically label Cornelius Jansen's work *Augustinus* (1640) heretical, it did condemn the book for contravening Pius VI's earlier Bull *De Auxiliis* (1618) imposing silence on debates concerning grace. *In eminenti* likewise forbade discussions on grace, free will, and predestination on pain of excommunication and condemned a long list of pro-Jansenist works. Officials used this bull to remove Antoine Arnauld from the Sorbonne when he broke the "law of silence" two years later. But few in France paid it much attention.

So in 1653, Innocent X, claiming to be guided solely by the Holy Spirit, issued the Bull *Cum occasione* to condemn five heretical propositions allegedly found in the *Augustinus*. By so doing, he hoped to upstage the Gallican bishops as the sole decision-makers on policies curbing Jansenism in France, demonstrate his superiority to the doctors of theology at the Sorbonne, boost the prestige of the Jesuits, and buttress his claim to infallibility. Instead, he unleashed a firestorm of protest during which most Jansenists admitted that the pope had the *right* to condemn the five propositions as heretical, but asserted that in *fact* those propositions could not be found in the *Augustinus*. This "right/fact" distinction and the appeal to "respectful silence" represented the response of most Jansenists when confronted with the new Formulary.

This new "oath of orthodoxy" constituted the heart of Alexander VII's Bull *Ad sacram* (1656), which condemned the five propositions "as Jansen meant them" as "impious, blasphemous, heretical, anathema, false, calumnious, and injurious to the goodness of God."[25] Yet because these propositions could also be interpreted as orthodox (if seen through Augustinian lenses) or as semi-Pelagian (if examined through Jesuit lenses), this bull reaped a whirlwind of debate and opposition across France. Many bishops opposed it while the Jansenists, asserting that the pope had misunderstood Jansen's thought, continued to use the right/fact distinction for refusing to sign the Formulary.

So Alexander VII issued a second bull—*Regiminis apostolici* (1665)—which once again condemned the five propositions and declared the right/fact distinction meaningless. This bull required the laity to take an oath of orthodoxy and the clergy to sign the Formulary. But when the bull reached France, Parlement balked at registering it, 40 bishops denounced it, and Jansenists *still* refused to sign the Formulary.

Under pressure from Louis XIV and Philip V, therefore, Clement XI, after fasting three days, released the Bull *Vineam domini* (1705), which condemned the position of "respectful silence" concerning the five propositions and affirmed the pope's infallibility when speaking on matters of faith and doctrine. Although Parlement and the General Assembly of the Clergy voted their approval and Louis XIV expressed his conviction that the bull would crush the Jansenists, in reality it gave political Jansenism a much-needed shot in the arm.

Consequently, when Clement XI issued the Bull *Unigenitus* (1713)—a belated condemnation of 101 propositions in Pasquier Quesnel's *Moral Reflections* (1672)—it faced a firestorm of opposition from the General Assembly of the Clergy, Parlement, the Sorbonne, Archbishop of Paris Noailles, and Procurer-general D'Aguesseau. Long after Louis XIV's death in 1715, *Unigenitus* cast a baleful shadow over church–state relations and was arguably the most divisive political issue during Louis XV's reign. Ironically, as if to prove that those who forget the lessons of the past are condemned to repeat them, in 1718 Clement XI issued yet a third bull—*Pastoralis Officii*—excommunicating those who refused to accept *Unigenitus*, including 3000 French bishops. But this bull offended the Regent (the *duc* d'Orléans) and the pro-Jansenist *parlementaires* refused to register it. Consequently, it never became a law in France.

12. The Growth of Toleration

While constantly seeking acceptance for their own views, Jansenists in the seventeenth century seldom showed toleration for others. In their writings, they opposed Protestants (as heretics), Jesuits (as their enemies), mercantilists (for promoting greed), ultramontanists (for favoring papal infallibility), and bishops (for dominating priests). In 1685, for example, Antoine Arnauld rejoiced at Louis XIV's edict revoking the Huguenots' civil and religious rights and banishing their pastors from France. Although expressing reservations concerning the dragoons' brutality in enforcing it, he felt this "strong measure" would force the "rebels" to convert. Ever the entrepreneur, he saw the Revocation as an opportunity to distribute copies of his book *Apology for the Catholics* among the "new converts" and help ease their return to Catholicism.[26]

Ironically, two years before, Arnauld had told Prince Ernest of Hesse-Rhinfels that tolerance was the most reasonable, equitable approach rulers could take toward schismatics and heretics, for "this is the law of the Gospels."[27] Obviously, Arnauld did not believe this "law of the Gospels" applied to the Huguenots, but then, neither did most other Catholics. The seeds of tolerance would require decades to mature.

After Louis XIV's death, the *duc* d'Orléans (1715–1723) watered that seed by recalling the bishops who had been exiled for opposing *Unigenitus*, releasing scores of imprisoned Jansenists, and inviting hundreds of fugitive *appelants* to return to France. In the 1730s, Minister D'Argenson, believing that toleration often succeeded in cases where persecution failed, moderated government pressure on the Jansenists. During the 1770s, as Jansenists embraced popular social and political causes, society became more tolerant of them as well. Their campaigns to expel the Jesuits, abolish the Inquisition, and soften penal codes against heresy won them many friends. Writers for the *Ecclesiastical News* praised Joseph II for his tolerant laws toward Lutherans and Calvinists in Austria, Bohemia, Hungary, and the Austrian Netherlands; after 1775 they favored granting French Protestants their civil and religious rights.

During the 1780s, Jansenist writers like Clément de Boissy, Robert de Saint-Vincent, Charles

Adrien Le Paige, and the *abbé* Grégoire argued that Louis XVI should follow the example of Joseph II and grant full legal rights to Protestants, Jews, and Negroes. They supported the Declaration of 1787 (the "Edict for the Non-Catholics") restoring the Reformed to full French citizenship. The *Ecclesiastical News* asserted that granting these groups equality with Catholics demonstrated "zeal for the public good, good faith, and good sense." Such a policy would bring positive benefits not only to Jews and Protestants but also to France.[28]

Finally, during the French Revolution, many Jansenist deputies urged the Constituent Assembly to abandon religious toleration in favor of religious liberty. In a bold speech reminding his colleagues that toleration had often led to persecution, deputy Rabaut de Saint-Etienne declared:

> It is not the old tolerance that I wish to reclaim; it is liberty. Tolerance! Support! Pardon! Clemency! These ideas are supremely unjust to dissidents, to the extent that it will be true that differences of religion and opinions is not a crime. Tolerance! I demand that it be proscribed among us; and it must be, for this unjust word presents to us citizens worthy of pity, as guilty ones whom we pardon.[29]

Saint-Etienne's moving speech carried the day. When the Assembly voted in favor of religious liberty, the *Ecclesiastical News* printed its resolution, including the phrase that "no one must be disturbed for his religious beliefs."[30] After 150 years of suffering, Jansenists, it seemed, had finally learned to grant others the same rights they themselves had struggled to obtain.

CHAPTER 1
Who Were the Jansenists?

"[Christians must] uphold the truth, not by resisting, but by suffering; not by shedding others' blood, but by giving their own."—*Antoine Arnauld*[1]

Over a decade ago, Jansenist scholar J. D. Crichton asserted that "The bibliography of Jansenism (and anti-Jansenism) is enormous, probably over 100,000 titles."[2] In Paris alone, the Bibliothèque de Port-Royal on the *rue* St. Jacques holds 15,000 documents, the Bibliothèque Nationale de France contains 956 titles, and the police records in the Archives de la Bastille at the Bibliothèque de l'Arsenal fill over 2,300 green cartons. The Archives Nationales houses an equally rich collection. Even the seldom visited Bibliothèque de la société de l'histoire du protestantisme français on the *rue* du Saint-Pères, which many years ago purchased the Charles Sainte-Beuve Collection, contains rare original sources on two centuries of Jansenism in Paris and throughout France.[3]

Despite this gold mine of source material, much confusion has existed over the years regarding who the Jansenists were and what they believed. Some writers have denied that Jansenism existed, calling it a "phantom" or straw man resurrected by the Jesuits. Marxist scholars have seen it as the ideology of an upper middle class of magistrates and *parlementaires* in France. Other historians describe it as the religious manifestation of the robe nobles' reaction to the economic and social crises of the seventeenth century, including the Fronde and the state's attempt to replace venal officials with *commissaires*. Still others have focused on Jansenist *parlementaires'* links with Gallicanism.[4]

Despite this disparity of views, historians agree that one cannot understand seventeenth-century France without comprehending the relationship of Jansenism to its religious, social, political, and intellectual landscape. H. G. Judge (1960) believed that the "major internal problem of the French Church in the second half of the century was that of Jansenism."[5] Pierre Chaunu (1962, 1998) saw French Jansenism as the heart or hub of "a synergy of opposing forces" intersecting other major "streams" of thought—Cartesianism, Augustinianism, Richerism, Convulsionism, Gallicanism—that one must understand in order to fully grasp "the crisis of the European conscience."[6] Philippe Loupès (1993) described it as "the tree which hid the forest,"[7] while David Bell (2001) called Jansenism "the most powerful force in French intellectual life in the decades around 1700."[8] Still other writers have referred to it as "a current with multiple facets"[9] and "a ferment of social transformation" which, by encouraging individualization, "accelerated the rise of the bourgeoisie and contributed to the decline of the Old Regime edifice."[10]

Most scholars, however, agree that the real roots of Jansenism lay in the Catholic Reformation of the late-sixteenth and early seventeenth centuries and in the crucial role that religion played in the daily lives of men and women. In Early Modern Europe, religion was the superstructure of life, the "crown of all realities"; it lay "at the heart of both the individual's conscience and of the collective conscience. It determined the finality and the modes of existence." Life eternal in heaven was what really mattered for most individuals; earthly existence was merely a step toward eternal life. Therefore, religion permeated every level of life—parish, town, and kingdom. Lay society and religious society were coextensive.[11]

But religion was also a profitable business. The annual revenues of the Gallican Church from its tax-free *dîmes* and *rentes* reached 100,000,000 *livres* in 1662 and 150,000,000 *livres* by 1674—while the revenue of the Crown in 1662 amounted to only 75,000,000 *livres*.[12] And as Humanist scholars and Protestant reformers emphasized, such wealth corrupted the Church at all levels and compromised the piety and zeal of its officials from parish priests to popes.

Jansenists opposed this "worldliness" and sought to reform the church. As Catherine Maire (1998) asserted, the taproot of Jansenism drew nourishment from the Council of Trent's (1545–1563) redefinition of doctrine in reaction to Protestantism, especially its new picture of God as all powerful, above all, and everywhere present.[13] From Saint Augustine, the movement inherited two streams of thought regarding salvation. The first was a pessimistic view of human nature, profoundly marked by original sin and man's inability to change. Therefore, God alone decided an individual's eternal destiny by an absolute decree of his omnipotence (predestination). The second stream was an optimistic view of God's efficacious grace as the divine solution to the human dilemma: God could save those he predestined. Calvinists and Lutherans emphasized the weak human will, whereas Christian Humanists and the Society of Jesus emphasized man's free will. The Council of Trent steered a middle path through this theological minefield by condemning one group's over-emphasis on free will while attacking those who denied that human will could be empowered by God.[14]

To strengthen parishioners' moral will, the seventeenth-century Gallican Church insisted that all Catholics attend Easter Communion; it urged priests to post the names of absentees on church doors and to threaten them with excommunication. Bishops tried to make the celebration of the Mass uniform. Reformer Vincent de Paul claimed that he had watched seven priests perform the service in seven different ways. Church leaders attacked corruption in some of the older religious orders (like the Benedictines and Clunisians) and regularized church appointments, eliminating nepotism, simony, and appointing children as young as four to eight years of age as abbots and abbesses. Finally, noting that many priests "could not read, write or sing, and their prodigious ignorance was often accompanied by such scandalous lives that nobler persons felt degraded to enter church offices,"[15] a campaign to raise the educational level of ecclesiastics was begun.

As "Disciples of Saint Augustine," rejecters of the humanism of the Renaissance, and defenders of the Council of Trent, Jansenists supported these reforms. From their beginnings, Jansenists were dogmatic, moralistic, and ascetic. They preached a different view of God's grace from that propounded by the Jesuits. The Society of Jesus promoted a Renaissance view of man's mental powers, his self-confidence, and the perfectibility of his reason. They taught that humanity had "sufficient grace" and "free choice." But Jansenists, more pessimistic, insisted that the tragic fall of Adam and Eve in the Garden of Eden brought sin and anguish to all humanity in an incomprehensible universe. Only God's grace, granted to the predestined Elect, could save them from sin. Jansenists, who drew their morality from Christ's Sermon on the Mount, sought to restore first century apostolic purity in the Church and to regenerate politics with Christian faith and mysticism. Wishing to curb the alarming spirit of independence (libertinism) in society, they urged obedience first to God and conscience and second to king and pope.[16]

Although Jansenism did not originate in France, its peculiar blend of Gallicanism, Richerism, and conciliarism (as explained below) soon made it a distinctly French brand of Roman Catholicism—what historian Robert Remsberg (1940) called "Gallican Roman Catholicism" or the "patriotic religion" of France.[17] And because from its medieval origins Port-Royal, a community of Cistercian monks consecrated to prayer, had been a microcosm of piety and zeal, it became, after its reform by Angélique Arnauld in 1609, the crown jewel of the Catholic Reformation. Its *soeurs* (sisters) and *messieurs* (brothers) lived lives of penitence, silence, and manual labor and shared a community of goods in separation from the world and obedience to their superiors.[18]

But not all Jansenist religious separated themselves from the world like cloistered nuns and monks. By the early eighteenth century, historian David Hudson (1984) estimated that roughly 6000 of the 200,000 priests in France (3%) had adopted Jansenism as their creed. In addition, between 1717 and 1735, the theological faculty of three universities (Paris, Rennes, Nantes) and the members of five religious congregations (Benedictines, Oratorians, Chartreux, Camaldules, and Feuillants) identified themselves as *jansénistes*.[19]

Yet few people in seventeenth-century France understood who these *jansénistes* were. The term "Jansenism" itself did not appear in print until 1641, a year after the publication of Biship Cornelius Jansen of Ypres' book *Augustinus*; it identified the followers of Jansen (or Jansénius) and their peculiar Augustinian views on grace. But the term lacked negative connotations until the papal bulls *In eminenti* (1643) of Urban VIII and *Cum occasione* (1653) of Innocent X condemned five propositions in the *Augustinus* as heresy.[20]

Even so, no consensus existed on what to call these followers who espoused Jansen's ideas. The *curé* Guy Droppier in a letter to his friend André Rivet in 1642 referred to "the *Janseniens* [who] bestir themselves here very actively."[21] In his 1645 work *Continuation of the Examination of the Doctrine of the Former Abbot of Saint Cyran and His Cabal*, Abra de Raconis attacked *Jansénistes*, *Cyranistes*, and *Arnaudistes* as "innovators" and "domestic factions."[22] The Jesuit François Vavasseur called them both *Janseniani* (followers of Cornelius Jansen) and *Calviniani* (followers of Jean Calvin) in 1650.[23] In a "Letter to a friend concerning Jansenism" (1651), a certain Mersenne, describing "this sort of people whom they call *Jansénistes* after the name of Jansénius their founder," provided the most widely accepted name for the group for the next two centuries.[24]

Jansenism, however, did not constitute a monolithic system of thought. It included "moderates" like Arnauld d'Andilly and the Bishop of Comminges; "centrists" like Antoine Arnauld and Pierre Nicole; "monastics" like Saint-Cyran, Martin de Barcos, Antoine Singlin and the Port-Royal sisters; and "extremists" like the *abbé* Le Roy and Jacqueline Pascal.[25] In a letter to Pasquier Quesnel in 1688, Louis du Vaucel, a Jansenist agent at Rome, defined three types of Jansenists: those holding to the Five Propositions in the *Augustinus* ("very few in number"); those zealous for good morals and severe self-discipline ("a very great number"); and those who hated the Jesuits ("an infinite number").[26]

The enemies of Jansenism, however, lumped these groups together and attacked them with vituperative propaganda. As early as 1654, the historian François Pinthereau called them a "party [faction] of St. Augustine."[27] Richelet's *Dictionary* for 1695 defined Jansenism as a "sect"; *The Art of Thinking* referred to them as "a sect of liars."[28] The word *secte* retained its pejorative meaning well into the eighteenth century. In the preface to *Jansen Condemned by the Church* (1705), the Jesuit Jacques-Philippe Lallemant promised that his book would "arm the Faithful against the artifices of the Partisans of the new Sect" of Jansenists. These "innovators," he declared, "seduced" people into believing "dangerous doctrines."[29]

Yet who these "innovators" were and what "dangerous doctrines" they taught remained unclear to many as the eighteenth century dawned. The writer Jacques Fouillou admitted in his *Chimera of Jansenism* (1708) that for the past sixty years, everyone had spoken of Jansenism but none could agree on what it was. Various groups saw them as innovators, heretics, disobedient Catholics, or criminals. Fouillou himself considered them "pretended Jansenists," but recommended that "it is better to pray for them than to war against them."[30] Two year later, the author Silvester Jenks quipped: "It was a great pity so important a matter as Jansenism should be so universally talk'd of and so little understood."[31]

Those labeled "Jansenists," however, consistently rejected the title. One of their leaders,

Pasquier Quesnel, author of a French New Testament, stated: "My name is *Christian*; my surname is *Catholic*; my party is the *Church*."[32] The so-called Jansenists, he declared, "are eager for orthodoxy and they have a horror for the spirit of schism and everything that resembles it."[33] Quesnel's contemporary, Pierre Nicole, even published a book entitled *Letters on the Imaginary Heresy* (1665) to prove that Jansenism did not exist.[34] Robert Arnauld d'Andilly assured Anne of Austria that Jansenism was only a chimera, a phantom, a ghost. "The crime of which I am accused, Madame, is that of being a Jansenist. I want to assure Your Majesty that this alleged Jansenism is such a chimera that I swear to Your Majesty that before God and upon my salvation, I do not know what it is. . . . I am, Madame, as Catholic as it is possible to be."[35]

No one defended the orthodoxy of Jansenists so vehemently as their chief theologian and writer Antoine Arnauld, whose works fill 43 volumes. In his "Letter to a person of high estate" (1655), he asserted that Jansenists were not heretics but "truly Catholic persons . . . truly disciples of Tradition & the Church." "Neither persecution, nor injustice, nor false brothers, nor enemies, nor the world, nor hell can separate them from the love & indissoluble union" of the Church, which is their "holy mother & revered mistress."[36] In his *First and Second Letters to a Duke and Peer* (1655), Arnauld called Jansenists "truly Catholics . . . nurtured in the fold of the Church on the milk of her breasts; [they] have always been members of the body of Jesus Christ . . . and have never had any other leaders or Fathers than those of all the faithful believers, namely the Sovereign Pontiffs of Rome & the Archbishops of Paris." To call them heretics or schismatics libeled their good name and denied their catholicity.[37]

To emphasize the nonexistence of this alleged heresy, Arnauld repeatedly used the term "phantom." "The furor of our enemies [the Jesuits]," he told the Bishop of Coutances in 1656, is directed against "a phantom."[38] The "disciples of St. Augustine," he asserted in his *Apology for the Religious of Port-Royal* (1664), have never been convicted of any error in Catholic orthodoxy. They are not "new Dogmatists" or heretics, and to condemn them as such based on rumors and slander violated church canons and rules.[39] He regretted in 1682 that "[n]o one seems to be able to help the King [Louis XIV] understand that the specter he fears under the name of Jansenism is only a phantom" which can never "offend his conscience or render him guilty before God."[40] His letters in the 1680s and 1690s frequently refer to the "chimera," "chimerical heresy," "were-wolf," "great mystery," and the "phantom" of Jansenism.[41]

Yet after thirty years of rumors and slander against this "phantom," he told Prince Ernest of Hesse-Rhinfels in 1686, no legal judicial court had proved "that any one person . . . holds to this heresy," despite "widespread noise [from the Jesuits] that France is full of these new heretics."[42] Attacks from the Society of Jesus had caused divisions in the Roman curia and at the courts of Spain and France, increased censorship and persecution of "pious ecclesiastics" suspected of Jansenism, and led to "ceaseless scandal."[43] His definitive work on this topic—*The Phantom of Jansenism* (1686)—declared that "Jansenism was only a phantom because there was no one in the Church who defended any of the Five Propositions [of Jansenius]."[44]

But Arnauld was being somewhat disingenuous in his definition of heresy. In the index to his 43-volume *Oeuvres*, he defines *Heresie* not as error, but as stubbornness in holding error. He compares heretics to pagan philosophers: they are dishonest, use deceit and artifices to avoid the truth, and their lives are full of vices (heresy is like adultery, he explains). Since the ascetic "disciples of Saint Augustine" did not fit this description, then surely they were not heretics. Moreover, proven heretics should be converted, not killed; persuaded, not persecuted.[45]

Arnauld's smokescreen concerning the phantom of Jansenism set the tone for the apologists who followed. In his *Abridged History of Jansenism* (1698), Jacques Fouillou asserted, "It is true that . . . Jansenism is a Phantom."[46] A decade later, he declared in 1708 that "[o]ne cannot deny that Jansenism is only an empty phantom & a purely imaginary heresy"; consequently, "there are neither Bulls nor Mandates that can give reality to a chimera." In fact, he added, Jansenism is Augustinianism, which the Church has taught for over 1300 years.[47]

Some recent historians concur with this assessment. In a study of Jansenist doctrines, Jean Carreyre (1934) explained that since the Church never declared Jansenius a heretic, his teachings could not properly be considered heresy.[48] In her work on the *convulsionnaires* of Saint-Médard, Catherine Maire (1985) agreed with Carreyre that Jansenism was not a heresy but "the essence of Catholicism," the "bastion of anti-papal gallicanism" which unfortunately became "a phantom of the absolute monarchy" in its rivalry with the *parlementaires* in the eighteenth century.[49]

Those who disliked the term "Jansenist" advanced more acceptable substitutes. As early as 1655 Antoine Arnauld suggested the descriptors "true Catholics" and "Thomists" (after Thomas Aquinas) which defined their unity with the Church and their adherence to the Augustinian doctrine of grace.[50] He also used the term "disciples of Saint Augustine,"[51] which Jansenist theologians liked. Others preferred the name *amis* (friends) because friendship constituted a private link among them, a free, voluntary association independent of any authority that (unlike a faction or sect) offered no threat to the state. Hence in different settings they became *Amis de la Verité* (Friends of Truth), *Amis de Port-Royal* (Friends of Port-Royal), *Amis de Saint Augustin* (Friends of Saint Augustine), and *Amis des libertés de l'Eglise gallicane* (Defenders of the liberties of the French Church). But in a hierarchical, absolute monarchy that refused to permit transverse structures to exist unregulated, this growing group of "friends" appeared to threaten the state.[52]

The real essence of Jansenism, however, lay in its defense of certain neglected truths, such as the doctrine of efficacious grace. Hence the most frequently used term in Jansenist writings is *Verité* (Truth). Antoine Arnauld believed that Truth had been revealed by God to the Church and should be lovingly yet vigorously defended—even at the cost of personal suffering.[53] In 1649 he declared that "truth has the misfortune of being often beaten down; yet it also has this advantage, that it is always victorious. In the end it will triumph over falsehood."[54] Defending the Truth encouraged Jansenists to develop strong, independent minds because their theology emphasized the importance of the individual's conscience and the necessity of listening to "the voice within."[55]

Defending truth in a land where king and Church defined orthodoxy often brought persecution. Yet no one enjoyed suffering like a Jansenist. Jansenism, Pierre Chaunu (1998) asserted, was fundamentally both masochistic and sadistic: its adherents took pleasure in the suffering they imposed on themselves and others (sparse diets and lifestyles, severe penance) and prided themselves on their degree of self-denial. While asceticism especially appealed to the Port-Royal *soeurs* and *solitaires* and surfaced in the bizarre behavior of the *figuristes* and *convulsionnaires*, it remained a fundamental aspect of life for all who chose to live as Jansenists.[56]

Ironically, because of Jansenists' defense of truth and ascetic lifestyles, the public continued to conflate Jansenism and Calvinism to the end of the *ancien régime*. A *Secret Memoirs* in 1787 declared: "It is well known that Jansenism and Protestantism are first cousins."[57] As late as 1798, the Tuscan prelate Giovanni Marchetti compared Jansenism to the Danube River: "It begins Catholic, becomes protestant, and ends Turk."[58] With tongue in cheek, the historian Jean Carreyre (1933) said that "a Jansenist is a Calvinist saying the mass."[59] In their Augustinian emphasis on the sinfulness of humanity, the grace of God, and predestination, David Bell (2001) asserted, Jansenists truly were the "Catholic cousins of Calvin."[60]

This doctrinal resemblance intrigued seventeenth and eighteenth-century commentators. In his short treatise *The Jansenists Identified as Calvinists* (1652), the Jesuit Jean de Brisacier argued that Jansenists were really "disguised Calvinists" because of their separation from the Church, Augustinian emphasis on grace and predestination, conciliarism, and disobedience to the authority of popes. Like the Huguenots, they had formed a sect to reform the Church, mocked the popes' bulls, published their own catechisms and Bibles, and formed "cabals and intrigues" behind a façade of virtue.[61] Four years later, the papal nuncio Nicolo di Bagno went even further, accusing French Jansenists of being in league "with the body of Calvinists and other heretics" to form "a type of republic."[62]

Oddly enough, their similarity to Protestants often earned Jansenists the sympathy and even admiration of Calvinist leaders like Pierre Jurieu.[63] Writing from exile in Holland, he praised Antoine Arnauld for preaching that the Ten Commandments can be kept only by God's grace; that humans have free wills and can resist God's grace; and that human merit or works have no salvation power.[64] During the 1720s and 1730s in Paris, the popular collective memory also linked the prophetic, miraculous, and convulsive behavior of the former Camisards of the Cévennes (1685–1710) with the current bizarre activities of the Jansenist *convulsionnaires*. Police spies warned *lieutenant-général de police* Hérault that street gossip suggested that the two groups might forge an entente against the Church and state.[65]

All too often, however, the public's misperceptions of the two religious faiths backfired in hostile actions toward one or the other group. In 1740 during the funeral of M. de Grimaudet du Landru, a Jansenist in Anjou, one woman shouted that since both Jansenists and Huguenots were heretics, they should toss Landru's body into the river. Instead, onlookers agreed to bury him face down in his coffin.[66] A decade later, in their pro-Jesuit critique of Pierre Quesnel's *Moral Reflections on the New Testament* (1754), L. Patouillet and D. Colonia declared that Jansenism "is principally the dogma of Calvin" and that both "are the source of all that is most abominable in sensual Quietism." Both heresies, they asserted, attack faith and morality, destroy free will, promote vice and crime, and worship a cruel God.[67]

While such propaganda proved patently untrue, the striking similarities between Calvinism and Jansenism have intrigued historians to the present day. In their lifestyles, both groups rejected worldliness, stressed individualist tendencies, sought to return the Church to apostolic purity, gave more power to priests (Richerism) and pastors (presbyterianism) than to bishops, and favored the authority of councils and synods over papal bulls and bishops' mandates. Both reflected an Augustinian strain of piety, saw life as a constant conflict between the forces of good and evil, and in resisting evil, both became suffering communities persecuted by the same enemies (king, Jesuits, and bishops).[68]

In building their doctrinal foundation, both Jansenists and Calvinists placed scripture well above tradition or papal pronouncements. Both published vernacular Bibles in French (the Geneva Bible and the Mons Version) and established schools (the *petites écoles* for the former and academies and colleges for the latter) to teach their children the tenets of their faith. In their understanding of holy writ, both shared an Augustinian view of God's free and abundant grace, man's weak and sinful will, and God's right to save or damn whomever he wishes (predestination).[69]

However, if the "Jansenists were the Puritans of the Catholic Church" (as Robert Palmer once quipped[70]), the Church saw the Huguenots as heretics and the Jansenists as schismatics. Why? While both groups tried to reform the Church and both were excluded from it eventually, Jansenists never accepted their expulsion. Unlike the Protestants, they never renounced the authority of the Roman Catholic Church, but continued writing appeals (hence their nickname "appellants") to popes and councils to clear their name. They also raised doctrinal questions that many thought had been put to rest. Moreover, although they, like Calvinists, sought perfection and absolute goodness in their lives and shared Augustinian viewpoints on God, grace, and human will, they never embraced Protestantism.[71]

Yet many of their leaders came from families who had once crossed the line from Calvinism into Jansenism, especially the Arnaulds and Le Maîtres.[72] The grandfather of the Jansenist theologian and writer Antoine Arnauld and his sister Angélique Arnauld (reforming abbess of Port-Royal)—Antoine de la Mothe-Arnauld—had been born a Catholic. Converted to Calvinism in 1559, he reconverted to Catholicism in 1572 out of fear and duty after Catherine de Medicis protected him at her Court during the atrocities of the St. Bartholomew's Day Massacre. While three sons and two daughters followed him into the Church, the other eight members of his family by his second wife Anne Forget remained Protestants. Grandfather Arnauld's conversion hastened his promotion to the Chamber of Accounts in Paris—but an intemperate speech accusing the Jesuits of "plots more horrible than their bacchanals" and urging their expulsion from France earned their undying hatred toward the Arnauld offspring.[73]

While Protestantism had largely died out among the Arnauld grandchildren by 1640, Angélique had two Calvinist aunts who visited her at Port-Royal and urged her to leave the abbey and convert to the Reformed faith. According to this story (which seems apocryphal), she considered running away to the Huguenot stronghold of La Rochelle, but an attack of malaria which left her gravely ill for two months prevented this. The marquis d'Eucourt, grandson of Isaac Arnauld, remained a Calvinist, however, and in 1685 fled to England with his three sons rather than be forced to convert to Catholicism during the Revocation.[74] Nonetheless, their Protestant roots left a mark on generations of Arnaulds, both positively and negatively. This heritage influenced their preference for plain living and their distaste for conspicuous consumption. But it also contributed in a significant way to their "travails of conscience" as they found themselves not only opposing Louis XIV and the Catholic hierarchy, but also enmeshed in gender conflicts and theological disagreements within their extended family. For, in a very fundamental sense, the Arnaulds—like all Jansenists—were "protestants": they thrived on conflicts with popes, kings, Jesuits, and even one another.[75]

The theological similarities between the two faiths begs the question as to whether Cornelius Jansen read Jean Calvin's works and if so, to what extent his theology was shaped by them. Although many writers have hypothesized that Jansen's teachings on grace, free will, and predestination in his *Augustinus* prove that he was influenced by Calvin's *Institutes*, certain facts cast doubt on this theory. First, Jansen cited Calvin only once in his three-volume *Augustinus*. Second, he quoted directly from the works of Saint Augustine; he did not filter these quotations through Calvin's works. Third, questions regarding grace, human will, and predestination interested all theologians in the seventeenth century, not just Jansenists. Finally, in his views on the Church and its authority, Jansen reflected the Baianism (see the discussion of Michel Baius below) prevalent at the University of Louvain rather than what Calvinists had to say on the subject.[76]

Likewise in their view of the world, Jansenists differed significantly from Protestants. While Calvinist merchants embraced the life of trade and mercantilism, Jansenists rejected the world and secular lifestyles and sought solitary, contemplative lives apart from the materialism around them. Unlike the Huguenots with their emphasis on salvation by faith, for Jansenists, the gap between a radically corrupted world and the sphere of divine perfection remained unbridgeable, even through faith, because no one could penetrate the purposes of God.[77] They felt that "the narrow road of asceticism was the only one for Christians."[78]

In their relationship to the Church and the Council of Trent, the two groups were polar opposites. While Protestants attacked the papacy, its councils, and the Catholic Church in general as "Babylon" (corruption), Jansenists supported the Catholic Reformation. In a 1688 letter to a friend in Rome, Antoine Arnauld spoke reverently of "that which God's Spirit said to the Council of Trent."[79] Like the Puritans in the Church of England, the Appellants remained within the Catholic fold, hoping to reawaken an interest in Augustinian theology and reform the lifestyles of Church officials and laity.[80]

In their attempt to reclaim Saint Augustine, Jansenists felt that they deserved the gratitude of the Church. They wondered why the Church allowed the Jesuits to preach ideas previously condemned as heresy in the Semi-Pelagians while they themselves faced persecution for repeating the words of Augustine.[81] Moreover, in the face of Protestant attacks, they boldly defended the saints, images, and relics, and upheld the real presence in the Eucharist, urging members to spiritually examine themselves before partaking of this sacred rite.[82]

Despite all their apologetics, however, Catholic officials feared that accepting Jansenists into the Church would drastically transform it. In his *Inconveniences of Jansenism* (1653), Léonard de Marandé, almoner to Louis XIV, argued that to receive them into the fold would bring doctrinal novelties and confusion; introduce old heresies and errors (like Arianism, Nestorianism, Donatism, Pelagianism, and Calvinism); and spawn many new sects. He worried that such a move could overthrow the work of Church councils for 500 years and change the relationship of Church and state. By introducing more representative (plenary) councils, the Jansenists might even transform the Church into a republic, which would bring chaos.[83]

Marandé's fears underline another fundamental difference between these two persecuted groups: their attitude toward toleration. While the Protestants in France sought civil toleration (that guaranteed rights to someone who did not share the national religion), Jansenists wanted ecclesiastical toleration (which protected dissidents within the Church against exclusion from communion). Ironically, the Catholic clergy tried to force the Reformed to partake of the sacraments they rejected while denying the Jansenists the right to the Eucharist they so earnestly desired. The latter's more narrow definition of toleration obviously excluded heretics such as the Calvinists.[84] In fact, most Jansenists rejoiced in 1685 when Louis XIV revoked the Edict of Nantes (1598), stripping the Huguenots of their civil and religious rights. On October 20 when the edict was made public, Antoine Arnauld called it "great news" and rejoiced at the prospect of rapid conversions to Catholicism it would bring in its wake.[85]

To assist in this work of conversion—and to defend themselves against the attacks of their enemies—Jansenist theologians and apologists generated a blizzard of books, pamphlets, and other controversial literature. In fact, the print culture in Europe, with its growing number of presses and increasingly literate public eager for reading material, helped spread Jansenism. This "civilization of the Book" (as Bruno Neveu has called it) made it nearly impossible for the Church to impose uniformity and orthodoxy on its members and equally difficult for the state to censor Jansenist works pouring forth from underground presses. How could any institution control ideas and words that multiplied so rapidly.[86]

For example, in their *Dictionary of Jansenist Books* (1754), Patouillet and Colonia list 1,063 Jansenist works by 181 male authors from 1643 to 1751—a publication rate of more than ten titles each year (and this list ignores the significant literary output of the Port-Royal *soeurs*).[87] Equally male-centric, a manuscript in the Fonds Sainte-Beuve shows that sixteen leading Jansenist writers from 1645 to 1734 produced 1,127 works—again, about ten per year.[88] "Silent Jansenists" did not exist: being a "Friend of the Truth" compelled one to be a writer.

Unfortunately, most of the early Jansenist scholars, theologians, and apologists of the seventeenth century have long been forgotten by all but specialists in Early Modern European religious history. Because the lives, writings, and contributions of the following fourteen figures are crucial to an understanding of Jansenist ideals and teachings, short biographical sketches (arranged roughly in chronological order) are provided for the non-specialist.

Michel Baius (1514–1589)

Michel de Bay (or Baius) prepared the fertile soil in which Jansenism sprouted and grew. He was a professor of theology at the University of Louvain, then one of the leading centers of learning in northern Europe, situated in the midst of the struggle against Protestantism on the frontier of Catholicism in the Low Countries. Here raged disputes about grace, original sin, and justification as each side in the debate hurled epithets of "Pelagianism" and "Lutheranism" at the other. Beginning in the 1550s, Baius began studying the Bible and patristic sources in the original languages without filtering them through the lens of scholasticism. An emphasis on Saint Augustine led him to focus on grace, perfect union with God, moral living, and the natural endowment of humans with immortality, integrity, and sanctifying grace. Baius agreed with Augustine that humans could not overcome the corruption of Original Sin by their own efforts or merits ("works"); they could be saved only by God's grace. He therefore held an optimistic view of human nature but a pessimistic concept of human willpower, weakened by millennia of sinning. Rejecting the Council of Trent's teaching on mankind's preternatural innocence and free will, Baius denied the possibility of achieving spiritual and moral perfection in this life because humans lacked free wills.[89]

Despite being a theologian to the king of Spain, Baius came under fire for what many saw as ancient Pelagianism or modern Lutheranism. In 1560 the Franciscans debated his Fourteen Propositions before the theology faculty at the Paris Sorbonne. Pius V's Bull *Ex omnibus afflictionibus* in 1567 and Gregory XIII's Bull *Provisionis nostrae* in 1579 condemned 79 propositions attributed to him as false and heretical. Bowing to the will of the pontiff, Baius retracted his views and was accepted back into the Church. But at the University of Louvain, his writings would later be read by professor Jacques Janson—who would teach them to his disciple Cornelius Jansénius.[90]

Luis de Molina (1535–1601)

But condemning Baius' theses for minimizing the role of human effort and exaggerating the role of God's grace in human salvation required more damage control than papal bulls could accomplish. Eight years after Baius' retraction, the Spanish Jesuit professor Luis de Molina countered with the idea of God's "sufficient grace" which, though granted to everyone, became "efficacious for salvation" only with the individual's consent, which God must respect (limiting God's predestination to foreknowledge).[91]

As the Spanish Armada churned the waters of the English Channel in a futile attempt to conquer England, Molina wrote *The Reconciliation of Free Will with Free Grace* (1588) putting forth "a middle way" (called Molinism") between Baianism and Catholicism. God's grace, he asserts, is sufficient to save everyone—but not everybody will accept it. Those who do, however, find it efficacious to achieve their salvation. But God's foreknowledge of who will accept and who will reject his grace does not determine their choice or the success or failure of their efforts in the sense of predestining their salvation or damnation. Therefore, humans, who are free to work out their own salvation with God's help, should be proactive in seeking his grace, which is "efficacious" for those who cooperate with him and "inefficacious" for those who resist him.[92]

But if Baius' teachings had landed him in the frying pan, Molina's theology put him in danger of the fires of the Inquisition. Although the recently founded Society of Jesus eagerly adopted Molina's theology, the Dominicans in Spain's universities accused him of Pelagianism and urged the Inquisition to burn him as a heretic. When word reached Rome, Clement VIII in 1597 established a special commission (*De auxiliis divinae gratiae*) to examine Molina's teachings. Paul V, who defended Molina despite the fact that he could not understand "subtle and complex [questions] on the method of divine action" in salvation, dissolved this commission in

1607 and forbade further public discussion regarding grace. The Jesuits considered this a victory in their favor.[93]

Edmond Richer (1559–1631)

Thus, even before the birth of Cornelius Jansen, the theological line in the sand had already been firmly drawn, with Saint Augustine and Baius on one side and Molina and the Jesuits on the other. At the turn of the new century a man appeared who added to this debate a volatile mixture of Gallicanism and conciliarism called "Richerism."

Trained in logic and philosophy at Hénault by Jesuit professors, Edmond Richer went to Paris at 18 to attend the College of Cardinal Lemoine. Tonsured at 19, he received his M.A. in Theology at the Sorbonne in 1585 and a doctorate in 1592, after which he returned to LeMoine to teach. An avid scholar, he ruined his health through study, his sparse diet, and lack of exercise. Yet his brilliance and hard work soon paid dividends as he climbed the ladder of academic success and became grand master and then syndic (equivalent to a modern dean) of the Faculty of Theology at the Sorbonne between 1608 and 1612.[94]

Although his published oeuvre covers a broad range of topics—theology, grammar, a history of Paris, a biography of Joan of Arc, a history of Church councils—the most famous work attributed to him is the *Libellus de Ecclesiastica et Politica Potestate* in 1611 (*Book of Ecclesiastical and Political Power*). In it he advanced several significant ideas that impacted French church–state relations for the next two centuries. French kings, who are sovereign by divine right, are also independent of all other authority, including the pope. The Church has spiritual authority to "cure souls," but no power to constrain the state, because kings appoint bishops ("princes of the Church" with delegated powers) within the Gallican Church. Moreover, the "church community" is aristocratic, not monarchical: the exercise of power rests with the "body of pastors" (bishops, archbishops, cardinals) gathered in general councils (the only infallible authority in the Church), which are superior to the pope (who is the "elected president" of the Church). Even bishops (descendants of the 72 disciples sent forth by Christ) should be elected by the clergy, gathered together in synods, then confirmed by the king and the people. Finally, papal interpretations of law can be modified by councils.[95]

Obviously, this potent mixture of Gallicanism, conciliarism, and democracy met with stiff resistance from ultramontanists across Europe. Since his more democratic vision of the Church contradicted the hierarchical model of the Council of Trent as explicated by the Jesuit Bellarmine, Richer's former mentors in the Society of Jesus bitterly attacked him as "an enemy of all kings and monarchical states." The Jesuits and Louis XIII charged Richer with heresy and removed him from his position as syndic. Paul V placed his *Libellus* on the Catholic Index of Forbidden Books in 1613. Although demoted and declared a heretic, Richer enjoyed the protection of the prince de Condé. During his active retirement, he wrote defenses of Gallicanism and attacked Oratorians and ultramontanists. But during Conti's revolt, Richer was briefly imprisoned at Saint-Victor, then released in 1622 after he recanted; his disciples were removed from the Sorbonne. In the 1620s he tried but failed to make a comeback with a declaration showing that his beliefs agreed with many at the Sorbonne. Abandoned by Cardinal Richelieu, condemned by popes, Richer retracted his views in his *Spiritual Testament* of 1629 and died two years later from nephritis at 72.[96]

But condemning Richer's book did not kill the ideas it contained. Instead, ecclesiastical censorship helped spread the ideals of *richérisme* and further prepared the soil for the growth of Jansenism, a potent blend of political Gallicanism and ecclesiastical Richerism. Jansenists would consistently oppose the Jesuits, whose fourth vow of implicit obedience to the pope made them avid ultramontanists (a word signifying appeals to the pope in Rome "across the [Alps] mountains").[97] Jansenists, like many other Catholics, never accepted the infallibility of popes; denied papal power over kings and the distinction of cleric and laity; and refused to adopt the Vatican's pompous Baroque style in art, architecture, and music. Instead, they advanced a tripartite Gallicanism: episcopal (for bishops to preserve their authority *vis-à-vis* popes and kings); royal (for kings to be independent of popes); and parliamentary (for Parlement to be free from the domination of Rome). These three Gallicanisms sometimes clashed, leading strange bedfellows to pair off against one another.[98] By the eighteenth century, Gallicanism in one form or another would lie behind nearly all the appeals against the Bull *Unigenitus* of 1713 registered at the Sorbonne, at French universities, and in the Parlement of Paris. Although separate in the seventeenth century, Richerism and Jansenism would fuse in the eighteenth century *parlementaire* resistance to the absolutism of Louis XIV and Louis XV—and Gallicanism would be the glue that bonded them together.[99]

Cornelius Otto Jansénius (1585–1638)

Born at Leerdam, Holland, the fifth child of Catholic peasant farmers who protected fugitive priests in this Protestant region, Cornelius Jansen (Latin Jansenius) attended primary school at Culemborg and college at Louvain, taking first honors in the Arts. At the College St.-Jerôme in Utrecht, he studied philosophy and the humanities from Catholic professors and rhetoric with Protestant ones, gaining some carpentry skills on the side. Returning to the University of Louvain in 1602, he studied theology at the College of Lys and the College of Pope Adrian VI (1604–1609); after being tonsured and appointed a deacon, he studied for the priesthood at the College of Faucon (run by the Jesuits). When his best friend Othan Zilly joined the Society of Jesus in 1604, Jansen tried to enter its ranks as well, but the Jesuits rejected him because of his poor health and negative temperament. Angered by this "bloody affront," he organized his friends (which included the future *abbé* de Saint-Cyran) into an "Augustinian Party"; they used the ideas of Michel Baius to oppose the Society of Jesus. Leaving for France in 1604, Jansen was appointed principal of the College of Bayonne in 1612 and ordained to the priesthood two years later. He often visited the nearby home of his friend Jean Duvergier de Hauranne, the future *abbé* de Saint-Cyran. Returning to Holland in 1617, he entered the Collège of Adrian VI (directed by the pro-Baius, anti-Jesuit Jansonius), and earned his doctoral degree (his thesis attacked Protestantism). He next was elected principal of the newly established College of Sainte-Pulchérie to train Dutch Catholic clergy. Twice (in 1623–24 and 1625–26) the University of Louvain sent him to Madrid to block the Jesuits' attempt to teach theology at the university. After he appealed his case to Philip IV, the king ordered the Infanta (who was governor of the Spanish Netherlands) to forbid the Jesuits to teach theology. His appointment as canon of the collegial church at Saint-Pierre de Lille brought him 1000 florins a year, making him financially independent.[100]

While he lived, Jansen enjoyed widespread popularity and promotions. Chosen regent of the faculty at the University of Louvain in 1628, he also occupied its prestigious Regius Chair of Theology and established a new library and archives. During the 1630s he became rector (a position combining today's president, academic dean, and treasurer) and canon of the collegial church. When the Bishop of Ypres (in Flanders) died in 1634, Philip IV, with Urban VIII's approval, appointed Jansen to that office, making him the spiritual shepherd of 130,000 Catholics in 105 parishes. In 1635 he finished his controversial *Mars Gallicus*, an attack on France's alliance with the Protestant German and Dutch states in the Thirty Years' War (1618–1648). Finally, in 1638, after more than twenty years' labor, he completed his magnum opus, the *Augustinus* (dedicated to Urban VIII); with his dying breath, Jansen charged his chaplain, Réginald Lamée, to make sure an exact copy was printed after his death. That same year, while ministering to those afflicted by the bubonic plague, Jansen died at 53. The *Augustinus*, published with the approval of the *conseil privée*, appeared one year later.[101]

To the very end, Jansen claimed to be a faithful son of the Roman Catholic Church, declaring that "he would uphold or reject, condemn or anathematize, all that Rome had sustained, rejected, condemned, or anathematized, and that he wished to live and die in the communion of that Church."[102] Yet his personality and love of controversy often caused trouble. Although a recent Jesuit biographer described Jansen as pious, honest, pure, ascetic, and fervent in worship, his hard-working nature and total devotion to the truth made him at times petulant and impetuous.[103] As a boy growing up in a Protestant area, Jansen had a penchant for attacking heresies. Later, after being rejected by the Society of Jesus, he wrote diatribes against the Jesuits. In his controversial pamphlets, he often expressed "sincere indignation" at his opponents' claims and then transformed his accusers into the accused, enmeshing them in their own arguments to embarrass them.[104]

He employed this technique in *Mars Gallicus* (1635), a direct attack on the policies of Cardinal Richelieu and Louis XIII during the Thirty Years' War. Although Jansen is considered primarily a theologian, he took a keen interest in politics and international affairs. Although his adversaries considered him "too much a friend of the French," Jansen strongly disliked Richelieu's policies towards Spain and the Low Countries. As a loyal citizen of Flanders, he opposed the attempts of Richelieu and the Dutch *stadtholder* the Prince of Orange to dismember it. Furthermore, he recoiled at the thought of a Catholic nation (France) allied with Protestant powers (Sweden and some of the northern German states) against another Catholic power (Spain).[105]

Consequently, in 1634–35 he penned what Jean Orcibal has called "a bloody pamphlet" (actually 88 chapters and 452 pages) against Cardinal Richelieu's political aims in Flanders.[106] In it Jansen debates the justice of wars and the inappropriateness of ecumenical alliances. Wars, he states, must be fought only for "just causes" and backed by the king's "best intentions." Therefore, if a monarch takes up arms against a Catholic state, his subjects have no obligation to obey him. Jansen concludes by urging Louis XIII to sever his alliances with the Protestant Germans and Swedes and with the Turks.[107]

While Jansen's *Mars Gallicus* created a tempest in a teapot in the Sorbonne and among the *dévots* and *politiques* in France, his *Augustinus* unleashed a hurricane of controversy across Europe. In 1640, as the Jesuits celebrated the centennial of the founding of their order by Ignatius Loyola, the *Augustinus Cornelii Jansenii Episcopi seu doctrine sancti Augustini et humanae naturae sanitate aegritudine, medicina, adversus Pelagianos et Massilienses, tribus tomis Comprehensa* was released.[108]

Its content, defending Saint Augustine and attacking Pelagianism and Molinism, represented the fruit of over twenty years of careful thought and reading. In 1618 Jansen had purchased a new library containing the works of almost all the Church Fathers. The following year, he focused his reading on the question of grace—Adam's and Christ's—and the two states of human nature. To keep his research secret from the Jesuits, he used the code word "Pilmot" in letters discussing his project with friends. In 1621 he studied Pelagian, Molinist, and scholastic thought to refute their errors; from 1622 to 1627, he focused on Augustine's writings.[109] In the preface to his *Defense of Monsieur Jansenius* (1644), Antoine Arnauld claimed that Jansen read Augustine's published works "ten times from beginning to end" and his writings about grace "more than thirty times."[110] Frequent discussions with Saint-Cyran concerning God's grace and human will in 1625 and 1626 and writing two previous pamphlets attacking modern Pelagianism had set the stage for completing this magnum opus.[111]

Although written entirely in Latin, the *Augustinus* (in Jean Orcibal's words) is "one of those rare works that escape the general mediocrity of seventeenth-century Belgian writings." Jansen's style is frank, expressive, picturesque, sometimes lyrical and energetic; he sets forth his penetrating ideas with certainty and erudition.[112] Jansen had once declared: "It is possible to ignore many things without prejudicing the Catholic Faith, but in that which concerns Original Sin, the Incarnation of the Son of God, and the two human natures by one of which we are captives to sin and by the other redeemed from our sins—it is in these things that the Christian religion properly consists."[113]

Every one of the 1,300 pages (with two columns each) of the *Augustinus* reflects a deep admiration for Augustine's thought concerning grace, sin, human will, salvation, and predestination. Jansen praised the Bishop of Hippo as the "Foremost of the Doctors, . . . the leading ecclesiastical writer after the canonical doctors, Father of the Fathers, doctor of the doctors, subtle, sound, ineffably admirable." In a letter to Saint-Cyran, he exclaimed, "I love him uniquely and it seems to me that there are none among the Ancients or Moderns who can come within one hundred leagues of him."[114] Jansen considered Augustine's oeuvre to be "the fifth gospel" (after the New Testament gospels of Matthew, Mark, Luke and John). In the *Augustinus*, he calls the saint "angelic, seraphic, excellent, admirable beyond all comparison."[115]

It is important to recognize Jansen's reverence for St. Augustine because nearly all Jansenists shared this admiration. For them, Augustine's thought was the touchstone of orthodoxy even more than the theology of St. Thomas Aquinas (Thomism). As Martin de Barcos stated: "The truth of M. d'Ypres [Jansen] was the truth of Saint Augustine," but "the truth of Saint Augustine" was not necessarily "the truth of the church." Rome held the doctrine of St. Augustine as "a privileged reference, not a doctrinal norm." Consequently, the popes did not authenticate the presence of Augustinianism in Jansen's *Augustinus* on the subject of grace; instead, they allowed Church theologians to examine the book and pronounce on its orthodoxy. Therefore, subsequent Bulls like *In eminenti* and *Unigenitus*, which condemned Jansen's and Quesnel's works as heretical, did not in any way diminish the Church's respect for St. Augustine or his theology.[116] But Antoine Arnauld, in his *Second Apology for Jansenius* (1645), asserted that Jansen's doctrines conformed not only to Augustinian theology, but also with Thomistic (Thomas Aquinas) teachings regarding sin, grace, free will, conversion, and justification.[117] The Calvinist writer-in-exile Pierre Bayle concurred. In his famous *Dictionary*, he asserted: "It is clearly obvious to anyone who examines things without prejudice . . . that the doctrine of St. Augustine and that of Jansenius, Bishop of Ypres, are the same."[118]

Recent scholars have agreed with Bayle. Bruno Neveu (1994) stated that the *Augustinus* was not a "critical history of theology," but a "work of positive theology," an exposition of the truths of Christian dogma, and a doctrinal commentary that "selectively nourished only a part of the Augustinian tradition." Although it is the best example of patristic, fundamental Augustinianism, it is not objective in tone, as certain apologetic presuppositions color its methodology. In essence, it is Jansen's *cri du coeur* (heart cry)—a "doctrinal manifesto" against the pelagians and semi-pelagians of his age.[119] Fabian Gastelier (1998) described the *Augustinus* as a "work of combat," employing Augustine's views on grace and predestination to fight those advanced by the Jesuits and Molinists.[120] Daniella Kostroun (2000) has also shown how Jansen used Augustine's doctrines on grace, free will, and salvation to combat the Molinism of the Jesuits (whom he saw as the modern Pelagians).[121]

Reading the 1,300 pages of the *Augustinus* in Latin (or French) is a formidable task. Its 25 "books" present a history of the Pelagian heresy and attack scholastic philosophy in many areas. Topics like human free will, original sin, man's primeval nature (a "state of innocence"), predestination, God's grace, the limits of human reason, Christ's atonement, the state of nature before and after the Fall, and reprobation are covered exhaustively. The addendum highlights recent heresies (Molinism and semi-Pelagianism) regarding free will, predestination, and efficacious grace.[122] Jansen considers the Pelagians (ancient or modern) heretical for teaching that human nature is inherently moral; that free will banishes the need for God's grace; that grace can be acquired by human merit; and that predestination demonstrates both God's absolute and conditional will. The Scholastics' errors included an over-emphasis on human reason and pagan virtues and an under-emphasis on Christ's saving grace, love of truth, the corruption in human nature, and the errors of the Manicheans. Human free will, he explains, comes only through God's grace—which comes in two varieties: sufficient and efficacious.[123]

Unfortunately for the Bishop of Ypres, the Church hierarchy did not agree with these views. While Jansen believed that Saint Augustine should be the doctrinal norm for Catholic orthodoxy, Catholic theologians saw his writings as only "a privileged reference point." Therefore, papal and episcopal attacks on the *Augustinus* did not in any way diminish the Church leaders' or members' respect for Saint Augustine himself.[124] For example, whereas Jansen taught that God had given Adam sufficient grace to live a sinless life before his Fall, but that original sin had deprived him of it, the Jesuits taught that God gave sufficient grace to every person after the Fall. And while Jansen taught that the only way humans could break free of sin and corruption was to accept God's efficacious grace, the Jesuits and Molinists emphasized the role of human merit and works in preparing the soul to receive this grace.[125]

Equally unfortunate for Jansen and his later followers, Pius V's pontifical decisions (*De auxiliis*) from 1611 to 1625 had imposed silence regarding the very issues discussed in the *Augustinus*. Even those Church officials who did not find anything heretical in his work nonetheless deemed it imprudent and disturbing to the Church's peace and unity.[126]

But many found both error and heresy in the *Augustinus*. The assistant general of the Jesuit Order in France, *Père* Annat, member of the Council of Conscience and Louis XIV's confessor, led the campaign to condemn it. He persuaded French bishops to oppose it and the Sorbonne to censure it. In the 1650s Annat published six books and wrote numerous letters against Jansen's ideas. He even asked the pope to condemn the *Augustinus*. As a result of Annat's lobbying, Innocent X issued the bull *Cum occasione* on 31 May 1653 declaring five propositions in the work to be heretical.[127] Bishop Jacques Bossuet, one of Louis XIV's favorite Court preachers, agreed with the pope that the five condemned propositions "are the heart of the book" and that those who denied this practiced "pure chicanery."[128]

One form of "chicanery" often advanced by the Jansenists (following Antoine Arnauld's lead) was to distinguish between *droit* (right) and *fait* (fact). This tactic, for example, permitted them to agree that the pope had the right to condemn as heretical the so-called "five propositions" while denying that those same heretical theses could in fact be found in the *Augustinus*—or in any of Jansen's writings for that matter. Thus, while the pope had the right to define doctrine and condemn heresy, Arnauld asserted that he could not define "facts" (i.e., impute heretical beliefs to Jansen when none actually existed in his writings). As chapters 2 and 3 will show in greater detail, this clever ploy enabled many Jansenists to walk the tightrope between orthodoxy and heresy for over a century.[129]

Yet by condemning Jansen's theology, Rome painted itself into a corner. Responding to a growing tidal wave of anti-Jansenist criticism, the papacy faced the necessity of clarifying the Church's position *vis-à-vis* Saint Augustine and fifth-century Pelagianism. But seventeenth-century popes claiming to be infallible did not know how to make pronouncements against the rulings of their fifth-century predecessors, so they attacked Jansen instead, overlooking the fact that some of his points concerning Augustine and Pelagianism might in fact be accurate.[130] Recognizing this trap, the Jesuit *Père* Annat quipped: "In condemning the five propositions, the pope did not carefully consider whether he was likewise condemning St. Augustine or not."[131]

Paradoxically, although Jansen's posthumously published work was condemned as heretical, Jansen himself died neither as a heretic nor as a leader of any heretical movement—including the one named after him. Despite his inability to solve the dilemma of grace and free will to the later satisfaction of Jean-Paul Sartre ("If man is free, then God is not" and "If God exists, then man is not free"[132]), Jansen died "in the odor of sanctity" and Catholic orthodoxy. Although not quite the ultramontaine that some have called him, he considered the pope as the universal bishop of the Church and recognized his ex cathedra authority. Ironically, however, unlike his devoted followers, the Bishop of Ypres opposed Richerism and remained hostile toward royal Gallicanism throughout his life.[133]

Sébastien Zamet (1587–1655)

As Bishop of Langres, Zamet had a well-deserved reputation as a Tridentine reformer of the Cistercian Order at Tart. Strongly influenced by Cardinal de Bérulle and the Oratorians, he was pious and deeply spiritual, though not mystical.[134] His connection with the famous Arnauld family began in 1622 when Robert Arnauld d'Andilly heard Sébastien's older brother Jean Zamet's last confession. Two years later in 1624 Sébastien met Robert's younger sister *Mère* Angélique Arnauld, the abbess of Port-Royal des Champs; she admired his zeal and pragmatic spirituality. Both shared a reformist mindset; both had known François de Sales as their confessor. Zamet became her spiritual advisor; beginning in 1625 he visited Port-Royal frequently and they corresponded regularly. Beyond giving her "holy counsel," he (and Angélique's mother) helped her find larger quarters for her 84 *soeurs* (nuns) in the *faubourg* Saint-Jacques in Paris when their rural retreat proved unhealthful.[135]

As his influence over *Mère* Angélique grew, Zamet spearheaded further changes at Port-Royal between1626 and 1636. He persuaded the abbess to transfer jurisdiction from the Cistercians to his newly established Institute of the Holy Sacrament (which followed the Augustinian Rule). Following the earlier pattern of the Daughters of Blessed Mary at Geneva, Zamet created the Daughters of the Blessed Sacrament to unify the sisters at the abbey of Port-Royal with those of Tart. In 1627 Urban VIII gave this new Institute his approval; in 1630 Louis XIII became its protector. In the 1630s, despite opposition from the jealous Carmelites, the Institute enjoyed the enthusiastic support of Archbishop Gondi of Paris and of the lay-led Company of the Most Holy Sacrament.[136]

In addition to his ecclesiastical office, however, Zamet was also *duc* de Langres and a peer of France, and his noble status influenced his interpretation of religious life at Port-Royal. A man of Baroque spirituality, he loved incense, floral bouquets, perfumed rooms, splendid linens, refined manners, and majestic music. His fundraising ensured that the sisters' new lodgings in Paris were sumptuous, with beautiful furnishings, neat clothing, and a varied cuisine of well-spiced foods. As he labored to increase the level of piety among the postulants, he also insisted that each one learn to read and write correct French. He invited only the most popular clergy to preach and celebrate Mass in the chapel. Such fashionable surroundings, he hoped, would attract the support of the wealthy, elite families near Paris, because in order to grow, Port-Royal must recruit the daughters of the Court nobility and rich bourgeoisie. To set them apart from other orders, Zamet designed fine white linen habits with scarlet scapulars for them to wear.[137]

Although Angélique Arnauld considered Zamet a "man of God," she disapproved of these compromises in pursuit of financial success. By 1636 she saw him as "a dangerous innovator." Then, amidst their quarrels over lifestyle issues, she discovered that he was smuggling letters from discontented sisters out of the convent and secretly visiting nuns in an exterior parlor provided by Madame de Pontcarré, a lay boarder at Port-Royal. In short, Zamet was undermining her authority.[138]

Given her proclivity for asceticism, Angélique felt drawn toward the "doctrine of self-abasement" presented by someone the exact opposite of Zamet. In fact, in his secret letters to Cardinal Richelieu, the jealous Zamet accused the *abbé* de Saint-Cyran of being "violent and inflexible" in defense of the Truth, "cold and moderated in his actions," "loving to dominate others" whom he treated "condescendingly."[139] But the abbess of Port-Royal considered him a godsend.

Abbé de Saint-Cyran (1581–1643)

Born at Bayonne into a prosperous merchant family, Jean Ambroise Duvergier de Hauranne was tonsured at ten in 1591. As an adolescent, he studied philosophy and theology and mastered Latin, Greek and Hebrew under the Jesuits at Bayonne, Agen, and Paris. After completing a Master's Degree in Paris, he returned to Louvain to earn his Bachelor's in Theology in 1604. He then went to Bayonne to manage the family estate at Comps-de-Prats. Cornelius Jansen joined him there in 1611 and the two became best friends. Between 1608 and 1620, he became canon at the Cathedral of Bayonne, principal of the local college, grand vicar, and finally *abbé* of Saint-Cyran with an income of 1,800 *livres* a year. He taught the young Henri de Guise. His growing popularity soon brought him to the attention of the royal family. Anne, the Queen Mother, made him her almoner in 1622. His close friendship with members of the Arnauld family led to his meeting Angélique Arnauld in 1625 and subsequent invitations to visit Port-Royal. Appointed Bishop of Bayonne in 1630, Saint-Cyran broke his ties with *Père* Joseph and Richelieu—a move that would cost him dearly. But in 1635, as Zamet's star declined, Saint-Cyran accepted Angélique's invitation to be her spiritual director. He helped establish the *petites écoles* (Little Schools) at Port-Royal in 1637 and wrote *Familiar Theology,* one of their textbooks.[140]

During his meteoric rise, however, Saint-Cyran made many powerful enemies. Although educated by the Society of Jesus, he became one of its severest critics, a *malleus Jesuitarum* ("hammer of the Jesuits"). Originally a friend of Richelieu, he refused a bishopric at his hands because he knew the cardinal would try to dominate him. For much the same reason, he declined offers to be royal almoner for Marie de Medicis in France and for Queen Henrietta Maria in England, telling Robert Arnauld that he would not be anyone's "performing dog." His independent attitude offended Richelieu. Then his friend Zamet—whom he had defended in print in 1635 against clerical attacks of "bad doctrine"—turned against him. Zamet, no doubt jealous of Saint-Cyran's rising influence at Port-Royal, denounced his "dangerous propositions" in a memoir to the Bishop of St. Malo and in letters to Richelieu.[141]

Consequently, although investigators found nothing suspicious (politically or doctrinally) in his papers, Richelieu sent Saint-Cyran to the chateau de Vincennes for six years (1638–1643). On 6 February 1643, the day of his release, the sisters at Port-Royal hosted a huge victory dinner in his honor. But eight months later on 11 October, weakened by the rigors of his imprisonment, Saint-Cyran died. Six bishops led his funeral and buried him at Saint-Jacques du Haut-Pas near Port-Royal des Champs.[142]

As spiritual director of Port-Royal, Saint-Cyran had instituted a more ascetic lifestyle than Zamet. Confessions, voluntary privations, and penitence increased. Eucharistic sermons emphasized God's "terrible grandeur," the small number of those saved and the vast majority who would be damned. Although Angélique Arnauld embraced this lifestyle of self-denial, many of her nuns (led by Sister Anne de Jésus) resisted it at first. Only after Zamet withdrew from Port-Royal in 1636 could Saint-Cyran implement his reform program.[143]

Saint-Cyran transformed Port-Royal into a Jansenist stronghold. Before the *abbé* became the convent's spiritual director in 1636, Jansen's Augustinian theology existed primarily in the realm of intellectual thought and debate, locked away from most readers in its heavy Latin tome. But after 1636, Saint-Cyran had a community where he could shape Jansen's doctrines to fit the spiritual needs of the *Soeurs* and *Solitaires*. It was this combination of *Mère* Angélique's monastic reform ideals and Saint-Cyran's Augustinian theology, as Daniella Kostroun (2000) correctly asserts, that marked the true origins of "the phenomenon known as 'Jansenism.'"[144]

Although Saint-Cyran could not read the *Augustinus* after his release from Vincennes in 1643 due to his poor eyesight, he apparently scanned its table of contents and urged Antoine Arnauld to defend it in print, which he did. Jansen and Saint-Cyran had been close friends for years, conferring together at Louvain (1621) and Péronne (1623) and corresponding regularly between 1617 and Jansen's death in 1638. Consequently, in their frequent discussions of the patristic writings, Saint-Cyran, the elder by four years, strongly influenced Jansen's thought; many saw him as the "master" and Jansen as his "disciple."[145]

Yet Saint-Cyran was a complex man full of paradoxes. Defending himself against charges of contradictions in his writings, he once declared that he had a "celestial temperament wherein two contrary qualities, fire and ice, mix, which makes me sometimes self-contradictory."[146] While one side of his temperament was cordial, happy, and kind, the other side tended toward austerity and melancholy. He was a somber man with a joyous heart, brilliant but excitable, pious yet not a visionary, brilliant and at the same time affectionate. Women found him fascinating; children loved him. An associate described him as "that friend of a thousand creases." Strong-willed and heroic, he was physically weak and often ill. An inflexible defender of doctrinal truth, he could be subtle and calculating in his political dealings with Richelieu. He took as his motto: "To speak little, to tolerate much, and to pray always." Yet this man of deep spirituality had "no taste for the confessional"; in his entire life he heard no more than 30 confessions.[147]

Like Cornelius Jansen, Saint-Cyran never appealed to a larger public by promoting his writings. He left their propagation to his friends and disciples after his death.[148] But unlike Jansen's Latin magnum opus the *Augustinus*, Saint-Cyran wrote ten short works in French. His major book—*Christian Thoughts on Poverty*—is 240 pages long; the other nine treatises are 11 to 72 pages in length. These pamphlets discuss Catholic services (the Mass, Confirmation, Eucharist); devotional topics (conversion, prayers, spiritual mysteries, rules for religious life); and Christ's life (especially his poverty and sufferings). Perhaps his best known work—*The Familiar Theology* (1643)—a catechism composed for Jérôme Bignon, son of the advocate-general, explores the history and logic of Catholic doctrines (God, creation, the Fall, redemption, penitence, the Eucharist, etc.). Its rigorist theology reflects Saint-Cyran's Augustinian views on grace, confirmation, confession, and communion.[149] Although the Archbishop of Paris banned this last work as a "false catechism," the Archbishop of Sens, seventeen French bishops, and eight doctors of theology at the Sorbonne signed an affidavit giving their approval.[150]

Between 1629 and 1643 Saint-Cyran wrote 135 letters to his friends and admirers. Some are only a paragraph long; others cover twelve or fifteen pages. Most of them, interestingly enough, he sent to abbesses, mother superiors, and nuns. Despite the fact that Richelieu had sent him to prison without formal charges and given the suffering he endured at the chateau, not once in his letters does Saint-Cyran mention his physical discomforts or refer to the political situation in France. Instead, he instructs his readers how to live the Christian life (50% of the letters); offers them consolation in death, illness, and misfortune (25%); and discusses a wide variety of practical topics (25%, which deal with temptation, running convents, family life, charity toward the poor, etc.).[151]

Reading his letters and pamphlets helps one understand the complexity of Saint-Cyran's personality and religious experience. Like many other seventeenth-century religious figures, he was a moral rigorist: he opposed Jesuit casuistry and preached the strict observance of such Catholic practices as the Eucharist, confession, and fasts. Born during the Catholic Reformation, he was by nature a reformer, calling everyone to a higher plane of moral conduct and sanctity. Also like his contemporary Blaise Pascal, Saint-Cyran was a melancholy man and at heart a *solitaire*. He preferred the life of meditation and prayer, although unlike Pierre Nicole, he was not a true mystic, but like Moses in the Old Testament, a prophet who descended from his mountain of meditation at times to warn the people to change their lives.[152] He redefined Catholicism around two poles: the Eucharist and the priesthood. As a Jansenist, he believed that humanity, corrupted by original sin, was incapable of meritorious acts without God's efficacious grace.[153] This pessimistic view of human nature even included the clergy. "In an era when the number of good ministers is so rare," he declared, "I do not think that those who love the Church tenderly can show a greater devotion to her than to weep continually."[154]

By contrast, he rejoiced at the godly lives of his friends at Port-Royal, whom he called "the Elect," "God's servants," and "the flock of Jesus Christ." His reforms at Port-Royal aimed at transforming the *soeurs* and *solitaires* into "divine hosts" and helping them imitate the first century saints. In his sermons, he emphasized renunciation of sin and contrition (rather than attrition), love of God's immutable rules, fear of punishment, charity toward the poor, and suffering as the beginning of the Christian's life.[155] He warned *Mère* Angélique in 1647: "That which you occasionally suffer in the present is a just punishment for the faults you have committed in the past."[156] This "Cyranian spirit" pervaded Port-Royal in the 1630s. Like their Cistercian forebears, sisters arose at 2 a.m. for matins; extended their devotional time; focused their meditation on salvation, predestination, and grace; and minutely traced their spiritual journeys to grasp their deeper meanings. Saint-Cyran himself benefited from this experience.[157] "When God leads a soul to his director," he said, "he at the same time touches the heart of the director."[158]

So who really was Saint-Cyran? His contemporary, Antoine Singlin, considered him "the most enlightened of all my friends."[159] Modern biographers have debated whether he was only a simple innovator, a reformer, or a revolutionary. Jean Laporte (1922) questioned whether he added anything unique to Jansenist doctrine.[160] He probably did not. Yet by combining the theology of Saint Augustine and the ascetic reforms of Angélique Arnauld, he transformed Port-Royal into a Jansenist bastion capable of withstanding the combined assaults of Church and state for nearly a century.

Martin de Barcos (1600–1678)

When Saint-Cyran died of apoplexy in 1643, his nephew, Martin de Barcos, became the new *abbé* de Saint-Cyran and spiritual director of Port-Royal (demonstrating that even Jansenists could embrace nepotism). That same year he penned the preface for Antoine Arnauld's *Frequent Communion* in which he asserted that Saints Peter and Paul were "two heads that make but one." Because the Jesuits thought Barcos questioned the primacy of Peter, Innocent X summoned both men to Rome to defend themselves. When they refused to go, the pope condemned the *Frequent Communion* in 1645.[161]

In his relationship with Port-Royal from 1643 to 1661, Barcos' letters reveal that he took asceticism even further than his uncle had. Believing that some of the *soeurs* and *solitaires* enjoyed "too much liberty" to live as they pleased, he required greater submission and deeper penitence, especially of their local directors Antoine Singlin and Angélique Arnauld. Rigidly anti-Thomistic and anti-Cartesian in thought, he longed to devote his life to otherworldly pursuits. Yet this strong advocate of silence and solitude supported Antoine Arnauld's battle within the Church over *droit* (right) and *fait* (fact) in Jansen's *Augustinus*. The man who hated "the Church militant" (especially the Jesuits) and who believed that "the true ecclesiastic has no greater enemy than the political man," nevertheless led his Port-Royal charges in refusing to sign the Formulary which stated that the five propositions could indeed be found in the *Augustinus*. Like his uncle, Barcos' life demonstrated that he too lived with contradictions and paradoxes.[162]

After the death of *Mère* Angélique in 1661, however, his influence at Port-Royal and in the Paris region declined. His opposition to what he perceived as the compromises leading to the "Peace of the Church" in 1669 brought a rupture between him and the nuns, so with a couple close friends, he retreated to his abbey at Saint-Cyran, dying there in 1678, a peripheral figure to the growing movement. Barcos' contributions have largely been ignored by modern historians of Jansenism like Sainte-Beuve, Gazier, Laporte, and Orcibal.[163]

Antoine Arnauld (1612–1694)

No historian of Jansenism, however, can ignore the outstanding contributions made by Antoine ("The Great") Arnauld. In the sixteenth century, his great-grandfather, Henri, seigneur de la Mothe of Auvergne, had been a Huguenot. His grandfather, Antoine I Arnauld, however, became a Catholic in 1572 to save his life during the St. Bartholomew's Massacre. His father, Antoine II Arnauld, an *avocat* in the Paris parlement who owed his advancement to Henri IV's and Sully's favor, took an active role in the campaign to expel the Jesuits from France in 1594 and in 1603 (after they returned), wrote a *Frank and True Discourse* against them. The Society of Jesus considered this affront "the sin of the Arnaulds which no sacrament can erase"; it inspired their undying hatred for all the family. And there were many of them, for Antoine II (who died at 103) and his wife Catherine Marion had 20 children. Ten died young, but every one of the four sons (who became lawyers and magistrates) and six daughters (who became Port-Royal nuns) that survived became strong supporters of the Jansenist movement. Indeed, over a period of several years, Antoine II's wife, two of his sons, all six of his daughters, five granddaughters, one grandson, and so many of his nieces and nephews abandoned the world to live at Port-Royal that the convent became family property. Under Louis XIII (1610–1643), the Arnaulds grew wealthy, influential, ambitious and aggressive in promoting their family's objectives.[164]

Born in 1612, the last of 20 children, Antoine III allegedly received the nickname *le grand* ("the great") in jest for his diminutive size. His parents, however, devoted more attention to his religious development than that of their other children. François Sales blessed the young Antoine and Saint-Cyran guided him spiritually. He attended the Collège de Calvi, trained in law, but entered the priesthood in 1641. He then completed a doctorate in theology at the Sorbonne (where he later taught). As a theologian and "defender of the Jansenist faith," his printed works today fill 43 folio volumes. As a magistrate, he became essentially Port-Royal's defense attorney, fending off the attacks of Church and state against his relatives' rural enclave.[165] To the first Saint-Cyran, he declared: "I understand what is expected of me in the defense of truth."[166]

Saint-Cyran, in fact, played a major role in shaping Antoine's future career. As spiritual advisor for the whole family in matters theological in the 1620s, the *abbé* had already become a close friend of Antoine's older brother Robert Arnauld d'Andilly and of his sister Angélique. In the 1630s he became Antoine's confessor, directing his conscience and guiding his theological studies. The youth considered his mentor to be "the oracle of our century."[167]

This congenial five-year relationship began in 1638–39 when Antoine wrote to Saint-Cyran, calling him "My Father" and begging him to be his spiritual director. "Allow me to call you this name, since God has given me the desire to be your son," he implored. Promising "to separate myself from all attachments to the world" and study St. Augustine more faithfully, Antoine begged for "instructions for salvation." He assured Saint-Cyran that his counsel "will be received as coming from the Spirit of God who speaks in you."[168] When Saint-Cyran accepted, Antoine's happiness knew no bounds. He promised his mentor that he would live in solitude, cultivate "purity of heart," and bear "persecution . . . in defense of the truth" even if it meant becoming a martyr.[169] In all his letters and books, Arnauld praises his confessor's patience amidst persecution, love for the Church, devotion to the Holy Sacrament, pious writings, and even his exemplary death.[170] After Saint-Cyran's death, Arnauld wrote the lengthy *Apology for Sir Jean du Vergier de Hauranne, abbé de Saint-Cyran* (1644) to defend his reputation against Jesuit libels.[171]

Saint-Cyran's tutelage so changed Antoine's character that his older sister Catherine (wife of Isaac LeMaître) described the transformation as "this second rebirth," calling him "my new brother."[172] He had grown bolder, telling Paolo Walloni (papal nuncio to France): "I am a man of the world who is unable to constrain himself, and to speak with his mouth that which is not in his heart."[173] But he had also become more pious, declaring that "the glory of God and the prosperity of his friends" would guide his actions.[174]

Arnauld's "holy boldness" pleased some of his contemporaries and offended others. President of the Paris Parlement de Lamoignon called him "one of the leading ornaments of our century."[175] But the list of his enemies grew as the century progressed: the Jesuits, the French Court, the Holy See, the archbishop of Paris, Louis XIV and his confessor *Père* La Chaise.[176] "The Grand Arnauld" was less a great theologian than a leading controversialist who enjoyed arguing with everyone; having little diplomacy in his makeup, he could not be "a party man." Even his theological works reflect his legal training: they read like a lawyer's brief, subdivided into main proofs and subordinate proofs and making fine distinctions between *droit* and *fait*. For him, being a Jansenist meant arguing against someone or some cause. He refused to be silenced or ignored; consequently, he spent 30 years in exile.[177]

This legalism (which J. D. Crichton called the "Arnauldist vice"[178]), however, proved useful when the need arose for Jansenists to defend themselves with petitions, appeals, tracts or books. Yet it could also cause rifts within the Jansenist camp, as in the debate over signing the Formulary. While some Jansenists felt that one could sign it even if he did not believe that the five condemned propositions were found in Jansen's writings, Arnauld, believing such "sophisms" dishonest, argued that conscience and Christian sincerity prevented one from signing. Instead, he counseled his friends to maintain "a respectful silence." This, he felt, would stop all debates, demonstrate submission to ecumenical councils, and protect the individual's conscience. But if forced to sign, one should add the caveat that while recognizing the five propositions as heretical and acknowledging the pope's right to condemn them, the signer nonetheless declared that they could not be found in Jansen's *Augustinus*.[179] While this legerdemain helped the Port-Royal nuns survive decades of harassment, it did not save Arnauld's neck: in 1656 the Faculty of Theology at the Sorbonne voted to expel him from its ranks.[180]

Nonetheless, he never forgot the oath he had taken when he received his Doctor of Theology degree: "To defend the truth and even give his life for it if necessary."[181] For him, the best way to "defend the truth" was to write. When the Jesuit Isaac Habert attacked Jansen's *Augustinus* as Calvinistic in his *Defense of the Faith of the Church*, therefore, Arnauld fired back with both barrels in his *First* (1644) and *Second Apology for Jansénius* (1645). Accusing Habert of being one of those "vipers who tear at the breast of their mother [the Church]," he assures readers that Jansenists oppose Protestants as heretics. Whereas Calvin held God responsible for man's corrupt nature, Jansenists blame humanity for sin's existence. Moreover, Jansenists, who agree completely with St. Augustine, are more in harmony with papal pronouncements on grace than most other

Catholic groups. Finally, Arnauld clarifies doctrinal issues such as attrition and contrition, predestination, and sufficient grace. Accusing Habert of "not having read either the titles or the text" of the *Augustinus*, Arnauld cleverly shows that Habert disagreed, not with Jansen, but with Augustine's teachings.[182]

Furthermore, he declares, after eight of the "most qualified Theologians in Rome" spent six months examining Jansen's work, they have "found nothing that was not in conformity to St. Augustine's writings, & consequently more worthy of approbation than censure."[183] The Archbishop of Philippi had declared the *Augustinus* to be "the orthodox, solid & Catholic doctrine of St. Augustine . . . very useful to those who love true piety & . . . true Christian humility."[184] Moreover, several Doctors of Theology at the Sorbonne have found the work "full of science, full of the most true & pure Catholic doctrine; a work very perfect & complete, which God has caused to be born at this time for the consolation of the faithful & the good of his Church."[185] The real problem, Arnauld asserts, was that the Church itself—influenced by the Jesuits—has drifted from its emphasis on an Augustinian theology of grace.[186] "But time is the Father of truth & the enemy of lies," he exclaims optimistically.[187]

Arnauld saw a recent papal bull as contributing to the misunderstanding regarding Jansen's teachings; using legalistic logic, he endeavored to reinterpret it. Urban VIII's bull *In eminenti* (1643), he explained, used the term *prohibemus* (prohibited), not *damnamus* (damned), "which shows clearly that the doctrine in this book [*Augustinus*] is not condemned as error or heresy." Although the bull forbade discussion and debate about Jansen's work "on pain of excommunication," it labeled none of its eighteen propositions as "heretical, erroneous, false, or rash."[188]

Furthermore, as mentioned above, Arnauld advances the distinction between *droit* (right) and *fait* (fact) regarding the allegedly heretical Five Propositions in Jansen's writings. Throughout his *Oeuvres*, he consistently argues that while the Church has the *right* to judge matters of faith and doctrine, and therefore the *right* to condemn as heresy the Five Propositions, these heretical statements *do not in fact* appear anywhere in the *Augustinus*. Therefore, whereas the Church is infallible in matters pertaining to faith and doctrine, it is fallible in pronouncing on matters of fact. After condemning the Five Propositions "in whatever book they are found without exception" as contrary to "the faith & doctrine of the Church," Arnauld cleverly suggests that these propositions can be found in certain Jesuit works which "are full of errors & heresies."[189]

Ever suspicious, Arnauld blames the Jesuits as being the current leaders in a conspiracy to turn the Church against Jansen and, by extension, away from Augustinian theology. He asserts that since Jansen's writings have never been carefully examined either at Rome or in France; neither Urban VIII, Innocent X or Alexander VII have condemned them as heretical; no doctors of theology have proven "with solid reason" that they contain heresy; therefore, the matter remains doubtful.[190] Furthermore, since "facts" require "rules [proofs] to determine their certainty," "no human authority can force one's belief in a doubtful fact." The Church herself, he declares, "has never enforced a belief in facts not divinely revealed." Indeed, "God alone is able to command faith . . . because he can remove, by his command, all human uncertainty."[191] Therefore, he accuses the Jesuits of inspiring popes to issue "careless" and "provisional" bulls to make the name of Jansen "odious." They are guilty "of the heresy of domination." The secret "Jesuit plan," he intones, "is to create a situation favorable for the recognition of papal infallibility," to make the pope absolute and independent of all checks by councils, assemblies, cardinals and bishops.[192]

This fear of a Jesuit conspiracy and papal infallibility explains why Arnauld (and all Jansenists) uncompromisingly defended Gallican liberties. Because he considered general councils superior in authority to popes (in his 1657 *Writings on the Bulls of Alexander VII and the Formularies of the French Clergy*), he recognized papal infallibility in matters of faith *only* if the pope's decrees had been approved by Church councils. A decade later, in *Ten Memoirs on the Cause of the Bishops Who*

Distinguished Fact from Right (1668), he argues that Gallican bishops have the right to examine and criticize papal bulls; to abrogate this right would "entirely ruin the Liberties of the Gallican Church." Bishops, he asserts, "are not simply executors of everything that it pleases the pope to ordain"; they are "the Judges established by Jesus Christ" to insure that the pope conforms to the faith and canons of Church law. Far from being obliged "to submit blindly to the popes' Constitution," he declares, bishops "must obey God first." As such, they are the "ecclesiastical police" to maintain unity, order, and doctrinal truth in the Church. It is they—and not the popes—who have the right to judge in matters of faith "in the first instance," to convene councils and condemn their errors, to establish new churches, and to examine papal bulls.[193]

Naturally, Arnauld's aggressive defense of Jansen and Gallicanism proved unpopular in Rome and Paris. On 14 January 1656, by a vote of 124 to 71, the Faculty of Theology at the Sorbonne censured him and then expelled him from their ranks.[194] Fearing imprisonment, he fled to Port-Royal des Champs and the protection of his younger sister, *Mère* Angélique Arnauld. Writing "from the desert" to Queen Anne (the Queen Mother), he begged her to protect him and his friends ("disciples of St. Augustine" who "love the truth").[195]

Although Arnauld recommended that Jansenists maintain "a respectful silence" toward papal bulls condemning the Five Propositions,[196] he himself could not remain silent even in exile. In a letter to the canon Father Salesse, he bemoaned the fact that Alexander VII's bull *Ad sacram* (1657) "more and more oppresses the Catholic truth of the Grace of Jesus Christ" and teaches Molina's doctrine of grace, thus "arming the semi-pelagians of our century."[197] Three years later, he defied efforts to force him to sign the Formulary, telling an assembly of bishops: "You have no authority or jurisdiction over me . . . There is no law that obliges me to sign the Formulary, neither to coerce others to sign it in my diocese, as you are neither my superior nor my judges, everything that it pleases you to order in your assembly has no force of law over me."[198]

Arnauld saw the bishops and popes as puppets in this conspiracy to crush Jansenism; the Jesuits pulled the strings backstage, led by Louis XIV's confessor *Père* Annat. In a letter to the *abbé* de La Lane in 1663, he called Alexander VII's bull "a new outrage against the innocence & truth we have received" perpetrated by "the bad faith of the Jesuits." The Jesuits, he exclaims, "are the imposters, and they very much deserve to be eternally outwitted." He hopes that their "trickery" will cause a backlash in France, engendering stronger unity and opposition to papal decrees.[199] In the meantime, however, the "disciples of St. Augustine" should maintain "respectful silence" and show due submission to the Church.

The nature of their submission, however, worried many Jansenists. Should they give "exterior deference" (outward compliance) to keep the peace and avoid punishment? Could they in good conscience show "interior approbation" (consent that the pope's judgment conformed to truth and justice)? Or might they give written consent (sign the Formulary) in order to avoid "disorder & confusion." Arnauld and the Port-Royal *Soeurs* and *Solitaires* felt that the first and third choices violated their consciences.[200]

For Arnauld, all of these issues coalesced in 1641 when a dispute arose regarding the frequency of observing Communion. The *princesse* de Guéménée, guided by Saint-Cyran, felt that the *marquise* de Sablé, whose confessor was the Jesuit Pierre de Sesmaisons, erred in taking Communion the same day she had attended a Court ball rather than to observe several days of penitence between confession and the Eucharist. To set her straight, the princess gave the marquise the "rules of conduct" Saint-Cyran had prepared for her. When the marquise shared these guidelines with her confessor, Sesmaisons published a refutation of them. Saint-Cyran, recently released from the Bastille and too ill to reply, asked Arnauld to combat Sesmaisons' lax position. Within two years, Arnauld, with the help of Saint-Cyran, his nephew Martin de Barcos, and Port-Royal teacher M. de Sacy, completed the famous *Frequent Communion.*[201]

In the preface to *La Fréquente* (as contemporaries referred to it[202]), Arnauld declared: "I wrote the book . . . solely for the love of the truth & a desire to save souls . . . and [nothing] shall prevent me from defending the truth."[203] By August, 39 censors had approved it; many praised it for its "solidity, force and eloquence, its clarity, elegance and nobility of style."[204] The future Alexander VII, Fabio Chigi, then Bishop of Narni and papal nuncio to Cologne, wrote two letters in Latin recommending the book.[205] It gained the approval of five archbishops, 22 bishops, and 24 doctors of theology; most of the delegates to the General Assembly of the French Clergy praised its merits. Five archbishops and at least twelve bishops told Urban VIII and Innocent X that they had "recommended it to all the faithful" in their dioceses.[206] The writer Honoré de Balzac, who praised *La Frequente* as "a learned, wise, eloquent book," asserted that it was "so solid and strong on all sides that I do not think that all the machines in the arsenal of the Society of Jesus can erase a single line of it."[207] Its admirers included high Court ladies, French bishops and priests, and Roman cardinals.[208]

Yet its appearance three months after the death of Louis XIII signaled "the point of departure for open combat between the Jansenist party and its adversaries."[209] Even the Jesuit *père* René Rapin recognized its significance. "Nothing contributed more to the reputation of Jansenism," he confessed, "than the book *Frequent Communion*," due to its "spirit of moral severity."[210] It constituted both a defense of the ideas of Saint-Cyran and a manifesto for the Port-Royal nuns.[211]

Frequent Communion criticized the laxism of the Jesuits by emphasizing the need for perfect contrition for one's sins (attrition was "imperfect confession"), a "responsible conscience," and making "appropriate preparation" in one's heart and life before taking Communion. Citing scripture, the church fathers, papal decrees, councils' decisions, saints' pronouncements, and church traditions, he asserted that Catholicism had become lax in administering the sacrament of penitence, which must be proportionate to the sin, given after confession but before absolution. Furthermore, the Eucharist—which some took daily—should be observed far less frequently, following the pattern set by the apostles in the first century. Only those who had made "proper spiritual preparation" (by both interior conversion and exterior penance) should receive it. Daily or weekly observance—a recent trend—made the rite too common.[212]

In contrast to the Jesuit position (laxism) of taking Communion as often as one wished, Arnauld advanced the position of rigorism, or extreme severity in applying the rules of morality and religion in the administration of the sacraments.[213] Believing that the best rule to follow was "to observe what conforms to Antiquity, to the Traditions of the Saints & to the old customs of the Church," he discovered that first century Christians celebrated Communion infrequently. Such a practice, he felt, would inspire greater respect, awe, love, and honor for the rite today. The Council of Trent, which advised believers to celebrate it frequently—even daily—showed its "prodigious ignorance" of this tradition and thereby dishonored the Holy Spirit. Frequent observance diminished reverence, reduced awe of holy things, and left believers cold-hearted. [214]

But Arnauld went further in his recommendations. Those who commit mortal sins should be forbidden to partake of Communion until, by severe penitence, "they show themselves worthy of partaking again." If they do not repent, they should be excommunicated.[215] Otherwise, he said, priests and bishops would be guilty of blasphemy for encouraging those "who lead lives totally corrupt and pagan" to receive "the Holy of Holies in their mouths full of filth and corruption." Such a course constituted "a strategy of the devil" and those who followed it would, like the citizens of Sodom and Gomorrah, suffer "divine vengeance."[216]

Instead of taking Communion often, Arnauld recommends both frequent confession and penitence "to cleanse the soul." These sacraments, he states, are "ordained to make us pure in soul." Therefore, he exhorts, pray often, confess often, do penitence often, fast often, weep often, and give alms often—but take Communion infrequently, only when the heart and soul have been carefully prepared.[217]

The ink had hardly dried on *Frequent Communion* before its detractors swarmed to attack it. Two examples will suffice. In his *Examination and Judgment of the Book Frequent Communion* (1644), Charles François d'Abra de Raconis, Bishop of LaVaur, hastened to defend the frequent observance of the Eucharist and expose Arnauld's "new Dogmatics and artifices" as threatening Church unity. Frequent Communion, he declares, often prepares the way for true conversion, not the other way around. He attacks Arnauld's "sinister interpretations," faulty judgments, lies, misquotation of Church fathers, poor theology, weak historical interpretations, and all his "scandalous and injurious propositions." Arnauld misunderstands confession, the relation of absolution to Communion and to public penitence, and why frequent Communion is preferable, he asserts. Finally, he accuses Arnauld of dangerous tendencies toward illuminism.[218]

Councilor of State and royal almoner Léonard de Marandé, in *Inconveniences of Jansenism* (1653), accuses Arnauld of libel, abuse, bad faith, and preaching "new doctrines" that will have "dangerous consequences." In *Frequent Communion*, he asserts, one can find Lutheranism, Calvinism and Jansenism as well as an unwholesome mixture of "dangerous maxims, novelties, and heresies." Marandé charges its author with opposing Church doctrine, falsifying Christian Antiquity, and destroying the foundations of the faith (prayer, contrition, penitence, baptism, the Eucharist, etc.).[219]

Although the king's almoner might attack Arnauld with impunity, Louis XIII found himself caught on the horns of a dilemma. If he took the side of the Jesuits, he risked alienating the bishops and doctors of theology at the Sorbonne. If he backed Arnauld, he risked offending the Jesuits. Fortunately for him, the grim reaper solved the problem by snatching him away in 1643, the year *Frequent Communion* appeared. Louis XIV's first minister Cardinal Mazarin sided with the Jesuits, but the Sorbonne and the University of Paris remained sympathetic to Jansenism and hostile to the Society of Jesus.[220] Meanwhile, Paris Archbishop Hardouin de Péréfixe and *Père* de La Chaise opposed Arnauld. In his letters, Antoine recognized that both men "have tried to prejudice the King against me" as a writer of books "pernicious to Church & State." Péréfixe especially "wants me to perish," he told his friend Du Vaucel.[221]

Arnauld still had highly placed friends in Rome, however. In 1690, Cardinal Tanora, internuncio at Brussels, declared that, following a close examination by the Papal See, the *Frequent Communion* "had been judged undeserving of any Censure."[222] In addition to the pope, Arnauld stated that cardinals on the Inquisition "have spoken with praise for the book."[223] In 1695, Cardinal Jean Grimaldi, papal nuncio to France, used his influence at Rome to defend the book and protect Arnauld's reputation.[224]

It should not be surprising, therefore, that *Frequent Communion* exerted a tremendous impact on the European Catholic Church at the end of the seventeenth century. For one thing, Jesuit attacks on Arnauld as a "scorpion," "serpent," and "lunatic leader" of "the Jansenist party" only increased readership of his book. In Paris, the number of Catholics taking weekly Communion declined sharply after the 1640s.[225] Arnauld interpreted this trend as vindication that the Church had adopted "the doctrine of the Church Fathers" regarding infrequent Communion.[226] His friend Pierre Nicole agreed, asserting that the doctrines taught in *Frequent Communion* "were more and more authorized & practiced in the Church, whereas . . . the errors of the Jesuits had been formally censured."[227] In a letter to Cardinal Cibo in 1677, Arnauld rejoiced that, despite Jesuit censorship and book burnings in some places, his work, "blessed by God," had reached every diocese in France.[228]

Even the Society of Jesus had been forced to modify some of its teachings and practices regarding Communion and absolution in response to the book's popularity. Recognizing that

Arnauld was correct in asserting that infrequent Communion had been Church tradition for centuries past, they gradually stopped attacking his book and, in some cases, recommended less frequent observance of the rite and delaying absolution to those whose outward lives disqualified them from partaking of it.[229]

Henri Arnauld (1597–1692)

This did not mean, however, that the Jesuits stopped hating the Arnaulds for the role they had played in the order's expulsion from France a century earlier. If they despised Antoine for his numerous attacks on them in print, they disliked his older brother Henri for his close ties to Port-Royal, that "hotel of Jansenism." As Bishop of Angers for 42 years (1650–1692), Henri played a decisive role in the *querrelle janséniste* in France. Yet while Antoine loved the hustle and bustle of Paris, his brother enjoyed the pastoral life of his rural diocese. If Antoine preferred vigorous debates with numerous rivals in print, Henri favored charitable work for the poor and basked in the adulation of the Port-Royal community, whom he continued to visit well into his nineties.[230]

But the bishop could also defend the Jansenist cause vigorously when the need arose. In an undated "Reflections on Jansen's Book," he praised the *Augustinus* for its organization, sound theology, and practicality; it reflected "the love of God." After summarizing its teachings on grace, original sin, and freedom of the will, he appended the favorable papal bulls of Alexander VII and Innocent X.[231]

Robert Arnauld d'Andilly (1589–1674)

Henri's and Antoine's older brother Robert Arnauld d'Andilly would also use his considerable influence to defend Port-Royal. Known for his probity, honesty, and piety among Jansenist friends, he was equally admired for his eloquence, brilliance, and "lively spirit" at Court. A clerk for an *intendant* of finance at fifteen, his career really took off after he married Catherine le Fevre de la Boderie, whose father had been ambassador to Rome, Brussels, and London. Robert became *intendant-général* for the *duc* d'Orléan's household until Louis XIII appointed him *intendant* of the army during the Thirty Years' War. At Catherine's untimely death in 1637, however, he relinquished his posts and retreated to Port-Royal des Champs to live the life of a solitaire near his children (his daughters and one son lived there). At Port-Royal he prayed, read, gardened, and wrote. His correspondence with the influential Calvinist Anne de Rohan led to her conversion to Catholicism. As an intermediary for Port-Royal at Court, he wrote 80 letters and several books defending its way of life during the troubled 1650s; consequently, Mazarin promised to protect the community in 1655.[232]

Robert's circle of friends included St. François de Sales, Jansen, and Saint-Cyran. In 1625 Jansen, then living with Saint-Cyran in Paris, wrote Robert a letter, praising him for being "untainted . . . by the great corruption of our times" and for his "profession of the truth . . . in the Courts of Princes." Jansen, who had heard much about Robert's "good virtues" and "worthy judgment," thanked him for imitating Christ's love in a wicked world.[233] In 1645, two years after Saint-Cyran's death, Robert assembled his letters and published them in four volumes with a glowing recommendation to French archbishops and bishops. Saint-Cyran, he exclaimed, "had a general affection & a Catholic charity for the common Mother of the Catholic Church, [and] a particular love & charity for the Gallican Church." His "pure & sincere" motives, his "respect for your Apostolic Order," and his "zeal for the Hierarchy . . . of the Princes of the Church" rendered him worthy of esteem and praise by Church leaders.[234]

As an apologist for Jansenism, Andilly proved himself particularly useful by defending those under attack. When the Jesuits censured his younger brother's *Frequent Communion* in 1643, Robert penned a series of letters to Cardinal Bentivoglio and sent him a copy of the book. The cardinal, though ill in bed, read it "with great satisfaction" and praised Antoine's "rare & excellent pen" which reflected the author's eloquence, piety, and logic.[235]

As an "ambassador at large" for Port-Royal, Robert vigorously defended the interests of the community at Court, sending letters to the queen, Mazarin, M. de Bartillat (an officer of the queen's household), the Bishop of Coutances, the *duchesse* de Chevreuse (Port-Royal's protector), and other influential friends. Repeatedly, he emphasized that the *soeurs* and *messieurs* submitted to the authority of the Church and state, obeyed Mazarin's orders, and desired peace in the Church. He also asserted that they could not sign the Formulary because the Five Propositions were not found in Jansen's *Augustinus*. Robert also defended his brother Antoine from the Sorbonne's accusations, negotiated a shorter exile for himself, and tried (but failed) to prevent the dispersion of the Port-Royal community in 1656.[236]

Writing to the *duchesse* de Chevreuse, Robert declared that the "enemies of this House [Port-Royal des Champs] have tried to give bad impressions of it to His Eminence [Mazarin]." But it is only a small monastery with only three priests and fewer than a dozen sisters employed in domestic and charitable duties. Pledging on his honor that the convent is loyal to the king, he begs the princess' protection against the "great lies" of its "blind, unjust, and angry" enemies.[237]

He could be equally insistent in his appeals to Mazarin. Less than two weeks later, he wrote "to inform Your Eminence of the truth of what passes here." Contrary to rumors of a Jansenist stronghold, he assured the first minister that Port-Royal des Champs "has neither rule, nor vows, nor constitutions, nor community, nor society, nor cells, nor anything that approaches this; and it does not form assemblies." Only ten or twelve women and seven or eight boys (scholars at the "little school") lived there—and they "have done nothing contrary to the laws and ordinances of the Kingdom." Therefore, he urged Mazarin to disregard "the evil intentions of our enemies."[238] A year later, as "violent and angry" reports spread questioning Port-Royal's loyalty, Robert again assured Mazarin that the community did not harbor enemies of the king (such as the *duc* de Luynes), but served Louis XIV wholeheartedly.[239]

Andilly also wrote to Queen Maria Theresa. Promising her that his unjustly attacked brother Antoine and all his Jansenist friends were orthodox Catholics and loyal subjects, he requested the queen's protection against their enemies in the Church. He hoped that God would "touch your heart in favor of our oppressed innocence."[240]

Three weeks later, Mazarin assured him that "his complete submission to the wishes of His Majesty" and his "entrusting this matter into the Queen's hands" could only result in "your contentment" if "you continue as you have begun."[241] Robert thanked the minister for "dissipating my incredible anxiety" by his "kind and favorable reply." Despite royal favor, however, Andilly had to leave Port-Royal des Champs for his estate at Pomponne in what Mazarin hoped would be "repose and tranquility." A week later, Robert thanked the first minister for "all the favors you have done for me" and assured him of "my zeal for the good of the State and my ardent passion for the service of their Majesties [and] of Your Eminence."[242]

But a Jansenist's idea of "tranquility" in exile did not include silence. Robert continued to defend himself, his brother, and his Jansenist friends. To Mazarin, he explained Antoine Arnauld's views as consistent with those of St. Chrysostom and St. Augustine; his brother was not a heretic, but innocent of the charges leveled against him.[243] In a letter to his friend the Bishop of Coutances, he blamed "the passion and animosity of the Jesuits against my brother" for his censure at the

Sorbonne. Their "impostures and calumnies" brought "shame to Christianity"; he anticipated the day when the state will have cause to regret the "evil actions" and "poisoned maxims" of the Society of Jesus.[244]

In the meantime, Robert saw other impending threats to the Church. In his frank letters to Claude Auvry, Bishop of Coutances, he warns of a "cabal" against Jansenism led by the Archbishops of Toulouse and Rouen and the Bishop of Montauban. This, he predicts, will lead to "a new war more violent and more obstinate than ever before." The "artifices," "illusions," "libels" and "bad designs" of these "diabolical" clerics and other "insolent ones" must be exposed, he asserts, so that "peace in the Church" can be restored. "There was never a lie so black . . . so full of malice . . . as these diabolical artifices . . . and abominable crimes" against the truth. He promises to take up his pen and reply to "a thousand impostures against us," even at the cost of life itself. He fears that "the fury of the Jesuits [will] send me to the Bastille."[245] Fortunately for him, he was wrong. He died peacefully, surrounded by friends, at Port-Royal des Champs on 27 September 1674 at the age of 85.[246]

Pierre Nicole (1625–1695)

Another defender of Port-Royal and a close friend of the Arnauld family, Pierre Nicole was born at Chartres into a family of robe nobles that included numerous lawyers, bailiffs, procurers and magistrates. The only boy among three sisters, he felt socially and spiritually isolated as a child. During the 1640s, he earned a bachelor's degree in theology and a master's degree in philosophy at the Sorbonne. Unlike other Jansenists, however, he at first accepted Jesuit casuistry and signed the Formulary in 1645. Naturally timid and modest, Nicole nevertheless demonstrated exceptionally deep thinking and writing skills.[247]

These skills soon attracted like-minded friends within the Jansenist camp. In 1654, Pierre made a friendship pact with Antoine Arnauld; they agreed to support each other in defending truth and battling the Society of Jesus. They collaborated in writing the *Four-Part Dissertation* (1656) and the powerful *Apology for the Religious of Port-Royal* (1665). For the next 25 years, living in close proximity, they conversed, dined, attended Mass, and recited the breviary together at the close of the day. Because the Jesuits sometimes blamed Nicole for anonymous works Arnauld had written, the two friends shared the insults of their opponents throughout life.[248] Nicole's friendship with Saint-Cyran's nephew Martin de Barcos pulled him into Port-Royal's orbit, where he met Antoine Singlin, spiritual advisor to the sisters there. Soon he began teaching philosophy and the humanities at the *petites écoles* in Paris, where he became friends with Le Nain de Tillemont, teacher, and Jean Racine, pupil.[249]

During the "Peace of the Church" (1669–1679), his fame grew. Following a formal dinner at the Archbishop of Sens' palace in Rome, Nicole and Antoine Arnauld were presented to the papal nuncio as "the Ecclesiastics of France who were the most worthy of his honor and friendship & the protection of the Holy See." The nuncio, who complimented Arnauld on being the man with "the golden pen," expressed his "satisfaction & esteem" at meeting them. When word of this honor reached France, Louis XIV invited Arnauld to Court.[250]

Years later, in a letter to Prince Ernest, Landgrave of Hesse, Arnauld praised Nicole as "one of the Port-Royal writers who is best known and highly regarded."[251] Indeed, even his private diary (c. 1649) demonstrates that in his twenties, Nicole could reckon historical dates using the Hebrew chronology, begin a paragraph in French and finish it in Latin, and think deeply about such abstract topics as man's sinfulness, God's love, and how to live a blessed life.[252]

Then in 1668, with Arnauld's coaching, Nicole wrote a major defense of Port-Royal. The

Clarification of Several Difficulties of the Religious of Port-Royal Concerning the Signing of the Formulary was intended to solve all the community's problems by showcasing their good deeds and pure motives. But the "Peace of the Church" ended the following year and persecution resumed.[253]

Two years later, Nicole published his famous *Treatise on the Education of a Prince* (1670), a brief 77-page manifesto for Christian education. Princes, he declares, are "children of God . . . instruments of God's mercy or anger upon humanity." They must receive the best Christian education possible so as to lead their people to salvation. They should study languages (French and Latin), grammar and writing, history, mathematics, science, geography, and jurisprudence—not only from textbooks, but also from everyday life. More importantly, however, the Christian prince will learn discernment ("good sense and reason"), taste, good manners, civility, and honesty as well as morality and the Christian virtues (truth, honesty, charity, etc.). His tutors will help him live purposefully, achieve self-control, defend the truth, hate violence, love Christ, and build a strong character.[254] As chapter 3 demonstrates in greater detail, Nicole's treatise on Christian education helped establish the blueprint for the "little schools" of Port-Royal.

Despite his Jansenist connections, Nicole's treatise won widespread approval from Church and state institutions, including the doctors of theology at the Sorbonne, who found in it "nothing but what conforms to the Apostolic & Roman Catholic Religion." Louis XIV granted it the coveted "Privilege of the King," permitting publishers to "print, sell, and circulate it" for seven years.[255]

Equally well received, Nicole's 600-page *Treatise on Prayer* stressed its importance in the life of the Christian:

> Prayer is the first & principal part of the vocation of every Christian. Thus one can say that a Christian Prince is a man who prays & governs the State; that a Christian General is a man who prays & leads the army; that a Christian Magistrate is a man who prays & renders justice to people; that a Christian artisan is a man who prays & works at his trade; that a Christian laborer is a man who prays & who tills the soil; that the mother of a Christian family is a woman who prays & who guides her family. Prayer enters into every vocation and it sanctifies all of them.[256]

But this life permeated with prayer required preparation and "continual vigilance." Beginning early each morning, one must read scripture and meditate on it, praise and adore God, and resist temptation. By focusing one's thoughts on the life and death of Christ, the Christian will soon come to reflect Jesus' attitude of charity, humility, trust, and perseverance in good works.[257]

In the second volume, Nicole gives instructions on the do's and don'ts of prayer. The Christian should *not* ask God for temporal blessings or harbor illusions concerning the worldly benefits to be gained from praying. On the other hand, he or she *should* ask for divine blessings, salvation, more love and Christian virtue, deliverance from temptation, greater zeal in God's service, and inner peace. Contrary to some Catholic theologians, Nicole maintains that silent prayer (what he called "mental prayer" or "thinking good thoughts") was as effective as spoken prayer—and, from the examples he gives, this had been practiced by the saints from apostolic times.[258]

Pasquier Quesnel (1634–1719)

Unlike Nicole, Pasquier Quesnel, the son of a bookseller on the *rue* Saint-Jacques, grew up in humble surroundings. But like Nicole, he had been trained by the Jesuits in the humanities at the College of Clermont and in philosophy at the College of Lisieux before taking a master's degree in theology at the Sorbonne and entering the Congregation of the Oratorians (where he remained from 1657 to 1681). Also like Nicole, he became a priest in 1659 and signed the Formulary that repudiated the Five Propositions in Jansen's *Augustinus*. For several years he taught at and directed the Oratorian Seminary of Saint-Magloire before returning to the Congregation on the *rue* Saint-Honoré in 1669. Following Quesnel's retraction of his signature on the Formulary and publication of his famous *Moral Reflections on the New Testament* (1692), the Archbishop of Paris banished him (and 40 other Oratorians) from Paris and he fled, first to Orléans and Mons and then to Holland and Brussels from 1685 to 1703.[259]

But the long arm of French justice extended even to the Low Countries. Louis XIV issued a *lettre de cachet* (secret royal arrest warrant) and on 30 May 1703, with the cooperation of Philippe V of Spain (Louis XIV's grandson and ruler of the Spanish Netherlands), police apprehended Quesnel near Brussels. A week later, the marquis de Bednor (Spanish governor of the Pay-Bas), charging him with leading a cabal against the government and causing schism in the Church, seized his papers and imprisoned the septuagenarian in a damp, dark, unheated chamber with fungi growing on the walls.[260]

Quesnel's plight inspired widespread sympathy. In France, where the poet Boileau enjoyed favor at Court, someone composed the following quatrain:

> Against Quesnel Rome and Versailles unite in vain,
> For him all of France has the eyes of Noailles [Archbishop of Paris],
> The Ignacean League [Jesuits] so keen to censure him,
> The public, revolting, obstinate to admire him.[261]

Fortunately for Quesnel, his admirers rallied to his defense. His good friend Antoine Arnauld, who a year before his death in 1694 had bequeathed him an annual pension of 120 *livres*,[262] denied that Quesnel was involved in any "secret cabal" against the state or the Church. Arnauld protested his friend's innocence, blaming his arrest on the Jesuits and particularly on Louis XIV's confessor *Père* La Chaise.[263]

Taking pen in hand, Quesnel vigorously defended himself as well. In a 60-page letter to La Chaise, he protests his innocence and denies the Jesuits' "false accusations" that the Jansenists are rebels, heretics, or schismatics. Far from being involved in a cabal, he declares, they sought to advance "truth, justice & innocence."[264] In a subsequent letter, he assures Louis XIV that "I have never said, written, or done anything contrary to the respect and obedience that I owe and have shown all my life to Your Majesty." His writings bear witness, he declares, that he has always "defended the sovereignty of kings & their inviolable rights." Even in his dank dungeon, "where the violence of my enemies has forced me to retire," he promises always to be loyal "to your sacred person."[265]

After four months of suffering, however, Quesnel decided he had had enough of Spanish prisons. On the night of September 12–13, 1703, with the help of his brother William, Pasquier escaped from his dungeon cell in Molines disguised as a woman and fled to Liege in Holland. There, refusing to remain silent, he penned some 4000 letters and several polemical works defending himself, attacking the new Bull *Unigenitus* (1713), and defending his Jansenist friends. His writings ignited the flame of the second wave of Jansenism and gave new life to the movement in the eighteenth century.[266]

Quesnel's works also reveal the strong undercurrent of Richerism and Gallicanism that permeated Jansenism for over a century. Even at the age of 85 when he penned his "Last Testament" in December 1719, he defended these "truths." His final "profession of faith" recognized the Roman Catholic Church as the only repository of truth and the pope as Christ's vicar on earth. One last time he protests his innocence, declaring that he has "never pretended to say, write, or think anything contrary to what the holy Catholic Church believes and teaches." If unknowingly he has written anything "against the beliefs of the Church," then "I retract and detest it and submit myself in advance to whatever the Church decides concerning my writings and my person." Quesnel then appeals for a future council to vote on the orthodoxy of the Bull *Unigenitus*, to end "the spirit of schism and division" within the Church, and unify the faithful defenders of truth.[267]

Ironically, Quesnel's *Christian Instructions* (1671) and his *New Testament in French with Moral Reflections on Each Verse* (1692) ignited that division within the Church. When it first appeared, however, *Christian Instructions* enjoyed the patronage of the powerful. It had been approved by Cardinal Noailles, Archbishop of Paris, and granted the coveted "Approval & Privilege of the King." The Bishop of Châlons recommended "this holy book" for all the priests, vicars, and *curés* in his diocese. He praised its author as "a disciple in the school of the Holy Spirit," and promised that God would bless all who read it with "pious reflections," "great inner purity," and "a sincere desire to love our Lord Jesus Christ."[268]

Christian Instructions demanded a high level of commitment from every Christian. Daily reflections, meditating on scripture, listening for the Holy Spirit's guidance, and focusing on death keep the soul pure. "Meditating on death," Quesnel states, "has always been seen by the Saints of the Old and New Testaments as the most certain preservative against sin." Another sure "remedy" is to dwell on Christ's passion and death. "A great number of pious persons nurture their devotional life [by dwelling on] the death of Jesus Christ," he adds. This constituted the pathway to truth.[269]

Moral Reflections, although not published until 1692, was an expanded and conflated version of his commentary on the four Gospels (written in 1672) and his commentary on Acts, the Pauline Epistles, and Revelation (written in 1687). In 1677 the earlier commentary had received a 30-year publication approval from the Council of State; Louis XIV himself signed the letters patent on 27 March forbidding anyone from pirating Quesnel's work on pain of 6000 *livres* fine. A decade later, the doctors of theology at the Sorbonne, "finding that it contains nothing contrary to the Roman Apostolic Catholic faith," gave the book their hearty approval, recommending it as "useful to the public."[270] Antoine Arnauld praised *Moral Reflections*, finding it "full of edifying thoughts [which] raise the heart to God." He added that it was "as good as a catechism" for explaining doctrinal truths and morality and "very useful for training a young ecclesiastic."[271] Over the next 35 years it went through 40 editions and, despite its controversial nature with the Jesuits, became a devotional bestseller.[272]

While most of the propositions in *Moral Reflections* agree with Catholic orthodoxy, the tone of the book, with its Jansenist emphasis on Christocentrism, is undeniably partisan. Organized into "epistles," "lessons," and "gospels" to be read in Church during the liturgical year, the three-volume work includes an extended commentary on Matthew, Mark, Luke and John. Quesnel interprets each verse in a paragraph, adds a Latin gloss in the margins, and supplies textual cross-references. He comments extensively on the origin and nature of sin, justice, and fear; on grace and predestination; on belief, penitence, communion, and charity. But by highlighting the prophetic role he expected the Jews to play in last-day events by their conversion and restoration to Israel, Quesnel introduced the element of Figurism that would become so prominent in eighteenth-century Jansenism. Like Edmond Richer, he also exalted the authority of the lower clergy against that of the bishops and favored lay involvement in electing pastors, confirming doctrines, and excommunicating members. In addition to this "Presbyterian spirit," he introduced such liturgical innovations as using the local dialect or language for baptisms, weddings, and funerals; suggested that psalms be sung in French; and composed several new prayers.[273]

Although Quesnel quoted extensively from the Vulgate and cited the Church Fathers at length in his *Moral Reflections*, these "Quesnellisms" got him into serious trouble with the Church hierarchy. His caustic remarks about the Jesuits (calling them "enemies of the state" for "crying cabal" against the Jansenists) did not help matters either. His book's potent mixture of Richerism, Gallicanism, conciliarism, and Jansenism won him enemies in Rome and France. In 1711 Louis XIV informed Clement XI that he wanted the work condemned in a papal bull—and if the pope refused to do so, the General Assembly of the French Clergy would. After two years of negotiation and debate (as chapter 5 shows), Clement XI in 1713 issued the Bull *Unigenitus* condemning 101 propositions in *Moral Reflections*.[274]

That Pasquier Quesnel—a proponent of royal Gallicanism and a strong supporter of the Catholic Reformation—should be condemned by both his king and pope presents a double paradox. He was certainly neither a hypocrite in his theology nor a Machiavellian in his politics. Yet as Catherine Maire so aptly said, "It is precisely because Quesnel is an ardent defender of divine right in Church and State that he will be perceived as a heretic and a seditious person. Such is the truth about the chimera of Jansenism!"[275]

But the ghost of Jansenism, given new life by Quesnel, proved impossible to suppress either by royal declarations or papal bulls. Although Quesnel himself hid his convictions in coded letters to his friends,[276] *Quesnellisme* spread rapidly in France. It permeated the pages of the eighteenth-century underground Jansenist newspaper *Ecclesiastical News*, echoed through the halls of the Oratorians' sixteen seminaries and 27 colleges and at the convent schools taught by sympathetic Benedictines, Genovesians, Barnabites, and others. Jansenist bishops propagated it in their mandates; rebellious priests advanced its ideals when they stood for "Gallican liberties" and opposed papal infallibility; and the laity experienced it in daily worship services emphasizing piety and devotion to the cross (rather than to the sacred heart of Jesus, the Jesuit's focus).[277] Like a raging river in spring, the floodtide of Jansenism could not be contained between the orthodox banks of Church and state.

Blaise Pascal (1622–1662)

Once described by Antoine Arnauld as "one of the brightest minds of the century, & a man of singular piety,"[278] the writer Blaise Pascal had many connections to Jansenism. His family (including his father Guillebert and his sister Jacqueline) were "disciples of Saint-Cyran"; they attended services at Port-Royal in Paris from 1646 to 1648 when they came to the city for medical treatment. Influenced by its spiritual director Antoine Singlin, Jacqueline asked her father's permission to join the community, but he refused. After his death in 1651, however, she entered Port-Royal in January 1652, and Blaise assisted Robert Arnauld d'Andilly at the service in which she took her vows and donned the habit of a novice (henceforth to be "Sister Sainte-Euphémie"). Completing her novitiate, she became a nun and teacher of novices in 1653. As sub-prioress at Port-Royal des Champs after 1659, Jacqueline wrote some guidelines for religious education and continued teaching until her death in 1661. Blaise's nephew Etienne Périer studied at the *petites écoles* for nine years from 1651 until they closed in 1660. His niece Marguerite Périer, also a novitiate at Port-Royal, became famous when in March 1656 she experienced a miraculous healing after touching her face with the "holy thorn." When Blaise himself had a deeply emotional conversion after a near death experience in 1654, he retreated to a cell at Port-Royal des Champs and began writing the famous *Provincial Letters* (1656–57) defending Jansenism and attacking the Jesuits.[279]

Pascal had once assured his Jansenist friends: "I have read your books and those of your adversaries: may it be sufficient for you to know that I am of your sentiment."[280] During his two-month sojourn (November 1654–January 1655) with the *solitaires*, this literary giant, famous throughout

Europe, "walked the talk" by living the ascetic lifestyle at The Grange. Lodged in a tiny cell with a hard bed, a chair, a table, and a single crucifix on the wall for decoration, he arose at 5 a.m. to assist at Prime. He said his prayers, attended all the other religious services (except Matins at 2 a.m.), fasted, and followed the spiritual direction of Singlin and Le Maître de Sacy.[281] Jacqueline, who had been "sad when I saw that you were in the world," expressed her "joy at finding you happy in the solitude."[282]

Although Pascal left The Grange at the end of January to attend to urgent business in Paris, in a spiritual sense, he brought Port-Royal with him. He released most of his servants, stripped his walls bare of tapestries, avoided sensual pleasures, and prepared simple meals for himself, dispensing with the gourmet foods he loved. Even his writing changed. In place of secular poetry and prose, he penned treatises on grace and a short sketch of Christ's life. And whenever he could, he returned to Port-Royal, making short visits in January 1656 and August 1659.[283]

His friends there would always be dear to his heart, as his writings attest. When others questioned the genuineness of his niece's miraculous healing in 1656, Pascal defended Port-Royal as "the sanctuary of [God's] graces" where he had "poured out his favors" through a miracle to defeat the "calumnies" of its detractors.[284] Yet he admitted that these detractors were correct about one thing: this religious community had been "a secret cabal for thirty-five years [1625–1660], over which Monsieur de Saint-Cyran and Monsieur d'Ypres [Jansen] have been the leaders."[285] Although a very sick man during the last five years of his life, Pascal boldly defended his friends in the "Jansenist cabal" against the Jesuits and all who maligned them until his death on 19 August 1662.[286]

R. A. Knox (1950) has suggested that Pascal's bilious illness affected his temperament as well, giving him a jaundiced view of people toward the end of his life. In his *Thoughts* and *Provincial Letters*, this "Christian pessimist" seemed obsessed with original sin, human corruption, and Christ's redemption for a contemptible world. He taught the Jansenists to be gloomy, Knox asserted, and helped to fix in them that "mood of despair" and pessimism so different from their earlier attitude of lightness and humanness set by Sébastien Zamet in the 1650s.[287] Perhaps, but not entirely so. As this chapter and the following ones show, pessimism concerning human nature and contempt for the world entered Jansenism decades before Pascal wrote his *Provincial Letters*. It was a legacy from Saint Augustine as reinterpreted by Cornelius Jansen, Saint-Cyran, and Antoine Arnauld. Pascal perhaps intensified the virus within the soul of Jansenism, but he did not plant it there.

His truly original contribution was in applying the rigor of geometrical reasoning to the principles of Augustinian theology in his *Provincial Letters*, an apologetic work defending the teachings of Port-Royal.[288] Recognizing the incendiary nature of these letters, Pascal covered his tracks by adopting pseudonyms ("Louis de Montalte" and "Guillaume Wendrock") and supplying a fake publisher's name ("Pierre de la Vallée" for Daniel Elzevier) and city (Cologne for Amsterdam) for the book's place of origin.[289] In reality, Antoine Arnauld and Pierre Nicole collaborated with Pascal in writing these nineteen letters. They each provided him with information and quotations, and together drafted a general plan for the work. They also proofread the letters before handing them to friends of Port-Royal (Nicolas Vitart, the *intendant* for the *duc* de Luynes, and Baudry d'Asson, a nobleman from Bas-Poitou) who took them to Amsterdam to be published.[290]

The immediate cause for writing these letters occurred on 1 February 1655 when the vicar of Saint-Sulpice in Paris refused absolution to the *duc* de Liancourt, a noted Jansenist and friend of Port-Royal. When Monsieur Olier, the local curate, defended the vicar's action, Antoine Arnauld entered the fray. He protested with his *Letter of a Doctor of the Sorbonne to a Person of Rank* (24 February) and a *Second Letter of a Doctor of the Sorbonne to a Duke and Peer of France* (10 July), defending Liancourt's orthodoxy as a faithful follower of Saint Augustine. When the Sorbonne expelled Arnauld from its Theology Faculty, Pascal defended his innocence by writing the first three *Provincial Letters* in January and February 1656.[291]

Yet these letters served a wider purpose as well. Because they constituted a defense of Arnauld in the court of public opinion, they changed the terrain of combat from a theological squabble at the Sorbonne to an appeal for public intervention in behalf of an innocent man maligned by corrupt accusers. Pascal underlines not only the innocence of Liancourt, Arnauld, and the Port-Royal Jansenists, but also the moral corruption of those telling falsehoods about them. These "enemies" include the Jesuits, certain Sorbonne theologians, Louis XIV, and even Popes Innocent X and Alexander VII who, by their bulls of 1653 and 1656, forced the Catholic clergy to sign the Formulary.[292]

Letters 1–3 (appearing on 23 and 29 January and 9 February 1656) defended Arnauld against charges leveled by the Sorbonne. With wit, logic, clarity, and cunning prose cloaked with religious sincerity, Pascal's skilled composition persuaded the public of Antoine's innocence. The success of these first three letters emboldened Pascal to attack Jesuit morality and their theology of grace in Letter 4 (March 1656), a clever conversation among a Jansenist, a Jesuit, and the author. Letters 5–9 (20 March–3 July, 1656), a response to the Spanish Jesuit Escobar's *Moral Theology*, ridiculed the casuistic arguments and doctrines of probability, equivocation, mental reservation, and direction of intention advanced by the Society of Jesus. Letter 10 (2 August 1656) further attacked the Jesuits' preference for attrition (regret for wrongdoing based on fear of hell) over contrition (regret based on love for God) and their denial that a believer must experience inner conversion in order for the sacrament of penance to be efficacious.[293]

In Letters 11–14 (18 August–23 October 1656), Pascal opposes the moral philosophy of the Jesuits and defends himself against their accusations that his letters make a jest of holy things. In Letters 15–16 (25 November and 14 December 1656), he defends his friends at Port-Royal against Jesuit charges of slander and calumny. By Letters 17–19 (January–April 1657), his tone had become more conciliatory, as if seeking reconciliation between the Jansenist and Thomist theological positions. Addressing himself directly to Louis XIV's Jesuit confessor *Père* Annat, he appeals for a truce between Church and state and Port-Royal, which he declares is not a heretical community. Although in Letter 17 he asserts, "I am not from Port-Royal," these letters, taken together, comprise his strongest defense of that ascetic community and in favor of his goal—peace and truth.[294]

Although neither the Sorbonne nor the Holy See officially condemned the *Provincial Letters*, the Inquisition placed them on the Catholic Index in 1657 because Pascal had discussed litigious and doctrinal issues only savants had the need to know. By writing in French, he had aired the Church's dirty laundry before the public, enabling non-theologians—and especially women—to debate serious issues pertaining to salvation.[295] The *Letters*, in fact, gave Jansenism the shot in the arm it needed, and probably won more converts to Jansenist morality than any other contemporary work. By attacking the Jesuits morally, theologically, and socially as the chief enemies of Port-Royal and Gallicanism, Pascal also helped persuade public opinion that the Jansenists constituted the chief defenders of Gallican liberties.[296]

Pascal's *Letters*, translated into Italian, Spanish, and Latin, sold thousands of copies across Europe. Applauded for their witty style, they influenced Molière and Bossuet, providing a model for French literature during the Classical Age. Despite being on the Index, the *Letters* found their way into the Vatican where cardinals read them during the conclave of Alexander VIII. They inspired further attacks on Jesuit probabilism and laxism, intensifying the conflict between Jansenism and its growing number of enemies. Their eloquence and ridicule appealed to the public and helped turn the tide of opinion in favor of Port-Royal and against the Society of Jesus.

Within a few years, Popes Alexander VII and Innocent XI would condemn over 100 casuistic propositions—the long-term fruits of Pascal's *Provincial Letters*.[297]

Paradoxically, however, some Jansenists expressed delight and others dismay at their appearance. Antoine Arnauld bragged that the *Letters* had "made a great impression on minds & changed for a long time the face of Jesuit affairs." They had "excited the zeal of the *curés*," called forth ecclesiastical assemblies to discuss the issues Pascal had raised, and inspired numerous authors to attack the Jesuits. "Over the past two hundred years," Arnauld exclaimed, "there has been no book as widely known and read around the world in French or Latin as the *Provincial Letters*."[298] Pierre Nicole agreed with Arnauld that Pascal had written a "just defense of truth." But Antoine Singlin and *Mère* Angélique Arnauld, while grateful for that defense, felt that the tone and style of Pascal's prose did not constitute a model of Christian charity or piety.[299]

Others, however, remembered Pascal's piety after his passing. Before he died on 19 August 1662, Pascal confessed and received the sacraments from Monsieur Beurier, a *curé* at the Jansenist Church of St.-Etienne-du-Mont in Paris.[300] Then an anonymous engraver carved his epitaph: "To the Glory of God, Here lies Blaise Pascal, Esquire. If piety is immortal, he will live forever."[301]

Jean-Baptiste Racine (1639–1699)

Jean Racine, another famous literary figure whose family was connected with Port-Royal, would also (like Pascal) become one of its greatest defenders. Suzanne des Moulins, his paternal great aunt, had lived at Port-Royal from 1625 until her death in 1647. She had in turn influenced her sister-in-law Marie Passart to enter the convent. In addition, several nephews had matriculated at the *petites écoles*.[302]

After his mother died in 1641, Jean lived with his Aunt Agnès, but the following year, she entrusted the three-year-old to the care of the sisters at Port-Royal de Paris. There he "learned to know God in his infancy." In their *petites écoles*, he also studied grammar and literature under Pierre Nicole, Claude Lancelot, Jean Hamon, Robert Arnauld d'Andilly, and Antoine LeMaître (who became a father figure to him after his own dad died in 1649). Then in 1653 he entered the College of Beauvais (whose teachers were Jansenist sympathizers). Here, while playing a rough game of "the Fronde," he was struck in the face by a stone that left a permanent scar. In 1655 he returned to Port-Royal des Champs to study drama and literature under Lancelot and Le Maître. When the lieutenant-civil closed Port-Royal a year later, however, Racine transferred to the College of Harcourt to study philosophy with the Jesuits (whom he detested).[303]

Molded by the Jansenist philosophy of education for two decades, Racine would always remember his school days at Port-Royal. His great love of poetry and Greek tragedy, encouraged in the *petites écoles*, bore fruit in his famous dramas *Esther* and *Athaliah*.[304] Despite his reservation that even religious dramas could not be truly "edifying," Antoine Arnauld praised Racine as "one of the best friends we have among the men of the world."[305] In April 1692, Louis XIV awarded Racine a generous pension of 4000 *livres* as one of the "famous men of letters" in France (the other being the poet Boileau). On at least one occasion, the king invited him to Versailles as an honored guest—one of the few times the king favored a Jansenist.[306]

Despite his fame as a member of the Académie Française and his good fortune as the king's historian, Racine remained humble. In his final will of 10 October 1698, he requested the privilege of being buried at Port-Royal in a tomb donated by his old teacher Jean Hamon. "Although I recognize that I am unworthy by the scandals of my past life and by the poor use I have made of the excellent education I received in former times at this school," he nonetheless begged the abbess "to grant me this honor." To prepare the way for her consent, he sent a gift of 800 *livres* with a further request for the prayers of the whole community. His request was granted.[307] After her husband died in April 1699, Madame des Moulins Racine retired to Port-Royal des Champs where she was "very much loved" to the day of her death.[308]

Racine is, of course, justly famous for his tragedies and his insightful commentaries (beginning in his adolescence) on famous Classical philosophers and dramatists (such as Plato, Aristotle, Euripides, Sophocles, Virgil and Lucien).[309] But four years before he died, he also wrote *An Abridged History of Port-Royal*, a powerful defense of the principles and individuals who had made that community a beacon of Jansenism for half a century. Although written in 1695, it was not published until 1742.[310] During his lifetime, therefore, Racine's letters did more to advance Jansenism and defend Port-Royal than his apologetic history. As one who moved in the highest Court circles at Versailles, Marly, and Fontainebleau, Racine corresponded with Louis XIV, Madame de Maintenon, the poet Boileau, *Père* La Chaise, and a host of princes, dukes, ambassadors, and military figures. Prince Henri-Jules de Bourbon-Condé was one of his generous patrons. Racine also wrote to many archbishops, bishops, abbots and clerics, providing each with a favorable image of Port-Royal.[311]

The public relations efforts of these Jansenist proponents were desperately needed by the end of the seventeenth century (as chapter 4 explains) as public stereotypes concerning Jansenism crystallized Most people saw it as a cauldron of errors—Baianism, Calvinism, Richerism, Gallicanism, and conciliarism—and its proponents as a heretical party, sect, or cabal.[312] Yet given the diverse personalities of its defenders, it would be impossible to speak of Jansenism as monolithic. It was a patchwork quilt that included Angélique Arnauld—judgmental, over-dramatic, always on the edge of tears and seeking martyrdom. It accommodated Saint-Cyran— self-centered, patronizing, often clannish in his attitudes toward other Catholic groups. It made room for the combative Antoine Arnauld, the great controversialist, arguing with everyone in defense of the truth. It included the legalistic Pierre Nicole who, with a lawyer's mind and methods, split hairs over "fact" and "right" in opposing the Five Propositions. But it also accommodated the pessimism of Blaise Pascal, obsessed with Original Sin and bequeathing a mood of despair to late-seventeenth century Jansenism.[313]

Because not every proponent interpreted Jansenism in exactly the same way, the movement also represented diverse protesting groups. While most of them shared a core of common beliefs, a few stretched various points of Jansenist theology to the breaking point, developing curious and, in some cases, even bizarre interpretations of their own. Chapter 2 examines both their commonly held beliefs and some of their diversity.

CHAPTER 2
What Was Jansenism?

"I hope God will continue to guide you along the path of affliction and suffering so you will come to love [his] sufferings."—*Agnès de St. Paul Arnauld*[1]

When Agnès Arnauld wrote the above words to her older brother Robert in 1635, she had just become abbess of Port-Royal in Paris. While Robert moved in high Court circles, his sister had voluntarily withdrawn from fashionable society to enter the cloistered world of prayer, meditation, and fasting. Yet at the end of her letter, she invited Robert to embrace the sufferings of Christ for the "good effects" they would bring in his life. For "when we lack all things," she added, "then we will discover our true and unique consolation" in God's grace.[2]

Although nearly all Jansenists would have agreed with Agnès that suffering benefited the soul, not all of them followed her example in leaving the secular world behind. As chapter 1 shows, even the prominent leaders in the movement did not always agree on how best to live the tenets of their creed. In part this was true for two reasons: first, because those who embraced Jansenism came from many different backgrounds, and second, because several "streams" of Jansenism existed. This chapter will explore the consensus and diversity within the movement by examining the sociology and teachings of Jansenism in France.

Half a century ago, the neo-Marxist historian Lucien Goldmann, in his book *The Hidden God* (1955), posited four distinct groups of Jansenist sympathizers along a continuum from liberals to extremists. The more liberal "Third Party" (including Robert Arnauld d'Andilly and the Bishop of Comminges) sympathized with Jansenism but made reluctant accommodations to secular society because they wanted to advance within it and therefore had no firm ascetic ideology of their own. The "Centrists or Moderates" (such as Antoine Arnauld and Pierre Nicole) sought a balance between compliance to authority and a demand for justice; in their struggle for goodness and truth, they created for themselves a more restricted sphere within the world. The "Rejecters of the World" (like Saint-Cyran, Martin de Barcos, Antoine Singlin, and Angélique Arnauld), who embraced ascetic lifestyles either at home or at Port-Royal, steered an uneasy course between showing deference for secular and ecclesiastical authority and rejecting everything they considered worldly. Finally, the "Extreme Ascetics" (embracing Jacqueline Pascal and the *abbé* Le Roy), who made no concessions to Church or state authority as "outside the Truth," proclaimed goodness and right in an evil world they knew would persecute them.[3]

Despite all their talk of suffering and persecution, however, most of those who embraced Jansenism came from society's higher ranks and enjoyed the benefits of wealth, education, and a network of powerful friends. By the eighteenth century, many hailed from the upper bourgeoisie and robe nobility, the rich and cultured society of France's bankers, merchants, lawyers, judges, and *parlementaires*. In their struggles against Church and state inroads upon their Gallican liberties, they admired the movement's spirit of insubordination and moral austerity, which reinforced their opposition to royal absolutism, papal infallibility, and aristocratic extravagance. Many in the Paris Parlement had sisters, daughters, or nieces at Port-Royal. The robe and Jansenists usually agreed on issues relating to Gallicanism, opposition to papal bulls, conciliarism, and rejection of the Formulary.[4]

Yet as Albert Hamscher (1977) emphasized, "early Jansenism [in the seventeenth century] was not the ideology of the robe." Indeed, when Louis XIV after 1661 sided with Parlement in his conflict with the pope over the *Regale* and other issues, the robe's support for Jansenism diminished rapidly. Even in the eighteenth century, the judges became reluctant allies with Jansenists (though few converted to their teachings) because they needed their support in conflicts with the king, pope, and Catholic clergy.[5]

The Jansenists themselves enjoyed the support of some powerful allies, not only in France, but internationally as well. These highly placed friends demonstrated their loyalty by writing letters of support on behalf of persecuted Jansenists, sending their sons and daughters to Port-Royal, and liberally financing the community's endeavors. These benefactors, who came from France, England, Scotland, Ireland, Italy, and the Spanish Netherlands (Belgium), frequently provided refuge for French Jansenists harassed by the Church or the state. Antoine Arnauld, Pasquier Quesnel, Nicolas Le Gros, the *abbé* Etémare, and many of the *solitaires* found safety with Jansenist sympathizers in Brussels, Utrecht, and Amsterdam.[6]

Still others fled to Poland and the protection of its queen, Louise-Marie de Gonzague. Before she married King Wladislas-Sigismond, Louise-Marie, then *princesse* de Mantua, had lived in France, where Saint-Cyran and Antoine Singlin had given her spiritual guidance. When the latter advised her to move closer to Port-Royal so that she could forget the amours of her former life (including Gaston d'Orléans and Cinq-Mars), she did so, believing that Singlin "cared deeply about my salvation." During the controversy surrounding the *Frequent Communion* (1643), she often visited Port-Royal and corresponded regularly with both Antoine and Angélique Arnauld. For two decades (from 1646 when she left France until her death in 1667), Louise-Marie wrote scores of letters to her friends at Port-Royal. In letters to Pope Alexander VII, she defended the community against the Jesuits' charges of heresy and disloyalty.[7] Before Angélique (her "Holy Mother") died in 1661, Poland's Queen declared that she would not accumulate earthly wealth so that "if I become a widow, I would have only enough goods to be received by Mother Angélique at Port-Royal."[8]

While Port-Royal depended on the influence and financial support of royalty and nobility from all over Europe, not all of the great ones who visited the convent received a hearty welcome. When Queen Henrietta Maria, exiled wife of the former King Charles I of England, came to see her friends madame de Guéménée and madame de Sablé, who lived near Port-Royal, she also visited the convent, creating quite a stir. "I am glad the visit of the Queen of England passed off well enough," *Mère* Angélique sniffed. "But I would to God that by his grace he will preserve us from her return."[9]

Within France, however, the Jansenists enjoyed the support of a host of influential men and women who frequently enjoyed the hospitality of Port-Royal. Both the prince de Conti and the prince de Condi became devout sympathizers and defenders of the community, moving nearby after the Fronde. The latter, perhaps hoping to turn his servants into Jansenists, enforced a strict code in his household: no immorality, drunkenness, gambling, card playing, novels, theater attendance, quarrels or duels—on penalty of immediate dismissal.[10]

Many highly born Jansenist sympathizers, however, would have found Condi's code impossible to keep, primarily because their position in society required them to live in two worlds. Anne de Rohan, the wealthy *princesse* de Guéménée, enjoyed a close, supportive friendship with the Andillys and Arnaulds for 40 years, but vacillated between notorious love affairs and religious seclusion. Finally in 1641, she and her two sons left their luxurious apartments at the Place Royale and moved to Port-Royal. The blonde, blue-eyed marquise de Sablé, worldly wise and beautiful, shared Angélique's confidences during the 20 years she lived near Port-Royal but kept "one foot in the world" through her connections at Court. Likewise, the young and ravishing Elisabeth de Choiseul, *comtesse* du Plessis Guéngaud, wife of a secretary of state, supported her Jansenist friends while entertaining wealthy nobles at her Paris salon. Madamoiselle de Montpensier, cousin of Louis XIV, did not allow the king's hatred of Jansenism to curtail her frequent visits to Port-Royal. In contrast with her life in Paris, she found the sisters "devoted, naïve, simple, and lacking worldly manners," more ascetic than the nuns in other convents she had visited. For her support at Court, Le Maître de Sacy dedicated his book *Imitation of Christ* to her. Louise Séguier, the *duchesse* de Luynes, sent two daughters to Port-Royal and with her husband the duke, built a small chateau close by to "adore God in secrecy."

Other women, however, rejected the world and embraced ascetic lifestyles. The marquise d'Aumont, a generous benefactor of the convent, moved closer to be near Angélique. The wealthy, fun-loving madame de Longueville, who had traveled Europe and acted in plays, experienced a dramatic conversion and built a chateau near the convent. Her generous charities and powerful influence protected the sisters and helped establish the "Peace of the Church" from 1669 to 1679. Similarly, madame de Sevigné, an amateur Jansenist, gave up her worldly life, came to Port-Royal seeking salvation, and used her wealth to support the "Friends of the Truth." Madame de La Fayette, a novelist and biographer who held the *soeurs* and *solitaires* "in great veneration," lived in high society in Paris and Rambouillet far from her husband in Auvergne. But when her health failed, she moved to Port-Royal in 1692 and protected the community during its final years. Finally, madamoiselle Marguerite de Joncoux, called "the new Deborah," wrote letters defending the convent during its final struggle to survive against Church and state persecution (1699–1710).[11]

Wealthy noblemen also forsook worldly pleasures and embraced the life of self-denial, often leaving their noble titles behind when they arrived at Port-Royal. Roger du Plessis, the marquis de Liancourt, who came to hear Singlin's sermons, sought spiritual counsel from Saint-Cyran during the latter's imprisonment at Vincennes. He and his wife Jeanne de Schomberg, believing that "the Court is not a proper refuge for our salvation," remained close to Port-Royal even during the Fronde. Thomas du Fosse, controller of accounts at Rouen, resigned his position, gave all his possessions to the poor, and with his wife, joined the community to finish their days in prayer and good works. Some nobles, in fact, became servants there. Monsieur de Gibron, son of a seneschal at Narbonne, worked in the kitchen. Monsieur de Pont-Chateau, the brother of the *duchesse* d'Epernon, dirtied his hands weeding the communal vegetable garden. Many other examples of this "negation of self" could be provided.[12]

Port-Royal also benefited from the close friendship of the upper bourgeoisie, especially among the judges and magistrates. Jansenist sympathizers among the *parlementaires* included prominent members of the Marion, Arnauld, Pascal, Bagnol, Bernière, Molé, Bignon, Briquet, Saint-Beuve, and Daguesseau families.[13] Jean Le Nain, the father of Sébastien Le Nain de Tillemont (former student at Port-Royal, priest, and writer), a *conseiller* in the Paris Parlement and legal counselor for the *duchesse* de Longueville, defended the legal rights of Port-Royal in the 1650s and 1660s. Le Nain frequently attended services there, corresponded with its directors, bankrolled the community during the Fronde, and gave thousands of *livres* to its Little Schools and charitable endeavors to the day of his death at 89.[14] Guillaume du Gué de Bagnals, another Paris *parlementaire*, gave not only his wealth (some 18,000 *livres*), but himself to Port-Royal. A frequent correspondent with de Sacy, Singlin, and Angélique Arnauld, Bagnals also wrote letters to the pope to defend the interests of Port-Royal. In 1646 at the age of 30 he converted to Jansenism, abandoned his career, and devoted his life to penitence and charitable works (including another

40,000 *livres* given to the destitute). Although he died in 1657 at 41, this "procuror-general of the poor" left behind an endowment to provide dowries for impoverished demoiselles wishing to join convents.[15]

If good works and a desire to live a holy life attracted many seventeenth-century robe nobles to Jansenism, opposition to the Jesuits drew wider support from the upper bourgeoisie in the eighteenth century. As later chapters show, between 1713 and 1765, many *parlementaires* supported the Jansenists in their on-going battle with the Society of Jesus. For example, they refused to register the Bull *Unigenitus* in 1714, supported the lower clergy against Archbishop Vintimille's attack on the St.-Médard miracles in the 1730s, and denied Archbishop de Beaumont's authority to refuse last rites to those without *billets de confession* (tickets of orthodoxy) in the 1750s. Likewise, these same magistrates and lawyers rejoiced when in 1764 the Jesuits were expelled from France.[16]

Indeed, Jansenist supporters sometimes appeared where one would least expect to find them. Despite Louis XIV's use of the police to suppress the movement, the chief of police in Rouen in the 1640s embraced Jansenism, as did many other magistrates, physicians, gentlemen and bourgeois in that city.[17] In Paris during the 1650s, 38 out of 68 *curés* (56%) were Jansenists who championed moral rigorism, opposed laxism in the Society of Jesus, and used Richerist arguments to exalt the role of priests and curtail the authority of their bishops.[18] Despite their different social backgrounds, perhaps the one golden thread that bound Jansenists together was personal loyalty. Neither Saint-Cyran, Pascal, or Racine probably read Jansen's *Augustinus* in its entirety, but all remained fiercely loyal to its ideals in combatting the Jesuits and in their support of Port-Royal.[19]

The ideals of Jansenism, however, could be interpreted in different ways. Indeed, as several writers have pointed out, over the course of 150 years, "many Jansenisms" arose. Even in the 1620s and 1630s, well before the release of Jansen's *Augustinus* (1640), a nascent form of Jansenism existed in the expressions of the *dévot* movement. Led by Catholic enthusiasts like Pierre de Bérulle, founder of the French Oratory, the *dévots* espoused an Augustinian theology, opposed the Jesuits, defended the rights of the bishops against the authority of the pope, and urged Louis XIII to make policy decisions based on religion. Because of the far-reaching influence of the *dévots* and Oratorians, by the end of the seventeenth century, nearly half of the Catholic clergy in France, Belgium, Spain and other Mediterranean countries had become "infected" (Pierre Chaunu's term) with Augustinian piety, mysticism, Richerism, asceticism, and reforming zeal.[20]

Despite the remarkable variety in the patchwork quilt of Jansenism, Antoine Arnauld saw Augustinianism as the "glue" that bound its supporters together. In his *Apology for the Abbot of Saint-Cyran* (1644), Arnauld defined "Jansenists" as "an infinite number of Prelates, Theologians & Religious in all kinds of Orders who . . . revere with Monsieur Jansénius . . . the heavenly doctrine of St. Augustine concerning Grace."[21] A decade later, in his "Remonstrance to the Jesuit Fathers" (1651), he argued that the term "Jansenist" was, in fact, a misnomer, since his followers really deserved to be called "Augustinians" (just as the Jesuits, he asserted, should be labeled "Molinists").[22] Likewise in the *Second Letter to a Duke and Peer* (1655), Arnauld argued that the use of the term "Jansenist" implied the existence of a sect whose members followed Jansen, when in fact they followed the teachings of Jesus Christ as interpreted by St. Augustine. He accused the Jesuits of originating the term "Jansenist" and equating it with a sect responsible for splitting the Church. On the contrary, Arnauld asserted, "there is nothing more pure, more Catholic, and more holy than the words & meaning of St. Augustine himself."[23] To the end of his life, in the *Difficulties Proposed to M. Steyaert* (1691), he opposed the term "Jansenist" as "a secular word most equivocal, insidious, and most often used [by Jesuits] to abuse & lie about those who are good & faithful Catholics."[24]

In addition to their adherence to Augustinian theology on issues relating to God's grace and human nature, however, Jansenists shared a certain austere mindset often described as moral rigorism, "a severe and psychologically demanding form of Christianity." Their religious attitude encompassed a gloomy predestinarianism on the one hand and a concern for spiritual reform and renewal on the other. Their puritanical view of uncompromising virtue and saintliness did not circumvent their acts of Christian charity toward those who failed to live up to their creed. Nor did their strict penitential discipline and thorough-going gravity prevent them from establishing progressive schools for boys and girls who, as alumni, treasured their early educational experience at Port-Royal. Although pessimistic regarding the sinfulness of mankind and the corruption of society, they did what they could to help those in physical and spiritual need of their assistance.[25]

Their rigorist mindset also led them to implement the Council of Trent's reforms in the daily lives of the clergy and laity. Through doctrinal instruction, prayer, liturgical services in the vernacular, and writing books of meditation, they hoped to elevate the moral tone in each parish. Among all levels of the clergy, they attacked immorality, pluralism, and absenteeism and advocated lifestyles of sobriety and piety. They urged priests and bishops to explain the sacraments in the language of the people, to visit parishioners frequently, and to establish schools to educate the children (girls as well as boys) in their districts. Jansenist parishes were characterized by accurate record keeping, regular catechism classes, evangelistic efforts for the unchurched, a strong emphasis on scripture, as well as faithful care of the poor and sick and a rigid daily schedule of prayers, Bible reading, and meditation. Such parishes also placed more emphasis on public penance and contrition, focused on the Eucharist and the cross (rather than on the sacred heart of Jesus), and encouraged believers to suffer in defense of the truth. Despite widespread popular resistance, Jansenist clergy tried to curtail dancing, taverns, festivals, gambling and hunting; likewise, they opposed superstition and folklore.[26]

If moral rigorism transformed the visible lifestyles of its adherents, it also changed their inner lives. Eager to revive in the Church the virtues, zeal, and purity of apostolic Christianity, Jansenists sought within themselves a deeper spiritual piety through hours of meditation, prayer, and self-examination. Many of them embraced solitude, either within their own homes or at Port-Royal des Champs. Although the sisters and solitaires at Port-Royal rejected mysticism per se, by their example and writings, they encouraged their followers to devote considerable amounts of time every week to prayer, meditation, and fasting.[27]

This habit of withdrawing from secular society bred within them an attitude of suspicion and opposition that most outsiders saw as combativeness. In their speeches and writings, Jansenists opposed Protestants (as heretics), Jesuits (as their enemies), ultramontanists (for favoring papal infallibility), mercantilists (who promoted greed), and episcopal authority (bishops v. local priests). Like the Friends (Quakers) of England and America, they also opposed everything worldly.[28]

Paradoxically, attacking worldliness required them to remain in contact with the society they hoped to enlighten and reform. But citing John 2:15–16 ("Love not the world, neither the things that are in the world"), Jansenists typically manifested a contempt for the pleasures of secular society. In Christian monasticism, *contemptus mundi* (contempt for the world) had a long history stretching from the original ascetic orders like the Benedictines to recent ones such as the Society of Jesus. Yet when French Jansenists adopted *mépris du monde* (scorn for the world) as their motto, they consciously set themselves in opposition not only to worldly (i.e., sinful) pleasures, but also to much of the cultural progress of the age. They clearly despised Classical and Baroque art, music, dance, literature and theatre because these creative forms rested on sham and illusion, aroused the baser passions, and distracted the faithful from the task of seeking salvation. Jansenist priests routinely denied actors access to the sacraments. They also opposed dueling, usury, simony, gaming, and hunting.[29]

In its rejection of worldly values and secularism, however, this Jansenism which "never learned to smile"[30] also turned its back on the Renaissance. Jansenists opposed the seventeenth-century "Cult of Antiquity" for exalting Greek and Roman paganism. They distrusted human reason because it fostered pride and vanity. They boycotted the plays of Corneille, Molière, and Racine—even though the latter wrote some religious dramas (*Athaliah* and *Esther*) and defended Port-Royal. They rejected any form of luxury and self-indulgence as being a poor use of God-given talents and means and inevitably nourishing pride—a mortal sin. Although Jansenists themselves evinced no evangelistic fervor for saving sinful souls, they attacked Jesuit attempts to convert the Chinese and Native Americans, accusing them of making cultural compromises between Catholicism and libertinism.[31]

This disapproval of everything worldly led Jansenists to adopt austere lifestyles. Like solitary voyagers on the path to heaven, they sought a deeper experience in Christ by focusing their attention on the cross. They made the sufferings of their Savior their own by adopting lives of constant self-denial. By fasting they denied themselves nourishing food; through hours of prayer and meditation they denied themselves adequate sleep. With consciences sensitized to their own sins and faults, they resolved (as Corneille phrased it) "always to love, always to suffer, always to die."[32]

Two early testimonies from Jansenists who left the world behind and embraced lives of self-denial will illustrate this point. In 1637 at the age of 30, Sieur le Maistre, an advocate of the Paris Parlement and a Councilor of State, "deeply impressed by God . . . renounced all his goods and all his earthly fortunes to spend his time weeping for his sins in a profound solitude." Resigning his prestigious position, he retired to Port-Royal des Champs, took the name "Charles of the Cross," and "began a penitence that did not end until the day of his death."[33] Following a similar profound conversion experience, the *duchesse* de Liancourt withdrew from high society and penned her "Disposition to Live More Like Christ." In it she resolves every day "to give God my first thoughts. I will adore him, give him thanks, and resign myself to His will." Doing God's will involved spending half an hour daily in prayer and meditation. In addition, she promises to read good books, attend Mass often, fast, and spend an hour in "holy conversation" each day. She will contribute liberally to charities, upgrade her servants' moral and spiritual lives, and choose only "the most innocent entertainment" (like walking and painting) while avoiding those "which lead to hell." Finally, she will place "all affairs in God's hands" and obey his will regarding the disposition of her wealth and property.[34]

Such dramatic conversions, surprisingly common in the seventeenth century, demonstrate how adopting Jansenism brought social consequences both positive and negative. On the positive side, Jansenism represented a rigorous morality, an ascetic lifestyle, a form of presbyterian democracy (Gallicanism and Richerism), an emphasis on penitence and the Eucharist, and strong support for education (the *petites écoles*) and charities (hospitals, orphanages, food and clothing distributed to the poor).[35]

The public, however, seemed more inclined to see the negative features in Jansenism. It made unrealistic demands on the believer concerning penance and communion. For over a century, the Jansenist controversy with the Jesuits would tear the Church apart. Jansenism also seemed to oppose everything—humanism, mercantilism, materialism, secularism—that represented cultural progress in the seventeenth century. Its emphasis on ecclesiastical democracy (Richerism, conciliarism, Gallicanism) led kings and popes to label its adherents republicans subverting good order in the body politic. And while Jansenists' inward-looking piety helped improve the spiritual condition of the Church to some extent, their lack of concern for Christians and pagans outside the Catholic fold led them to criticize Jesuit missionaries even while the latter risked their lives for their faith in North America.[36]

In essence, the Jansenists wanted to turn the clock back and restore the Church to its apostolic purity. Peering through rosy-tinted lenses at the first century, writers lauded the early Christians for their many virtues—faith, hope, trust in God, charity, piety, humility, patience, justice, and temperance—virtues sadly lacking, they felt, in the contemporary Church. In their sermons, tracts, and books, Jansenists emphasized a litany of themes designed to revive these virtues within the hearts of seventeenth-century Catholics. The Christian's purpose on earth is to seek salvation, which is difficult to obtain, so most people will be damned to suffer eternally in hell. Only God's efficacious grace—not any merit on the believer's part—can save one from damnation. Christ provided the pattern for all to follow; his law and doctrine will guide the faithful to eternal life. But while here on earth, one must practice the virtues of love, piety, goodness, and charity toward others. The best way to accomplish this is to live in poverty, avoiding the accumulation of wealth ("the riches that damn") and mortifying the body through frequent penance, fasts, and physical labor.[37]

An omnipotent God, sinful humanity, redemption through divine grace for only a few—these constituted the anchor points of hard-line Jansenism. And behind this rigorist Augustinian theology lay a view of God somewhat harsher than that cherished by other Catholics. Jansenist writers seldom portrayed the loving side of God the Father or Jesus Christ the Son. Instead, they emphasized God's justice: he could save or damn as he wished, for he was high, remote, unaccountable and terrible in his judgments.[38]

By contrast, human beings, corrupted by Original Sin, were evil, weak, and headed for damnation. As a result of Adam and Eve's fall from grace in the Garden of Eden, nothing upright remained in human nature. In contrast to the Jesuit view that Adam's sin had destroyed only the supernatural within mankind, leaving human nature with its original innocence, Pascal and Nicole's gloomy view denied human beings even their free will to choose right from wrong. Humans were sinners, living out their short lives in this world of pain and suffering, then condemned to eternal punishment in hell.[39] Contrary to the promise of John 3:16 ("that whosoever believes in him [Christ] shall not perish, but have eternal life"), Jansenists—like Calvinists—limited the saved to an Elect few. To graphically illustrate this teaching, the Jesuits accused the Jansenists of creating their own crucifixes with Christ's arms extended vertically (to show that he died for a chosen remnant) rather than horizontally (to show that he died for all)—a myth that endured for three centuries.[40]

As Christ died on the cross to save humanity, so Christians must contemplate his death and (as Saint-Cyran phrased it) "die to self all the days of our lives." Jansenists viewed death in a positive light as the great leveler, teaching all to be humble. The sick, they believed, enjoyed advantages over the healthy, for their suffering prepared them spiritually for death on this earth and eternal life beyond. In their writings, they called suffering and death "our last penitence," "our purgatory in this world," "our sanctification," and that "double grace" that prepares one for eternity. Believers, who lived each day as if it were their last, prepared for "a good death," knowing that such preparation cleansed their souls of sin's stain.[41]

No matter how good one's death, however, the only way to cross the divide from earth to heaven came through the grace of Jesus Christ. And like their Augustinian "cousins" the Calvinists, Jansenists believed God dispersed this grace to the elect few. As Jean Vallier, Louis XIV's *maître d'hôtel*, expressed it: "The matter of grace is very delicate and comprises an abyss so deep that it is dangerous to approach too near it."[42] Jesuits and Jansenists, in fact, approached that abyss by different routes. The former declared that attrition (regret for having offended God from fear for eternal damnation) was sufficient for receiving grace, whereas the latter insisted that contrition (regret for having offended God from love for him) was essential for salvation. Jansenists considered attrition to be "imperfect contrition" because it fell short of the mark of a perfect repentance inspired by love for God, good, truth, and righteousness. From Jansen to

Quesnel, this insistence on contrition infused the works of Jansenist leaders and formed the dogmatic cornerstone of Port-Royal, their heaven on earth.[43]

To recreate this community of contrite saints meant reviving first-century Christianity and transplanting the "primitive Church" to seventeenth-century France. When Jansenists contemplated early Christianity, they conjoined eight elements to describe the apostolic community as a minority church, a persecuted church, a church of martyrs, a church full of God's miracles, a poverty-stricken church, a democratic church, a scripture-based church, an ascetic and severely moral church.[44] When they compared this pastoral utopia with modern Catholicism, the evangelical fervor and rigorous theology of the former contrasted sharply with the moral laxity and doctrinal compromises they saw in current Catholicism. To combat this decline and decay, they posited a model of the Church militant not unlike that portrayed in the New Testament book of Acts. This Church formed a united brotherhood of heroes willing to live and die for their faith. These "persecuted saints," resisting the state's encroachment on sacred matters, accepted martyrdom for the cause of Truth.[45]

The tremendous influence of first century Christian Antiquity, and the Jansenists' claim to interpret it correctly, gave them great authority in seventeenth-century France. They effectively denied popes and bishops the right to be the sole interpreters of the Church Fathers and ecclesiastical tradition. In fact, Jansenist writers often accused recent Church leaders and theologians (especially the Jesuits) of "obscuring the Truth" and compromising the legacy bequeathed by the Apostles. For them, human history since the first century represented a sharp decline from the purity and zeal of the early church.[46]

But the papacy saw things in a different light—and the chair of St. Peter was not a university chair, obligated to consider all sides of an argument and rule accordingly. Instead, the Holy See could—and did—rule dogmatically, positively or negatively, on matters of doctrine and the writings of the Jansenists on theological and ecclesiastical issues. Popes, who by the late seventeenth century saw themselves as infallible, issued bulls to promote or suppress certain ideas and expected their decrees to be obeyed.[47]

Antoine Arnauld, and the Jansenists in general, wrestled with this increasingly popular view of the pope as an absolute, infallible authority. Given their roots in Gallicanism, Richerism, and conciliarism (as explained in Chapter 1), it is not surprising that they almost universally opposed the teaching of papal infallibility. In the 1650s, Arnauld limited the pope's infallible authority to questions of faith and doctrine. In temporal affairs (such as enforcing the Formulary), the pope should consult a general assembly of the clergy, for he has no jurisdiction in France except by the united consent of the bishops, who cannot be forced against their will.[48] Any papal attempt to coerce agreement would be "prejudicial to all the Liberties of the Gallican Church" and would establish "a true Inquisition" in France, Arnauld declared. Only spiritual persuasion, not force, should be used in spiritual matters.[49]

In his "Pastoral Letter from the Bishop of Alet" (1668), Arnauld goes even further, asserting that popes cannot be absolute rulers because bishops, never "simple executors" of their wishes, have the right to examine their bulls and briefs to determine if they agree with scripture and tradition. Moreover, decisions binding on the Gallican Church require long discussion, wide consultation among the bishops, and the consensus of believers as expressed in church councils.[50] By 1681, however, faced with the growing power of Louis XIV's divine right monarchy, Arnauld struggled to balance the rights of the Holy See and Church councils on the one hand with the growing might of the French state. In his *Considerations* (1681), he longed for the day when pope, king, and Church councils, recognizing their limits and boundaries, would cooperate "to the glory of God."[51]

While Arnauld punned in 1683 that the "infallibility [of the pope] is not a point of faith which is infallible,"[52] he feared that if the Jesuits had their way, the pope would be declared infallible in France. Therefore, throughout his writings, although Arnauld shows deep respect for the Holy See, he provides checks and balances on papal authority. Yes, he declares, the pope is the Vicar of Jesus Christ, the successor of St. Peter, the Primate of divine law, and the Chief Minister of the Church. As Universal Bishop, he has unlimited power to teach and edify the faithful; as Sovereign Judge, his decrees must be obeyed. Yet at the same time, he is "first among equals"—a brother, colleague, and co-bishop with all the other bishops in the Church. As such, he exercises "servant leadership" over the Church. His decisions can be enforced only through representative councils.[53]

This emphasis on representation, liberty, and individualism sprang from the very roots of Jansenism. As Michel Dupuy stated: "The most profound intuition of Jansénius had been to make [human] liberty the essential premise for an encounter with God."[54] A generation later, the *abbé* Guillaume Le Roy expressed this spirit of independence in his "Letter on Constancy and Courage" (1665). "A single man, a single priest, a single bishop who would express this independence under present circumstances [the crisis of the Formulary] . . . would be stronger than a multitude, than the entire kingdom. He would rule over those who reign. He would be above earthly kings as once were the prophets who rebuked wicked and unfaithful kings oppressing God's people."[55]

Such radical sentiments led some to accuse Jansenists of republicanism. In his *Memoirs*, the *duc* de Saint-Simon called them "a republican party both in the Church and in the State."[56] But republican ideals did not make them anti-royalists. Both Arnauld and Quesnel clearly expressed in their writings profound respect for the monarchy and urged their followers to obey God *and* the king, for Christ himself had commanded it ("Render therefore unto Caesar what is Caesar's and to God what is God's"). Unlike the sixteenth-century *monarchomachs*, Jansenists did not preach the right of the people to rebel against their kings (who are "images of God"). Instead, in *Sovereignty of Kings Defended* (1696), Quesnel supported papal, royal, and imperial authority and opposed those who favored the overthrow of Louis XIV.[57]

Based on his reading of the Bible and St. Augustine, Arnauld agreed with Quesnel that subjects owed respect and obedience to their rulers. Desiring to differentiate the Jansenist position from that of the rebellious Calvinists, he wrote the *Treatise on the Sovereignty of Kings* which described monarchs as both sacred and secular. After being anointed by the Holy Spirit, they became mediators between the clergy and the people. Even if persecuted, subjects had no right to revolt against their rulers; instead, they owed them "heroic loyalty."[58]

Yet while Quesnel, Arnauld, and other Jansenists quoted political theorists like Jean Damat and Hugo Grotius, they did *not* cite the resistance rights theories of the *monarchomachs* (Theodore Beza, François Hotman, or Philippe du Plessis-Mornay) or the republican ideals of John Locke. Although the Jesuits portrayed them as rebels, *frondeurs*, and republicans—which they denied—Jansenists constituted an "opposition movement." If they were not republicans or democrats in the modern sense of those terms, their frequent remonstrances and frank criticisms of Church and state policies led many to accuse them of *lèse-majesté*. Politically, therefore, Jansenism could be defined as resistance to all forms of oppression. Given their impatience with authority (civil or ecclesiastical), it is little wonder that Louis XIV and his confessor *Père* La Chaise considered them "the enemy of all domination, spiritual as well as temporal," a cabal that made "too much noise" to be ignored. Absolute power, having suppressed the great nobles and the Huguenots, could not tolerate any independent force in the realm.[59]

The Jansenists' struggle for liberty, however, owed less to John Locke than to their fundamental belief that freedom of conscience was essential to the search for Truth. As Benoît Fourgon, a Lyon merchant imprisoned at Pierre Encize Chateau, told the archbishop during his interrogation in 1714, he believed he would be "damned by blind obedience," even to bishops and kings.[60]

In the salvation equation, following one's God-given conscience superceded submission to earthly authority, which could err.

Yet earthly rulers, Jansenists felt, should also be led by God and follow their consciences. Essentially, their political model replicated the medieval "mirror of the Christian prince" model. In his *Discipline of the Church Taken from the New Testament and Several Ancient Councils* (1689), Pasquier Quesnal stated that the prince must love his people and demonstrate courage, magnanimity, sincerity, faithfulness, prudence and simplicity in lifestyle. A Christian ruler will respect the Gospel and lead his people to observe its teachings.[61] Pierre Barral's *Maxims Concerning the Duty of Kings* asserted that such rulers, following Christ as their example, will put their duty toward God above all earthly considerations of power, ambition, or wealth. They will obey the laws and promote the common good.[62]

The Jansenist political model—which endured well into the mid-eighteenth century in the pages of the *Nouvelles Ecclésiastiques*—included several elements. It combined an image of the fourth century Primitive Church under the Christian emperors with a "Golden Age" or "State of Nature" myth. In this rural, largely agricultural utopia, priests and bishops shared equal power in a democratic church. The freedoms enjoyed by all arise from Christian principles guiding both Church and state. Jansenists hoped to project the innocence and happiness of the pre-historical "State of Nature" into present society by positing a "Christian contract," voluntarily signed by all, as a hedge against the greed and corruption they found in the modern state. In their "New Canaan," farmers, fishermen, and artisans would prevail over bankers, merchants, and manufacturers. Like the Luddites of nineteenth-century England, the Jansenists opposed mercantile greed and technological progress for corrupting the human spirit; their ideal remained the quiet rural community of Port-Royal des Champs.[63]

Jansenists, therefore, were not republicans in the sense that the French Revolution would define that term in 1792. But neither did they favor blind submission to an absolute monarch. Instead, they took a middle ground. Their brand of monarchy, based on Gallican and Christian principles patterned after the Early Church, promoted the ideals of egalitarianism and cooperation. Rulers who followed this model of the "Christian monarch" need not fear rebellion.[64]

For the most part, however, Jansenists denied the right of revolt. For every firebrand like the *abbé* Le Roy who advocated the overthrow of despotic princes, moderates like Martin de Barcos and Jean Racine counseled submission on the grounds that God held earthly monarchs to account. And towering over all stood Antoine Arnauld the centrist, who spoke cautiously of the right of passive resistance to corrupt rulers.[65]

Early on, in his "Letter of a Doctor in Theology to One of His Friends" (1644), Arnauld had expressed deep concerns regarding the combination of Church and state. He asserted: "It is still more strange that we mix State & Religion so easily, & that the Court takes an interest in these quarrels which do not concern them, & which can only be resolved by those to whom God has given the care of souls & the dispensation of [divine] mysteries." When kings meddle in doctrinal disputes, they often precipitate "the most dangerous of all evils, civil wars."[66] While Arnauld recognizes the absolute power of monarchs in temporal affairs, he denies their right to issue judgments in matters of theology, the province of bishops and church councils. In all other areas of life, however, subjects must obey their rulers and not revolt against them.[67]

Yet obedience came in two flavors—positive and negative submission. In *Writings on the Bulls of Alexander VII* (1657), Arnauld explains that taking an oath to obey an ordinance constitutes positive submission. But promising publicly not to resist or obstruct an ordinance is negative submission. Because Christians cannot sin against their consciences and act contrary to what they believe to be the truth, this latter kind of submission is acceptable when legitimate authorities try to coerce the conscience. Such "non-resistance," he says, "conserves the good order of States."

This argument, like a double-edged sword, was employed in succeeding years both to resist the popes' efforts to compel Jansenists to sign the Formulary and to block Louis XIV's attempts to coerce the bishops and *parlementaires* to enforce papal bulls in France.[68]

Such sentiments led many outside the movement to question Arnauld's loyalty and impugn his patriotism. Pained by this, he told Mme. de Fontpertuis in 1692 (two years before his death) that "[a]ll those who know me recognize on the contrary that I have a love for my country & for my King which many people think is excessive."[69] While Arnauld, like all Jansenists, disapproved of Louis XIV's pomp, extravagance, and meddling in church affairs, he never forgot—even in exile—his duty to submit to his king insofar as conscience allowed.[70] Yet under rare circumstances, even conscience could be compromised. When a Monsieur Perrier wrote asking whether he should accept the post of royal tax farmer, Arnauld advised him to take the position. Although most tax farmers, he admitted, make "such great profits and immense gains" that it "imperils their consciences," he knew that Perrier had eight children to support. Therefore, Arnauld urged him to accept the position but to be "very honest" in his duties.[71] As Christ had once been an honest carpenter, Peter an honest fisherman, and Zacchaeus an honest tax collector, so the Jansenist ideal for all—prince or peasant—meant following one's conscience in whatever position one filled in life.

From the Jansenists' perspective, however, one group in France did not embody their belief that Christianity could be lived without compromises or concessions—the Society of Jesus. The enmity between these two religious groups waxed so hot that Cardinal Giovanni Bona once defined a Jansenist as "a Catholic who does not like Jesuits."[72] Although one could despise the Jesuits and still not be a Jansenist (many Gallican bishops and parish clergy accused them of enjoying "special privileges" as the popes' favorites),[73] one could not favor the Jesuits and remain a Jansenist. Why?

Basically, their mutual enmity reflected sharp differences between the two camps, which each side emphasized in its apologetic literature. While the Jansenists preached moral rigorism, saintliness, and severe self-denial, the Jesuits advocated a lax moral theology. If the Jansenists promoted a penitential ethic, acts of charity, and internal reform, the Jesuits appeared to favor an *honnête homme* morality. Whereas the Jansenists emphasized an Augustinian, predestinarian theology premised upon a sinful, limited human will, the Jesuits preferred a Molinist free will model. The Jansenists exalted the authority of the secular clergy (priests and bishops) as opposed to the Jesuits backing the authority of the regular clergy (abbots and monks). Jansenists admired the pure theology, holy zeal, and homogeneity of the first century Apostolic Church, whereas the Jesuits praised the theological and ecclesiastical progress made by popes and Church councils over the centuries.[74]

The two groups held divergent attitudes about a wide range of theological, social, and ecclesiastical issues. Jansenist theologians favored the "historical perspective," accumulating scripture quotations and citing the Early Church Fathers; Jesuit theologians employed a "speculative theology," basing their exegesis on humanist arguments and reason to adapt themselves to the times. Jansenists therefore accused Jesuits of being "modernists" and "casuists" who bent their principles to fit a changing world; Jesuits saw Jansenists as "primitivists" whose rejection of the world made them impractical spiritual guides for contemporary Christians. If the Jesuits, with their optimistic emphasis on human abilities, freedom of the will, and focus on a this-worldly religion made church membership easier, the Jansenists, by their pessimistic emphasis on human helplessness, limited grace, and other-worldly asceticism made it harder.[75]

By the same token, each group defined "Church" differently. The Jansenists saw themselves as the heirs of the real traditions of Catholicism and blamed their opponents as the innovators. If the Jansenists had prevailed, the French Catholic Church would have been an honor society of the spiritual select, a community of the elect who had attained exceptionally high standards of personal morality. But it would also have been a sect of the devout, an inward-looking church indifferent to the spiritual needs of a dying world. On the other hand, the Jesuits saw themselves as the proponents of the organic development of Catholic tradition and truth that evolved over time. If the Jesuits had prevailed, the Gallican Church would have become the club for all human kind, keeping entrance requirements low and dispensing benefits to those who paid their dues. The Jesuits might have lowered the standards of morality and devotional requirements, but they also would have required more frequent communion and confession.[76]

Anyone who spends much time immersed in Jansenist polemics—whether in the seventeenth or eighteenth century—can easily recite their lengthy list of complaints against the Society of Jesus. Theologically, they hated the Jesuits for their Molinist position on grace and free will; for their formalism regarding devotional exercises and frequent communion; for their laxity that subverted moral and religious principles. Socially, they disliked their "spirit of domination," their "ambition for conquest," and their "grand design" to take over the world. Politically, they distrusted their tolerance for contrary dogmas, their love of hierarchical authority, their alleged plots to dethrone kings and undermine subjects' obedience to their rulers. Economically, they despised their imposing tributes on other religious groups in Catholic countries. Philosophically, they abhorred their advocacy of casuism, by which a Catholic could perform an evil action (murder, theft, lying) for a worthwhile end. First introduced by the Spanish Dominican Bartolomé de Medina in 1577, casuism taught that if 100 theologians agreed on the safest course of action, but one theologian provided an easygoing alternative, then a Christian could follow that alternative in good conscience.[77]

Possibly more than any other Jesuit practice, the red flags of casuistry and probabilism[78] inspired the special ire of Jansenist writers from the very beginning. In his provocative "Digest of Several Propositions Taken from a Book Entitled *Apology for Casuists against the Lies of the Jansenists*" (1657), Georges Pirot painted Jesuit laxity in the darkest hues. The Jesuits use casuistic logic to justify murder for honorable ends, to promote the spiritual benefits of simony, and to permit usury in rents to benefit one's heirs. They make calumny only a venial sin; grant absolution without contrition to those who profane the sacrament of penitence and to others who refuse to renounce their vices; and label the senses morally neutral so that one may eat and drink without guilt. They permit poor servants to steal from their masters, judges to accept bribes, unwed couples to have sex by mutual consent without parental approval, and women to gamble away their husbands' wealth. Finally, the Jesuit teaching of probability allows one to follow two opinions at the same time or to choose the least probable one without sinning.[79]

Although modern readers will recognize the exaggerated propaganda in this and similar pieces of Jansenist literature, contemporary Jansenists accepted it as gospel truth. Before Marie des Anges left Port-Royal des Champs to visit the convent at Maubuisson in 1626, Angélique Arnauld warned her to have nothing to do with the Jesuits in the area.[80] A quarter century later, complaining to the archbishop of Paris that the Jesuits' "defamatory libels" concerning heresy and disorder at Port-Royal slandered her nuns' pious reputations, Angélique pleaded for justice against them.[81]

This visceral hatred by the Arnaulds against the Society of Jesus had been smoldering for almost a century. As shown in chapter 1, Antoine II Arnauld had believed during the reign of Henri IV that the Jesuits threatened the throne and had worked for their expulsion. In print he had called them "thieves, corrupters of the youth, regicides, conspirators against the state, the plague of republics, and disturbers of the peace." He wanted them "exterminated from the face of the earth." His vituperative and flamboyant words had earned him a special "Act of Recognition" from the Sorbonne—and the undying hatred of the Society of Jesus.[82]

It was only natural then that his son, Antoine III ("The Great") Arnauld, imbibed his father's hatred of the Jesuits. Attacks against the Society permeate his books, letters, and sermons. In "Considerations on the Letter of M. de Vabres" (1650), he accuses them of condemning St. Augustine himself when they attack Jansen's *Augustinus*.[83] His "Remonstrance to the Jesuit Fathers" (1651) charges them with teaching the "wicked doctrine" of parricide and regicide.[84] In a rare ecumenical moment, he makes some favorable remarks about *Père* de la Croix (a Jesuit imprisoned by the Society for his Augustinian views) and about an alleged order of "Jesuitesses" in Italy later suppressed by Urban VII in 1631.[85]

For the most part, however, Arnauld is consistently hostile toward the Jesuits and everything they represent. He opposes their stance on papal infallibility as "this new heresy."[86] He finds their libels that he is in league with Oliver Cromwell, Nicolas Foucquet, or other "enemies of the state" utterly ridiculous.[87] In his *Moral Practices of the Jesuits* (1683), he attacks their casuism, probabilism, worldliness, immorality, and permissiveness.[88]

Likewise, in personal letters to family members and friends, Arnauld regularly defames the Society of Jesus as a group who will "ruin the church."[89] In his litany of name calling in the 1680s, they are liars, false politicians, idolaters, persecutors, intriguers, and murderers.[90] He accuses them of hypocrisy, vanity, and apostasy; of printing libels and spreading disorders; and of fomenting persecution in regions where they constitute the majority.[91]

Even at the end of his life in the 1690s, Arnauld refused to bury the hatchet. Writing to Cardinal Paolo Walloni at Rome, he called the Jesuits "the pests of the church," the "new heretics," a "cabal" within Christianity.[92] In his *Moral Practices of the Jesuits* (reprinted in 1734), he warned of the "dangers" of the Jesuits and highlighted their "darkest and most unreasonable impostures."[93] Responding to a letter from his friend Madame de Fontpertuis in 1692, Antoine provided some fascinating insights to explain his life-long war against the Society of Jesus:

> They tell me that I should not find it strange when I am asked, for the good of the peace, not to write against the Jesuits. I would like to be able to comply; but I cannot promise it because I am obliged to do it for the good of the truth & for the Church, which are dearer to me than anything else. [Furthermore] it would not be reasonable to obligate me not to write against them unless they agree not to write against me and treat me as a heretic [which is] an atrocious injury . . . [After all], what does His Majesty care about these theological disputes so long as the theologians continue to live within the borders of the Church?[94]

Unfortunately for Arnauld, the Jesuits did not consider Jansenists to be faithful sheep worthy of dwelling within the borders of the Church. When Jansen's *Augustinus* appeared on the centennial of the founding of their Order, the Jesuits took it as a personal affront. In 1641, the Society at Louvain, citing Paul V's decree forbidding anyone to write about grace or Baianism, attacked the book for resurrecting ancient Pelagianism and the propositions of Baius which had been condemned by the Council of Trent.[95] A generation later, *Père* Annat, Louis XIV's Jesuit confessor, called for the faithful to "burn all their Writings" which "are full of impostures, calumnies & errors." Calling Jansenists "illegitimate & defective" Catholics who sowed "discord & division" in the Church, he suggested they go to Geneva to recruit their ministers rather than to "amuse the world with their so-called imaginary Heresy." After all, he asserted, they are really "Calvinists in disguise" regarding grace, predestination, and free will. Although he considered them heretics unworthy of participating in the Mass, Annat nevertheless denied rumors of a Jesuit plot to destroy them, for "our views of the Jansenists are those of charity and zeal for the defense of the Faith & the authority of the Church."[96]

A century later, however, as the campaign to expel the Society from France gathered momentum, such charitable views evaporated. In their four-volume *Dictionary of Jansenist Books or Those That Favor Jansenism* (1754), the Jesuit authors L. Patouillet and D. Colonia reached new depths of vituperation in their attack on this Catholic "heresy," which they saw as a renewal of Baius' errors.[97] They labeled Saint-Cyran "a hypocritical Reformer, a heretic . . . a Manichean, Lutheran, and Calvinist" whose books contained "monstrous errors and detestable dogma" and whose letters spread "astonishing blasphemy." They accused him of advocating Arianism, Manicheanism, Lollardism, Quietism, Illuminism, Phariseeism—and parricide.[98]

Patouillet and Colonia considered Saint-Cyran's nephew Martin de Barcos "dangerous." His writings included the "venom" of "innumerable errors," particularly concerning grace, predestination, and the equality of Peter and Paul. Aside from the fact that Barcos' "scandalous, impious, and blasphemous false doctrines" brought "injuries to God," his smokescreen that Jansenism was only a "phantom" flew in the face of numerous papal bulls and decrees labeling it a heresy.[99]

In the same vein, they attacked Le Maitre de Sacy's *Illumination of the Famous Almanac of the Jesuits* (1654) as full of errors, satires, and libels against the Church Fathers, finding his version of the Ten Commandments "Calvinist." His *History of the Old and New Testaments* (1669) presented "pernicious portraits" of several Jesuits and "falsified Scripture," being a "scandalous" departure from the Vulgate. His other writings, presenting many "heresies" on grace, free will, and the sacraments, were deemed equally "dangerous."[100]

Patouillet and Colonia considered Jansen's *Augustinus* "barely watered-down Huguenotism [Calvinism]." Although they—like Jesuits everywhere—remained certain that heretical statements could be found in his book, they treated him gently because they believed that "several hours before he died," Jansen had "submitted himself and his book to the judgment and decisions of the Roman Church."[101]

The Jesuits, however, showed less forgiveness toward the Arnauld family. As Patouillet and Colonia colorfully phrased it, "The Huguenot blood that courses through the veins of the Arnaulds has made all their family members manifest an implacable and hereditary hatred for this Society."[102] Interpreting Antoine Arnauld's *Frequent Communion* as a threat to the whole sacramental system that would eventually undermine the power of the clergy, the Jesuits refuted his writings in their sermons, pamphlets, and books.[103] Calling him a "liar & a traitor," an "enemy of the [Church] hierarchy & of the State," and a "criminal," they demanded his condemnation.[104]

More than half a century after Arnauld's death, Patouillet and Colonia embellished these Jesuit charges in their *Dictionary*. Labeling Antoine "a bad subject," "a child of iniquity," and a "disturber of the public peace," they condemned him for propagating "detestable heresies" regarding sufficient grace. Throughout his life, Arnauld the "rebel" had led "a stubborn revolt against the Popes & their decisions," just as Martin Luther had done in the Holy Roman Empire. The authors called him "one of the greatest imposters" in history.[105]

Not too far behind came Pasquier Quesnel, whom they accused of heresy, hypocrisy, and schism, charging him with spreading Pelagianism and Lutheranism in his works. Even some of his relatively harmless writings contained "contradictions," "errors," and "schismatic history," and were therefore suspected of "spreading his poison further." The Jesuits saw both Arnauld and Quesnel as leaders in a rebellion against Church and state. They both manifested a "proud, arrogant, and . . . heretical spirit," being by nature stubborn and insolent.[106] Quesnel's *Moral Reflections* (1693), they feared, "not only attacks faith, [but also] strikes at the foundation of all morality, both Christian and natural, for by destroying free will it weakens all Laws & virtues . . . and gives absolution to all crimes & vices." Jansenism, they claimed, is really "Calvinism and sensual Quietism"; these "false dogmas" would only create more hypocrites in the Church.[107]

For his attacks on the Sorbonne, the Dominicans, and the Society of Jesus in the *Provincial Letters*, the Jesuits called Blaise Pascal "insolent," "outrageous," "malicious," and a heretic full of "defamatory slander [who] spreads lies all around." Never ones to appreciate satire, especially when directed against themselves, the Society charged Pascal with promoting "slander and violence" in his letters.[108] Concerning the Port-Royal teacher Claude Lancelot, Patouillet and Colonia quoted the *comte* de Brienne's description of him as "the most stubborn and pedantic Jansenist that I have ever met," adding the coup de grace that Lancelot was also a very bad cook![109]

Because Pierre Nicole so steadfastly defended the teachings and lifestyle of the sisters and solitaires of Port-Royal, the Jesuits labeled him a "heretical and dangerous fanatic" as well. His "pernicious" theological writings "scandalized the simple," while his *Apology for the Religious of Port-Royal* (1665), full of "impudent lies" and "seditious maxims," constituted a "revolt against the Church & the King."[110] Likewise, they found Jean Racine's *Abridged History of Port-Royal* (1695) so "pernicious" that they forbade the faithful to read it. Racine's theological views, which they found heretical and Calvinistic (on grace and predestination), also deserved condemnation as both "absurd and erroneous."[111]

One did not have to be a Jansenist per se, however, to invoke the wrath of the Society of Jesus. Because they saw Cardinal Noailles as "the great Protector of Jansenism" in France following Louis XIV's death, the Jesuits accused the archbishop of Paris of "encouraging Schism" in the Church. Enraged by his refusal to accept the Bull *Unigenitus* (1713), they asked the pope to strip him of his red hat. They rejoiced when various popes condemned many of his pastoral instructions and mandates.[112]

Finally, against Port-Royal itself—that "nest of Jansenism"—the Jesuits directed their hostility. Because some of the solitaires made shoes there, the Capuchins and Jesuits derided them as *sabotiers* (clog wearers).[113] Jealous of the growing reputation and success of the *petites écoles* (as described in Chapter 3), the Jesuits resolved to close these "schools of Jansenism" by destroying Port-Royal itself. When Louis XIV accomplished that in 1709–10, Jansenists everywhere blamed the Jesuits for the community's demise.[114] Gladly accepting the credit, the Society staged street pageants depicting its triumph over Jansenism. In Maçon, scholars dressed in white pulled a chariot with a beautiful woman (actually a cross-dressing boy) carrying a sign reading "Sufficient Grace," while behind came another chariot with a young man tied, veiled in black and wearing a paper miter symbolizing "the defeat and shame of Jansénius."[115]

Unfortunately for the Jansenists, their enemies multiplied like mosquitoes as the seventeenth century progressed. In addition to the Jesuits, Antoine Arnauld blamed various popes (for bulls condemning Jansenism), Louis XIV and the Council of State (for persecuting Port-Royal), his Jesuit confessors La Chaise and Le Tellier (for *lettres de cachet* imprisoning Jansenist leaders), and the Archbishop of Paris (for harassing Port-Royal).[116] But the circle of those who hated Jansenism spread even farther than these men, powerful though they were. A closer examination of the most prominent opponents of Jansenism will help clarify the role each played in the persecution of Jansenism and in the eventual downfall of Port-Royal.

Ironically, when Jansen's *Augustinus* was first released in France in 1641, it faced no significant opposition; in fact, the Sorbonne at first approved the work. Because of the silence imposed on theological controversy by the papal decree of 1625 (reiterated in Urban VIII's 1643 bull *In eminenti*), no anti-Jansenist movement yet existed in France. Even with the release of Antoine Arnauld's doctoral dissertation *On Frequent Communion* in 1643, it took another five or six years before the Theology Faculty at the Sorbonne became the axis of the struggle to condemn the alleged heresy in Jansen's *Augustinus.*[117]

Consequently, during this decade-long pause before the storm, Jansen's ideas spread rapidly. In France, they owed much to the brilliant leadership and writings of Antoine Arnauld and to the prosperity of both Port-Royal and Port-Royal des Champs, led by his sister Angélique Arnauld. Outside France, Jansen's ideals spread to Spain, Italy, Belgium, and the Netherlands, elevating morals, promoting ascetic lifestyles, and advancing truth. Initially, his followers benefited from the ineffectiveness of the Jesuits' opposition, often employing second-rate writers, bishops, and university officials untrained in theology to attack the perceived heresies in Arnauld's writings.[118]

But in Cardinal Richelieu, they met their match. The first minister of France, who deeply respected the pope's authority in religious matters, had by 1625 embraced the Jesuits' views on theology. Consequently, he favored the position that sorrow for sin based on the fear of hell (attrition), while inferior to sorrow based on regret for offending God (contrition), provided an adequate basis for sacramental absolution. Likewise, he agreed with their stand promoting frequent communion and devotion to the Holy Sacrament.[119] He detested Jansen for attacking his international diplomacy in *Mars Gallicus*.[120] He had Saint-Cyran, whom he once referred to as "more dangerous than six armies," imprisoned at Vincennes.[121] But Richelieu died in 1642 before he could confront the rising tide of Jansenism. His successor, Cardinal Mazarin (1641–1661), would confront the Jansenists—and their protégé, the Cardinal de Retz—during the Fronde.

Antoine Arnauld accused Mazarin of being the chief plotter against Jansenism. Because the first minister favored the Jesuits, hated Retz, and wished to ingratiate himself with the pope, he hoped to use the Jansenists to destroy Retz and "to make himself necessary to Rome."[122] Since so many of the Paris *curés* who supported Retz also espoused Jansenism, Mazarin viewed them as "Jansenist agitators," Richerists, and rebels. He resented their attacks on Jesuit laxism and immorality at Court, their close ties with Port-Royal, their rigorist philosophy, and their opposition to the Formulary. Since the voting records of 38 of the 68 Paris *curés* (58%) who attended the General Assemblies between 1653 and 1662 demonstrated their sympathy with Jansenism, Mazarin had some basis for believing that they acted corporately. Far from "withdrawing from the world" of politics, they exhibited to his mind "a mentality of revolt."[123]

Yet Cardinal de Retz—who hoped to use the Jansenists for his own ends—ridiculed them as "the weakest people in the world in matters of intrigue and affairs of State." "They know nothing," he asserted, "about meddling in them; and far from having received any aid from them, they have disgusted several persons in my party and have refused absolution to those who were a part of it."[124] Perhaps one reason why Mazarin saw them as "rebels" and "intriguers" was because his inside sources were biased. His personal agent to Pius V, *Père* François Duneau, as well as the French ambassador to Rome, Le Bailli de Valençay, were both Jesuits. Therefore, while Mazarin viewed the pursuit of Jansenism as part of a wider effort to restore the middle ground of entente between France and Rome and regain the balance of power for France following war with Spain and a new alliance with Oliver Cromwell, the Jesuits saw the Jansenists as enemies to be eradicated from the Catholic fold.[125]

In the eyes of both Church and state, the Jansenists' association with those involved in the Fronde further tainted their reputation. While historians agree that the parlementary, noble and peasant phases of the Fronde lasted from 1648 to 1653, a further extension (known as the "Religious Fronde") from 1652 to 1662 drew many pro-Jansenist *curés* into what Richard Golden (1992) has called "a mentality of opposition" to Mazarin and Louis XIV through their close ties with known *frondeurs*. When the pro-Jansenist *duc* de Luynes (whose mother, the *duchesse* de Chevreuse, strongly supported Port-Royal) rebelled, Louis XIV blamed Jansenism as the root cause. Likewise, when many Paris ecclesiastics supported Retz in his on-going battle with Mazarin, the king held Port-Royal responsible.[126]

But despite their close ties with several *frondeurs* (the *princesse* de Guéménée, the *duchesse* de Chevreuse, the *comte* de Chavigny, the *duc* de Liancourt, among others), the solitaires of Port-Royal did not participate in the early Fronde. Yet their emphasis on individualism, their opposition to Court immorality and Jesuit casuism, and their constant appeal (through their writings) to public opinion made them a magnet for those resisting royal policies. The *dévots* who opposed the government's war policy; the *parlementaires* who hated Mazarin; Richerists who supported priests against bishops; those who wrote scurrilous *mazarinades* (over 5000 pamphlets attacking Mazarin)—all found a sympathetic ear among the *amis de Port-Royal*.[127] Granted, Jean Racine (a pupil in the "little schools" at the time) declared that "it was the doctrine of Port-Royal that under no conditions could a subject in good conscience rebel against his legitimate prince."[128] True, Blaise Pascal resisted attempts to recruit his talents on behalf of the Fronde. Moreover, Port-Royal's spiritual advisors refused to absolve those known to oppose Louis XIV. Nonetheless, given the highly charged political and religious climate of the 1640s and 1650s, many Jansenists, at the very least, acted indiscretely.[129]

As might be expected, the Arnauld family positioned themselves at the center of the controversy. At Port-Royal des Champs, Angélique Arnauld welcomed refugee nuns victimized by soldiers' violence during the Fronde. While she admitted that "we are always threatened," she remained confident that "M. le Cardinal Mazarin does not wish to persecute us."[130] Perhaps she felt that her brother Henri's service as Mazarin's ambassador to Rome and her nephew Simon's career as *intendant* of the king's army in Catalonia would protect her community.[131]

Angélique's brother Robert Arnauld d'Andilly, on the other hand, wrote two *mazarinades* in 1649 and 1652. As a first clerk for his uncle Isaac Arnauld (an *intendant* of finances), superintendent of finances for the *duc* de Schomberg, *intendant-général* for Gaston, *duc* d'Orléans in the 1620s, and *intendant* for the Army of the Rhine in the 1630s, Robert knew fiscal corruption first-hand. In 1643 he sent Queen Anne two *Memoirs* calling for the abolition of duels, benefices, venality and luxury at Court and pleading for tax relief and fiscal reform. Jealous of Mazarin after his appointment as tutor of the future Louis XIV (a position d'Andilly had coveted), he found other reasons to attack the first minister.[132]

The vigor and quality of expression place his "Political Advice to the Queen concerning the Government of Her Regency" (1649) and "The Truth Laid Bare" (1652) well above the mediocre quality of most other *mazarinades*. D'Andilly's passion, eloquence, and dialectic clarity make these two pamphlets (30 pages and 26 pages respectively) models of the genre. His polemical tone, patriotic ardor, and righteous indignation reflect Jansenist ideals. He attacks Mazarin's fiscal incompetence, urging Queen Ann to dismiss him. He strongly opposes venality of office and the war with Spain, and portrays the Fronde as God's punishment for France's sins. Then he calls for national repentance and the restoration of morality and honor.[133]

But spiritual solutions for France's fiscal problems did not appeal to Jean-Baptiste Colbert, who saw deeper issues at stake. In a 1657 letter, Colbert informed Mazarin that "all these sorts of religious affairs are fought with so much ferocity in Paris that we cannot doubt that the Jansenists, the friends of the Cardinal de Retz . . . are deeply involved and carry along the *dévots*; the ill-intentioned join them and nearly everyone follows."[134] For both Colbert and Mazarin, the Cardinal de Retz—whom they suspected of Jansenism—represented the key figure in the religious Fronde. Therefore, they resolved to destroy him and undermine his Jansenist base of support.

Born in 1613 into a Tuscan family living in France, Jean François Paul de Gondi studied under Vincent de Paul and at the Sorbonne prior to being ordained as a priest. At 30 he served as coadjutor to his uncle, the Archbishop of Paris, and soon gained a reputation as a popular preacher, Court confidante, military advisor, and something of a demagogue with the people.[135] As late as 1652, Mazarin praised Gondi's "passion for the Queen's service" and his desire to "serve the Queen in all ways without any reserve." Such devotion earned him Mazarin's support in appointing him Archbishop of Paris.[136] But during the revolt of the nobles, Retz opposed the policies of the Regency and clashed (verbally, at least) with Queen Anne and Mazarin, who then tried to have him condemned at Rome. But the cardinal enjoyed Alexander VII's support, making him a threat to Mazarin if he chose to use his influence in Rome and in Paris to have the first minister dismissed.[137]

From 1652 until Mazarin's death in 1661, therefore, these two antagonists treated each other as bitter enemies. In a letter to procurer-general Nicolas Foucquet, Mazarin warned: "It is essential to be on guard with him [Retz], because assuredly he has nothing good in his soul, either for the King, for the State, or for me."[138] He complained to Chancellor Le Tellier that Retz had "bad wishes toward me." He "is incapable of doing anything to the advantage of the King and the State" because his actions "will always be full of hidden poison and directed toward wicked ends."[139] In short, Mazarin accused the cardinal of plotting to overthrow him.[140]

Given the cardinal's onus toward the first minister, that charge seems valid. In his *Memoirs*, Retz calls Mazarin a cheater, a coward, and a dishonest social climber. "I never knew a man who respected truth so little as Mazarin," he declares. He accuses him of breaking all his promises and of "turning religion into a jest."[141] Satirically he acknowledges that Mazarin "must be a man of great skill, to deceive people, in a manner so useful to him."[142]

Such accusations could not go unpunished. On December 18, 1652, as he left the Queen's apartments at the Louvre, Retz was arrested for "dissimulating" against the monarchs and taken first to Vincennes and fifteen months later to Nantes. But in August 1654, he escaped and fled to Spain, then by ship to Rome, where Innocent X and Alexander VII received him gladly. After months of charges and countercharges from both sides, Louis XIV in April 1655 issued a *lettre de cachet* forbidding anyone to write to or associate with Retz, whose "pernicious designs" and "evil intentions" made him a "bad subject." Another *lettre de cachet* in September 1656, charging him with treason (conspiring with the Spanish troops in Italy to invade France), called for his immediate arrest "wherever he may be in the realm."[143]

But in their sympathetic biography of Retz a century later, Louis-Adrien Le Paige and J. B. F. Du Rey de Meinières presented a different picture. They accused the king of arresting and imprisoning the cardinal to please Mazarin, to ruin Retz's reputation among the Jansenists, and to exercise his royal arbitrary authority. By not following regular judicial procedures, Louis XIV caused much suffering and internal bickering between judicial and ecclesiastical authorities.[144] Certainly Retz's arrest, trial, and detention brought suffering to the Jansenists, who thought of him as their protector. A contemporary anonymous manuscript declared that thanks to Retz's "favor," Jansenism "has grown to a formidable grandeur."[145]

But the cardinal protected Jansenism when it suited *his* purposes and withdrew his favors when granting them proved disadvantageous to *him*. While this Machiavellian attitude baffled the Jansenists, they did not reject him. For awhile, Retz protected Antoine Singlin at Court, but when this friendship hurt his cause, he broke with him; the two reconciled years later in 1664. The solitaires believed that the Cardinal spoke favorably of them to Alexander VII in 1665; that he approved of their refusal to sign the Formulary; and that he helped arrange the "Peace of the Church" (1669–1679) between the Jansenists and Clement IX.[146]

Yet Retz experienced a variable relationship with Jansenist leaders like the Arnaulds. During his 45-year friendship with Antoine Arnauld, the cardinal shared his "greatest confidence." He thanked Antoine for rendering him "several services" and found his writings "edifying" in his final years.[147] But in his *Memoirs*, Retz poked fun at Robert Arnauld d'Andilly who, he says, conjured up a devil to frighten Anne de Rohan, *princesse* de Guéménée, into behaving more spiritually during her stay at Port-Royal. She quit curling and powdering her hair for awhile, until "I conjured up another devil on my side under a more benign and agreeable form," the Cardinal chuckled, and "this devil got her away from there."[148]

In 1657, as Mazarin negotiated a treaty with Oliver Cromwell, Retz found himself in a position to play both sides to his advantage. The Jansenist envoy, Baudry d'Asson de Saint-Gilles, approached him with promises of substantial monetary support from powerful friends if he agreed to plead their case at Court. But Retz, who longed to have his abbeys, estates, and archbishopric restored, had already promised "perfect fidelity to the King," to Queen Anne, and to the Gallican Church in hopes that His Majesty would grant him a public trial to clear his name. In return, he allegedly agreed to help crush the Jansenists.[149]

With little knowledge of his behind-the-scenes machinations, the Jansenists continued their flattering appeals to Retz. In 1658, while the Cardinal lived in exile at Rotterdam, Arnauld d'Andilly assured him: "Your reward in heaven, Monsignor, is assuredly well-deserved, since you seek no other recompense in the zeal that leads you to employ all the authority God has entrusted to you for His service and His glory."[150] Jansenist leaders helped Retz publish his manifestos and pamphlets; they pulled strings to get him restored as archbishop of Paris.[151] In 1659, Mazarin and Chancellor Le Tellier, convinced that Retz conspired with the Jansenist *curés* in Paris, even feared he would return to the capital and "cause some grand revolution."[152]

To allay those fears and hasten his return to Paris, the Cardinal in 1661 wrote a letter to Alexander VII affirming his submission to the papal bulls of 1653 and 1656 condemning Jansenism; he declared that "while I have breath in my body, I shall continue to obey the decrees of the Holy See." He even promised that, if restored as archbishop of Paris, he would repress the Jansenists.[153] Finding Retz's "declarations of orthodoxy" satisfactory, the pope cleared him of the charge of Jansenism, informing the French envoy D'Aubeville that while the Cardinal might have used the Jansenists to serve his purposes, he was not one of them. As they had sent him hundreds of thousands of *livres* to plead their cause in high places, so he had used his connections with them to influence public opinion in his favor.[154]

Yet despite his Machiavellian maneuvers, in the end, Retz had to resign as Archbishop of Paris in February 1662. His submission, however, paved the way for his return to France in 1664 after twelve years in exile.[155] Invited to Versailles, the Cardinal bowed before Louis XIV, who remarked, "M. le Cardinal, your hair has grown whiter." Retz replied: "Sire, one grows whiter quickly when one has the misfortune of being in disgrace with Your Majesty."[156] Once restored to royal favor, Retz lived "a retired & exemplary life" for another twelve years, dying in 1679 still a cardinal, but never again Archbishop of Paris.[157]

In the final analysis, the Jansenists gained very little from their courtship with Cardinal de Retz. Retz's father had befriended Saint-Cyran and publicly protested his imprisonment; his uncle, the first Archbishop Gondi of Paris, had protected Port-Royal in the 1620s after Urban VIII transferred it to his jurisdiction. But although Retz became friends with many Jansenist leaders, his interventions—largely opportunistic—failed to protect the movement from Church and state persecution even during his lifetime.[158] Yet in 1652, a quarter of a century before his death, Retz had counseled the papacy to handle the Jansenist threat with great care. "The Court of Rome should take care not to light a fire in France which might be difficult to extinguish," he warned, "and which, in the end might even involve Rome itself in a yet more dangerous fashion."[159] Imminent clashes between the papacy and Louis XIV on the one hand and Port-Royal and Jansenist leaders on the other would highlight the wisdom of those words.

This temporary liaison with the Cardinal de Retz, which represented a significant departure from their credo of *mépris du monde*, damaged the public image of Jansenism for generations. Long after the Fronde ended and he returned to power, Mazarin continued to see the Jansenists as *frondeurs* (intriguers). This cloud of suspicion hung over the Arnauld family, who felt compelled to defend themselves. In March 1655, Robert Arnauld d'Andilly assured Mazarin "that there have never been individuals more faithful to his Majesty [nor more eager to give him] the obedience that God requires us to render to the King as His living image" than the Arnaulds and their

Jansenist friends.[160] In August he declared that his brother Antoine's writings reflected his "sincerity and good faith" and that Antoine had "kept the peace ordered by your Eminence" until verbally attacked by the Jesuits.[161]

After the Sorbonne censured Antoine Arnauld, Robert insisted that the first minister should intervene to clear his brother's name. In a 12 February 1656 letter concerning Antoine's hearing, Robert told Mazarin that the Jesuits (with their "animosity . . . and furor . . . against my brother") had engineered his trial and condemnation, for they wanted "his blood and his life." The Society of Jesus—and not his brother—had "lit the blaze" which threatened the Church.[162] One month later, in a letter to his friend the Bishop of Coutances, Antoine portrayed himself as a victim of "the injustices, violence, persecution [and] the furor of the Jesuits."[163]

After Robert agreed to leave Port-Royal des Champs in March 1656 and return to Pomponne, however, Mazarin reassured him that "Your complete submission to His Majesty [and the] esteem and affection which the Queen has for you [should reassure you that] the matter can only have successful results to your satisfaction."[164] Following five weeks of "happy solitude" on his estate, Robert wrote to Mazarin and to Queen Anne ("the greatest queen in the world") in early May to thank them for allowing him to return to Port-Royal des Champs, on which "the repose of my life depends."[165] Mazarin assured him that "I am overjoyed with satisfaction that you have returned to your solitude and I esteem myself happy for having had the joy of contributing something to it." Then he added, "I do not doubt that in the repose and tranquility you will enjoy there, you will still show the same zeal for the service of the King."[166] Four days later, Robert thanked "the greatest Minister of the most just King on earth" (even Jansenists could use "worldly" flattery), promising him "my passion for the service of Your Eminence." In return, Arnauld begged Mazarin to be "the protector of this Holy House [Port-Royal des Champs] and of the innocence of my relatives and friends."[167] Two years later, in a letter to the Bishop of Coutances expressing his "esteem and affection" for Robert, the first minister promised to "give him some proofs [of my esteem] with pleasure in his person and that of his son."[168]

Despite this entente cordiale between Mazarin and the Arnauld family, the flood of Jansenist propaganda in the 1650s impelled the government to suppress Jansenist printers. In 1659 Mazarin complained to Chancellor Le Tellier that clandestine presses "are altering the calm and repose that His Majesty desires to see among all his subjects" by criticizing the religious establishment with their "seditious libels." Since "the Inquisition is not recognized in France," the lieutenants civil and criminal should destroy Jansenist presses, he said; their owners must be sent to the Bastille. Ultimately, he hoped, the Jesuits "will thereby gain the advantage over Port-Royal." He expected that Louis XIV would soon issue a declaration against that community.[169]

Before the axe fell, however, Mazarin urged Angélique Arnauld in March 1660 to persuade the sisters and solitaires to sign the Formulary. "It brings me great displeasure," he wrote, "to learn that the religious ones who until now have been considered as among the wisest and the most spiritual group in the Church are now divided in so foreign a manner." He exhorted them to submit to the Holy See.[170] This long struggle to force the men and women at Port-Royal to sign the Formulary is discussed in chapter 3.

On his deathbed in 1661, Mazarin urged Louis XIV "not to tolerate the sect of the Jansenists anymore," but to "engage all [his] efforts and all [his] authority" to crush them.[171] Other counselors over a quarter of a century had been giving him the same advice. His mother Anne of Austria, who had raised him to be devoted to God and to the Roman Catholic Church, favored the Jesuits at Court and hated Jansenism. His early governors and tutors (the *duc* de Villeroy, the marquis de Sénecy, the Bishop of Rodez, François de Mothe le Voyer, Pierre de la Porte)—all hated the Jansenists and Port-Royal. His first confessors—*Pères* Paulin, Louis Dinet, François

Annat—openly despised Jansenism and reminded him that Port-Royal represented a threat to the Church and to the monarchy. Louis XIII's first minister, Cardinal Richelieu, had seen Jansen as "a dangerous heretic" and the Jansenists as a subversive sect; as we have seen, he sent Saint-Cyran to Vincennes. His successor, Cardinal Mazarin, who viewed the Jansenists as conspirators and *frondeurs*, continued Richelieu's anti-Jansenist policies by enforcing the popes' bulls against Jansenism.[172]

Therefore, Louis XIV grew up hating Jansenists for a variety of reasons. They did not conform to Roman Catholic orthodoxy. They represented a divisive element within his kingdom. They offended his royal dignity and authority. Because some of their leaders had ties to the Cardinal de Retz and the Fronde, he saw them as "rebels" and "intriguers." Their Richerist, democratic spirit clashed with his love of hierarchical authority and arbitrary power. The asceticism of those at Port-Royal implicitly condemned the pomp and worldly luxury at Versailles.[173]

Yet the king knew that the eradication of Jansenism would require the cooperation of a host of institutions—popes, bishops, Parlement, the Sorbonne—often at loggerheads with one another. When he took the throne in 1643, he could hardly have envisioned the hundreds of bulls, *mandements*, *placets*, and *lettres de cachet*[174] that would be required over the next seven decades in his war with Jansenism.

At first, the papacy proved eager to assist Louis XIV in his holy crusade against Jansenism, which, in the eyes of the Church, stood triply condemned. Theologically, Jansenists were heretics; ecclesiastically, they were insubordinate; politically, they were factious rebels. Therefore, this multiform error (Richerism, Gallicanism, Jansenism) sapped Catholic doctrine and undermined Tridentine reforms. Jansenists stood before the bar of St. Peter condemned as heretics, schismatics, and rebels.[175] As early as 1567, Pius VI's Bull *Exomnibus afflictionibus* had condemned 79 propositions in the works of Michel Baius. Subsequently, in 1607 and 1625, Rome had imposed silence on any discussion regarding divine grace.[176]

Consequently, when Jansen published his *Augustinus* in 1640, Rome saw this as "breaking the law of silence" imposed fifteen years before. Fearing that the book would revive the propositions already condemned in Baius and provoke a scandal in the Church, Urban VIII issued the Bull *In eminenti Ecclesiae militantis* on 6 March 1641. Essentially, this bull reproduced the texts of three previous bulls by Pius V (1567), Gregory XIII (1579), and Paul V (1611) condemning Baius' propositions and forbidding the printing of any work concerning *De Auxiliis* without Rome's approval. But the new bull also contained a long list of condemned pro-Jansenist writings on the subjects of grace, free will, predestination, and apologetics for Jansen.[177]

Ironically, however, the 1641 bull condemned the *Augustinus* for contravening Pius VI's Bull *De auxiliis* imposing silence on discussions of grace; it did not articulate the precise errors within the book. Two years later in France, it became the "club" used to beat Antoine Arnauld for issuing his *Frequent Communion*—and thus once again breaking the "law of silence" imposed by previous popes.[178]

In eminenti stirred up a hornet's nest in France. Saint-Cyran, fearing for his life, fled Port-Royal for his rural retreat. Antoine Arnauld, questioning its legitimacy, penned his *Observations on the Bull* (1643), a manifesto for those in opposition. Although the Archbishop of Paris, Jean-François de Gondi, welcomed the bull and published it, many Gallican bishops did not accept it. When on November 27 the Faculty of Theology at the Sorbonne received a *lettre de cachet* ordering them to register the bull, they expressed dismay, for this was not their normal role *vis-à-vis* papal decrees. Wishing to preserve their freedom to discuss, dispute, and write on such matters, they voted on 15 January 1644 not to receive or publish the bull.[179]

As debates among the French bishops, Jesuits, and theologians concerning *Frequent Communion* grew hotter, Innocent X believed that many of the charges against Antoine Arnauld seemed "greatly exaggerated." Therefore, in the interests of keeping the "peace of the Church," he decided in 1646 not to condemn the work.[180] In the same spirit, five years later the Archbishop of Paris proscribed *Père* Brisacier's *Jansenism Confounded* for its libels against the nuns of Port-Royal, calling them "impenitents, asacramentaries, and incommunicants." Contrary to these "lies and impostures," stated the archbishop, the sisters "are pure and innocent," living lives of "good manners" and integrity. Published widely and pasted on every church door in Paris, this broadside provided the Jansenists much-needed support.[181]

As the Society of Jesus mounted a campaign to crush them, they would need all the help they could find. Both in Rome and Paris, the Jesuits boasted of their successes in defeating opponents in the battle over Jansen's disputed propositions. Indeed, they had already engineered the discharge of pro-Jansenist faculty at the University of Caen and at the College of Montaigu. They hoped to persuade the pope to issue a bull condemning these propositions.[182]

But exactly how many propositions deserved condemnation as heretical remained in dispute, especially at the Sorbonne. Staunchly Gallican, pro-Richerist, and anti-Jesuit, the theology faculty resented efforts by the king, the chancellor, bishops, and regular clergy to control their decisions regarding Jansenism.[183] Then in July 1649, all their pent-up frustration erupted when Nicolas Cornet, a former student of the Jesuits at Amiens and now the syndic of the theology faculty in Paris, submitted seven propositions he deemed heretical in the *Augustinus*.[184]

As syndic, Cornet supervised the content and orthodoxy of theses presented to the Sorbonne. He had often complained about the plethora of "new opinions" espoused by these theses. So when on July 1 he alerted the faculty to several subversive propositions in Jansen's work, they expressed concern. However, following several days of debate, the doctors of theology reduced his seven propositions to the following five:

1 It is impossible to keep several commands of God because despite the will and best efforts of just men, they lack the grace that makes obedience possible.
2 In the state of man's fallen nature, he cannot resist interior grace.
3 To be deserving or undeserving in a state of fallen nature, it is not necessary that man possess a freedom exempt from inner necessity; it suffices that his freedom of choice be exempt from restraint.
4 Semi-Pelagians admitted the necessity of an inner grace preceding every particular action and for faith to exist; they were heretical for stating that the human will could resist or obey this grace as it wished.
5 It is semi-Pelagian to say that Christ died and offered His blood to cover the sins of all humanity.[185]

Even so, the faculty remained divided: 60 theologians found nothing heretical in the five proposals, while another 85 urged Innocent X to condemn them.[186] When Parlement prohibited the Sorbonne from further debates on these propositions, Cornet resigned as syndic in October 1649.[187]

No doubt his faculty colleague, Antoine Arnauld, rejoiced at Cornet's demotion. Arnauld had long suspected the syndic of being in league with the Jesuits to promote their theology in the Sorbonne. He also disliked Cornet personally, calling him "the leader & chief of all the enemies of St. Augustine's doctrine." Consequently, he considered the syndic's "fabrication" of the five propositions as "a plot, long planned, to crush the doctrines of St. Augustine by surprise & by cabal." To his mind, the Jesuits had masterminded "this cabal" to divide the faculty of theology and bring "trouble & ruin" on the Sorbonne.[188] Arnauld's sister Angélique agreed, declaring that Cornet (and Vincent de Paul who had helped him find the seven propositions) had shown "zeal without science."[189] More seriously, Louis Gorin de St. Amour, a theologian at the Sorbonne and delegate to the Holy See, accused Cornet of wreaking "dreadful mischief" in the Church, "wholly disturbing the peace" in France, and dividing the faculty at the Sorbonne.[190]

Finally, 85 French bishops asked Innocent X to intervene and issue a bull condemning the five propositions. The time seemed right, for in 1653, a rare entente existed among the French king, the pope, and the Gallican clergy.[191] As few in France had paid much attention to the 1643 bull *In eminenti*, the pope hoped that by issuing another bull (*Cum occasione*), he could accomplish several goals. First, he wanted to upstage the Gallican bishops as the sole decision-makers on policies curbing Jansenism in France. Second, by claiming that the Holy Spirit had guided him in drafting this bull, he demonstrated his superiority to the learned doctors of theology at the Sorbonne. Third, condemning the *Augustinus* boosted the prestige of the Jesuits both in France and at Rome, where they boasted of their influence with the pope. Finally, although not a theologian, Innocent X hoped this bull would buttress his claim to infallibility.[192]

Antoine Arnauld (and the Jansenists in general) questioned the pope's double claim to inspiration by the Spirit and infallibility. Although Arnauld complimented Innocent for his "common sense," the fact that he had no theological training rendered somewhat dubious his "ability to rule on matters of doctrine and faith . . . by the enthusiasm of the Holy Spirit."[193] Direct revelation without deep research and wide consultation, he warned, "has been rejected by all Catholics as an open door to all kinds of errors." Heretics for centuries had claimed direct inspiration for their aberrant views.[194] For the pope "to judge the most difficult questions of faith . . . without knowing any Theology," claiming that "the Spirit will enlighten him and make him understand things which he has never studied," was the height of "pretentiousness," he scoffed.[195]

Beneath this pious claim of being led by the Spirit, Arnauld asserted, lay a more sinister reason why Innocent X issued his 1653 bull without consulting anyone: He wished to advance the new doctrine of papal infallibility. Such a claim would enable him to bypass the College of Cardinals, the Faculty of Theology at the Sorbonne, even the General Assembly of the French Clergy. And instead of convening a Church council, reading canon law, or searching the writings of the learned doctors of centuries past, Innocent declared that he would "consult his Crucifix" and pray for the Spirit's inspiration.[196]

Yet the pope could never hope to succeed in his "war against Jansenism" without the help of Louis XIV. Despite their disagreements concerning the Regale and other Gallican prerogatives, Louis did believe in papal infallibility—despite warnings from his advocate-general Omer Talon that it threatened his crown. Louis backed the pope because he, too, needed powerful outside help in his campaign against Port-Royal.[197]

Therefore, when twelve French prelates informed Urban VIII in 1651 (and subsequently Innocent X in 1652) of the need for a "new discussion of Augustinianism and grace," the latter appointed a congregation of five (later increased to seven) cardinals (led by the Dominican Francesco Albizzi) to closely examine the *Augustinus*. As these cardinals made no claim to divine inspiration, they consulted French deputies (both pro- and anti-Jansenist) and German and Spanish theologians at several universities. After twenty sessions among themselves and ten meetings with the pope, they drafted the bull *Cum occasione* in May 1653. Heaping adjectives atop one another, it condemned the five propositions as "impious, blasphemous, heretical, anathema, false, calumnious, and injurious to the goodness of God."[198]

As Lucien Ceyssens (1971) observed, however, the bull fulfilled the prophecy given by Hosea: "For they have sown the wind, and they shall reap the whirlwind" (Hosea 8:7).[199] Prior to the publication of *Cum occasione* in June, French prelates warned Innocent X that the five propositions could be interpreted as heretical (if seen through Lutheran or Calvinist lenses), as orthodox (if viewed through Augustinian lenses), or as semi-Pelagian (if examined through Jesuit lenses).

Drawing up a chart in three columns, they attempted to convince the inspired but unlearned pope that the Council of Trent and previous popes had interpreted the doctrines of grace, works, and salvation favorably in their bulls.[200]

In France, the Jansenists—who objected to the bull's lumping together St. Augustine, Baius, and Jansen, to the disadvantage of the latter—also published a "Writing in Three Columns" in 1654 to explain the differences between Augustinianism, Pelagianism, and Molinism. While they agreed that the pope had the right (*droit*) to condemn the five propositions as heretical, they argued that in fact (*fait*), none of the five could be found in Jansen's *Augustinus*. Therefore, they asserted, the pope's bull did not condemn the entire book, but only certain misunderstandings of Jansen's thought. Because Innocent X's bull nowhere specified the chapter and verse in the *Augustinus* where the five heretical statements could be found, Jansenists for generations argued that the pope in reality had not condemned Jansenism per se.[201]

But Church officials across Europe saw things differently. In France, the Holy Roman Empire, Spain, Austria, and Poland, the bull received enthusiastic receptions. Only in Flanders—the birthplace of Jansenism—did many Catholics reject it.[202] In France, Mazarin believed *Cum occasione* helped to "clear the air" of theological confusion. If before 1653, many saw "Jansenism" as merely a pejorative term, after the pope's bull, they recognized it as a heresy. "Before the Pope's decision," he declared, "no one in France or Flanders had ever doubted that the five propositions contained an abridged version of Jansénius' doctrine."[203] To prevent future generations from becoming confused by the Jansenists' *droit* v. *fait* hairsplitting, Mazarin added the words "extracted from Jansen's book" to his *Mandement* of 4 July 1653—something no papal bulls had done.[204]

For French Jansenists who advocated silence as the best response to the controversy, the General Assembly of the Clergy responded in the negative. By declaring that the *Augustinus* did indeed contain the five propositions, the bishops asserted that anyone who put their signature to the Formulary would be acknowledging that as *fact*.[205] This effectively removed any neutral ground the Jansenists might have occupied. After 1653 one either belonged to the Holy Apostolic Roman Catholic Church—or one was a heretic, a member of a subversive party, considered an enemy of the Church and a threat to the state.[206]

Although 85 bishops on the General Assembly of the Clergy believed the bull condemned the five propositions "in the sense used by Jansenius," four courageous bishops did not. Like the four Hebrew worthies in Babylon who defied King Nebuchadnezzar's order to kneel before his golden image (Daniel 3), the Archbishop of Sens and the bishops of Angers, Beauvais, and Comminges refused to accept the Bull of 1653. Instead, they argued that because Innocent X had not consulted the College of Cardinals or the General Assembly of the French Bishops, the bull lacked validity in France. Furthermore, they agreed with the Jansenists that the *Augustinus* did not contain the five heretical propositions. Therefore, they submitted to the pope "with reservations," which he graciously accepted.[207]

Likewise, the Faculty of Theology at the Sorbonne refused to issue a blanket condemnation of Jansenism as Innocent X and Louis XIV wanted. Instead, like theologians everywhere, they spent days debating each of the five propositions. They labeled the first heretical; the second, contrary to scripture; the third, heretical; the fourth, false (first part) and heretical (second part); and the fifth, false and scandalous.[208]

Meanwhile the Parlement, more concerned with protecting Gallican liberties than ensuring orthodox praxis, simply refused to register *Cum occasione*. Mazarin, distracted by the Fronde and the interminable war with Spain, decided not to press the matter. Consequently, this 1653 Bull lacked legal status in France.[209]

In 1654, when a total eclipse of the sun threw Paris into consternation, an ecclesiastical almanac predicted that this portended either the utter destruction of Jansenism or the end of the world within the next two years.[210] Neither occurred. But the outlook for Jansenism darkened considerably when in 1655, Jean-Jacques Olier, the *curé* of Saint-Sulpice, advised Charles Picoré, his vicar, to refuse absolution and communion to a Jansenist sympathizer, the *duc* de Liancourt (whose granddaughter was a pensioner at Port-Royal). Angered by this action, Antoine Arnauld penned two "Letters to a Person of Rank" attacking priests who, "without authorization, take unto themselves the power of removing from the communion of the Church the Messieurs of Port-Royal." His colleagues at the Sorbonne demanded that he retract his views and submit to the pope's judgment condemning Jansen as a heretic. When he refused, they censured him and removed him from the Faculty of Theology (without the required two-thirds vote) in February 1656. Louis XIV threatened to issue a *lettre de cachet* to arrest anyone who opposed his suspension. Although Arnauld subsequently complained of his mistreatment as "persecution," he had in fact refused a hearing by his peers as "dishonorable." In August, the pope placed all of Arnauld's works on the Index of Forbidden Books.[211]

Following Arnauld's condemnation, Church and state officials took a harsher attitude toward Jansenism. In 1656, the Formulary, drafted by the General Assembly of the Clergy "to stop the course of one of the greatest evils afflicting the Church," began to be enforced.[212] Although Jansenist works had been censored intermittently in the 1640s, Chancellor Séguier, who clearly favored the Jesuits, began cracking down on printers and colporteurs in Paris and Rouen (two Jansenist centers) who distributed these works in the 1650s. He struggled in vain, however, to curtail the flood of literature illegally entering the realm from Holland.[213] Perhaps, he mused, another papal bull would do the trick.

Unfortunately for Séguier, however, Alexander VII, the pope in 1657, distrusted Mazarin and hesitated to crush the Jansenists if that would strengthen the first minister's power. An "obsessed anti-Jansenist," Alexander also exhibited anti-French inclinations. In a letter to the General Assembly of the Clergy in March 1656, the pope urged the bishops to help bring peace in the Church—a position contrary to Mazarin's desire to crush the Jansenists and continue the war with Spain.[214]

In response, the General Assembly asked the pope for another bull denouncing Jansenism. On 7 November 1656, after only six weeks' deliberation, Alexander VII issued the bull *Ad sacram* at Rome; it appeared in France on 31 March 1657—one week after Pascal's last Provincial Letter. Like Innocent X's *Cum occasione* four years earlier, *Ad sacram* condemned the five propositions "as Jansen meant them" and affirmed that they could indeed be found in his *Augustinus*. Furthermore, this new bull closed the loophole for those who wished to make clever distinctions between "right" and "fact."[215]

When the bull reached France in 1657, the General Assembly of the Clergy issued a circular letter ordering that it be published and enforced in every diocese as a demonstration of "the truth of the Faith." All Church prelates must sign their names to show their submission within one month.[216]

But when the bull reached the Sorbonne, its members refused to register it. So on 4 April 1657, Louis XIV issued a *lettre de cachet* commanding his "Dear and good friends . . . to receive it with the respect and submission that is due to the holy See" and thereby "purge the Church of a doctrine so dangerous and so pernicious to our religion."[217] When presented to Parlement later in April, the bull met a wall of opposition. Colbert had warned Mazarin that registration would be difficult because "the Jansenists have inflamed minds in Parlement . . . against the bull."[218] Angry, Mazarin pressed the magistrates, but their defense of Gallican liberties and fear of establishing an Inquisition in France stymied his efforts to present Louis XIV with a fait accompli when the king returned from the Dutch war. Finally, at a *lit de justice* on December 19, Louis, with Mazarin by his side, forced the recalcitrant *parlementaires* to register both the 1653 and 1657 bulls as law in France.[219]

The forced registration of *Ad sacram* and the insistence that all clerics sign the Formulary deeply concerned Jansenists everywhere. From Port-Royal des Champs, Isaac Le Maistre wrote a letter describing "the inquisition that is to be established in France." The Church, he feared, would be stripped of its Gallican liberties; bishops and *parlementaires* would lose their authority.[220]

One of the groups the Jansenists feared most was the Company of the Most Holy Sacrament. From 1630 until its dissolution in 1666, this largely lay organization, opposed to all "theological novelties," promoted ultramontanism, piety, morality, and Catholic orthodoxy in France. After the release of Innocent X's bull in 1653, the Company purged its ranks of all Jansenists. Its adherents, who favored the Society of Jesus, denounced priests suspected of Jansenism.[221]

At first, its members admired the reforms Angélique Arnauld had introduced at Port-Royal des Champs from 1618 to 1626. After all, Sébastien Zamet, her spiritual advisor, belonged to the Company of the Holy Sacrament. But after the publication of *Augustinus* in 1640, the two groups drifted apart as the Jansenists advocated Gallican liberties and the Company promoted ultramontane policies. In 1643 the Company denounced Arnauld's book *Frequent Communion* as "designed to destroy the Mass and the Communion." During the 1640s and 1650s, they sided with the Jesuits in the "war of libels" against Jansenism. Believing that in his *Provincial Letters*, Blaise Pascal had attacked them as well as the Jesuits, they resolved in 1657 to ruin Port-Royal, close its "heretical seminary" (the *petites écoles*), and scatter its members. Largely through their influence, Louis XIV issued the Declaration of 7 June 1659 stipulating that only regular houses, monasteries, seminaries, and communities with royal letters patent could continue to exist. As chapter 3 shows, this law sealed the fate of the "Little Schools" at Port-Royal.[222]

Throughout France, the Company loved staging spectacles showing the defeat of Jansenism. For example, in Caen, its members led a parade with a float featuring a statue of the Virgin Mary with a serpent (labeled "Jansenism") wrapped around her leg. Catholics along the parade route chanted, "Flail of the Jansenists, Pray for us; Destroyer of the Jansenists, Pray for us." Soon children repeated this prayer in the streets.[223] Back in Paris, the Jesuit preacher Jacques Nouet, using similar colorful language, called Antoine Arnauld "a snake with a three-pronged tongue," "a monster," and "a wolf in sheep's clothing."[224]

But in its efforts to crush Jansenism, the Company of the Holy Sacrament overplayed its hand, especially in Normandy and around Paris. Ironically, the Jansenists themselves helped topple their enemies' house of cards. Between 1658 and 1660, Pierre Nicole, Blaise Pascal and others denounced them as an "occult" group in league with the Jesuits against the regular clergy, the Oratorians, and the *dévots*. Their hierarchical organization and ultra-secrecy, many felt, threatened the state. Convinced by this propaganda, in 1665 Louis XIV ordered the Company to disband. Jansenism, at least for the moment, was saved.[225]

In her own way, Pascal's niece, Marguerite Périer, helped save the Jansenist cause in 1656 just as the tidal wave of persecution seemed about to crush it. The ten-year-old daughter of Monsieur Périer, councilor at the Court of Aids in Clermont, lived as a pensioner at Port-Royal in Paris with her aunt, Sister Jacqueline, a sub-prioress and supervisor of novices. For over three years, she had endured the pain caused by a cancerous ulcer in the corner of her left eye. As it grew, the ulcer consumed the cartilage in her nose, broke through her palate, and leaked its foul pus into her throat. The slightest touch to the side of her face brought excruciating pain. Although several of the best doctors, oculists, and surgeons had treated her, she found no relief in their remedies.[226]

Then on 24 March 1656, as the nuns recited the introit for the Mass ("Perform a sign in my favor so that they can see . . . "), something dramatic happened that changed Marguerite's face forever. Sister Flavie Passart, the nun who cared for her, urged her to touch her sore eye with the convent's most valuable relic—a thorn allegedly taken from Christ's crown of thorns worn on the cross. She felt immediate and complete healing. Subsequent examinations by Paris's finest surgeons (Dalencé, Guillard, Cressé) confirmed that the malignant cancer had disappeared. "God alone could have effected a healing so sudden and so complete," the doctors exclaimed. In the ensuing months, 80 more sufferers reported being healed by the "Miracle of the Thorn."[227]

Jansenists at the time—and some recent historians—considered this event a "Christian miracle" both for its instant healing in a religious context and for the positive results that followed. Yet a closer examination raises some questions. Flavie Passart, the nun who suggested the Holy Thorn remedy, had a reputation for being meddlesome, mischievous, turbulent—a trouble-maker with an obsessive interest in relics who loved to claim miraculous cures for herself and others. In some cases, illnesses were induced so that miraculous healing might occur. Therefore, her testimony must be received with caution. Did she apply some "wonder drug" or medication that, over time, eradicated Marguerite's cancer? Historians may never know the whole truth for certain.[228]

What is certain, however, is that most contemporary observers believed Périer's recovery had been a divine miracle. Jansenists saw "the miracle of the thorn" as proof positive that they had the truth and that God was with them and not with the Jesuits.[229] Quoting St. Augustine, Pascal exclaimed, "I would not be a Christian without the miracles."[230] To demonstrate his confidence in the genuineness of his niece's healing, he adopted as his seal the crown of thorns with rays of light emanating from it and beneath it the motto *Scio cui credidi* ("I know in whom I have believed").[231]

Even more significantly, the Queen Mother, Anne of Austria, certainly no friend of the Jansenists, allegedly believed that Marguerite's healing was providential. At any rate, she told Mazarin to cease persecuting the Jansenists.[232] During this hiatus, as miracle cures multiplied, Jansenists penned tracts defending them as proof that they possessed the truth. By the end of the seventeenth century, as Robert Kreiser (1978) has stated, "The expectation of miracles and other supernatural signs had become almost an integral part of the Jansenist worldview," bringing them "profound psychological consolation" amidst their persecution. The stage had been set for the convulsions in St.-Médard (see chapter 7).[233]

Persecution increased in the 1660s under the new Archbishop of Paris, Hardouin de Péréfixe. Determined to end the Jansenists' resistance, in June 1664 he ordered all clerics to sign the Formulary without reservations. To those who quibbled over "right" and "fact," he declared: "Demand divine faith for the Right and human faith for the Fact," but sign! Twelve prelates who refused to do so were scattered to other religious houses; the sisters and solitaires at Port-Royal des Champs were deprived of the sacraments.[234]

Eight months later on 15 February 1665, Alexander VII released another bull. *Regiminis apostolici*, like *Cum occasione* (1653) and *Ad sacram* (1657), condemned the five propositions in Jansen's *Augustinus* and declared the question of "right" and "fact" meaningless. Moreover, the new bull required every Catholic to take an oath (laity) or sign a new Formulary (clergy) confessing that Jansen had been in error.[235] But four clerics—the bishops of Alet, Beauvais, Angers, and Pamiers—refused to sign. In their mandates, they underlined the difference between *droit* and *fait* and denied the pope's infallibility. When Louis XIV in July issued an *arrêt* abrogating these bishops' mandates, nineteen more bishops joined the renegades in protesting the papal bull and the king's arbitrary action.[236]

As this chapter has shown, Jansenism, representing a kaleidoscope of beliefs and lifestyles, embraced liberals like Robert Arnauld d'Andilly, moderates like Antoine Arnauld, conservatives like Saint-Cyran, and extreme ascetics like Jacqueliine Pascal. Yet nearly all of its adherents, well-educated members of the upper bourgeoisie and robe nobility, shared a common set of beliefs. These included a love of (Augustinian) truth, contempt for the world, moral rigorism, and in many cases, the pursuit of ascetic and even suffering lifestyles that contrasted with their Jesuit opponents' lax moral theology, casuism, and free-will Molinism. Moreover, their stubborn refusal to sign the Formulary required by the Bulls of 1653, 1656, and 1665 brought them into conflict with Mazarin, Louis XIV, Archbishop Péréfixe, and Popes Urban VIII, Innocent X, and Alexander VII. In addition, their emphasis on conscience, individualism, and liberty exposed them to the charge of being "frondeurs" and "republicans." The stage had now been set for a decades-long conflict—and Port-Royal would be at the heart of it.

CHAPTER 3
Sunrise Over Port-Royal, 1600–1661

God touched me so deeply that, from that moment, I found myself far happier as a nun than I had been unhappy being one before."—*Angélique Arnauld*[1]

Seventeen-year-old Jacqueline Arnauld spoke the above words in 1608 following a dramatic conversion that transformed her from a pleasure-seeking girl of nearly eleven (when she first came to Port-Royal des Champs in 1602) to an ascetic, reform-minded abbess in 1609. How did this happen, and why? What long-term impact did the youthful *Mère* Angélique's conversion have on this isolated rural community—and on Jansenism as a whole? How did Port-Royal become the center of Jansenist resistance to Church and state? This chapter will answer these and other questions.

Modern historians have advanced various interpretations for the symbolism and reality of Port-Royal. Henri Lefebvre (1949) saw it as "a reactionary utopia" full of "internal contradictions." Although isolated from the world and medieval in spirit, its members retained control of outside properties; they also loved poverty, but did not love the poor.[2] While its members' rigorist lifestyles made it resemble Calvin's Geneva, Jean Orcibal (1950) asserted that in its emphasis on repentance, contrition, penitence, and the sacraments, the community truly reflected "the spirit of the Council of Trent."[3]

More recently, Perle Bugnion-Secretan (1991) captured the essence of Port-Royal as both a "monastery" and a "movement" in defense of Jansenism.[4] Bernard Chédozeau (1991) cautioned, however, that not until the 1690s did this rural community become "mainstream Jansenist" when it fought to prevent Louis XIV and the papacy from eradicating Jansenism. Combating this new "alliance of Throne and Altar" precipitated a "revolution" in relations between Port-Royal and the monarchy that brought about the "slow death" of the religious community.[5] For Pierre Chaunu (1998), this on-going war with the Church made Port-Royal "the archetype of the philosophical cabal" of the eighteenth century. In their defense of human liberty and their opposition to papal infallibility and bulls condemning Jansenism, the sisters and solitaires, he said, were Catholic first and Roman last.[6] In his preface to Jean Lesaulnier's *Images of Port-Royal* (2002), Bruno Neveu concluded that in reality, Port-Royal represented the "heart" of a "constellation" of Jansenist convents, Messieurs, aristocratic friends, students, and the Arnauld family—all of whom claimed Port-Royal as their "spiritual center."[7]

Paradoxically, this rural hub of Jansenism originated in a swamp. Although its etymology is uncertain, it appears that Port-Royal des Champs (or "royal door in the fields") derived first from *porra* or *porrois,* Low Latin for "stagnant pond," before becoming *Porregius* and then *Portus Regius* ("royal door").[8] Given the medieval fear of wild, untamed places, it is not surprising that contemporaries saw this isolated parish of Magny-les-Hameaux as "a frightful and savage valley."[9] Tourists today admire this "picturesque valley" eighteen miles southwest of Paris, nine miles south of Versailles, six miles from Madame de Maintenon's abbey of Saint-Cyr, and roughly three miles from the village of Chevreuse on the poplar-lined road to Dompierre. All that remains of the rural Port-Royal are The Grange (a six-room former school, now a museum), a cross-shaped canal, and a medieval dovecote that once held 5000 pigeons.[10]

But its sister convent at Port-Royal de Paris still stands at 121, boulevard de Port-Royal—as a maternity clinic! Here in the heart of the old *faubourg* Saint-Honoré, where celibate monks and nuns from eight different religious orders once gathered to worship, prospective mothers now come for checkups and advice prior to childbirth. However, visitors can still see the cloistered gardens and lovely little chapel where seventeenth-century religious walked and worshiped.[11]

But more than four centuries before that, as French knights rallied to the Fourth Crusade, Port-Royal arose in the Chevreuse Valley. In the thirteenth century, Milon de Voisins held from the chevalier Guillaume de la Ferté a fief purchased from the prior de Bonnelles in Porrois. In 1204, with the help of Eudes de Sully, Bishop of Paris, Mathilde de Garlande, wife of Mathieu I de Marly-Montmorency, bought this fief to establish a Cistercian priory with twelve monks to honor her husband's courageous service in the Fourth Crusade. In 1214, Bouchard I and Mathieu II de Marly transformed it into a Benedictine abbey, known by 1216 as "Port-Royal." Seven years later, the abbey received from Pope Honorius III authorization to receive laypersons who wished to live there without taking vows.[12]

As the centuries passed, its white-robed nuns farmed the land, catechized the peasants, and buried their sisters who died all too often from malarial fevers. By 1500 so many, in fact, had died on that unhealthful terrain that Port-Royal des Champs began to decline. Whereas ten abbesses led the abbey in the thirteenth century, and in the fourteenth century, another ten directed its affairs, only seven abbesses served throughout the fifteenth century while only two served during the entire sixteenth century. Without strong leadership, the nuns earned a reputation for living lives of idleness and scandal. Neglecting the Rule of St. Benedict, they seldom heard preaching, took communion only once a month, and wore costumes and masks at the local carnivals.[13]

But the winds of change, generated by the Council of Trent, were already blowing across France. Old monasteries and convents were reformed and new ones established. Between 1604 and 1650, at least 48 new religious houses for women sprang up in the Paris region alone—more than one every year. Whereas Paris in the 1590s had 30 convents, the capital by the 1650s had over 100 religious houses for women; mid-seventeenth century France had more nuns than the total of its monks and friars combined. The Church had been "feminized." This stunning burst of religious construction and spiritual asceticism witnessed a revival of the communal rites of penitence and ecstatic and apocalyptic spirituality.[14] The Oratorians (a group with close ties to Port-Royal's sisters and solitaires), founded in 1611 by Pierre de Bérulle, began holding spiritual "retreats" lasting one week to three months for priests, ordinands, and seminary students to encourage the clergy to live sanctified lives.[15]

In like manner, women in seventeenth-century France who practiced "heroic asceticism" as nuns or lay sisters sought outlets for their reforming zeal. But they faced formidable obstacles in a man's world. Hippocrates, Galen, and Aristotle had defined them as "deformed beings" (because conceived on the left side—Latin *sinistre*—of the womb). They had been condemned by the Church Fathers and canon law as "temptresses and seductresses" (from Eve's "original sin") who had not been created in God's image.[16] Consequently, the Church forbade women to teach doctrine. Nonetheless, they created new roles for themselves as catechizers of the laity and educators of children and the poor, often at schools established by charitable donors beyond the cloisters. As Barbara Diefendorf (2004) argues, elite women who enjoyed the patronage of French aristocratic women higher yet on the social scale took leading roles in advancing Tridentine reform goals. Their "heroic asceticism" set in motion a Catholic renewal across France.[17]

In 1591, as famines and epidemics ravaged France and war with Spain sapped its economy, one of those future "ascetic heroes" saw the light of day at Tours. The fourth child of Catherine and Antoine II Arnauld, Jacqueline became an unruly, rambunctious brat, frequently beaten for showing irreverence on feast days and for bullying her younger sisters Anne-Eugénie and Jeanne. While her parents granted her older sister Catherine permission to marry, they lacked sufficient dowries to see their other three daughters properly wed; they would become nuns instead. With her mother perpetually pregnant and her father immersed in his business, Jacqueline grew up feeling neglected and unloved. "My mother did not love me," she complained years later to her nephew Antoine Le Maître, adding, "she had an aversion for me." The unhappy little girl spent most of her time with her maternal grandfather, the wealthy merchant Simon Marion, who tutored her in French, Latin, writing, and math. Adoring her too much to let her marry, Marion made the decision to cloister Jacqueline nearby. Paradoxically, Catherine, who did marry, wanted to become a nun, while Jacqueline, who wanted to marry and have children, was forced to become a nun.[18]

Ever the strong-willed child, she protested loudly, but was sent to the convent of Maubuisson in October 1599 as a novice in her eighth year. Blessed by the *abbé* de la Charité, she took the name "Sister Angélique de Madéleine." The abbess, Angélique d'Estrées (the sister of Henri IV's mistress Gabriel d'Estrées), had herself borne twelve illegitimate children by different fathers. D'Estrées loved having the novices come to her boudoir to regale her with tales of their pleasures.[19]

Wishing to rescue his granddaughter from such a lax environment, Marion in June 1599 secured from Henri IV the right of nomination for the crumbling, disease-infected abbey of Port-Royal des Champs. The asking price was cheap, because the recent Wars of Religion had bankrupted the place both financially and spiritually. One abbess, Madame de la Vallée, had been removed in 1574 for lax discipline; her replacement, Jeanne de Baulehart, had served 25 years without a scandal, but also without reforming the abbey. Her Bernardine confessor, who spent his days hunting wild game, knew neither the Pater or the catechism. Instead, he read only his breviary. For 30 years, no one had preached a sermon there.[20]

As part of the arrangement, Marion planned to transfer Angélique from Maubuisson to Port-Royal des Champs. On the one hand, this would save the family the cost of a dowry; on the other, it represented a great investment for the Arnaulds, who would enjoy a steady income from this benefice, including the right (called *in commendam*) to appoint future abbesses. Their daughter Jeanne (now Sister Agnès), who had memorized her Psalter at nine, already paid her way as abbess of the convent of Saint-Cyr.[21]

But one obstacle stood in the way: Angélique refused to go. Years later, she recalled: "I had a horrible hatred for the convent. I was excitable and playful. All religious exercises displeased me." She called her vanity "this sickness in my soul."[22]

Had she known the conditions inside the abbey, she might have thrown another tantrum. Between 1599 and 1602, Port-Royal des Champs had only twelve nuns: one mentally retarded, one deaf, one senile, and nine pleasure-seekers who came from old noble families. Port-Royal, now a Cistercian abbey, had become a "cold, worldly, but decorous religious house."[23]

After much arm-twisting, Angélique agreed to go, but only if she could be abbess. The nine-year-old girl still loved bossing others around. But then the Arnaulds faced a new obstacle: when they petitioned Rome, the pope refused to allow her to become abbess, explaining that Jacqueline (her name used on the application form) was too young and had not yet taken her vows as a nun. The family's multi-generation hostility toward the Jesuits may also have played a role. Angélique's crafty grandfather solved the problem: in 1601 he signed a fraudulent application indicating that Angélique (the new name entered on the application form), now nearly eleven years old, was actually seventeen. Finally, on 13 May 1601, the pope issued the bulls granting his approval; on 14 February 1602, Henri IV gave his permission. But Angélique served first as *coadjutrice* (or associate abbess) with Jeanne de Boulehart until the latter died on July 4; on July 5, not yet eleven years old, she became abbess over fifteen nuns.[24]

But this child-abbess, now addressed as "Mother Angélique," had to submit to two higher authorities. Her mother, Catherine Arnauld, administered internal affairs while Catherine-Angélique Dupont, an older nun and prioress, controlled the finances and served as Angélique's governess and advisor. In effect, her parents ran the abbey: they established its daily schedule; they fired or transferred nuns according to their pleasure.[25] From the Arnauld family itself came at least three abbesses, four prioresses, and four solitaires (or "messieurs") who administered Port-Royal in the seventeenth century.[26] Meanwhile, the adolescent abbess who hated devotional literature and found convent life "an unbearable yoke" played games, took long walks in the countryside, visited with neighbors, entertained friends, occasionally read Plutarch's *Lives*, and led (in her words) "a pagan and profane existence."[27]

All that changed dramatically, however, in March 1608 when she heard a monk's sermon that touched her heart. Following *Père* Basile's homily on the incarnation and birth of Christ, Angélique experienced a deep conversion.[28] "God touched me so deeply that, from that moment, I found myself far happier as a nun than I had been unhappy being one before," she exclaimed.[29]

This heart-felt change soon led to her reform of the abbey. With advice from *Père* Pacifique and *Père* Bernard, she resolved to return Port-Royal des Champs to the ascetic ideals of the Cistercian Order. In 1609 she ordered the nuns to relinquish their personal possessions for the common good and to observe a strict seclusion from the outside world. As part of her reform, she tightened the rules, increased the frequency of prayers, augmented the sisters' duties, and encouraged charity toward the poor. These changes impacted five areas: simplicity (in church décor and personal lifestyle), continual silence (prayer and meditation), manual labor (gardening), evangelistic poverty ("holy poverty and humility"), and fraternal charity (sharing goods in common). Aside from three or four "spiritual conferences" each week, sign language replaced oral dialogue. "Silence frees the soul," the abbess insisted, "and makes it capable of hearing God's Word." Likewise, physical toil "frees the spirit," she told them, while ministering to the needs of others brings "spiritual joy." The sisters, however, experienced little joy when they tasted the changes in the refectory: two eggs per week, no meat, little butter, more fruit and vegetables—in short, they suddenly became fasting vegetarians.[30]

Although Angélique fasted right along with her nuns, she continued to read Plutarch's *Lives* and "other profane books." But the teenaged abbess began spending more time with devotional literature, listening to more sermons, requesting spiritual advice from the elderly priests *Pères* Pacifique and Bernard, and focusing more on serving God and developing patience and humility—virtues in short supply in the Arnauld family.[31]

In fact, far from supporting their daughter in these reform efforts, her parents felt that she had gone too far. When Angélique had asked her father's permission to reform the abbey, Antoine not only refused, but also insisted that she renounce any future ideas of reform (which threatened his proprietary rights over the convent). When the impetuous teenager threatened to reenter secular society, Antoine angrily prohibited her from doing so. Perhaps to spite her father, Angélique then decided "to serve God first" and proceed with the reforms. "They did not consult me by making me a nun," she allegedly declared; "I will not consult them now that I wish to live like a nun in order to save myself." When word of this reached her parents, Catherine objected strongly to the new dietary changes, while her husband threw a fit concerning Angélique's imposing *cloture* (closure) on the abbey.[32]

On 25 September 1609—the famous *Journée du guichet* ("Day of the Wicket Gate")—all these bottled frustrations exploded. Ignoring Angélique's imposition of closure, her parents, her brother Robert d'Andilly, and her sisters Anne-Eugénie and Catherine Le Maître (recently married to the Calvinist Isaac Le Maître) came to visit her. She had previously asked them *not* to come. When her father banged on the door, she at first refused him entrance. When he began shouting at her, she reluctantly admitted the family into a small side parlor. Antoine's reddening face betrayed his mounting anger; Catherine threatened never to see her daughter again; Robert called his sister "a monster of ingratitude." But she had won. By this courageous act of defiance, the youthful abbess had gained a victory over paternal authority, defeated the forces of "old corruption" (patronage, nomination, secular interference), and placed Port-Royal des Champs firmly in the camp of the Catholic Reformation. As Fabian Gastelier (1998) correctly stated: "Without that day of 25 September 1609, Port-Royal would not have existed"—certainly not as the center of ascetic Jansenism it would later become.[33]

In addition to the objections of outsiders like her father and mother, this plucky eighteen-year-old reformer also faced resistance from insiders. Her trusted advisor *Père* Bernard warned her: "Do not . . . reform your abbey. You have better things to do."[34] The elderly priest *Père* Pacifique called her reform program "pure folly." Even Catherine Dupont, the prioress at the abbey, viewed her reforms as "a novelty" and failed to see their point. She accused her superior of making an unnecessary fuss in a convent already "properly directed" by statute law.[35] Louis XIII agreed with that assessment. After all, the French crown, which had so far refused to implement the Council of Trent's reforms, had no central blueprint for reforming religious houses. While some followed the age-old practice of *commenda* or the patronage system by which the king, nobles or wealthy families chose the religious leaders of benefices they controlled, the nuns and monks at other convents and monasteries elected their own superiors. Given the prevailing misogynistic attitudes in seventeenth-century society, however, most Church and government officials preferred that even female religious houses appoint male directors, confessors, or spiritual advisors. But Angélique, who found reform-minded directors hard to come by, rejected this patriarchal model. Indeed, as Gastelier observed, her entire life could be summed up as a series of ruptures: with the world at eight, with her parents at seventeen, and with the king, popes, and archbishops throughout her career.[36]

Despite significant opposition, the nature and impact of her reforms cannot be underestimated; however, they brought both positive and negative results. Closure greatly improved the quality of religious life at Port-Royal, but forced Angélique to spend more time seeking benefactors to support the abbey's ascetic lifestyle.[37] Her new model of reform closely followed the character of Tridentine Cistercianism. As a radical reform of the Benedictine Order, it strongly emphasized contemplative prayer, liturgical services, poverty, simplicity, silence, solitude, discipline, and austerity—the "Ideals of Citeaux." But its extreme distrust of mysticism (a key component in Cistercianism) stifled charity and love toward others, which over the long run, made its focus on purity, truth, and prayer cold and sterile, lacking the flame of love to God and to one's neighbor in need. Eventually, as Port-Royal's liturgical life grew sterile, rigorous, and austere, it became an empty shell of its former being. Yet the abbess herself set an example for her nuns: she wore a simple, straight, sack-like serge dress; she slept on a hard, thin straw mattress; she gave up her perfumes, powders, soaps and bathing oils; she even sold the abbey's silver vessels and gave the money to the poor. She "mortified the flesh" by remaining silent all day, denying herself ruffles and lace and linen stockings, and dining on a Spartan diet of bouillon, omelets, and a piece of mutton (her parents feared she would starve). She also scrubbed floors, prepared meals, and changed bandages in the infirmary.[38]

Perhaps if she had changed her own clothing more often, she would have enjoyed a more healthful life. Believing that piety—not cleanliness—was next to godliness, Angélique seldom removed her clothes or shoes, even to sleep. As a result, her filthy body attracted fleas and frequently succumbed to preventable illnesses. This physical "suffering" became for her a sign of God's grace—a "test" of her devotion to God—but her relatives saw it as the penalty for her filthy habits. Behind this diseased asceticism, her father saw the influence of the Capuchins (whom he hated almost as much as he disliked the Jesuits), an order of friars he labeled "cockroaches, hypocrites, and bigots."[39] But sickness characterized the entire female side of the Arnauld family, not just Angélique. Over a thirteen-year period, Angélique's letters reveal that she, her sisters Agnès, Genevieve, Catherine, Angélique Thérèse, and Anne Eugenie, and their mother Catherine suffered repeated bouts of illness. The abbess encouraged them all to see their suffering as "blessings from God."[40]

Among those blessings that came through suffering, the young abbess and her nuns sought a continual growth in the "fruits of the Spirit." Her *Relation* (1655) emphasizes the need for more love, humility, docility, holiness, piety, and joy as well as more resignation to God's will, devotion to Truth, and reverence for the Holy Eucharist. She urges her nuns to manifest in their lives greater abstinence in diet, acceptance of suffering, simplicity, penitence, sweetness of disposition, trust in one another, even the willingness to suffer martyrdom.[41]

Both immediately and in the long run, these changes transformed Port-Royal des Champs. To show her consecration to this new task and to fulfill the pope's orders, Angélique retook her vows on 7 May 1610 before Dom Largentier, the Cistercian *abbé* de Clairvaux.[42] Word concerning the transformations wrought in her life and at the abbey spread quickly; soon, serious-minded women flocked to Port-Royal des Champs. From 15 nuns in 1600, their numbers grew to an average of 20 in the 1610s, to 42 in the 1620s, 50 in the 1630s, 68 in the 1640s, 92 in the 1650s, and to 112 by 1660, the peak year in the convent's "golden summer." This represents an astounding increase in the growth rate from 2–3% in the 1630s and 1640s to 10–14% by the 1650s. By 1661 (the year *Mère* Angélique died), both Port-Royals (in Paris and at Champs) housed 164 nuns, novices, and postulants.[43]

Angélique's fame as a reforming abbess soon brought her another commission: to reform the prestigious royal convent of Maubuisson. Here, where she had begun her career as an eight-year-old novice in 1599, corruption still reigned supreme. When at 27, Angélique returned in 1618, accompanied by three nuns (her sister Marie-Claire, Isabelle de Sainte-Agnès de Châteauneuf, and Marie de la Croix), she discovered that carrying out reforms could be hazardous to one's life. Although her former superior, the abbess Angélique d'Estrées, was away when the three arrived, they proceeded with their reform program anyway, bringing reason and discipline to what many considered a "rebellious convent." When d'Estrées returned in 1619 and learned that her nuns could no longer keep their possessions, take long walks in the countryside, or enjoy family visits, she insisted that Arnauld leave immediately. When the latter refused, stating that the *abbé* Boucherat of Citeaux had summoned her to Maubuisson and she would leave only by his orders, d'Estrées summoned the *comte* de Souzay and his armed men to evict her. When Arnauld refused to budge, the angelic abbess of Maubuisson grabbed the angelic abbess of Port-Royal des Champs by the robe, rebuked her for being so impertinent, and threw her out of the convent! But Louis XIII himself supported Arnauld as "the most capable of carrying out the reform of the said abbey." Knowing this, Angélique's lawyer-brother, Henri Arnauld, obtained an *arrêt* to imprison Angélique d'Estrées and reinstate his sister at Maubuisson. When Sieur Defontes appeared at the gates with the arrest warrant (and 150 archers), d'Estrées fled the scene, leaving the Arnaulds (and 50 archers) to restore calm.[44]

Over the next four years, *Mère* Angélique's reforms—including closure, silence, and all goods held in common—brought prosperity to Maubuisson. With the help of four sisters from Port-Royal des Champs (Anne Eugene Arnauld, Marie Anthoinette de Blond, Marie François

Grimoust, and Elizabet Ludgar de Paiot), she succeeded in "achieving better sanctity" there, turning Maubuisson into a little Port-Royal. Soon dozens of new postulants joined the convent; so many, in fact, that in 1623 Angélique persuaded 32 of them to return to Port-Royal des Champs with her.[45]

But those five contentious years at Maubuisson had taken a heavy toll on her physically and mentally. When at 32 she returned to the Chevreuse Valley, Angélique not only suffered from obesity, dropsy, a weak heart, perpetual headaches, and insomnia, but she had also barely survived an attack of smallpox.[46] Clearly, she needed assistance, and given the patriarchal nature of the Church hierarchy and its misogynistic attitudes toward women (as "Eves" and "Pandoras"), that help would most likely come from a man. Two previous directors (*Père* Archange de Pembrok and *abbé* de la Charmoie) and confessors (Dom Jean Catols and Etienne Maugier) between 1610 and 1614 had proved disappointing. The sisters had especially disliked Charmoie because he had persuaded their abbess to abolish meat from the refectory. Then during Angélique's five-year absence at Maubuisson, Port-Royal's director had been Marie de Medici's Jesuit confessor, *Père* Jean Suffren.[47]

In April 1619, however, while at Maubuisson, Angélique met the Bishop of Geneva, François de Sales. Charmed by his kindness yet firmness, his humility, patience, and confidence in God's goodness, she asked him to become her spiritual director. Sales taught her to embrace poverty, fasting, alms-giving, and spiritual obedience. He also rebuked her for her *préciosité*—a certain affectation in discourse—until she promised to expunge such prose from her letters. Sales' gift for organization and repugnance for disobedience helped Angélique reform Maubuisson.[48] While he remembered her as "my dearest daughter"[49] as he lay dying in 1622, she praised him as "pure and saintly."[50] Forty years later, as she lay dying, she told Queen Anne (the Queen Mother) that Sales' "pure and holy conduct" had taught her "entire consecration to God."[51]

Perhaps more significantly in light of future events, Sales had also shaped the abbess' political views. In private, he spoke with her about factions, inconsistencies, and incompetence within the Church. His political mentoring emboldened her to be more critical of those in authority. His letters condemned royal appointments to convents as "pure usurpation . . . against the right of election." He criticized Louis XIII's Jesuit confessors for encouraging the king to overstep his legal boundaries (granted by the Concordat of Bologna in 1516) and destroy "the spirit of piety" in convents. From him, she learned to despise the Society of Jesus as being "too political." In addition, Sales placed ecumenical councils above popes; he exalted the authority of bishops ("like the seraphim among angels") above that of the mendicant orders. Toward the end of her life, as the persecution of Port-Royal intensified, Angélique would demonstrate the political astuteness that she had learned from her mentor.[52]

After Sales died, however, she needed a new confessor. The Arnaulds knew and loved Pierre de Bérulle, a Cistercian (like St.-Cyran) who founded the Order of the Oratory to reform the French clergy in 1611, only two years after Angélique began reforming Port-Royal des Champs. Moreover, in the Saint-Jacques parish in Paris, close to Port-Royal, stood the Institution of the Oratory. The Arnaulds frequently wrote to and entertained members of this Oratory at their Paris hotel. In 1622, therefore, Jeanne de Chatal, a mutual friend, introduced Angélique to Sébastien Zamet, the immensely wealthy Bishop of Langres whom Henri IV had called "my moneybags cousin." Following a life-threatening illness, however, Zamet (like Angélique) had experienced a deep conversion and become a disciple of Saint Charles Borromeo. When in 1624 Zamet visited Port-Royal, she "fell under his charms." Finding him "totally devoted to God . . . full of zeal, self-mortification, and true devotion,"[53] she asked him to be her spiritual director.

Eager to create a new religious order devoted to the perpetual adoration of the Eucharist, Zamet agreed in 1625 to become her confessor if she in turn would help him establish this new institution. Wishing to break ties with the Cistercians (whom she described as "domineering intriguers" who mistreated nuns), Angélique agreed. By 1630, with permission from Urban VIII and Louis XIII, they founded the Institute of the Holy Spirit under the temporary supervision of the bishops of Langres, Paris, and Sens (eventually, the Archbishop of Paris became its principal superior). Day and night, through prayer and meditation, shifts of nuns ministered the Holy Sacrament at the altar. Even more important, the king granted the new order the "right of election" to choose its own abbess (something Louis XIV later regretted). Finally, Zamet designed a stunning new robe of white serge with a scarlet scapular for the Port-Royal sisters to wear.[54]

Although Angélique admired and respected Zamet, she disagreed with him in two important areas. While he wanted to admit only the daughters of the nobility to Port-Royal, she wished to accept poor girls without dowries if they proved sincere. Also, he admired the French Carmelites (with their wealth and refined lifestyles) while she favored the Spanish Carmelites (known for their poverty and humility). His vision of the religious life was that of "a select club" of the "fashionably penitent" drawn from aristocratic society (with Baroque music and formal services, flowers, incense and perfumes, and luxurious interiors). By contrast, her concept of religious devotion embraced a more ascetic lifestyle of poverty, silence, meditation, and service to the poor.[55] While Zamet valued his ties with influential friends at Court, despite its debauchery and self-indulgence, Angélique saw the Court as "the wicked world" of materialism, pride, and sin. To her, Paris represented an artificial life where "demons" lived amid noise and urban congestion, while "angels" dwelt in peace and solitude at Port-Royal des Champs.[56] Angélique deeply sympathized with her friend Madame de Ligny when she exclaimed: "How I pity my brother! I pray God that he be driven from Court, for I know not how it be possible otherwise for him to be saved."[57]

Searching for a confessor who shared her ascetic vision, Angélique encountered in the *abbé* de Saint-Cyran a spiritual twin to François de Sales.[58] Apparently her brother, Robert Arnauld d'Andilly, introduced them late in 1620, for in a 7 January 1621 letter to Robert, she thanked him "with all my heart for having found for me such a saintly friend."[59] For the next two decades, Saint-Cyran directed the spiritual lives of the nuns, teaching them how to obtain salvation through the practice of *renouvellement* (renewal or revival). For Saint-Cyran, external signs (weeks spent meditating, fasting, and giving alms) testified to one's genuine repentance and true conversion. Only after a nun had proved her "unction" or devotion to God would he grant her absolution.[60] Forbidden by the Archbishop of Paris to preach at the abbey, Saint-Cyran held informal "retreats" or "parlor conferences" in which he shared with the sisters his Augustinian views of human nature. He encouraged them to develop a deeper piety, to augment the time they spent in solitude, and to cultivate a "state of lamentation."[61]

By the 1630s, thanks largely to the influence of Saint-Cyran and Antoine Arnauld, a "new theology" had taken shape at Port-Royal. This French Augustinianism resembled Jansenism in its pessimistic attitude toward human nature, sin, grace, and predestination, but differed from the Jansenism of Louvain regarding the pope's infallibility and the meaning of individual liberty and God's truth. Because many perceived the rail of Jansenism as running parallel to the rail of Thomism (Thomas Aguinas' thought) on the tracks of Roman Catholic theology, at first, few doubted the orthodoxy of this new "theological school" of thought.[62]

Mère Angélique repeatedly expressed her delight with the spiritual "renewal" the *abbé* brought to her convent. In letters to her brother Robert, she called Saint-Cyran "such a holy friend," "a rare spirit," "an incomparable friend," and "this good Servant of God." She praised him for his "admirable science," his "virtue and singular devotion" to God and to the spiritual development of her nuns.[63] Even after his arrest and imprisonment at Vincennes in 1638, Saint-Cyran continued directing the spiritual life of the Port-Royal nuns through his correspondence with their abbess. Both Angélique and her sister Agnès, who bluntly called his detention "persecution," confidently expected God to deliver him.[64] Writing to her brother Antoine, *Mère* Agnès begged him to "ask God to manifest His power by the physical deliverance of M. de Saint-Cyran" from prison.[65] In a letter to her friend M. Macquet in 1640, Angélique asserted: "You have no more hope from men for M. de S. Cyran, but it is then that God delivers his greatest miracles."[66] Three years later, following the *abbé*'s release, she enthusiastically informed Macquet that "our good father M. de S. Cyran is at liberty by the grace of God with thanks to a large number of men of quality"; then she added, "He will yet do service for the Church."[67]

When death claimed the *abbé* within months of his release, Angélique blamed the Jesuits for harassing Saint-Cyran, censoring his books, and engineering his detention.[68] Grief-stricken, she lamented to the *princesse* de Guéménée that "this great privation" is "our extreme loss which we will feel to the day of our death."[69]

Yet another loss for Angélique and her nuns came with their removal from Port-Royal des Champs to Paris due to the miasmic conditions in the Chevreuse Valley. When in 1623 she had returned from Maubuisson to Port-Royal, Angélique had brought with her 32 poor sisters. By the end of 1624, however, half of them had died from malarial fever, unaccustomed to the mosquito-infested swamps surrounding the abbey. In 1625, a dozen more nuns perished—nearly one-third of the abbey's 84 residents. Obviously, leaving Port-Royal des Champs had become a matter of survival.[70]

Although Louis XIII, sympathetic to their plight, had issued letters patent in December 1623 giving the sisters his approval to move to the Saint-Jacques parish "for the glory of God" and "the grandeur and good order" of the convent," they had nowhere to live.[71] To complicate matters, Archbishop Gondi of Paris opposed allowing the Cistercians to gain a foothold in his archdiocese unless he had the right to inspect their enclosure, accept or reject applicants, discipline recalcitrant sisters, and control the nuns' movements to and from the capital. After negotiations with the Cistercian general granted him these rights, he welcomed the homeless sisters to Paris.[72]

Angélique's mother then provided a home for them. In the summer of 1624, Catherine Arnauld purchased the hôtel de Clagny in the *faubourg* Saint-Jacques for 24,000 *livres*. After jumping through the bureaucratic hoops to gain the approval of Bishop Nicholas Boucherat in 1624, Louis XIII in 1625, and Parlement in 1626, the sisters moved into their new domicile. The Arnauld family promised 10,000 *livres* annually to meet maintenance expenses; the Queen Mother, Marie de Medici, agreed to become their patron. Only Saint-Cyran objected to the move. Preferring the serenity of the rural abbey, he and a chaplain stayed behind.[73]

To sweeten the deal for the reluctant Jean-François de Gondi, the *abbé* of Citeaux, Urban VIII, and Louis XIII agreed in 1627 to transfer the now uninhabited abbey of Port-Royal des Champs from the Order of Citeaux to the jurisdiction of the Archbishop of Paris.[74] Then in 1628, during Marie de Medici's first visit, *Mère* Angélique asked her to intercede with the king to enable the sisters to elect their abbess rather than to have one appointed over them (by the king, archbishop, or a patron). This move altered Angélique's title from "perpetual abbess" (for life) to "elective abbess" (at triennial elections). In January 1629, Louis XIII granted her request; in February, the king's Council approved it; in April, Parlement registered this action. This proved to be a major coup in favor of autonomy. Thereafter, the choice of an abbess at Port-Royal proceeded independently of popes, bishops, kings, and family connections, all of whom surrendered their appointive right (*in commendam*). Ironically, Angélique, who had been instated as abbess by the commendatory system, sought to abolish it at both Port-Royals and reinstated the election of abbesses and prioresses by the sisters themselves. However, since France had never legally accepted the Tridentine reforms, Louis XIV later reclaimed his royal right of nomination by restoring the commendatory system.[75]

Consequently, their 38-year-old daughter looked forward to a brighter future. But if their rural retreat had provided them with ample but unwholesome space, the tiny convent on the *rue* Coquillière proved healthful but cramped for the eighteen sisters who moved there. Its dormitory, chapel, and choir proved much too small. So the nuns cleaned out the adjacent barns and moved in, creating spacious but malodorous rooms. Since all of them could not fit inside the refectory, they ate in shifts.[76]

The solution to this problem—at least according to former advisor Sébastien Zamet—would have been to admit girls from wealthy families whose parents could provide generous dowries to the abbey. But Angélique refused to take the easy way out. When three girls from rich families applied to Port-Royal, offering combined dowries of 40,000 *livres* (a tremendous sum), the abbess rejected them as unsuited for monastic life.[77] She much preferred poor but dedicated novices to rich, spoiled ones whose families abandoned them to convents when their prospects for marriage proved lean. Besides, pious girls from poverty-stricken backgrounds more easily adjusted to the ascetic way of life that Angélique promoted; God, she felt, could do more for them.

To all appearances, God intervened to help one twelve-year-old novice in 1627. Madéleine des Anges de Drui, Angélique's first cousin, had for three months suffered from high fevers, chest pains, and convulsions so violent that she beat herself and had to be tied to her bed. For eight months she had been unable to eat normally. The abbess summoned physicians, but they could do nothing for her. Finally, the nuns took the Holy Sacrament to her room. While partaking of the wafer and wine, Madeleine experienced immediate healing and began eating normally again.[78] This alleged miracle—and many others later—boosted the sisters' faith and assurance that God would bless them in their new location.

Fortunately for them, in September 1630, the king, gravely ill, also experienced immediate healing which he attributed to the Order of the Holy Sacrament recently established at Port-Royal de Paris. As this miracle occurred simultaneously with his victory over the Huguenot stronghold of La Rochelle, Louis XIII wanted to show his gratitude to God. When the pope suggested transferring Port-Royal from the jurisdiction of the Archbishop of Paris to that of the Archbishop of Sens (Octave de Bellegarde), the grateful monarch agreed. In 1633 he issued letters patent confirming that henceforth, the abbey would follow the Rule of St. Benedict, enjoy triennial elections, and submit to the authority of the Archbishop of Sens. Before long, Port-Royal became the largest convent in Paris with 150 nuns.[79]

Its prosperity, however, did not shield it from the disasters that struck Paris and France from the 1630s to the 1650s. With frightful regularity, famines hit the region in 1629–30, 1643–44, 1646–47, 1649–50, and 1651–52. Epidemics of tuberculosis, smallpox, and the bubonic plague ravaged north central France from 1628 to 1631 and again in 1636–37; throughout the 1630s, malaria killed many. During the Thirty Years' War (1618–1648), Angélique's brother Simon Arnauld died at the battle of Verdun.[80]

Back in Paris, Angélique faced her own battles, especially after the sisters elected Geneviëve Le Tardif as abbess in 1630. A proponent of Zamet, Le Tardif introduced changes at the abbey—more refined garments, more sumptuous food, a more elaborate décor in the chapel—that Angélique felt negated the principles of simplicity and austerity. The new abbess also decided to admit only the daughters of the nobility.[81] Although obligated to submit to the new mother superior, Arnauld's impatient nature bristled at what she saw as spiritual regress. As her brother Robert's wife quipped, Angélique resembled "the angels who terrify one at first and console one afterward."[82]

Perhaps to keep the peace, Arnauld left Port-Royal in 1633 and for three years, devoted her energies to building up the new Institute of the Holy Sacrament that she and Zamet (with the approval of Urban VIII and Louis XIII) had established in 1630. At this center of Eucharistic devotion, she participated in the eighteen daily Masses. When in 1636 she returned to Port-Royal as its new abbess, the king, delighted with her promotion of the Institute, persuaded Innocent X to transfer its title to the abbey in 1638. Henceforth, the convent would be called "Notre-Dame de Port-Royal du Saint-Sacrement." The nuns now discarded their old black robes and donned white scapularies with crimson crosses on the front.[83]

They also welcomed back their former spiritual advisor, Saint-Cyran, who reestablished unity and order at the abbey. Although Zamet had returned to Paris the year before, Angélique told her sister Agnès (abbess at the convent of Tard) that he should no longer visit Port-Royal. Saint-Cyran now enjoyed her full support in teaching the nuns his Augustinian principles, leading them to engage in introspective exercises, and shunning all worldliness.[84]

But the world itself intruded when *Mère* Agnès, as part of her devotional exercises, wrote a little book called *The Secret Chapelet* in 1627. Although strictly speaking, a chapelet is a rosary, a string of beads that one slides through one's fingers while reciting prayers, the term can also refer to the prayer itself. While adoring the Holy Sacrament, Agnès, then about eight years old, began recording her pious thoughts in a tiny booklet. Each of its sixteen sections, containing her mystical thoughts concerning one of the attributes of Christ, could be recited in praise services at the Eucharist.[85]

Her brother, Antoine Arnauld, who praised the *Chapelet* as "a book of piety & the spirit of grace," denied Jesuit charges that Saint-Cyran had influenced her to write it.[86]

In 1633, after the Sorbonne had condemned its "extravagances, impertinences, errors, blasphemies and impieties" as inspired by the devil, both Saint-Cyran and Zamet defended the booklet and even obtained "certificates of orthodoxy" so it could be printed.[87] But then the Jesuits stirred up a tempest in a teapot by accusing Agnès of promoting a "form of mysticism" that in reality verged on "dangerous quietism." They professed to find in this tiny handwritten work heresy and possibly even sorcery! Consequently, Urban VIII in 1634 ordered both the essay and the rosary destroyed "lest it cause idiots and simple-minded folk to act foolishly."[88] By contrast, Mlle. de Joncoux found the *Chapelet* "so unintelligible and so unimportant . . . that it did not deserve to be either attacked or defended."[89]

Important or not, the brouhaha over this devotional booklet had lasting effects on Port-Royal. First of all, it drove a wedge between the Oratory (who condemned the *Chapelet*) and the abbey (who defended it). Where previously amicable relations had existed, conflicts over teachings and lifestyles created a rift between their members. For example, the Oratorians refused to accept Jansen's *Augustinus* as the correct expression of Augustine's theology. Second, it pitted the Oratorians against the Society of Jesus in debates over organization, Church authority, and other politicized issues. Third, it inspired Richelieu—already angry with Jansen over his *Mars Gallicus*—to harass both the Oratory and Port-Royal. In 1638 he sent the Oratorian priest Séguenot to the Bastille and Saint-Cyran to Vincennes.[90] Consequently, although the "teapot" itself may have been small, the "tempest" it generated proved severe.

Angélique, overwhelmed by her younger sister's dilemma, described herself as "like a poor vessel tossed by the sea, unable to go where it wishes, but at the mercy of the winds."[91] To help the troubled abbess survive this tempest, Saint-Cyran kept his hand firmly on the rudder of Port-Royal's ship. Although imprisoned at Vincennes, he wrote her long letters and sent one of his disciples, a young priest named Antoine Singlin, to lead the sisters into deeper dependence on God, more frequent confessions, and a love for the truth.[92]

Thanks largely to the guidance of Singlin and *Mère* Agnès—whom the sisters reelected from 1636 to 1642 and again from 1658 to 1661—the abbey prospered. Most of its novices now came from well-to-do lawyers' families; they brought handsome dowries when they entered Port-Royal de Paris.[93]

Meanwhile, back at Port-Royal des Champs, a handful of men—known as the *solitaires* (solitary ones)—settled in during the 1630s and began transforming this disease-ridden swamp into a rural Eden. When the nuns left for Paris in 1625, Saint-Cyran invited socially prominent penitents (most of them with legal backgrounds) to join him in this sylvan retreat. Antoine Le Maître, Angélique's nephew and an advocate in Parlement, arrived first, followed by his brother, M. de Séricourt. Madame Le Maître, their doting mother, built them a house in the large courtyard. Soon they were joined by Monsieur Le Sec (an officer at the Hôtel-Dieu), Antoine Singlin and Claude Lancelot (both teachers), three more Le Maître brothers (de Sacy, d'Elmos, and de Valemont), the pious Monsieur Gaudon, Sr., and others. These dozen men met together to sing and pray and rebuild the crumbling abbey. They lived in solitude and penitence under the direction of Saint-Cyran, who helped them adopt rigorist lifestyles emphasizing silence, study, introspection, and a love of theological debates.[94]

Their writing and debating skills, however, soon gained them Richelieu's unfavorable attention. On 14 May 1638, he had Saint-Cyran imprisoned. On 12 July Chancellor Séguier dispatched a *lettre de cachet* giving the solitaires three days to pack up and leave. For about a week, they regrouped in Paris before fleeing to Ferté-Milon.[95] But they did not join other religious orders as dispersed nuns normally did because some were simply too old and infirm while others were too eccentric to fit comfortably into a regulated regime. All of them valued the freedom to come and go that they had enjoyed at Port-Royal des Champs. A handful had family, properties, or offices tying them to the world. Most wanted to structure their lifestyles around their own interests and abilities. In short, these free spirits refused to submit either their consciences or their lifestyles to any Church regimen.[96]

Meanwhile, back in Paris, the growing reputation of Port-Royal's sisters for purity of life and authentic Christianity attracted disciples. Some 400 lay associates and patrons—many from the nobility—moved near the abbey. Its 50 nuns in the 1640s would double to 100 in the 1650s, then double again to 200 by 1661.[97]

But the opening salvos of the Jansenist-Jesuit debate over the *Augustinus* did not leave Port-Royal unscathed. Its publication in France in 1641 delighted Parisian printers, who anticipated huge profits from the flood of Jansenist and anti-Jansenist pamphlets and books. The year 1644 broke all previous records for the number of books published.[98] The Arnaulds certainly did their part in this war of words. In October 1641, Bishop Henri Arnauld discussed the growing debate as to whether silence would be an appropriate clerical response to Urban VIII's bull *In eminenti*—or would it "be taken for tacit consent and approval"?[99] His brother Antoine Arnauld, who could never be silent, wrote three works—*Church Tradition on the Subject of Penitence and Communion* (1644), *Apology for Jansenism* (1644), and *Apology for Saint-Cyran* (1645)—to combat the sermons of the Jesuit preacher Isaac Habert. In 1645 Habert responded with his fiery *Defense of the Faith of the Church and of the Ancient Doctrine of the Sorbonne*—to which Arnauld responded with his *Second Apology for Jansenism* (1645).[100] As this debate heated up, the Queen Mother (Anne of Austria) reassured the anxious *princesse* de Guéménée, patron of Port-Royal, that the government would not trouble the abbey if someone could persuade Antoine to cease his aggressive attacks against the Jesuits.[101] Although there was little chance of that happening, the new pope—Innocent X—did his part to preserve an uneasy peace by refusing to condemn Antoine's *Frequent Communion*; instead, he merely censored Arnauld's reference to both Peter and Paul being founders of the Church.[102]

While Antoine Arnauld locked horns with Jesuit writers, his sister Angélique revisited the Chevreuse Valley in the fall of 1646. To her surprise, she found that the solitaires had drained the swamps. Confident that this restored environment would promote her sisters' health, she returned in May 1648, bringing 96 nuns with her. With hearts full of praise, they celebrated a

Te Deum in the chapel. While the Paris abbey remained the headquarters of the abbess, the rural convent became the seat of the prioress, dependent on the Paris house. Here in the country, Port-Royal des Champs had room to grow and prosper. The solitaires (or *Messieurs*) built on a nearby hill a farm and living quarters called The Grange. Here they farmed the land, meditated, and prayed; twice a day they joined the sisters in chanting the sacred offices.[103]

But storm clouds of religious dissent and civil unrest soon disturbed their idyllic existence. In July 1649, the syndic Nicolas Cornet led the Sorbonne in condemning seven propositions on grace and liberty in various theological theses. Antoine Arnauld, never one to remain silent, countered with his inflammatory *Considerations on the Enterprise of Master Nicolas Cornet.* Within six years, Arnauld's bellicose prose got him expelled from the Sorbonne. Unfortunately, his debates with his colleagues and with the Jesuits adversely affected his friends at Port-Royal. In a January 1650 letter to a friend in Poland, Angélique Arnauld complained that the Archbishop of Paris had forbidden her new spiritual director, Antoine Singlin, to preach at the abbey.[104]

When the Fronde (1648–1653) broke in Paris, however, far more than preaching ceased at both convents. To what extent did the inhabitants of Port-Royal—and Jansenists in general—participate in this bloody war? Antoine Adam (1968) asserted that although Louis XIV and his mother, Anne of Austria, identified Port-Royal as defenders of Cardinal de Retz (which association tainted them as *frondeurs*), in reality, the nuns, although hostile toward Parlement, remained obedient and staunchly loyal to the monarchy. But their close ties with Jansenist supporters such as the *duc* de Luynes and the *duchesse* de Chevreuse (considered "dangerous *frondeurs*") condemned them in the eyes of the Court as "intriguers."[105]

Moreover, as discussed in chapter 2, in 1649 and 1652, Robert Arnauld d'Andilly penned two of the pamphlets attacking the Queen Mother and Mazarin (hence called *mazarinades*) for financial mismanagement, poor appointments to political offices, and bungling the war with Spain.[106] Alexander Sedgwick (1977), in a discussion of Port-Royal's "*frondeur* mentality," highlighted the traits that made its nuns suspect. Their acceptance of persecution as a test of Christian faith, which strengthened their resolve not to compromise on "the truth," seemed suspicious to their opponents at Court. Their *dévot* idealism led them to oppose France's war policy with Spain and despise Mazarin's personal abuse of power. Their Richerist background made them sympathetic toward rebellious priests struggling to maintain their authority at the parish level against the incursions of powerful bishops. This philosophical attitude toward power and freedom caused them to defend the intellectual rights of individuals against any authority seeking to suppress them. In a rigidly hierarchical Church and state that valued submission and obedience, the Port-Royal mindset seemed dangerously democratic.[107] Two decades later in *Travails of Conscience* (1998), Sedgwick averred that Jean Racine was correct in calling the Port-Royal sisters indiscreet in choosing benefactors whose *frondeur* activities and ties to Retz cast aspersions on the abbey, but incorrect in claiming that the Arnaulds were not themselves *frondeurs*. As previously mentioned, at least one of them—Robert Arnauld d'Andilly—did write *mazarinades*.[108] Finally, Fabian Gastelier (1998) asserted that although the abbey accommodated fleeing *frondeurs* during the war, the nuns remained loyal to Louis XIV. They opposed Mazarin, not the monarchy.[109]

Despite their loyalty, the nuns at both convents suffered greatly during the Fronde. In January 1649, as civil unrest grew more intense in Paris, *Mère* Agnès moved 30 sisters into the private home of M. de Bernières on the *rue* Saint André des Arcs. Here, in cramped quarters, they did their best to hold worship services, keep silence, and carry on their spiritual duties as fighting raged in the streets. In a letter to Agnès, Angélique encouraged her to persevere amidst "great inconveniences & mental punishment."[110]

Because of the worsening situation in Paris, both abbesses saw wisdom in transferring all the nuns back to Port-Royal des Champs in the spring of 1649. "They tell us," Angélique wrote to the Queen of Poland, "that things will get much worse." The fact that Condé's troops blockading Paris had begun their "pillaging, cruelties and sacrilege" stiffened her resolve to leave the capital and "to die of starvation, if God ordains it, [rather] than to be exposed to the worst in Paris."[111] The rural priory opened its doors to refugees from nearby farms and villages; by the summer of 1651, nearly 120 persons found shelter there, with another 160 refugees living at Port-Royal in Paris. For months at a time, as long as they had bread, the sisters gave these homeless ones food, water, and shelter.[112] The 44 nuns and novices also nursed the sick and wounded. In September 1651, *Mère* Angélique, sharing her "very great apprehensions" about the war with M. de Fleury, rejoiced that among "so very many sick," not one had died.[113]

Given the Jansenist penchant for embracing suffering, it should come as no surprise that throughout her letters, Angélique sees "the evils that threaten us" as "God's chastisements." God, she asserts, is punishing us "for living so carelessly during the peace" as well as "for our sins."[114] But in 1652, after a fire destroyed one barn with all its cattle, horses, and fodder as the violence grew more intense, the abbess moved her community once more, this time to the *duc* de Luyne's fortified chateau. Guarded by 30 soldiers armed with swords, muskets, and pistols, the sisters knelt before the Holy Sacrament. Meanwhile, enlisting the aid of 250 laborers, the duke began fortifying Port-Royal des Champs to protect the horde of 1000 refugees squatting nearby. Poland's Queen sent 2000 francs; the duke's largess fed 500 starving souls; by May, 100 fleeing religious dined with the sisters.[115]

As atrocities mounted, Angélique cringed at the news that 300 religious had been "assassinated."[116] Updating Poland's Queen in the summer of 1652, she described France as "totally desolated" and Paris as "the most mistreated" city. "The villages all around are entirely deserted," she added; the inhabitants who had not been abused or killed by soldiers had fled into the woods. Abbeys everywhere had been pillaged; monks and nuns had been "indignantly treated" and even murdered. The troops had recently pillaged her brother Robert's estate at Pomponne. "All soldiers are possessed by demons!" she exclaimed.[117]

Despite these chastisements, however, she thanked God for protecting Port-Royal des Champs. Although nearby villages had been torched, their wheat fields and vineyards destroyed and their women raped, the army had left the abbey alone.[118] Men hired by the *duc* de Luynes had recently strengthened its walls and built eight 30–foot towers around its perimeter. In a solemn service on 1 July 1652, Angélique dedicated these towers to the Holy Sacrament, the Holy Virgin, and to saints Joseph, John the Baptist, Laurent, Louis, Peter, and Paul. "Every day new alarms are raised," she told Le Maître, yet "God is over all."[119] Despite the carnage all around them, by the summer of 1653, the solitaires had managed to complete the new dormitory for students at the *petites écoles*. The Queen of Poland sent 6000 *livres* to help the abbey with this project and to feed the hundreds of refugees who crowded onto the grounds.[120]

The abbess thanked her profusely, explaining that with wheat so scarce, the price of bread had skyrocketed to ten *sous* a pound. Port-Royal had bread enough for only five more days. In addition to the fleeing peasants, 400 religious from every order passed through the convent. The sisters fed as many as 182 of them at one time.[121] In the terrible summer heat, many of the abbey's servants succumbed to the plague, leading the abbess to lament, "Blessed are those who weep."[122] But weeping turned to rejoicing by mid-August when she could at last report: "Our Community is enjoying very great peace."[123] Finally, the Fronde had come to an end; Port-Royal des Champs had survived.

After the Fronde, the abbey and priory of Port-Royal thrived, in large part due to the strong support given by members of the Arnauld family. Although Antoine and Catherine Arnauld no longer controlled the convents as their private domain, in a very real sense, through their children, grandchildren, and even great-grandchildren, they continued to shape the future of both houses. And Port-Royal changed them as well. Before 1609, the Arnaulds' lives focused around events at Court and at the Palais de Justice; they entertained lavishly at their country estate and at their Paris apartments. But following the "Day of the Wicket Gate," Angélique gradually began to pull them into the spiritual orbit of Port-Royal. Perhaps, as Alexander Sedgwick has suggested, she felt that if she could spiritually transform her family, she might redeem herself in God's eyes for entering Port-Royal des Champs in violation of canon law. At any rate, as Angélique's reputation as a reformer grew in France, so did her influence over her family. Between 1609 and 1703, three generations of Arnauld women entered either the abbey or the priory.[124]

Jacqueline Arnauld herself, as Sister Jacqueline-Marie-Angélique de Sainte-Madéleine, served as abbess of Port-Royal des Champs from 1602 to 1633 and again from 1636 to her death in 1661. In 1610 her sister Jeanne Arnauld transferred from the convent in Saint-Cyr to Port-Royal des Champs and four years later took the name *Soeur* Jeanne-Catherine-Agnès de Saint-Paul. She served as abbess of Port-Royal in Paris from 1636 to 1642; Agnès also drafted the Constitutions of the abbey and wrote the *Secret Chapelet* described earlier. In 1615 Marie Arnauld, disfugured by smallpox at three, took her vows as Sister Marie de Sainte Claire at age seven; she first joined Port-Royal and three years later, helped Angélique reform the convent at Maubuisson. Angélique praised her as "a pillar in our choir." In 1620, Anne Arnauld, also scarred by smallpox, joined her two sisters as Sister Anne Eugénie de l'Incarnation at Maubuisson; later that year, following a significant dream, Madéleine Arnauld entered Port-Royal in Paris and took the name Sister Madéleine de Sainte Christine. Angélique's mother, Catherine Arnauld, recently widowed, came to Port-Royal as a novice in 1626 and, as Sister Catherine de Saint-Félicité, submitted to her daughter's authority. Until her death fifteen years later, she helped prepare meals, washed pots and pans, and did the laundry. Then in 1640, Angélique's sister Catherine Le Maître, exhausted after giving birth to thirteen children in a miserable marriage, became Sister Catherine de Saint-Jean at Port-Royal following her husband's death. Six of her daughters and three of her sons would follow her there.[125]

By the 1640s, the two convents became—spiritually speaking—a family firm. Ten of the 30 nuns (33%) singing in Port-Royal's choir hailed from the Arnauld family.[126] In addition to Angélique's mother and five sisters, she attracted six nieces to join either Port-Royal or Port-Royal des Champs.[127] One of the most famous—Angélique Arnauld d'Andilly—had, in fact, been named after her. Daughter of Robert Arnauld d'Andilly and Catherine Lefèvre de la Boderie, she was educated at Port-Royal. In 1641 she became a novice and in 1644 took her vows as Sister Angélique de Saint Jean. For 20 years she taught girls at the abbey. In 1653 she became sub-prioress at Port-Royal des Champs and in 1659, at Port-Royal in Paris. Beloved for her tenderness, energy, sensitivity and deep intellect, she penned over 800 letters and wrote the first significant history of Port-Royal. For her role in opposing the Formulary, Angélique spent ten months in detention at the Annonciades in Paris. Still, she refused to sign.[128]

In addition to her mother, sisters, and nieces, *Mère* Angélique attracted many of her brothers, nephews, and great-nephews to Port-Royal. Her brother Antoine ("the Great") Arnauld not only defended the interests of the abbey in his writings, but also took refuge there from time to time. Her brother Henri Arnauld d'Andilly, as Bishop of Angers, likewise lent his support to the abbey during the contest over the Formulary.[129] Saint-Cyran invited her brother Robert Arnauld d'Andilly (who had helped gain his release from Vincennes) to become one of the first solitaires at Port-Royal des Champs. Following a long career in law and in the army, Robert experienced a life-changing conversion in 1637.[130] His sister Angélique encouraged him: "Our good Fathers have all the hope of God in you," she exclaimed, calling him "the most assured friend of the Court, and the most powerful enemy—may you always be so for all just causes."[131] Then at the death of

Saint-Cyran ("whose friendship was for me a priceless treasure"[132]) in 1643, Robert retired from political life. He joined the priory in 1644 and spent the next 30 years studying patristic manuscripts, writing memoirs to the Queen Mother calling for a more virtuous government, and experimenting with fruit trees. Robert may, in fact, have been the only Jansenist remembered for his sense of humor, a rare trait among the disciples of St. Augustine; nonetheless, he sent all six of his daughters to Port-Royal.[133]

Well into the third generation, the grandchildren of Antoine II Arnauld continued visiting, supporting, and retiring to Port-Royal. His grandson Antoine Le Maître devoted his career to the Parlement of Paris, the Grand Council, and the Court of Aids; he even became a Councilor of State. But in 1638, at the age of 30, he renounced politics and joined the solitaires, declaring, "I am withdrawing into a life of solitude in order to do penance and to serve God the rest of my days." For 20 years, he studied sacred literature in "a very austere penance."[134] His younger brother Simon Le Maître de Séricourt, dissatisfied with his military career, sought solitude at The Grange.[135] He was soon joined by his brother Louis-Isaac Le Maître de Sacy, who as a boy, had been blessed by François de Sales, guided by Saint-Cyran, and taught by Claude Lancelot in the *petites écoles*. In 1645, complaining that "the world is nothing but an insane illusion," he retired to Port-Royal des Champs where he taught boys, confessed the solitaires, and published a French Bible (for which he spent two years in the Bastille—where he completed it).[136]

Three sons of Robert Arnauld d'Andilly also joined the solitaires at The Grange. Henri-Charles Arnauld de Luzancy, who had been educated at the Little Schools there, joined an army regiment but retired to Port-Royal in 1643. His brother Jules Arnauld d'Andilly, also a military man, spent his last years with the solitaires. Their brother Luzancy Arnauld d'Andilly, who built a house near The Grange in 1645, spent his time translating patristic works, restoring the convent gardens, and making love to his wife several times a night while asking God's forgiveness for indulging his carnal appetite.[137]

In addition to the support given by members of the Arnauld clan, Port-Royal in the mid-seventeenth century enjoyed the generosity of a growing circle of friends—*les amis de Port-Royal*. During its "golden age," upwards of 250 people—nuns, novices, servants, noble patrons, recluses, pensioners, solitaires, students, and teachers—clustered around the abbey and priory, seeking "upright and godly conversation."[138]

Between one and two dozen men—the solitaires or "hermits"—lived at or near The Grange farm at any one time. Although the earliest solitaires came from the robe nobility (lawyers and magistrates), later ones represented the bourgeoisie. Some (La Rivière, La Petitière, de Bessi, and Baudri d'Asson) had been soldiers; their skills proved useful in defending Port-Royal during the Fronde. In 1652 *Mère* Angélique told Poland's Queen that these 25 hermits "serve the Lord with great virtue and devotion." Already, they had remodeled the parlor and chapel and built additional rooms to accommodate 60 nuns and novices. If they had the funds, she added, they could erect more buildings to house 60 to 80 men. The *duc* de Luynes, who built a chateau nearby, also lived "with a humility and devotion quite extraordinary."[139]

As described at the end of this chapter, many of these men (among them Antoine Arnauld, Jean Hamon, Antoine Le Maître, Isaac Le Maître de Sacy, Claude Lancelot, and Antoine Singlin) served as tutors for the pupils in the *petites écoles*. Shortly after his tutor Saint-Cyran died in 1643, Singlin became the convents' spiritual director. His sermons packed the chapel. Angélique felt that his moral discourses "ravished the minds of all those who heard them." The prince de Guémenée agreed, boasting that Singlin "preached like a horse and reasoned like an angel."[140]

But Port-Royal's supporters also included men and women from the highest social circles in France, as chapter 1 shows. J. Bruggeman and A. J. Van de Ven's *Inventory* (1972) of 73 *amis*—obviously incomplete—lists two dukes and duchesses, one marquise, two counts and countesses, and many untitled "madams and mademoiselles." These nobles included many extremely wealthy Jansenist sympathizers who bankrolled Port-Royal with their incredible generosity. For example, Charlotte de Ligny gave 40,000 *livres*; Marie de La Chartie donated 30,000 *livres*; the *duchesse* de Longueville contributed £17,000. The marquise de Sablé, who drew many rich patrons to her "Jansenist salon" near Port-Royal in Paris (famous for its gourmet food and moral maxims) formed a lay auxiliary supporting the abbey. Thanks to their generosity, the abbey in 1658 enjoyed a net income of nearly 9500 *livres*. The sisters could also count on influential government officials—*intendants*, councilors, masters of request, secretaries, army and marine officers—to plead their cause. Friends within the Church included archbishops, bishops, abbots, vicars, priors, canons, and other clerics.[141]

They came to the convent for a variety of reasons. Some, like councilor of the Great Chamber of Parlement Benoise, simply wanted their hearts buried at Port-Royal des Champs.[142] Others, like Louis de Pontis, sought peace and solitude and a chance to repent of his bloody 60-year career fighting in the armies of three French kings.[143] Still others, like the poet Jean de La Fontaine, never actually visited Port-Royal, but defended it in their writings and envied its "profound peace that they taste in secret far from the noise of the world."[144]

No matter who they were or what their social status, however, this growing group of second generation friends proved invaluable allies in Port-Royal's growing battle against Church and state. As "resisters" to the "persecution" of Louis XIV, popes, bishops, and the Jesuits, these supporters stubbornly implemented methods of passive resistance centuries before those tried by Henry David Thoreau, Mahatma Gandhi, and Martin Luther King, Jr. In their letters, speeches, books, petitions, and memoirs, they upheld the values of truth, justice, liberty, charity, and grace while constantly opposing "blind obedience" to authority as harmful to one's Christian conscience.[145]

Their first real test came in 1653 in the form of Innocent X's Bull *Cum occasione impressionis libri cui titulus Augustinus* ("On the occasion of a book entitled *Augustinus*"). This bull opened a fresh debate between the Jesuits and Jansenists and between Port-Royal and the Party of the Dévots over whether the five propositions condemned as heretical in Jansen's book could actually be found there.[146] Obviously, the pope thought that Jansen had asserted all five propositions in his book. So did the Inquisition, which in 1654 condemned not only the *Augustinus* but also 50 other Jansenist works. *Père* Annat, Louis XIV's confessor, penned the *Chicanery of the Jansenists* to support the bull and condemn the Jansenists as too clever by half for maintaining the fact/right distinction (the pope was right in condemning the five propositions as heretical, but in fact, they cannot be found in the *Augustinus*).[147] As a result, in the 1650s, Louis XIV began punishing clerics who defended Jansen's work by denying them the income from their benefices.[148]

When news of the 1653 Bull reached Port-Royal, Angélique urged everyone "to wait on God's grace in silence and patience." Writing to her friend the *abbé* de Fleury in July 1653, she said, "The most humble submission to the Bull has astonished many who should have expected nothing less, because others had persuaded them that they would witness a terrible rebellion or schism, but that is one thing in this world that all true servants of God must abhor the most."[149] In August she reassured the Queen of Poland that "all the Disciples of S. Augustine have received [the bull] with the respect and perfect submission that is due to the Holy See, and there is no one in the world less desirous of causing a schism in the Church, which [we] believe is the worst of all crimes. Therefore, we must pray to God ceaselessly that he will give the spirit of submission and peace to all the children of the Church."[150]

Like most Jansenists, the abbess held that the five propositions, while heretical, could not be found in Jansen's writings. Consequently, she assured Monsieur de Fleury in Poland that the bull "does no harm to the doctrine of S. Augustine, which is that of the Church, and therefore cannot be abolished." Only "the disciples of Molina" (the Jesuits) would "create problems over it." But even they "are our brothers and we are obligated to pray often for them." She rejoiced that "so far not one of the disciples of St. Augustine has been harmed by it," recognizing in this God's "visible protection of the truth."[151]

As the year 1654 dawned, however, the abbess grew concerned that a "cabal" in Rome might persuade the pope to issue harsher condemnations of the five propositions that could bring "a revolt." If that happened, she promised Poland's Queen, then "we will write against it rather than receive it."[152] This passive resistance stance represents a paradigm shift from her earlier counsel that the friends of Port-Royal should "Pray, weep, groan: your tears will do more than your writings."[153] Clearly, her earlier policy of submission and trusting in God had been eroded by the increasing threats of "those who try to persuade the authorities to persecute us." Rumors spread that the abbess had been excommunicated, sent to the Bastille, or exiled from France. Realizing that all the above could happen to her, she prayed in June 1654 (when Louis XIV was finally crowned at Reims): "Lord, make this sovereign a saint."[154]

Throughout 1655, her letters expressed the growing fear that Port-Royal was being persecuted for refusing to accept the pope's bull. In February, she describes "all our troubles & threats" as "greater than ever."[155] Yet as the persecution increased, "God by his goodness prepares our hearts to suffer with as much humility & sweetness as we must."[156] Consequently, when Louis XIV's declarations threatened their existence, she "feared more [about] giving offense to God, for all other evils . . . are nothing if we have his grace to preserve us."[157] Her faith wavered later in March, however, when she told Poland's Queen: "We are pursued at Court with an extreme violence [by 22 Jesuits] to persecute us to the end." She worried that "our approaching ruin" would entail "the dispersion of all who are here."[158] Consequently, she persuaded the Queen to intercede with Innocent X to stop persecuting those who "are truly Catholics & very devoted to the Holy See [with] submission & obedience."[159] Despite the help of powerful friends, the abbess despaired of Port-Royal's survival. "This is the hour of the power of darkness," she intoned. "It is necessary to submit and to suffer from it as it pleases God."[160]

But silence and submission amidst controversy did not suit Angélique's brothers. In a January 1654 letter to Mazarin, Robert Arnauld d'Andilly defended the Port-Royal nuns as "innocent persons" who "will not be useless to the Church if they are left alone, to combat the animosity and injustice of those who seek to slander them with falsehoods and impostures."[161] A year later, Antoine Arnauld sent copies of his *Letter to a Person of Rank* (February 1655) and his *Second Letter to a Duke and Peer* (July 1655) to the pope. After reading them, Alexander VII praised Arnauld's "piety & erudition" and lauded Port-Royal as "a convent of great piety." Nevertheless, he admonished Arnauld and his friends to remain silent concerning the five propositions.[162]

Perhaps if Arnauld had taken the pope's advice, the Sorbonne would not have expelled him from its ranks in January 1656. Yet even if he had submitted, others refused to do so. Jacques de Sainte-Beuve, leader of a pro-Jansenist faction in the Sorbonne and for ten years Port-Royal's superior, sent the pope vigorous defenses of the five propositions.[163]

Therefore, on 16 October 1656, Alexander VII signed the Bull *Ad sacram beati Petri sedem* ("To the sacred throne of St. Peter") reiterating the condemnation of the five propositions found in Jansen's *Augustinus*.[164] To insure compliance, Archbishop Pierre de Marca of Toulouse and Louis XIV's confessor *Père* Annat drew up the following Formulary that all French clergy had to sign[165]:

> I submit sincerely to the Constitution of Pope Innocent X of 13 May 1653 according to its true meaning, which has been determined by the Constitution of Our Holy Father Pope Alexander VII of 16 October 1656. And I recognize that I am obligated in conscience to obey these Constitutions, & I condemn with heart & mouth the doctrines of the five propositions of Cornelius Jansenius, contained in the book entitled Augustinus which these two popes & the bishops have condemned, whose doctrines

are not those of Saint Augustine, which Jansenius has poorly explained compared to the true meaning of the holy Doctor.[166]

However, not *all* the bishops had condemned the five propositions. To keep from signing the Formulary, some Gallican clerics invoked the concept of "divine right," declaring themselves answerable only to God in matters of conscience. Popes could intervene in jurisdictional matters only if they were prepared to reject canonical norms and defined articles of faith. Far from ending the controversy over the five propositions, this pledge poisoned the life of the Church in France for more than a century.[167]

The debate over the Formulary also split the Jansenist community. Claude Lancelot argued that signing it condemned St. Augustine's and Jansen's doctrine of grace. Martin de Barcos, *abbé* de Saint-Cyran and Antoine Singlin, however, told the nuns to sign it unconditionally out of respect for Church authority. But Antoine Arnauld, Pierre Nicole, and the marquise de Sablé advised them to sign only with reservations (concerning the right/fact distinction). *Mère* Angélique, on the other hand, believed that to sign the Formulary even with this clever distinction would be to sin against St. Augustine. Instead, she advocated total silence, which Church officials could interpret any way they liked. She argued that to sign "in good conscience," the nuns would have to read Jansen's *Augustinus* in Latin. This they could not do because it would violate "God's order" (that men rule over women) and canon law (which forbade women to engage in theological debates). Port-Royal's sisters used this "theology of weakness" excuse to defy the "illegitimate use of authority" by Louis XIV, popes, and archbishops seeking to force them to sign the Formulary "against God's will." By taking this stand—and being willing to die for it—the nuns shaped the theological, legal, rhetorical, and gender-based argument for resistance advanced by Antoine Arnauld.[168]

In his *Writings on the Bulls of Alexander VII* (1657), Arnauld objected to the Formulary for several reasons. First, the Jesuits had written it; second, signatures to it were forced; third, it applied only to France and therefore contradicted "Gallican liberties"; fourth, some bishops in the General Assembly of the Clergy opposed it; fifth, it imposed "an unreal uniformity" on the Church. He believed that its ambiguous, compromising wording failed to clarify Jansen's true meaning, to distinguish orthodoxy from heresy, and to recognize the right/fact distinction. Instead, he feared, forcing this pledge on the Church would establish "a horrible Inquisition" in France.[169] The next year, in a lengthy letter to *Père* Feret at the Oratory in Lyon, Arnauld gave three reasons why he could not sign the Formulary: doing so would wound his conscience, go contrary to Church discipline, and condemn St. Augustine's doctrine (which, he asserted, is Roman Catholic doctrine).[170]

His friend Blaise Pascal agreed, stating that he could never sign the Formulary because its wording condemned "efficacious grace." No matter whether one found that teaching in St. Augustine or in Jansen's *Augustinus*, any papal bull, episcopal mandate, or pledge that forced one to repudiate truth violated one's faith and conscience.[171]

For the most part, the Jansenist nuns and solitaires adopted the intransigent position advanced by Arnauld and Pascal—and paid the price for their stubbornness. In March 1656, the government ordered the solitaires and their fifteen students to leave Port-Royal des Champs; lieutenant civil Dreux d'Aubray and two commissioners entered the priory on March 24 to insure that they had gone.[172] In a letter written that day to the Queen of Poland, Angélique Arnauld exclaimed, "All our Hermits have left here" (with the exception of her brother Robert, who departed shortly thereafter). "Our valley is truly a valley of tears."[173] Three days later, as the sisters wept for their departed brothers, she lamented to M. le Maître: "One day we will see, in the other world, & maybe yet in this one, some of God's reasons for allowing his servants & his truth to be oppressed

. . . I hope the devil will not gain anything from this dispersion."[174] To counteract the devil's designs, Antoine Singlin continued providing spiritual guidance to the solitaires in their scattered retreats, using coded messages and pseudonyms to frustrate the authorities. For example, Lancelot became "M. Dolibert" and M. de Saci, "M. de Gournay." Numbers were assigned to Robert Arnauld d'Andilly (900), *Mère* Agnès (923), *Mère* Angélique de Saint-Jean (924), and even to Paris Archbishop Péréfixe (992).[175] Only two months later in May 1656, however, all the solitaires received permission to return to Port-Royal des Champs.[176] Two events explain this sudden turnaround: the "Miracle of the Thorn" and the intervention of the Queen Mother.

All sincere Catholics credited inexplicable physical healing to divine intervention. Angélique Arnauld had told Saint-Cyran in 1652 regarding a woman declared incurable who had been healed following prayers: This "is a visible miracle of his [God's] intercession."[177] Four years later, Pascal's eleven-year-old niece Marguerite ("Margo") Périer, a novice at Port-Royal in Paris, suffered intense pain from a walnut-sized lachrymal fistula in her left eye that drained into her nasal cavity. After six months of hydrotherapy proved useless and her parents rejected a surgeon's recommendation for cauterizing the fistula, physicians declared her condition incurable. But when on 24 March 1656, at the urging of Sister Catherine de Sainte-Flavie Passart, Margo touched the fistula with a reliquary thorn allegedly taken from Christ's crown of thorns, she experienced healing. That evening, Margo declared, "My eye has healed. I no longer feel any pain in it."[178] Sister Flavie, after examining her and finding the wound clean and healthy, declared it a miracle. Eight days later, the physician M. de Chatillon and the surgeon M. Dalançé likewise called her healing "complete and miraculous." The latter exclaimed, "There have never been any miracles if this is not one." Three weeks later, as word spread, four more physicians and four surgeons examined her and pronounced her completely cured, using the terms "instant healing" and "miracle" in their reports.[179]

This perceived miracle ignited a firestorm of debate at Court, in the General Assembly of the Clergy, at all the convents and monasteries in Paris, and even in many of the salons.[180] If the niece of a prominent Jansenist writer residing at a notoriously Jansenist convent had indeed experienced divine healing, this would seem to indicate that God favored the Jansenist cause. After all, Blaise Pascal asserted, "miracles support religion. They have distinguished the Jews, Christians, saints, innocent ones and the true believers." Because "the Church has never approved a miracle among heretics," the healing of his niece proved the genuineness of her religious experience, and in this case, of Jansenism.[181] That is also how Antoine Arnauld portrayed the situation in his *Response to a Writing Published on the Subject of the Miracles which It Has Pleased God to Work at Port-Royal a Short Time Ago by a Holy Thorn from the Crown of Our Savior* (1656). Arnauld argued that Marguerite's healing constituted a genuine miracle; it brought "edification" to the Church and placed God's seal of "certitude" on Jansenism.[182]

His sister Angélique, who did not favor exploiting miracles to defend Jansenism, took a more cautious stance. She told one nun that "silence and humility . . . would be better for us and for the good of the cause than all the miracles in the world."[183] But silence proved impossible as miracles attributed to the thorn multiplied during the spring and summer of 1656. From near and far, 21 nobles, nuns, and commoners came to Port-Royal, touched their diseased bodies with the holy thorn, and walked away cured of colic, stomach ailments, paralysis, violent vomiting, fevers, cancerous growths, convulsions, tumors, and other physical disabilities. All had been declared hopeless and incurable.[184] "Miracles are occurring with such frequency," Angélique told the Queen of Poland, "that we are all astonished and confused. God knows what he is doing, and we await in peace whatever it pleases him to ordain." She hoped that these miracles would strengthen the faith of witnesses and hearers.[185]

Her brother Antoine hastened to assure her that this would be the case. The Holy Thorn miracles, he asserted, prove that "God provides the greatest protection to those he loves the most at the very moment when in the eyes of ordinary mortals, he appears to have abandoned them. In this way he strengthens the hearts of those whom he intends to save to make it possible for them to repel their enemies."[186] This proved true, for as miraculous cures multiplied in late 1656 and 1657, Port-Royal's enemies declared a truce with the convent.[187] Vicar-general Alexandre de Hadencq convened a commission of five theologians; after interviewing 25 witnesses, they sent a report to Mazarin declaring that through the Holy Thorn, God had worked several miracles. As a result, Anne, the Queen Mother, told the first minister to cease harassing Port-Royal.[188]

Her intervention, however, merely demonstrated her caution; it did not mean that she accepted Jansenism as orthodox. In fact, in 1659 the Queen Mother warned Robert Arnauld d'Andilly: "You are in the midst of Jansenists and instigators of heresy." To her, a Jansenist "is one who refuses to submit in all humility and without reservation whatsoever to the decision of the Holy See . . . [but] obstinately insists that Jansen's doctrine has not been condemned by the bull [of 1657]."[189]

Despite her lack of theological training, no one could have put the case more succinctly. And throughout the 1650s—despite all the healing miracles—the number of those exasperated by Port-Royal's passive resistance to Church and state authority grew. Ever since the Fronde when the Jansenists sympathized with the rebellious Cardinal de Retz, Louis XIV had sought ways to gain greater control over the archdiocese of Paris. Forcing priests, abbots, monks and nuns to sign the Formulary was one method of accomplishing that and at the same time, of uprooting suspected *frondeurs*.[190] His first minister, Jules Mazarin, agreed; as we have seen, he harassed various Jansenists during the Fronde for their "seditious activities" and expelled the solitaires from Port-Royal des Champs in 1656. Likewise, he strongly supported Alexander VII's Bull *Ad sacram* in 1657 and took steps to close Port-Royal's *petites écoles* in 1659.[191]

Riding the prevailing winds of government hostility toward Port-Royal, the Jesuits multiplied their attacks on Jansenism. In *Jansenism Confounded* (1651), Jean Brisacier maligned its nuns as "mad virgins" who did not believe in the sacraments and who refused to pray to the Virgin Mary or the saints.[192] The Society disseminated a scurrilous "Circular Letter from Port-Royal" (1657) purporting to explain the guidelines for followers of St. Augustine. The nuncio in Turin sent a copy to the secretary of state at the Vatican who handed it to Alexander VII. Although Antoine Arnauld called it a forgery "that stretched the patience of the human species," the Jesuits continued distributing it in various translations well into the nineteenth century.[193]

Consequently, as *Mère* Agnès lamented in 1657, "We are the object of the hatred of all the devout ones of the day."[194] Seeking friendlier pastures, a few Jansenist leaders even considered leaving for America in 1660. Perhaps among the Calvinist Puritans of the recently established Massachusetts Bay colony they would find sympathy.[195] But the sudden death of *Mère* Angélique Arnauld changed these plans.

On 25 May 1661, the septuagenarian abbess complained to the Queen Mother that she suffered from an illness so severe that she had requested the sacrament in the middle of the night, expecting "to appear soon before God." Despite her pain, she begged Queen Anne to protect the abbey over which she had served for 55 years ("though always unworthy"). In this her last defense, she argues that Port-Royal is not a "nest of error or heresy" (as the Jesuits charged). On the contrary, its sisters "have always desired to live in Christian simplicity, as humble daughters of the Church . . . wishing only to serve God in secrecy & silence." Despite "injurious accusations" to the contrary, the nuns submit to the pope and to the Catholic Church. In their defense, she cites the miracles by which "God has spoken in our favor." She begs Anne "to receive this letter as the last words of a dying person, who thinks more of the other life than of the one she touches."[196]

After lingering in pain for two months, Angélique Arnauld died on the Day of the Transfiguration—6 August 1661—a brilliant Saturday morning. Her final words to the weeping sisters gathered about her bed contained a warning: "I have understood death all my life and have always thought about it . . . But now all the world is less than nothing . . . It is necessary to prepare for this terrible hour."[197] Honoring her half-century of service as abbess of two convents, the nuns buried her body at Port-Royal de Paris and her heart at Port-Royal des Champs.[198]

The once rebellious novice left behind a proud legacy. Whereas most convents in late seventeenth-century Paris contained only 50 to 65 religious, Port-Royal in Paris had 124 in 1661 (63 pensioners, 5 novices, 14 converts, 12 postulants, 8 recusants, and 22 younger pensioners). That same year, Port-Royal des Champs had 66 religious (25 pensioners, 27 novices, 7 converts, and 7 postulants).[199] Through fervent prayer, strong financial support, and unflagging determination, by the time of her death, *Mère* Angélique had transformed two tiny, ramshackle convents into centers of Jansenism.

Yet even while she lay dying, the storm clouds of Church and state persecution gathered on the horizon. Haunted by the ghost of Cardinal de Retz and fearing the rise of a new Fronde, Louis XIV in 1661 asked his Council of State to impose a new Formulary to be signed by all Catholic clergy, religious orders, and lay teachers in France. This pledge would provide the litmus test of orthodoxy for every priest, monk, nun, abbot, abbess, and teacher in the realm, and would (the king hoped) bring unity in the Church.[200]

But there were several "formularies" floating around. Alexander VII's 1657 Bull *Cum occasione* inspired the first one, which the Port-Royal nuns refused to sign. So in the spring of 1661, the Archbishop of Paris had two vicars add a codicil to that Formulary recognizing the validity of the fact/right distinction. In June, with Antoine Arnauld's encouragement, the sisters signed this amended Formulary. But when Alexander VII condemned this codicil in August, the nuns signed the original version, adding a declaration that their signatures represented only respect for the pope's authority and not total acceptance of the "fact" that the five propositions existed in the *Augustinus*.[201]

Facing the imminent threat of closure from the General Assembly of the Clergy and the Council of State,[202] the nuns adopted a strategy that Daniella Kostroun (2003) has aptly called "the feminist paradox." Using gender as their trump card, the nuns claimed that their subordinate position in the Church rendered them incapable of passing judgment on Jansen's text. Therefore, they should neither be expected to understand the deeper theological issues involved nor required to sign a Formulary that implied that they did comprehend those matters. Citing centuries of misogynistic pronouncements by the Greeks, Romans, and Church fathers, they argued that since women were naturally the inferior sex, submissive to men, barred from reading and teaching theology, and thus incapable of heresy, they should not be required to take sides in the debate over Jansenism. Therefore, following Antoine Arnauld's lead in the right/fact distinction, they agreed (with the exception of Jacqueline Pascal) to "espouse absolutely and without reserve the *right* of the Roman Catholic Church [to condemn the five propositions as heresy] and . . . condemn all that it condemns." But they remained silent on the issue of *fact* (whether those heretical proposals could be found in Jansen's work).[203]

Consequently, *Mère* Agnès asked Arnauld to prepare an addendum to the Formulary so that her sisters could sign it and forestall their dispersal. Incorporating their gender submissive model, in November he wrote the following heading to the Formulary: "Considering our ignorance of those matters that are above our profession and our sex, the most we can do [by signing the Formulary] is give witness to the purity of our faith."[204] Their signatures testified solely to their obedience and submission to Church authority, not to their acceptance of the Church's teaching regarding Jansen's writings.

Their feminist strategy included three elements. First, they advanced the Catholic argument concerning women's natural weakness and ignorance in theological matters to prove that forcing them to sign the Formulary violated God's natural order for the sexes (females submissive to males). Second, to demonstrate their submission, they remained silent on the question of fact. Third, to show that God had given women the capacity to reason, they employed legalistic arguments in letters, tracts, and books to sustain their right to resist outside force in matters of conscience. Because they saw the command to sign the Formula as a threat not only to Jansenists, but also as a violation of everyone's freedom of conscience, they considered the popes' bulls and the king's orders as illegitimate uses of authority. In essence, by exalting their right of spiritual equality with men to follow their own reason and conscience, these submissive nuns, in their holy boldness, advanced a seventeenth-century form of feminism.[205] Moreover, this feminist strategy, although increasingly offensive to many Church and state officials, forestalled Port-Royal des Champs' dissolution for another four decades.

With the threat of dispersal temporarily delayed, life at the two convents returned to normal. But what constituted normalcy for Port-Royal differed somewhat from life at other religious communities. Jansenists typically harbored a suspicion of holy orders because the vows taken by monks and nuns were of human origin—and since human nature was weak and sinful, monastic life had no special holiness attached to it. The solitaires, for example, took no vows as priests or monks; they lived apart from the world but also outside the cloisters. Not a religious order nor a congregation nor an organized group, the *messieurs* could be likened to an academy of pious hermits who lived together at the hilltop farm called The Grange. In an era that considered manual labor socially discreditable if not shameful, these men grew fruit and vegetables and milked cows; they also read their Bibles, translated theological works, and taught students in the "Little Schools."[206] Antoine Le Maître, one of them, explained this paradox:

> They [the solitaires at Port-Royal des Champs] have no form of Community . . . No form or color of habit [religious dress] is affected there . . . No particular discipline [is] established, nor any stable dwelling place; no rule except the Gospel, no bond but that of universal Catholic charity, no special interest or common goal but gaining Heaven. It is only a place of retreat, totally free and voluntary, where one can come only if God's Spirit leads him and where one remains only because God's Spirit constrains him to stay.[207]

Unlike the solitaires at The Grange, the sisters at Port-Royal des Champs adopted a more ascetic lifestyle that embraced a triple solitude. First, through cloture, they separated themselves from the world; second, they isolated themselves from one another by living in sparsely furnished private rooms; third, they denied their selfish human nature through silence, meditation, and service for others.[208] Remembering the words of their recently departed abbess—that "the wind of vanity extinguishes lamps just as easily as the lack of oil"[209]—Port-Royal's sisters rejected the world. Human society—which represented the evil realm of Satan—contradicted the values of God's kingdom.[210]

Yet their retreat from social affairs did not lead them to condemn all human occupations, especially those—like farming, teaching, nursing, building, and helping the poor—most useful to others. Nor did they ignore important events at Court. The nuns regularly chanted *Te Deums* for the births of royal princes and princesses, and despite their pacifistic views, dutifully thanked God for the king's victories in battle. And the sound of royal hunts echoing across the priory's fields frequently reminded them that Versailles was only a few miles away.[211]

Yet the palace, with its pleasure-seeking courtiers, might as well have been located on another planet compared to the ascetic lifestyles practiced at Port-Royal des Champs. By withdrawing from secular society and embracing lives of self-denial, the sisters sought renewal—a new heart, some new grace, a new assurance of salvation—through penitence, meditation, prayer, and service. As God's true saints, his remnant "church within the Church," they felt called to live a deeper spiritual life of poverty, asceticism, and rigorous morality as an example to the world.[212]

Little wonder, then, that as the reputation of the two convents as centers of purer spirituality, higher virtue, deeper austerity, and greater suffering spread, the world beat a path to their door.[213] To those suffering from plague, famine, drought, or civil war, Port-Royal des Champs in the 1650s must have seemed like a utopia. Here solitaire philosophers and humanitarian nuns ate, worked, and studied together while reflecting God's love. But they were not always saintly: they expressed their individual moods and tastes, engaged in petty quarrels, and hatched their little plots.[214] Yet remarkably, for almost a century, these two sacred communities lived in harmony.

The "Constitution of the Convent of Port-Royal of the Holy Sacrament," however, was forged by tensions, both internal and external. First, Port-Royal was transferred from the jurisdiction of Citeaux to that of the Archbishop of Paris (1626); second, Zamet founded the Institute of the Holy Sacrament (1648); and third, conflicts over lifestyle issues caused Angélique to reject one confessor (Zamet) and choose another (St.-Cyran). This set of guidelines, drawn up by Agnès Arnauld, governed both houses and helped promote unity and protect their rights. The Constitution, a modification of Cistercian rules adopted in 1647, reflected the ideas and interests of Angélique Arnauld, St.-Cyran, and Antoine Arnauld for simplicity, austerity, poverty, and direct democracy by the sisters. It also established a clear chain of command. Each convent had a director (an abbess or prioress), a confessor (male), a chaplain (male), a sacristan (in charge of the chapel), a steward (to oversee the property), a PR agent, and a physician who lived nearby. A dozen servants helped with menial tasks like bringing in the wood, caring for the chickens and doves, and assisting visitors. The women and girls took turns working in the kitchen, laundry, infirmary, and gardens.[215] Basically, Port-Royal included four types of women. Those in the choir or chancel consecrated their lives to private prayer and choral chant (unaccompanied by instruments). Lay or "converted" sisters served the needs of the poor in the community. Novices, who wore religious habits and veils, spent a year preparing to become nuns (also called "pensioners"). Postulants lived in the community but attended services at the convent.[216]

The director—be she abbess or prioress—set the tone and shaped the direction of the convent. Through their letters to Port-Royal's network of friends and supporters, outstanding abbesses like *Mère* Angélique and *Mère* Agnès shaped its physiognomy and spiritual culture. By their personal example, they modeled the behavior they wished the sisters to adopt. Wanting her nuns—many of them daughters of the nobility—to embrace poverty, Angélique wore a habit patched from 40 pieces of cloth and slept on an old mattress with a tattered blanket in a tiny anteroom. Following her example, the nuns lived in cells containing a wooden table, a chair, a small bed, a water basin, and a lamp. Their beds were furnished only with a straw-filled mattress, a flannel blanket, two quilts, and a pillow. Their clothing consisted of a serge shirt, a tunic, a white robe, a white scapular with a red cross, a yellow leather belt, a white mantle, a linen hood, woolen bonnets, a black veil, and a headpiece (*toque*) that covered their shoulders and chest.[217]

Their daily schedule left little time for primping. Matins came at 2 a.m., rising at 5:30 a.m., prime at 6 a.m., *terce* or conventional Mass at 8:30 a.m., *sexte* at 10:45 a.m., and dinner at 11:30 a.m. In the afternoon, the sisters spent an hour with the abbess or prioress from 12:45 to 1:45 p.m.; rested, read, or worked in their rooms for another hour; attended *nones* at 2:30 p.m. and vespers at 4:00 p.m. before eating supper at 5:15 p.m. After dining, they attended *complines* at 6:30 p.m. and retired to bed at 8:00 p.m. And except for their conference with the director, they spent this entire eighteen-hour day in complete silence; internal communication consisted of handwritten notes.[218]

At The Grange up on the hill, the solitaires followed a similar schedule: Matins came at 3 a.m., prime at 6:30 a.m., *terce* at 9 a.m., *sexte* and self-examination at 11:00 a.m., then dinner at noon. After a brief rest, the solitaires spent four hours laboring in the orchards and gardens before eating supper at 6:00 p.m., attending *complines* at 7:00 p.m., with lights out at 8:00 p.m. During this long day, both groups dined only twice on bread, fruit, and vegetables cooked without sauces or seasonings and served on wooden or clay plates and saucers. They ate eggs from their own chickens, but no meat except fish, following the Rule of St. Benedict which forbade "eating the meat of quadrupeds."[219]

Despite their ascetic lifestyles, however, the sisters and solitaires were not so otherworldly as to be of no earthly good. If their schedules mandated much time for prayer, worship, and meditation, this did not make them physically lazy. They taught school, healed the sick, prepared meals, made candles, sewed garments, cobbled shoes, rebound books, scrubbed floors, trimmed trees and brush, picked fruit, and hoed vegetables. The sisters baked hundreds of loaves of bread (from whole grain, not white flour), cleaned endless windows, scoured greasy pots and pans, and made their own linens and vestments (but did not embroider them). Together, these men and women ran a 400–acre fruit and dairy farm.[220]

They also ministered to the needs of the sinful world beyond their borders. They regularly visited prisons and hospitals in the capital, taking food, medicine, and spiritual encouragement to the inmates. Their charity was legendary: Port-Royal des Champs alone gave alms totaling 27,000 *livres* every year. In 1656, the community donated 18,000 *livres* to establish the Hôpital-Général in Paris. As previously mentioned, during the Fronde, both houses sheltered, fed, and nursed hundreds of refugees.[221]

In many ways, therefore, these two institutions resembled scores of monasteries and convents run by other religious orders all around them. But important differences existed. For example, in an era when few religious (male or female) read the Bible, the Jansenists at Port-Royal studied it daily (in Latin and French), in addition to reading the patristic literature and great spiritual classics of the past. In contrast to the nuns in other orders, the Jansenist sisters frequently read (and wrote) poetry, memoirs, letters, and polemical works. Their verse ("poetry of the conscience") emphasized themes of truth, moral beauty, duty, suffering, and sacrifice. Although some nuns in other houses could not even read, much less write, there were no illiterate women at Port-Royal. Widely read and broadly educated, with reasoning abilities sharpened by frequent theological debates, these sisters were philosopher-saints to their supporters—and proud, stubborn savants to their enemies, who grew weary of their bold protests and self-justifying letters.[222]

Through the medium of education as exemplified in the "Little Schools," the sisters and solitaires bequeathed this intellectual heritage and combative strain to the next generation. The Jansenist *petites écoles* (for boys) and the *filles régentes* (for girls) must be seen in the context of the Catholic Reformation's efforts to apply Tridentine reforms to education and life in general. Forward-looking educators such as François de Sales, Pierre de Bérulle, Charles de Condren, Vincent de Paul, Benoît de Confeld, and Adrien Bourdoise transformed the curricula and teaching methodologies of schools taught by the Jesuits, Oratorians, Lazarists, Sulpicians, and Eudists. Originally, they wanted to better prepare young men to enter their seminaries where they would become better priests to serve the Church.[223]

By the mid-seventeenth century, the Jansenists also felt the need to train better priests. But more than that, they wanted to prepare educated Christians who could appreciate the "beauties of the Gospel" and resist the "false doctrines" of "false prophets" (non-Jansenists). To this end, they established 32 schools in Paris. In addition to the one at Port-Royal and its rural counterpart, Port-Royal des Champs, there were seventeen schools in the Saint-Antoine district, four in the Saint-Merry parish, three in the Saint-Etienne-du-Mont parish, two apiece in the parishes of Saint-Louis-en-l'Ile and Saint-Séverin, and one at Magny-les-Hameaux. Outside Paris, their

"Little Schools" could be found in Chesnay, Reims, Noyon, Troyes, Auxerre, Orléans, Lyonnais, Saint-Jean des Troux, Vaumurier, Sevran, and Toulouse by the early eighteenth century.[224]

The Jansenists established five different types of schools. The free charity schools—which took in infants, the poor, handicapped, and deaf-mutes—gave lower class children basic skills in reading and writing. Primary schools taught both boys and girls through the elementary grades. Secondary schools provided girls with pensions or scholarships with further education, while seminaries prepared boys for careers in the Church. Finally, the superior schools honed the skills of young men in canon law (at Saint-Josse) and oriental languages (at Utrecht).[225]

They were called *petites écoles* ("Little Schools") for several reasons. First, both their enrollments and classroom student/teacher ratios (six to one) remained small. Second, the vast majority of them offered only a primary education. Finally, the Jesuits had reserved the term *collège* for their schools and wanted no competition from the Jansenists or anyone else in the pedagogical market.[226]

In the light of the government's later hostility toward these schools, it is somewhat ironic that Jerome Bignon, Louis XIV's librarian and an advocate-general in the Paris Parlement, provided the impetus for their founding. He asked Saint-Cyran to establish a Christian school in Paris where his two sons, Jérome and Thierry, could be tutored. Their father wanted them to avoid the worldly "dangers" in other schools, preserve their innocence, learn Gospel truths and "chaste songs," read good books, gain control of their passions, and grow in piety.[227] So in June 1637, Saint-Cyran and Antoine Singlin started the first *petite école* with three students at Port-Royal des Champs. Because of the malarial environment, however, they moved the school to Port-Royal in Paris that fall. But when the Archbishop of Paris objected to youth living outside a regular monastery, the two men took their six students back to the rural priory in the spring of 1638. But after arresting Saint-Cyran, Richelieu dispersed them once again in July and they returned to various lodgings in Paris until the Archbishop of Paris permitted them to reassemble at Port-Royal des Champs following Richelieu's death in 1643. When Saint-Cyran died, however, three teachers—Claude Lancelot, Charles Walon de Beaupuis, and Pierre Nicole—moved the scholars in 1646 to the cul-de-sac Saint-Dominique on the *rue* d'Enfer in Paris. Here they remained until dispersed yet again in 1650, whereupon they reorganized into three separate groups. As harassment of Jansenists increased under Mazarin between 1656 and 1660, however, first the boys' schools (in 1660) and then the girls' schools (in 1661) were closed. Although some of them reopened during the "Peace of the Church" (1669–1679), Louis XIV ordered these schools closed forever in 1679.[228]

But why did Church and state officials persecute the *petites écoles*? After all, during their entire 23-year history, these tiny primary and secondary schools assembled only 27 teachers and at most 250 students.[229] What possible danger did they represent? Perhaps the *abbé* Grégoire expressed it best when he said that "everyone" knew that the *petites écoles* were "friends of liberty."[230] Both those who taught and those who learned saw themselves as "God's students," free to discover "God's truth" wherever the search might lead them—and it often took them down unconventional pathways.[231]

Unlike other Catholic schools at which only men (like Jesuit priests) or women (like Ursuline nuns) provided instruction, at Port-Royal, teaching represented a collaborative effort by the solitaires, sisters, preceptors, almoners, servants, and friends of the convent—some male, some female, some ordained, most not ordained.[232] The solitaires (perhaps 27 in number) who taught at the *petites écoles* came from varied careers—theology, law, business, education, scholarship, literature, farming—to mention only a few.[233] Of these two dozen solitaires, four men—the *abbé* Saint-Cyran, Antoine Singlin, Pierre Nicole, and Claude Lancelot—tower above the rest.

School founder Saint-Cyran once declared: "It is my desire to have the ability to serve the children . . . I strive always to take great care of them once I have begun to teach them."[234] Beloved for his charity, patience, and kindness, Saint-Cyran brought passion to his teaching. During their short life span, the "Little Schools" reflected his spirit and educational ideals: love, tolerance, piety, gravity, interior grace with exterior constraint. In the pursuit of excellence, he combined two irreconcilable currents: the optimistic idealism of the Stoics with the pessimistic realism of the Hebrews. He admired the excellence and potential of human beings as created by God, but recognized the corruption brought by original sin. Therefore, he tried to preserve the innocence of these children as long as possible in order to teach them how to strengthen their Christian characters and govern their consciences.[235] Students read his textbook *Familiar Theology* (1642), a catechism that imparted "vigor and originality" to the study of Church doctrines and set the tone for their highly theocentric education. Saint-Cyran's pedagogy emphasized the love of God as manifested in Christ and the student's dependence on God (for grace, peace, joy, and liberty) in the daily combat with "the world, the flesh, and the Devil." "The life of man is nothing but combat," he preached; therefore, frequent penitence was necessary to overcome pride, egoism, and worldliness. Consequently, he taught his pupils to speak little, to tolerate much, and to pray always.[236]

His earliest associate, Antoine Singlin, taught first at the Port-Royal des Champs school, then at the Port-Royal de Paris branch, and later at La Pitié Hospital. At the "Little Schools," famous for catechizing their students well in Augustinian theology, Singlin stood head and shoulders above the rest as a thorough teacher of the catechism from 1637 to 1646. When he died in 1664, his body was interred at Port-Royal.[237]

Equally inspiring, Pierre Nicole taught philosophy, Latin, and the humanities at the cul-de-sac St.-Dominique school in Paris from 1646 to 1653, during which he earned his Bachelor of Arts degree in Theology with a thesis on the Beatitudes, the trinity and grace. He taught next at The Grange school from 1653 to 1656, and then at the *petite école* at Troux from 1656 to 1660. When Mazarin closed the boys' schools, Nicole taught girls at Troyes and Chartres after 1660.[238] In 1670 he published his famous *Treatise on the Education of a Prince* reflecting the pedagogical methods employed at the "Little Schools." A balanced curriculum must include history, mathematics, languages, geography, politics, philosophy, and commerce. He stressed the importance of regular schedules and physical exercise. More than a century before Jean-Jacques Rousseau, Nicole emphasized the need to train the body, mind, and spirit equally in order to develop good taste, build virtuous character, avoid vice, and inculcate morality in the child. While other schools forced students to memorize without thinking, the *petites écoles* had them memorize "only that which is excellent," preferring that they learn practical skills and develop "honest curiosity."[239]

Claude Lancelot, Nicole's colleague and Saint-Cyran's former pupil and friend, demonstrated a real talent for instructing children. He taught Greek and mathematics at the "Little Schools" from 1638 to 1665; he also wrote twelve textbooks on how to learn Greek, Latin, Italian, Spanish, and French (most still published in the 1760s and 1770s). Like his peripatetic colleagues Singlin, Nicole, Le Maître, and Séricourt, Lancelot followed his scholars from Paris to Ferte-Milon, Port-Royal des Champs, Troux, St. Severan, and Chesnay as necessity required. After Mazarin closed the "Little Schools," Lancelot taught the sons of the prince de Conti and the *duc* de Chevreuse while participating in the "pamphlet war" to defend Jansenism. For his opposition, Louis XIV exiled him in 1679 to a Benedictine abbey in Brittany. Six years before he died there in 1695, he and the *duc* de Mazarin dined with another wanderer—James II of England—as the exiled monarch made his way to Versailles in 1689.[240]

As with the number of professors at the *petites écoles*, historians disagree on how many students attended from 1637 to 1660, perhaps because enrollment fluctuated in response to many factors (civil war, plague, persecution). Because each teacher had only five or six pupils in a class, probably one or two dozen youth studied at Port-Royal des Champs, at The Grange, in Paris, or at Chesnay at any one time.[241] Nonetheless, over a quarter century, the total enrollment may have reached as high as 250 students.[242]

Many of these pupils came from wealthy, upper class families. In his study of the *petites écoles*, Frédéric Delforge (1985) found the sons of the sword nobility: at least two dukes, four marquis, four seigneurs, four controllers, three army officers, and two presidents of the Grand Council. Many more came from the robe nobility: vicars-general, *parlementaires*, councilors of state, masters of requests, and *intendants*. Still others came from bourgeois backgrounds: physicians, priests, canons, writers, abbots.[243] Although nearly all came from Catholic families, the faculty accepted the son of a Calvinist (monsieur du Foi of Sedan) because his Catholic mother had sent him to Port-Royal in 1653 "to make him a Catholic."[244] Many alumni embarked on distinguished careers as councilors of state, magistrates in Parlement, and masters of requests; others became writers, poets, historians, teachers, and clerics.[245]

On the honor roll of distinguished alumni, certainly three names—Pierre Du Fossé, Le Nain de Tillemont, and Jean Racine—shine brightly. In 1643 when only nine years old, Pierre Thomas du Fossé and his two brothers entered the school at Port-Royal des Champs. At first terribly homesick, they soon grew to love their teachers (Saint-Cyran, Singlin, Le Maître, Séricourt, Nicole and Lancelot) who "raised us in piety, innocence, & simplicity."[246] Despite numerous moves to different campuses, Du Fossé mastered Greek, Latin, poetry, prose, and public speaking so well that he translated Ancient ecclesiastical documents for Chancelor Séguier. He later taught in the "Little School" in Paris.[247]

One of his pupils, Le Nain de Tillemont, with his brothers Sébastien, Claude, and Pierre, enrolled at the cul-de-sac school in Paris. As a child, he knew several members of the Arnauld family (Angélique, Agnès, and Antoine); his teachers included Nicole, Singlin, and de Sacy. Focusing his attention on Roman and early Christian history, Tillemont developed expertise in ecclesiastical history. Despite his penchant for minutia and his rather tiresome writing style, his six-volume *History of the Emperors* and sixteen-volume *Ecclesiastical History* earned him praise from Clement XI for its collection of original documents. Scholars for the next two centuries referred to these works.[248]

Orphaned at three in 1643, nine-year-old Jean Racine came to Port-Royal as a charity student with his recently widowed grandmother, Marie Des Moulins, in 1649. Like many pupils, his family had several ties to the abbey. His great aunt Suzanne Des Moulins had lived there as a nun (1625–1647); his aunt Agnès Des Moulins had entered the convent at 15 in 1642. From 1649 to 1653 and again from 1655 to 1658, Jean studied Greek, Latin, the Bible, and other Christian works. While still a boy, he filled his notebook with lengthy essays on such Greek figures as Homer, Plato, Pindar, Plutarch, Flavius Joseph, Basil the Great, Heliodorus, Diogenes the Cynic, Lucien, Polycarpe, Valentinian, and St. Denis of Alexandria. He demonstrated his skills at Latin in essays on Virgil, Horace, Cicero, Pliny, Quintillian, Tacitus, and Philo. Turning to the Bible, he wrote discourses on Queen Athaliah and the Israelites. As a teenager, he penned odes praising his "excellent education" at Port-Royal.[249] And near the end of his life, in his *Short History of Port-Royal*, this loyal alumnus praised his alma mater. "Never was there an asylum where innocence and purity were more protected from the contaminated atmosphere of the century," he exclaimed, "nor a school where the truths of Christianity were more solidly taught."[250] Although he admitted "the scandals of my past life," when he wrote his will in 1698, France's leading dramatist asked to be buried at Port-Royal des Champs. His gift of 800 *livres* no doubt paved the way for his burial there when he died in April 1699.[251]

Aside from their outstanding faculty and distinguished alumni, however, the true uniqueness of the *petites écoles* lay in their innovative curriculum and pedagogical methods. Unlike teachers at other French schools and universities, the Jansenists "broke once and for all with the spirit of mediaevalism." Rejecting Aristotle and the scholastics, they sought to apply the principles of French philosopher and mathematician René Descartes, English scientist Francis Bacon, and Moravian reformer John Comenius. Furthermore, for the first time in the history of boys' education, the "Little Schools" replaced the traditional Latin-based instruction with French. Oral instruction came first to teach the art of careful listening; written instruction came second to concretize learning. And while little scholars all over Paris wrote their essays with goose quill pens, those at Port-Royal composed theirs using the newly invented metal pen nibs. Their classes in anatomy, physiology and astronomy ventured outdoors in natural settings to learn from "God's second book" (nature) rather than from textbooks. Also unlike other schools, students and teachers at the *petites écoles* labored together in the gardens, fields, orchards, and vineyards, combining physical with mental labor. Recognizing that boys needed recreation, teachers had them build model forts, wage mock battles, and play useful games to strengthen bodies and minds.[252]

Perhaps surprisingly, in this highly religious environment, students were not required to attend Mass. Boys at all Jesuit schools and even marine officers in training at Brest, Toulon, and Rochefort attended Mass every single day—but not at Port-Royal. Why? Because the Jansenists believed that only those "with a sincere receptiveness to the spirit of the Eucharist," those who felt themselves "worthy of receiving the sacraments," should attend holy services—and that infrequently.[253] In an era that despised religious liberty and regimented religious observance, the *petites écoles* offered their pupils freedom of choice. While they sought to preserve the children's innocence, candor, and simplicity, teachers also wanted to develop their reason, self-control, and conscience.[254]

The accomplishment of these goals required small classes—only five or six students per teacher meeting in four classrooms. Tutors sought ways to make their instruction clear, following logical steps to make learning less difficult and more fun. Instead of memorizing Latin declensions, their pupils learned the universal rules of grammar that could be applied to the study of any language.[255] Although firmly based on an Augustinian theological foundation, the teaching methods at Port-Royal celebrated the freedom of the human will in the struggle against pride and egotism. Therefore, in addition to requiring some memorization, the teachers encouraged students to think, reason logically, and use their imaginations. Besides lecturing, they engaged their pupils in dialogues, debates, and discussions (in French, of course) to arouse their curiosity and deepen their analytical abilities—something other schools discouraged. However, being thorough Jansenists, they excised the arts (novels, theater, dance, painting) from the curriculum as manifestations of "worldliness" that fed human vanity.[256]

Of course, the tight, almost monastic schedules maintained at the *petites écoles*—dividing each day into hour and half-hour blocks—also militated against worldly vanity. The older boys rose at 5 a.m. (younger ones at 6 a.m.) for prayers and private preparation of their lessons until breakfast at 8 a.m. Lectures and studying followed until dinner at 11 a.m. and then recreation until time to study geography and history at 1 p.m. Sacred literature and poetry came next at 2 p.m., and further study time (with a brief snack break) until supper at 6 p.m., followed by recreation until study time at 8 p.m., prayers at 8:30 p.m., and bedtime at 9 p.m. They did not go to school on Sundays, but studied their catechism, attended Mass, read pious books, enjoyed promenades, gathered for vespers, and studied again before going to bed.[257]

While the Jasenists included many of the same courses offered at other Catholic schools, they approached them differently. As mentioned above, French—not Latin as in other schools—was the lingua franca for all instruction. Also, in all courses, students learned to read and write about that subject simultaneously (other schools emphasized only reading). Moreover, instead of reading portions of literary works and memorizing them, Port-Royal students studied the entire work, exploring the author's meaning and analyzing his thesis and supporting evidence. Teachers also gave more emphasis to geography and history (especially Ancient History)—at least one hour every day. They devoted much more time to mathematics (including arithmetic, geometry, algebra, astronomy, optics, perspective, mechanics, and music theory) than did the Jesuits (perhaps because the latter taught math in Latin). After studying the speeches of Greeks (Aristotle, Euripides, and Sophocles) and Romans (Cicero, Quintilian, and Seneca), students composed their own and delivered them. In addition to metaphysics and logic, philosophy classes encompassed morality and physics (although the curriculum included few laboratory sciences).[258]

In the study of languages, whereas most institutions focused exclusively on Latin, the brighter students at the "Little Schools" also tackled Hebrew (to understand the Old Testament) and Greek (to grasp the New Testament). The Jesuits, considering Greek a pagan language, disparaged those who studied it as "Hellenists" and suspected them of heresy. Given the prevalent anti-Semitism in France, those who studied Hebrew were also suspected of heresy. To help younger students master Latin declensions, Lancelot composed 261 six-line strophes as a mnemonic device; he also translated Roman names into French equivalents (Trebatius became M. de Trébace and Pomponius, M. de Pomponne). Another radical innovation was the teaching of modern languages such as Italian and Spanish.[259]

The small teacher/student ratios at the "Little Schools" also promoted a family atmosphere. In their efforts to preserve their students from the "miasma of the world," teachers built a spiritual wall around them by praying with them, exhorting them, and guiding their character development. The rhythms of daily life, their schedule of study, and their close association in working, eating, and playing together replicated a close family feeling. It also greatly reduced discipline problems. At the *petites écoles*, "discipline" meant helping children become "disciples of Christ," for the two words shared the same root (*discere*, to learn). Therefore, unlike other Catholic institutions, Jansenist schools rarely employed physical punishment. Instead, the faculty encouraged each boy to progress from dependence to autonomy by helping him develop self-discipline.[260]

At the *filles régentes*, the sisters taught self-discipline to their female students as well. Contemporaries praised the superior education girls received at the Port-Royal schools. Monsieur Cousin exclaimed: "The women are perhaps extraordinary, and assuredly as great as the men . . . in intrepidity of soul and depth of thought."[261] Racine believed that these girls had "edified the world by their wisdom and virtue."[262] Even the *abbé* Fromageau, charged by the Archbishop of Paris with inspecting female education, extolled the Port-Royal schools as "excellent": "One can find nothing to compare with the education they give the children," he wrote.[263]

In the seventeenth century, nuns taught the girls at Port-Royal des Champs and at Port-Royal in Paris. When Mazarin closed these schools in 1660, however, the Jansenists did not abandon the idea of female education. In the eighteenth century, they operated three schools in Paris. The Community of Sainte-Marthe, founded by Madame Théodon, opened in 1713 in the pavilion Adam on the *rue* Saint-Antoine. In 1726, this Community opened a free school for poor girls in Saint-Severin parish directed by Madame de Fleury (wife of the advocate-general). Somewhat later, Véronique Tabourin opened the Filles de Sainte-Geneviève (or Filles Noires) school, which taught reading, writing, and handcrafts to poor and bourgeois girls.[264]

If the original purpose of the *petites écoles* was to train better priests, the goal of the *filles régentes* was to prepare "perfect nuns or excellent wives and mothers." [265] The driving force behind these girls' schools was Jacqueline Pascal, sister to the poet Blaise Pascal and aunt to Marguerite Périer of the "Miracle of the Thorn" fame. Truly gifted, Jacqueline wrote poetry at eight, composed a five-act drama at eleven, and published a book of her poems at twelve. Invited to Court at thirteen, she charmed Richelieu and composed two poems on the spot for Queen Anne. But after nearly dying from smallpox in 1638, she wrote only austere, religious verse. Her poem "On the Conception of the Virgin" won her the Prix de la Tour award. When Jansenist folk practitioners allegedly healed her brother Etienne of a broken hip in 1646, the family began visiting Port-Royal. When her father died in 1651, Jacqueline entered the convent; guided by *Mère* Agnès, she took her vows in 1653 and became schoolmistress.[266]

Despite a busy teaching schedule, Sister Jacqueline de Sainte-Euphémie continued writing sacred poetry, a biography, an autobiography, letters, and devotional literature. The influence of the Bible, Catholic liturgy, patristic literature, and the guidance of individuals like Saint-Cyran, Antoine Arnauld, *Mère* Angélique and *Mère* Agnès are clearly visible in her style. Her poems emphasize feminine images of God—a radical departure from traditional Catholic portrayals of the divinity. Jacqueline's *On the Mystery of the Death of Our Lord Jesus Christ* (1651) matches each moment in Christ's passion with the virtues his female disciples should emulate. Her *Report of Sister Jacqueline de Sainte-Euphémie to the Mother Prioress of Port-Royal des Champs* (1653) provides a self-portrait of the writer's life and ideals. When *Mère* Angélique died in 1661, Jacqueline wrote her biography, portraying her as the ideal nun who feared God and espoused moral rigorism. The *Interpretation of Sister Jacqueline de Sainte-Euphémie* (1661) vigorously defends Port-Royal against charges of heresy. Her many letters (from 1647 to 1661) contest the right of males to overrule females' consciences.[267]

But Sister Jacqueline's most famous work—the *Rule for Children* (1657), composed at the request of the *abbé* Singlin—like Pierre Nicole's *Treatise on the Education of a Prince*, created the model for female education. Teachers, she states, must know the moral character of their girls and guide them in cultivating humility (the key virtue) and avoiding dishonesty (the chief vice). Because their salvation requires constant surveillance, classes must be kept small, the girls should meet with their teachers in biweekly conferences (where sisters recorded their behavioral improvements or transgressions), and the nuns must set high standards for "good confessions."[268]

Perhaps to a greater degree than the boys in the *petites écoles*, the daily schedule at the *filles régentes* integrated the girls more closely into the life of the convent. They lived, ate, and worshiped with the nuns; they even wore long robes with veils. The older ones, hearing the wakeup call "Jesus!", rose at 4 a.m.; the next older, at 4:30 a.m.; and the youngest, at 5:00 a.m. The girls said their prayers, kissed the floor, silently dressed in the commons room, and then prayed aloud together. At 6:00 a.m., they attended prime, where they prayed and recited the psalms while standing. After making their beds and washing their mouths with water and wine, they ate breakfast (in silence) at 6:30 a.m. as a nun read to them some martyr's tale. At 7:30 a.m., depending on their ages, they cleaned their rooms, played in pairs, or engaged in sewing, knitting, or needlework (silently). Readings by the schoolmistress followed at 8:00 a.m., *terce* at 8:30 a.m., and Mass (at which they knelt) at 9:00 a.m. Then (from 10:00 to 11:00 a.m.) they wrote their lessons, sang Gregorian chants (11:00 a.m.-noon), recited psalms and prayers at *sext* (noon), and ate lunch—again, in complete silence while a nun read aloud. After lunch, they enjoyed a couple hours of "serious conversation" in the commons or played knucklebones and badminton for exercise. Following prayer and admonition, they spent fifteen minutes confessing their faults before returning to their lessons and catechism. They sewed from 2:30 to 3:00 p.m., and then, depending on their ages, attended *none*, recited their catechism, or read in silence. Those under fourteen enjoyed a snack at 3:30 p.m., and attended classes at 4:00 p.m. while the older girls went to vespers. All convened for a silent supper at 6:00 p.m., followed by recreation in the garden until time for prayers and psalms at 7:00 p.m. (*compline*). Bedtime (like rising time) came earlier for the girls (8:00 p.m.) than for the boys (9:00 p.m.). Each girl slept in a separate bed to avoid the temptation of touching, kissing, and caressing one another. On feast days, the nuns allowed their pupils to sleep late (until 6:00 a.m.); although they still attended Mass and said their prayers and recitations, the girls sang French hymns and enjoyed more time to play. [269] As Sister Jacqueline declared (no doubt with utter seriousness), "Children simply do not have the strength to devote every hour in the day to God's service."[270]

Although their daily schedule shows that the girls devoted more time to "God's service" than the boys, they also studied their lessons, but separate from the boys. While the Jansenists provided a quality education for both girls and boys, they (like all schools at that time) did not integrate the sexes in the classroom. Both practical and religious, the curriculum for girls—though less ambitious than at the *petites écoles*—included lessons in theology, French hymnody, French and Latin grammar, reading the psalter, and writing. Their textbooks included traditional Catholic sources such as the *Imitation of Christ*, Louis de Granade's *Catechism* and *Sermons* (1602), St. Francis de Sales' *Introduction to the Devout Life* (1640), St. Jerome's *Letters* (1679), St. Theresa of Avila's *Meditations* (1665) and her *Path to Perfection* (1688). But they also studied Jansenist literature such as Antoine Arnauld's *Church Traditions* (1644), Saint-Cyran's *Letters* (1645) and his *Simple Theology* (1643), the *Hours of Port-Royal* (1650), and Arnauld d'Andilly's translations of *Christian Almsgiving* (1647) and *The Heavenly Ladder* (1652).[271]

Given their rigid daily regimen, lengthy reading list, close supervision, and the imposition of silence while they ate, worked, studied, worshiped, and exercised, discipline, as one might expect, presented few problems at Port-Royal.[272] As the rules forbade teachers from praising their pupils "excessively" and from showing favoritism, so they also prevented them from publicly rebuking or correcting the girls—especially in anger. "Postpone the punishment until [your] irritation is past," *Mère* Agnès advised, so that "they may realize that [you] love them no less when [you] punish them than when [you] praise them."[273] Non-corporal punishment often took the form of wearing a sign proclaiming a girl's offense ("lazy," "careless," or "liar") around her neck. Those breaking the rule of silence wore posters with large red tongues painted on them.[274] Shaming—not whipping—was the rule at Port-Royal des Champs.

Yet this educational regimen, which in the twenty-first century appears narrow and repressive, was for its time socially subversive. The Jansenists taught their girls Latin—the lingua franca of the Church, medicine, and law—so that they could read and understand the Psalter, the exclusive provenance of male priests. They insisted that they read their French Bibles every day—something very few priests, bishops, or popes did—and apply its principles to their lives. Even more radical, Port-Royal's girls studied Saint-Cyran's *Familiar Theology* even though this catechism had been condemned by the Archibishop of Paris in 1643. Furthermore, the nuns encouraged their charges to ask questions, participate in discussions, and seek to understand the deeper issues rather than simply memorizing words. While practicing the virtues of humility, respect, and love, the girls also learned to speak their minds in defense of truth—something that Church officials found hard to accept.[275]

One ten-year-old pupil, accustomed to speaking boldly, accompanied her mother to Court. Knowing that the countess' daughter had been educated at Port-Royal, Archbishop Péréfixe shared his impressions following his recent inspection of the convent. Then, turning to the little girl, he asked if she thought his report gave a true representation. Imagine his shock when the tyke replied, "I admire the profoundness of God's judgments for having given us a prelate as ignorant as you are!"[276]

Such holy boldness, especially when exercised in defense of a condemned heresy like Jansenism, aroused the animosity of Port-Royal's enemies, chief among them the Society of Jesus. They resented others' praising the "Little Schools" for providing "the most perfect education that one could give" to "cultivate the minds" of "honest men and good Christians."[277] Their hatred for heresy and their jealousy of the *petites écoles* as competitors in the educational market led them to view these schools as training camps for an anti-Jesuit militia (which, in a sense, they were).[278]

Jansenist and Jesuit education differed markedly from each other. The *petites écoles* never had more than 50 students at any one time; by contrast, the Jesuit schools in Paris alone had over 13,000 pupils. Whereas the Jansenists wanted their students to be disciples of Christ who loved eternal things and hated sin, the Jesuits wanted to produce brilliant students who would bring glory to their teachers and their alma maters.[279] To this end, all Jesuit schools followed the *Ratio Studiorum* ("Plan of Studies"), an educational manual published in 1599. Boys (the Jesuits did not teach girls), who entered elementary school at nine or ten, spent five or six years studying grammar, Latin, humanities, and rhetoric before graduating to the academy where they focused on philosophy, moral theology, and disputation for another two years. They sat in huge classrooms where proctors (older students) reported their misdeeds to the teachers. All discourse, both oral and written, was in Latin. The system, which discouraged freedom of thought as "a dangerous impiety," encouraged rote memorization and competition by dividing classes into groups, administering frequent exams, and giving winners lavish praise and tangible awards. Students read excerpts from books, focusing on style rather than content, and memorizing words rather than analyzing ideas.[280]

The two educational systems differed in other ways as well. Jansenist teachers, who valued the dignity of every child, gave the same education to rich and poor, showed them respect, and granted them significant responsibilities. The Jesuits, on the other hand, preferred teaching the children of the wealthy elite and saw little value in infants and children, whom they viewed as imperfect adults requiring firm control. The pro-Cartesian Jansenists taught students to think for themselves, whereas the anti-Cartesian Jesuits made them memorize words without understanding their meaning. Consequently, Jansenists granted their pupils more freedom and responsibility, while the Society of Jesus expected subordination and implicit obedience from their scholars. Whereas Jansenists saw Antiquity as only the first stage in the history of the world, which was changing rapidly, the Society of Jesus saw Antiquity as the "age of perfection" and Moderns as poor imitators of the Ancients. If the Jansenists condemned the secular creative arts (poetry, drama, novels, dance, instrumental music), the Jesuits encouraged them by awarding prizes to the best students in these areas. The "Little Schools" shunned fencing, horseback riding, and swimming, and permitted no debating clubs or theatrical plays—all activities avidly promoted at Jesuit schools. While Jesuit training aimed at developing well-rounded citizens and leaders in society, Jansenist education, through self-denial and self-discipline, created ascetic, polemical alumni.[281]

But as Monique Cottret (1998) so aptly stated: "The worship of poverty is an evangelical value which can easily become revolutionary."[282] Alumni of the *petites écoles*—with their talent for critical analysis, their taste for liberty, and their love of polemics—soon aroused the suspicions of a growing host of enemies. The Paris police, for example, who resented the nuns' and solitaires' confrontational attitude toward authority, saw Port-Royal's schools as hotbeds of rebellion.[283] In 1648, the lieutenant civil, investigating Jesuit rumors that students were being "nourished in heresy," visited the convent, but found the reports untrue. Five years later, however, another police inspector, professing to find heresy at the Saint-Dominique school, shut it down.[284]

With the publication of Pascal's sixteenth *Provincial Letter* in 1656 and Alexander VII's Bull *Ad sacram* in 1657, Jansenists and their schools came under increasing fire from Church and state officials. When Antoine Arnauld, seeking to defuse the situation, sent Queen Anne and Mazarin letters denying the harmful rumors against Port-Royal des Champs, the attempt backfired. By the Declaration of 7 June 1659, Louis XIV ordered the students dispersed. On 11 March 1660, lieutenant-civil Dreux d'Aubry arrived, *lettre de cachet* in hand, and within twenty-four hours, brought an end to the pedagogical achievements of the past twenty-four years. Aubry told the students to return to their families. In April he ordered all the pensioners, novices, and postulants to leave as well, then returned a month later to insure they had done so.[285]

But severing the head of the "hydra of heresy" (a favorite Jesuit metaphor) only produced more heads. In 1678 Pierre Nicole established a girls' school at Troyes. In 1709 Monsieur Tabourin founded a unique elementary school for both boys and girls at St. Etienne du Mont in Paris. The Sisters of Sainte-Marthe opened a girls' school in Paris in 1713 with Archbishop Noailles' approval. During the 1720s, the Vannist academies became important centers of Jansenist polemics. Far from disappearing, by 1789, according to Howard Barnard (1913), at least 32 Jansenist schools with 6000–7000 pupils existed throughout France.[286]

Despite being uprooted in 1661, therefore, the "Little Schools," like a fertile tree, dispersed their seeds far and wide during the following century. They would bear fruit, not only in the lives of its alumni, but also in the ideas that refused to die—liberty, individualism, hatred of the world, and defense of the truth.[287]

To keep these ideals alive, Jansenists everywhere grabbed their metal-tipped pens and wrote voluminously. On one occasion, the theologian Jacques de Sainte-Beuve told Bossuet that he refused to consult the nuns at Port-Royal des Champs because if he visited them, "there will be a book published against me immediately [for] they cannot keep themselves from writing."[288] Indeed they could not, for defending the truth required active pens. Censure, prison, exile—these only increased their self-confidence.[289] In his delightful manuscript, "The Literary History of Port-Royal," Clémencet describes Port-Royal's history as "a war full of battles between error and truth" for nearly a century.[290] Rumors flew that the convent had "a dozen sharp pens at the ready to refute all comers."[291]

Judging by their output, however, one might imagine that Port-Royal employed scores of apologists. Estimates differ regarding the number of their publications, but they are impressive nonetheless. The two-volume *Jansenist Library* (1740) estimated that from 1611 to 1740, Jansenists wrote at least 304 "suspected works"—about two each year.[292] But Dominique de Colonia, in his *Dictionary of Jansenist Books or Those Favoring Jansenism* (1752), counted at least 1067 Jansenist works between 1611 and 1752—almost eight per year.[293]

These publications took many forms: histories, biographies, autobiographies, theological treatises, letters, pamphlets, sermons, and funeral encomiums. In 1654, when Antoine Singlin asked Angélique Arnauld to write her autobiography, she penned the *Relation Written by Mother Angélique Arnauld about Port-Royal.* At her death in 1661, her niece Angélique de Saint-Jean gathered relevant documents and wrote a biography of her aunt—*Memories of the Life of the Reverend Mother Angélique de Ste. Madéleine Arnauld, Reformer of Port-Royal.* She also produced one of the first histories of the convent—*Memories of the History of Port-Royal*—as well as several necrologies of its nuns, solitaires, and friends. Throughout the 1660s, various sisters wrote apologetic *Relations* to answer charges against them and to defend the truth. Frequently republished in the eighteenth century, these accounts burnished the image of Port-Royal in the minds of those who remembered it as a pure community that defied Church and state. In the 1750s, for example, Charles Clémencet produced two influential works: a ten-volume *General History of Port-Royal* and a four-volume manuscript, the "Literary History of Port-Royal." More hagiography than history, these works extolled 228 nuns and 63 solitaires who stood for truth amidst persecution from 1643 to 1747.[294]

Another means of defending their way of life was by writing letters. As we have seen, the sisters were voracious letter writers. These letters, many of them lengthy epistles, proved useful in answering the charges levied against them and in recruiting powerful defenders to their cause. In her letters to the Queen of Poland and to her brother Antoine, for example, Angélique Arnauld frequently listed the "horrible impostures" and "defamatory libels" leveled against her convent and proceeded to refute them.[295]

Generally, these Jansenist polemics lack the analytical depth and erudite tone found in the works of their contemporaries, the Bollandists and Molinists. But the men and women of Port-Royal were neither great critics nor great theologians: they were apologists, writing to clear their names of heresy and to defend the truth of efficacious grace. If necessary, they would die for the cause. Their interminable appeals, petitions, and protests to God, the pope, and the king against every perceived act of persecution reveals their love for "playing the martyr." Refusing to blindly submit to male Church authority (as women religious were expected to do), they blended defiance and acquiescent suffering into a balancing act of passive opposition. Putting their consciences above conformity, they walked a fine line between martyrdom and rebellion—a line others did not see as clearly as they did.[296]

Certainly none walked that tightrope more gingerly than *Mère* Angélique Arnauld, abbess and defender of Port-Royal for half a century. Between 1620 and 1661, she penned more than 1,500 letters, most written late at night after a full day of spiritual and administrative responsibilities.[297] These letters reveal a great deal about her personally and about the heart and soul of Jansenism at Port-Royal. Among the many topics she discusses, five themes stand out: her defense of the truth, her sufferings, her submission to God, her role as defender of Port-Royal, and her inner fears and doubts.[298]

In a letter to a friend in 1643, Angélique stated: "[I]t is necessary to repulse with force and vigor that which is said with such insolence against the truth, but those who know the truth must not be slack in their defense of it. Forceful [arguments] that confuse the enemies of God and the Church are not unchristian."[299] Never a slacker herself, she assured Archbishop François de Gondi in 1653 that although "the slanders continue here against those who are called Jansenists, especially against us [at Port-Royal], yet . . . the truth is sufficient to enlighten them . . . "[300] Nonetheless, those "slanders," spread largely by the Jesuits, made her anxious a year later when she told M. de Fleury that "we have great concerns about the horrible efforts our adversaries are making to crush the truth; but in the end, it is God's truth and everlasting with him . . . .[We] must love it & defend it [even] at the cost of our lives."[301]

Angélique's "martyr's complex"—her joy in suffering—also comes through clearly in her letters. She told the *princesse* de Guéménée: "God established the Gospel by the blood of the martyrs. We will be so happy if our humiliations and our sufferings assist in making the truth known to others."[302] She assured her brother Antoine that "it is necessary to suffer for the truth and to teach the faithful by your persecution . . . the practice of penitence far more ably than teaching the theory of it in your book."[303] In 1644, long before Port-Royal felt the rod of persecution, the abbess embraced suffering as "a grand and singular grace that God gives us."[304] She told Antoine that "it brings great joy to my spirit and I find much happiness to have a part in such a delightful persecution," because "God has chosen our family to serve his glory in our suffering."[305] When in 1655 the Sorbonne censured Antoine, his sister assured him of "the natural love & tenderness that I have always had for my poor little brother." She comforted him with the thought that "there is more to be happy than sad about if we suffer the injustice of men, because it helps us to hope in God's mercy." She promised him that "God will be with you and you will better serve his holy truth by your sufferings than by your writings."[306]

Yet Jansenists believed that suffering—whether inflicted by one's enemies or by God—could strengthen the Christian's experience. In scores of letters, Angélique insists that suffering purifies the character, justifies the soul, develops humility and patience, brings greater blessings, removes imperfections, imparts grace, strengthens the will, and separates one from the temptations of the world.[307]

The proper response, then, both to divinely imposed suffering and human persecution was submission. In a letter telling her solitaire friend Isaac Le Maître about the dangers facing Port-Royal des Champs during the Fronde, the abbess declared, "We will submit to God's will, and he extends great mercy to the persecuted and not to persecutors."[308] Throughout her letters, she emphasizes the necessity of humility, obedience, and total dependence on God.[309] In 1661, as Church and state restrictions tightened the noose around Port-Royal, she reminded her friends that "this is the hour of man. The hour of God will come, which shall disclose many things, and avenge all."[310]

Yet waiting for God's hour to arrive did not come easily to the strong-willed abbess, who felt it her duty in "the hour of man" to enlist the aid of powerful patrons in defending her convent. In 1659, following the Peace of the Pyrenees, she asked Louis XIV's mother, Anne of Austria, to become Port-Royal's protector. The pious Queen Mother, convinced that Marguerite Périer's recent healing had been a divine miracle, defended the abbey against Mazarin's attempts to close it.[311] When in May 1661 Louis XIV sent a *lettre de cachet* ordering Angélique to disperse her nuns and novices, she wrote Anne a seventeen-page letter begging her to intervene with her son and save the nuns, who "are not engaged in error & heresy," from the king's "indignation." "Calm this tempest," she pleaded, and "protect our innocence."[312]

Yet at the end of her life, this suffering saint had serious doubts concerning her own innocence. As she lay dying in July 1661, she described her condition as that of "a criminal at the foot of the scaffold awaiting the execution of the judge's order."[313] In a final letter to her brother Henri, Bishop of Angers, she begged him to pray for her soul.[314] In her last letter to her sister Agnès, she lamented: "The time of the martyrs is long passed, but the time to suffer and be reduced to powder in body as well as in soul is with us always."[315] Angélique's will to suffer, declared her sister, was her greatest legacy to the nuns at Port-Royal. She persuaded those who feared persecution to see it as a sign of divine favor, that "God has chosen us to suffer for his truth."[316]

But she believed that some people should suffer silently. Although most Jansenists praised Blaise Pascal for writing the *Provincial Letters* attacking the Jesuits and defending Port-Royal, Angélique disapproved of them. "We should not mix jesting with holy things," she admonished.[317] "Silence would have been more appropriate and more agreeable to God who is more pleased with tears and repentance than by eloquence, which amuses more people than it converts."[318] In her voluminous correspondence, Angélique Arnauld makes not a single reference to Pascal's *Provincial Letters*, arguably one of the most effective defenses of Jansenism produced in the seventeenth century.[319]

She preferred the more pious apologetics penned by her brothers Isaac and Robert. In his famous book of meditations, *Rejection of the World* (1618), Isaac Arnauld discourses at length on "man's stupidity," the world's "false visions," and humanity's need of "eternal values." As with his sister Angélique's letters, Isaac's meditations focus on the themes of defending the truth, developing virtue, submitting to God's judgments, and accepting afflictions.[320]

Although Robert Arnauld d'Andilly filled his *Journals* in the 1620s with details concerning Court gossip and ceremonies, Parlement's debates, foreign battles and treaties,[321] by 1645 he, too, was ready to reject the world and embrace asceticism. At 57, he joined the solitaires, telling Angélique, "If you only knew how disgusted I am with the world, you would have even more impatience than I to arrive at God's gateway . . . .I want to spend the rest of my life praying to God." He spent his remaining years writing in defense of Port-Royal, which he called "a paradise on earth."[322]

Yet as this chapter has shown, Port-Royal was also a "reactionary utopia." More than a convent, it was a movement defending Jansenist truth, conscience, and human liberty. While its wealthy supporters praised its bucolic rural setting, ascetic lifestyles, *petites écoles*, and scholarly output, its enemies despised the sisters and solitaires for their refusal to sign the Formulary and opposition to papal infallibility and royal absolutism. In the 1640s and 1650s, officials tightened censorship of Jansenist publications; printers caught disseminating their works had their licenses revoked. Port-Royal's defenders had to publish their writings clandestinely or seek foreign printers in Holland.[323] Despite the brief respite they gained after the "Miracle of the Thorn" in 1656, Mazarin closed their *petites écoles* four years later. Perhaps, when they learned of the first minister's death on 9 March 1661, the remaining sisters and solitaires hoped for better days ahead. But as they would soon discover, Louis XIV harbored greater animosity than Mazarin ever had toward those he considered *frondeurs*. Port-Royal's days were indeed numbered.[324]

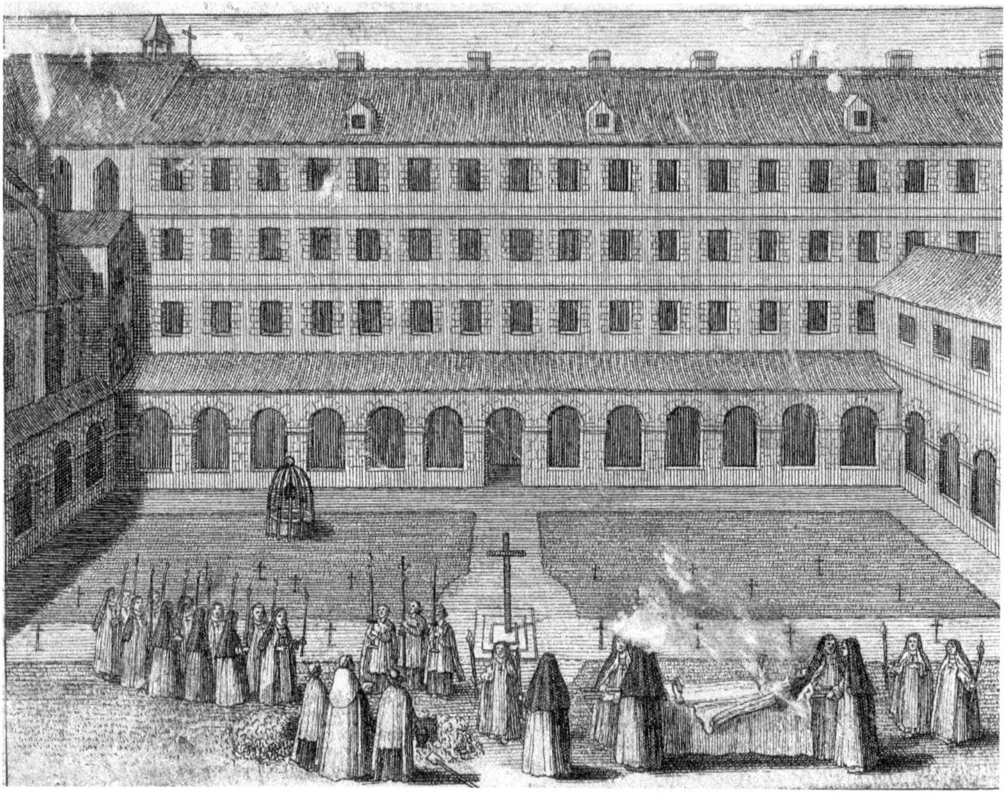

1 Cloisters and Cemetery of Port-Royal des Champs.

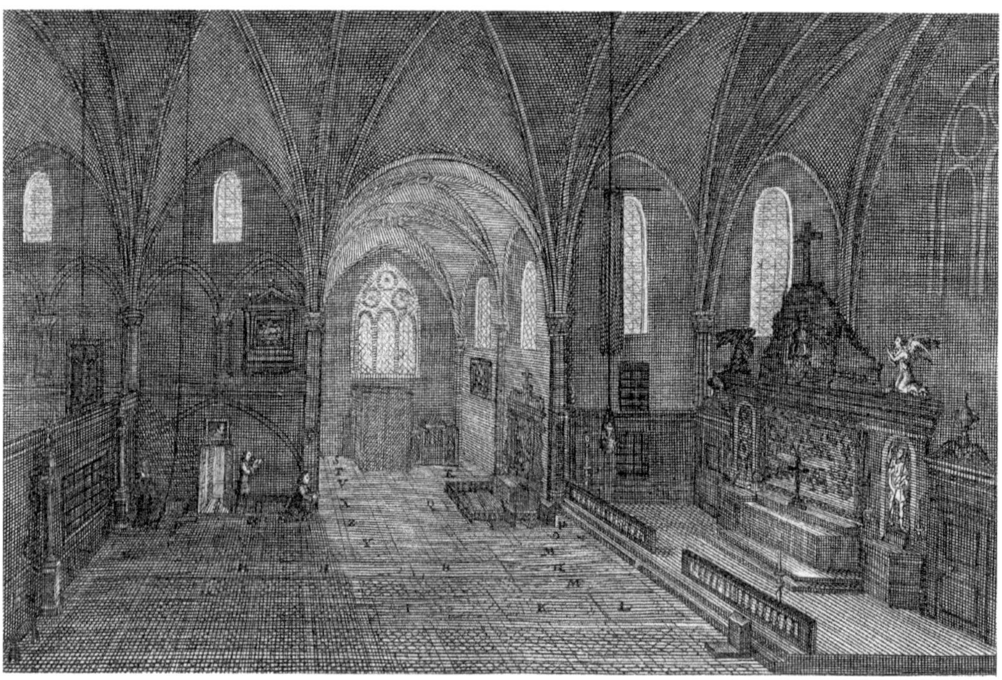

2 Church of the Abbey of Port-Royal des Champs dedicated to the Holy Virgin in the year 1230 AD under Pope Gregory IX.

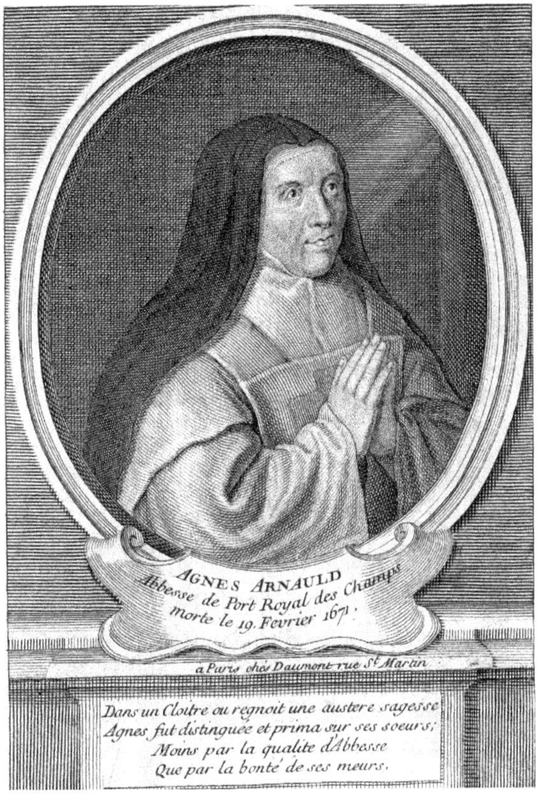
AGNES ARNAULD
Abbesse de Port Royal des Champs
morte le 19. Fevrier 1671.
a Paris chés Daumont rue St Martin
Dans un Cloitre ou regnoit une austere sagesse
Agnes fut distinguée et prima sur ses soeurs;
Moins par la qualité d'Abbesse
Que par la bonté de ses meurs.

3 Agnes Arnauld, Abbess of Port-Royal des Champs, who died on 19 February 1671.

4 The Nuns of Port-Royal des Champs ministering to the sick.

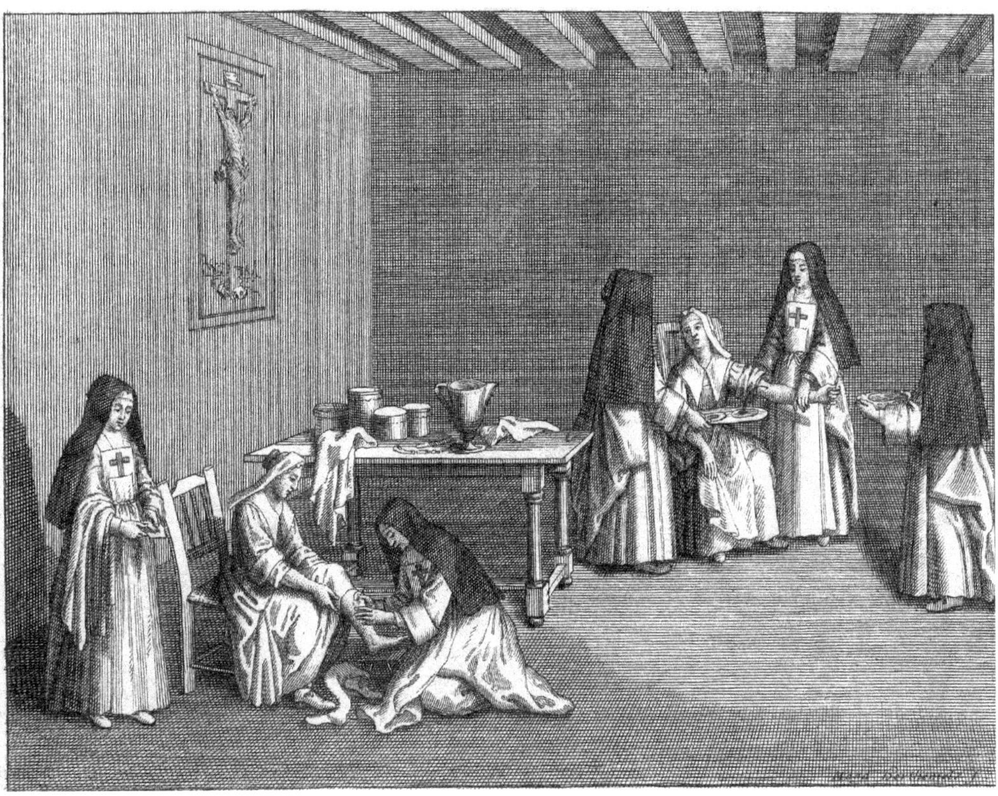

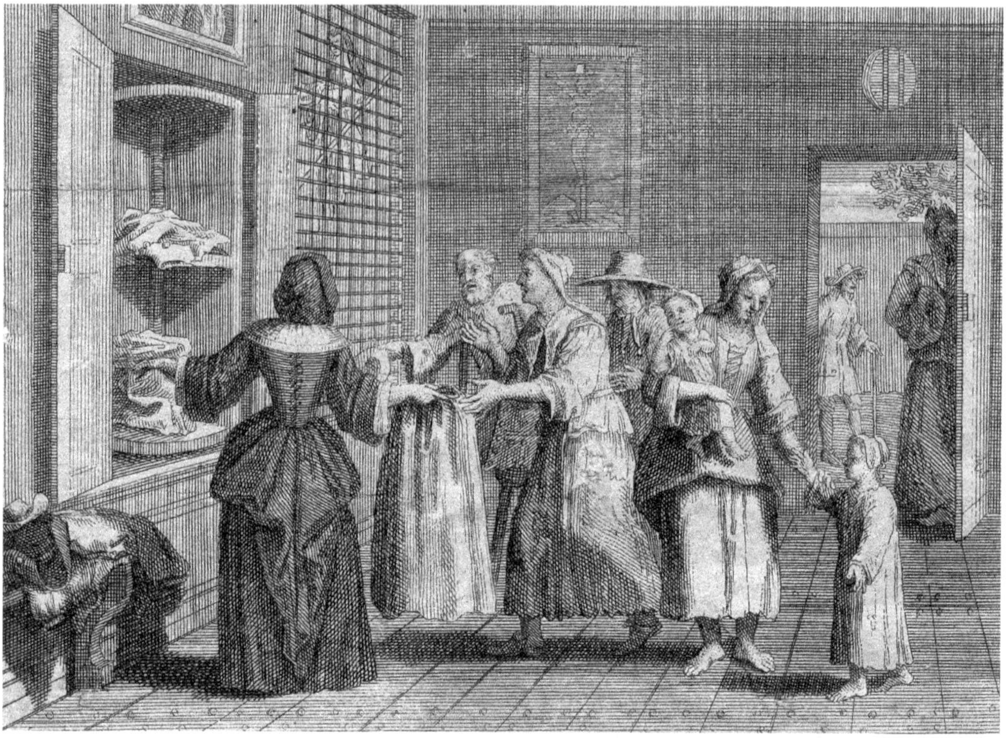

5 Distributing alms from Port-Royal des Champs.

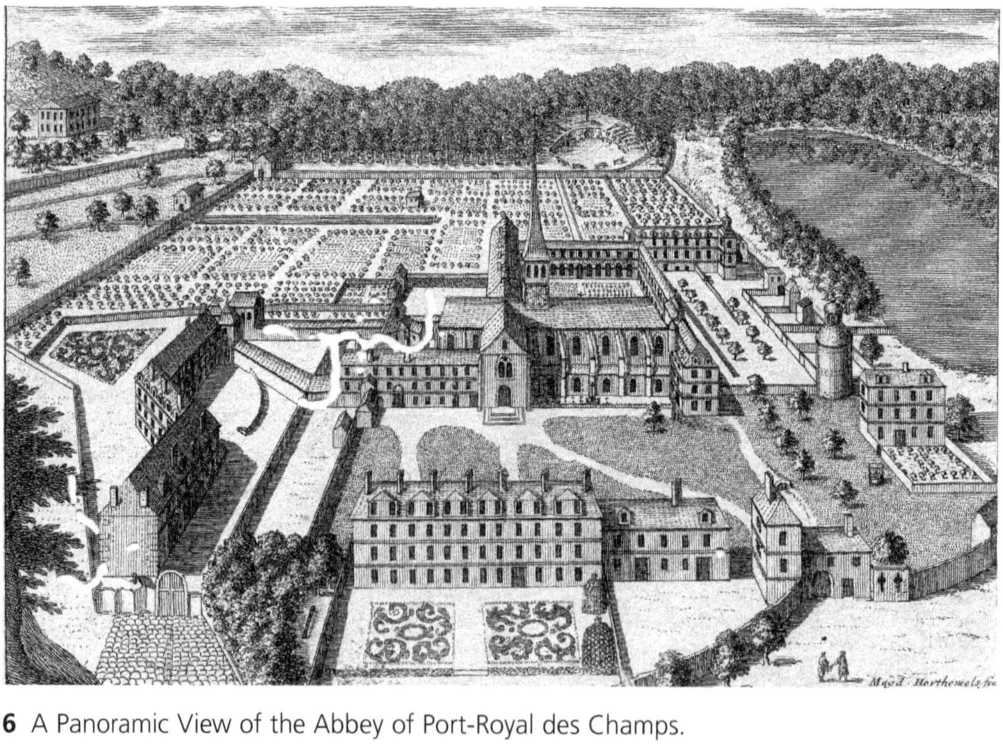

6 A Panoramic View of the Abbey of Port-Royal des Champs.

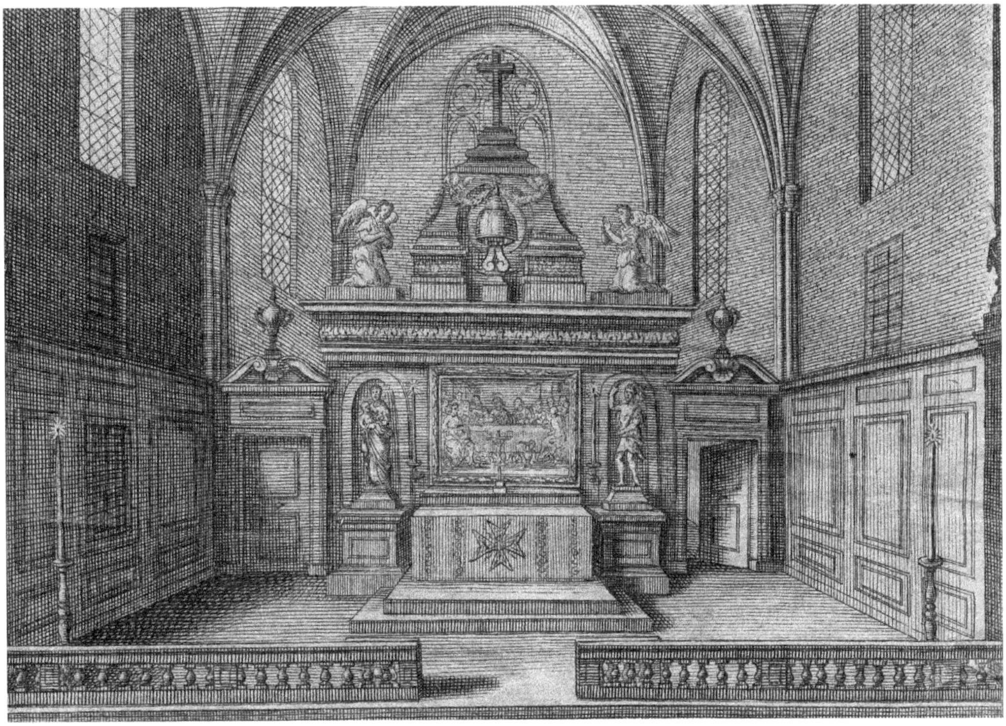

7 The high altar in the Church of Port-Royal des Champs.

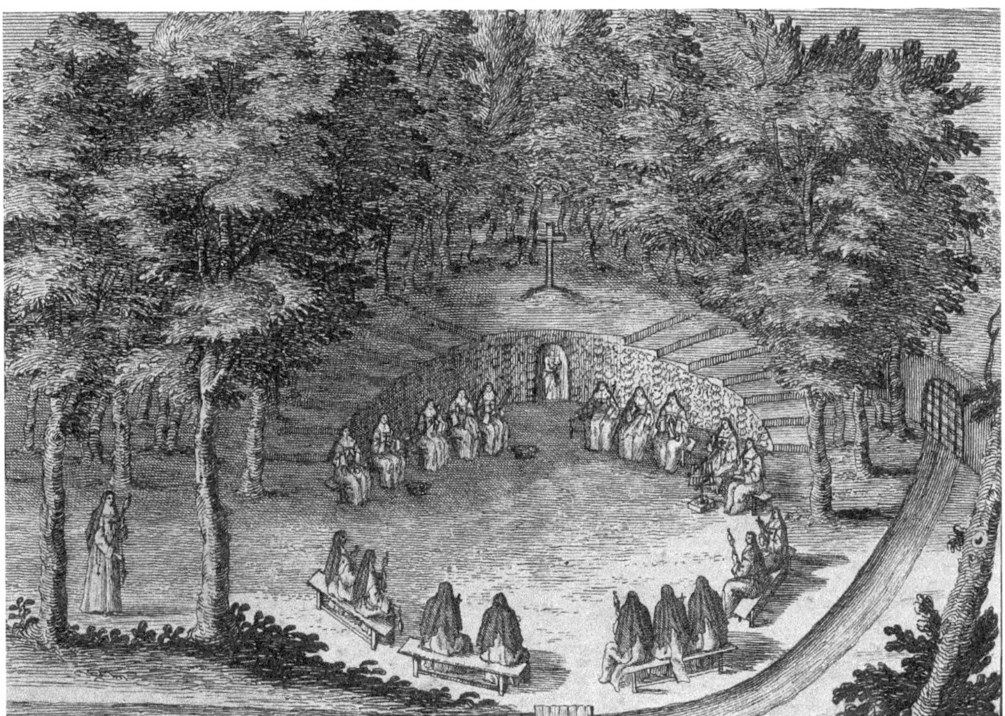

8 The Nuns of Port-Royal des Champs holding their Conference in Secrecy.

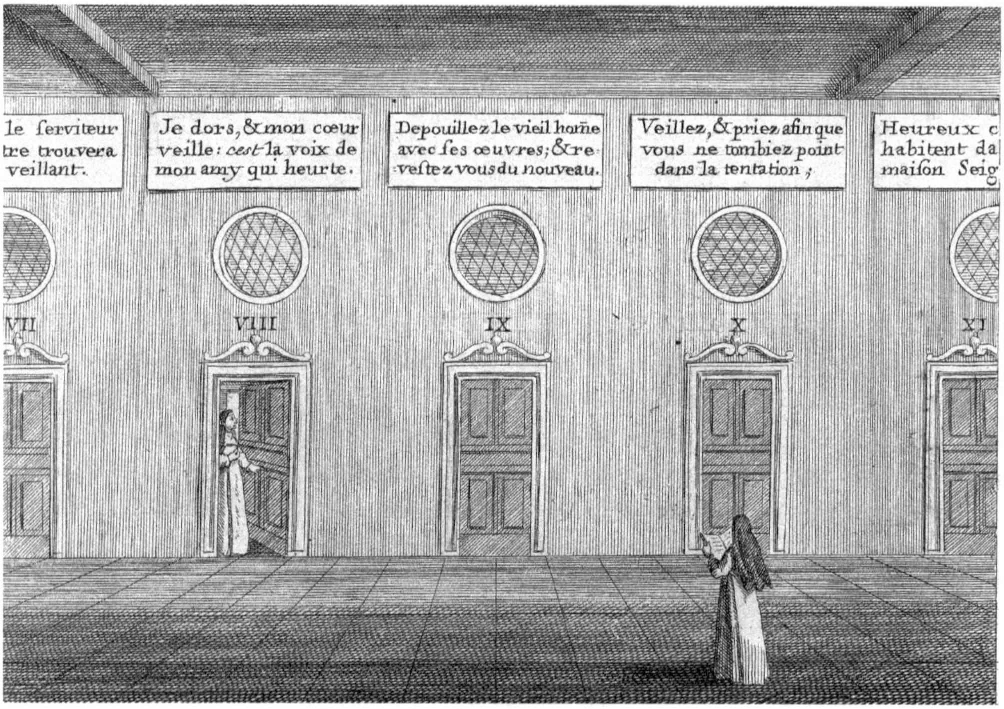
Je dors, &mon cœur veille: cest la voix de mon amy qui heurte.
Depouillez le vieil hoñe avec ſes œuvres; &reveſtez vous du nouveau.
Veillez, &priez afin que vous ne tombiez point dans la tentation;
VIII
IX
X

9 Dormitory of the Nuns at Port-Royal des Champs.

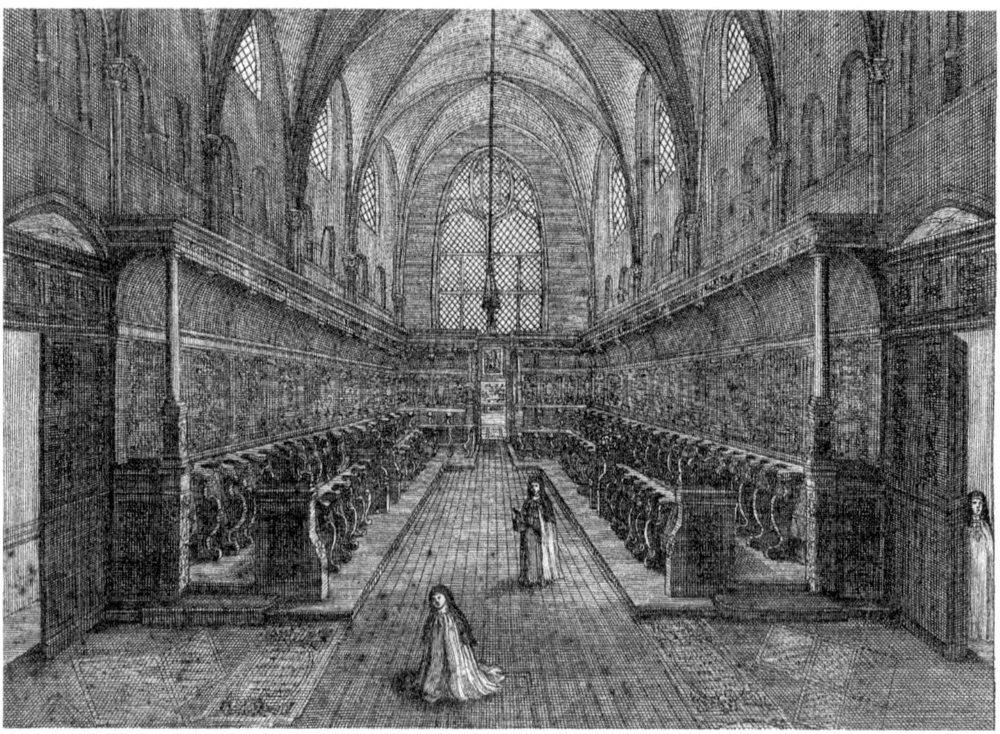

10 Choir of the Nuns at Port-Royal des Champs.

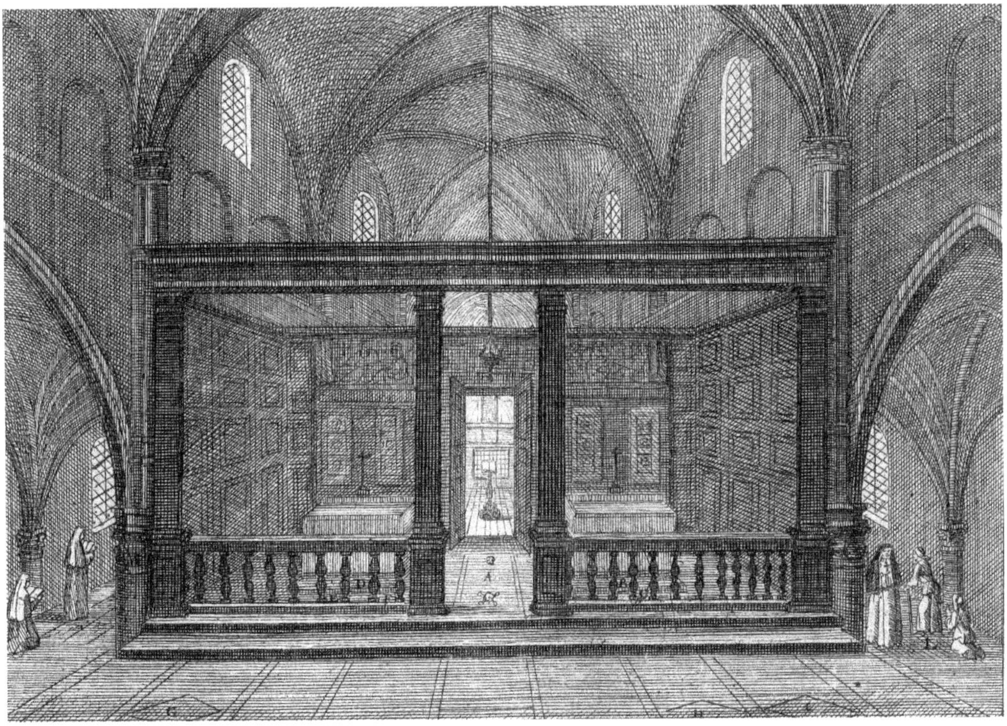

11 Burial Place of the Relics and the ten hearts in the Chapel of Port-Royal des Champs.

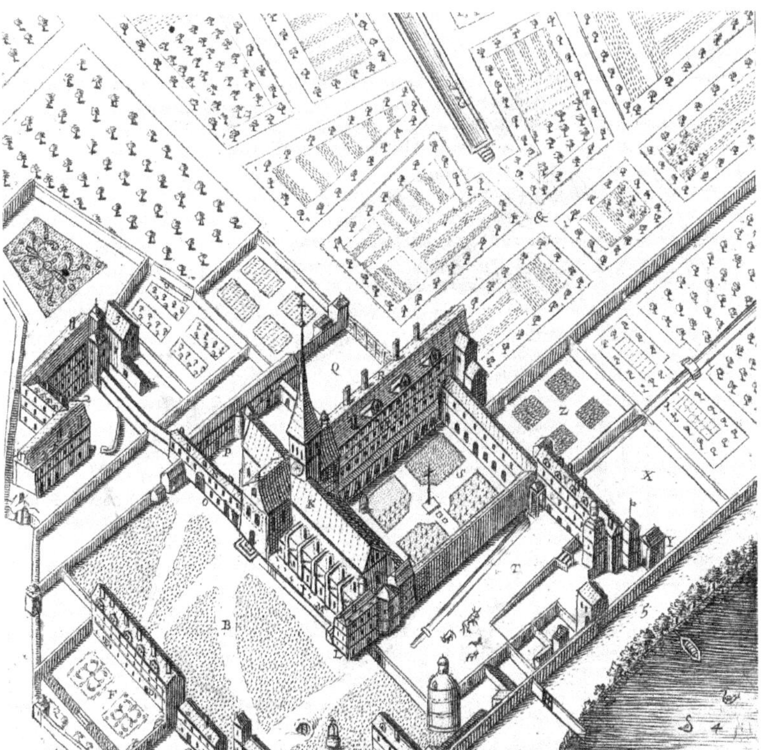

12 Architectural Blueprint of the Abbey of Port-Royal des Champs.

Chapter 4
Sunset Over Port-Royal, 1661–1711

> "I dedicated myself to destroying Jansenism and to breaking up the communities where this spirit of novelty was developing, well-intentioned, perhaps, but which seemed to want to ignore the dangerous consequences that it could have."—*Louis XIV*[1]

The year 1661—the *annus horribilis* for Port-Royal—witnessed the passing of Jules Mazarin and Angélique Arnauld, two key figures in the convent's history. But it also saw the commencement of Louis XIV's personal rule and the beginning of a policy of harassment that ended in the demolition of Port-Royal des Champs a half century later. When the year began, some 200 women lived at both convents; when it ended, only 90 women remained. What happened that year altered the course, not only of Port-Royal, but also of Jansenism as a movement.[2]

No longer merely a theological system espoused by a handful of women and men, Jansenism by 1660 had become a coherent ideal encompassing theological, social, moral, economic, political, and pedagogical dimensions. With powerful friends not only in France but across Europe as well, it had developed a complex character.[3] Yet it had also grown more rigid and extreme. In the 1660s, the *extrémistes intramondaine* ("extremists within the world"), a small but determined clique with one foot in the Court and the other in Jansenism, dominated the movement. Led by Guillaume Le Roy, *abbé* de Hautefontain, this "loyal opposition" favored negotiating with the state on some issues for reasons of political opportunism, but opposed compromise in other areas. For example, they absolutely refused to sign the Formulary. Their loyalty to truth, their willingness to suffer for it, and their refusal to remain silent, coupled with their indifference to creating schism in the Church, led them to welcome persecution as validation that they possessed the truth.[4]

Unfortunately for them, a growing number of enemies proved eager to dispute that claim. In Louis XIV's childhood, his first Jesuit confessor, *Père* Paulin, had planted in his mind the first "seeds of aversion" against the Jansenists and their theology.[5] His second Jesuit advisor, *Père* François Annat, watered those seeds. He wrote *Lies of the Jansenists* (1654) and *The Conduct of the Church and the King Justified in the Condemnation of the Jansenists* (1664) to prove to the young king that tolerating Jansenism encouraged the growth of illuminism, Calvinism, and rebellion in the realm. Jansenists should be punished for their "impostures, calumnies, and errors"; their "impertinence" in refusing to submit to papal bulls destroys the peace of the Church. These heretics, who have formed a "cabal" at Port-Royal, should be treated like Calvinists. Deny them absolution, access to the sacraments, and communication with true believers, Annat advised. If they refuse to submit to the Church, then destroy their writings and expel them from France.[6]

Consequently, when *Père* La Chaise became the king's next confessor, Louis XIV already disliked Jansenists. Although La Chaise allegedly stated that "Jansenism is my piss-pot. I place it where I must,"[7] he did not condone persecuting the movement. Although as a Jesuit, he disagreed with Jansenist theology, in several instances, he intervened to help Jansenists he felt had been mistreated. Moreover, he took no part in the final destruction of Port-Royal des Champs.[8]

The popular Court preacher Jacques Bossuet, Bishop of Condom, however, opposed both Jansenists and Calvinists in the 1660s. He considered the former "inexcusable deceivers" and the latter heretics. Bossuet wrote *The Perpetuity of the Faith* (1669) to condemn theological errors in Jansenism and Protestantism. Yet he also consulted with Jansenist prelates like Félix Vialart, seeking a "middle way" to unite Jansenists and Catholics against the Huguenots, their common enemy.[9]

But the king's intransigence undermined the plans of bridge-builders like Bossuet and La Chaise. "I do not think," Louis XIV once quipped, "that a Jansenist is capable of being a good man."[10] In his *Memoirs*, written for the Dauphin in 1661, the king described Jansenists as "obstinate schismatics" who by their piety "draw the populace after them," but who refused to submit to Church and state authority.[11] He hated the "noise" they made propagating their diverse views and despised them as a "religious cabal" that threatened the monarchy. His model of absolute divine right rule—premised on the existence of "one king, one law, one faith"—demanded religious conformity and the submission of one's conscience; it allowed no room for "pious individualism" to oppose the hierarchies of authority.[12] Resenting its spirit of independence and innovation, he called Jansenism "this cabal of the people in revolt against the decisions and opinions of the Church [which is] no less damaging to the state than to religion."[13]

Remembering the Fronde, Louis XIV equated Jansenism with rebellion. To his mind, by supporting the rebellious Cardinal de Retz, the Jansenists had brought division into the Church and disorder into the realm. In short, they were *frondeurs* and schismatics—possibly heretics.[14]

Consequently, in December 1660, the king shared with the General Assembly of the Clergy his resolution to "completely exterminate Jansenism" in France for the sake of his conscience, his honor, and the good of the state.[15] Perhaps, as the *duc* de Saint-Simon stated, his Jesuit confessors had poisoned his mind concerning the dangers of Jansenism. Or maybe it was his fear of hell, as the *princesse* de La Palatine maintained, coupled with his belief that anyone who disagreed with the Jesuits was damned.[16] Louis XIV's *Memoirs* also reveal his dislike of "novelties," his sense of insecurity regarding religious matters in general, and his compulsive need to justify himself.[17] Consequently, he did not always follow a consistent religious policy. For example, despite his harsh laws against the Huguenots in the 1680s, he permitted Duquesne and Turenne—both Protestant generals—to lead his army, but he never gave a military command to a known Jansenist. In 1706, when the *duc* d'Orléans asked permission for his friend Fontpertuis to accompany him to Italy, Louis XIV—believing Fontpertuis a Jansenist—refused, but acquiesced when his son explained that although his mother had been a Jansenist, Fontpertuis did not even believe in God![18]

Perhaps for all the above reasons, the king distrusted Port-Royal. "I hate that convent for its Jansenism," he complained to the *comtesse* de Gramont, whose recent visit there led him to strike her name from the list of invited guests at Marly.[19] According to the provisions in the Concordat of Bologna (1516), however, France's monarch had no authority over nuns or convents, which fell under the pope's jurisdiction. But Port-Royal's growing reputation as a "nest" of insubordinate sisters persuaded him that the time had come to bring them to heel.[20]

Doubtless the monarch hoped that forcing everyone to sign the Formulary would make the twenty-year controversy over Jansenism disappear. After weeks of debate and some coercion, the Sorbonne had approved the oath; the General Assembly of the Clergy voted to make it obligatory for all theology faculty and Church clerics to sign it.[21] But when Jansenist prelates refused, the Council of State published the Assembly's *arrêt* of 13 April 1661 declaring them "rebels, disobedient to His Majesty's orders, seditious and disturbers of the public peace."[22] Actions soon followed words when on April 23 civil lieutenant Dreux d'Aubray arrived at Port-Royal in Paris with a *lettre de cachet* ordering the 21 pensioners to leave within three days; the next day, he did the same at Port-Royal des Champs. In subsequent *lettres de cachet* for May 2 and 9, the king ordered the sisters not to accept any more novices or pensioners lest they "suffer our indignation."[23]

Complying with the letter of the law, Agnès Arnauld, the abbess at Port-Royal in Paris, sent the pensioners away but kept the postulants, reasoning that, after all, they were not nuns. Exasperated, the civil lieutenant returned with the *procureur du Roi* on May 13 and, without consulting the Archbishop of Paris, ordered all the postulants and novices to leave. The following day, "weeping and wailing," eight postulants and seven novices left the abbey.[24]

Agreeing with her brother Antoine Arnauld that "silence in the face of persecution is a bad remedy . . . because it has no other effect than to make our enemies bolder,"[25] Agnès on May 6 penned a strong letter to Louis XIV. She asked him to put in writing the reasons for his recent actions which "wound . . . the tenderness of our consciences." She defended her innocence, arguing that while she had complied with the king's initial command to send the pensioners home and accept no more novices, the royal order had said nothing about promoting long-serving postulants to novices. She hoped that His Majesty, "being informed of the innocent manner in which this action occurred, will not wish to destroy what was done in God's presence." With "confidence in the goodness of Your Majesty," Agnès pleaded with Louis XIV not to "extinguish one of the most ancient abbeys of your kingdom." She employed both flattery and tears to soften the ruler's heart, praising his "goodness" and avowing "respect" while begging him to see "the injustice of this action," to hear "their tears and prayers," and to consider "the affliction to which we have now come." After citing the two recent miracles (the healing of Marguerite Périer and Madéleine Boudrand) as evidence that God favored Port-Royal, she asked that the convent not be closed "without a solemn canonical judgment."[26] In effect, Agnès went over the king's head and appealed her case to the pope, confident that Rome would never help Louis XIV suppress a convent of annoying but harmless nuns who did not understand theology.[27]

While her assumption proved correct, her boldness brought the abbey further retaliation. Two days later, the civil lieutenant told Agnès that the king had refused her petitions and that by May 14, all postulants—new or old—must be sent home. The monarch also appointed the grand vicar M. de Bail as the convent's spiritual director and M. le Juge and M. Paulon as the nuns' confessors. In June, Louis XIV ordered all remaining males, including Antoine Singlin, Agnès' trusted friend and confessor for 23 years, to leave Port-Royal des Champs.[28]

Bowing to the royal will, the nuns at Port-Royal in Paris signed the Formulary on June 22. The sisters at Port-Royal des Champs, however, mulled the matter over five more months before agreeing to sign "this work of darkness and mystery of iniquity" on November 28.[29] But one woman refused to sign, even with reservations attached. In a letter to her sub-prioress (Angélique de Saint-Jean), Jacqueline Pascal explains that her integrity, her fidelity to the truth, and her willingness to die for it make it impossible for her to sign that "cowardly covenant with death." Conscience, she asserts, must always be supreme over authority. Forcing individuals to sign the "abominable" Formulary constitutes "a usurpation of power with the most dangerous consequences." Quoting Saint-Cyran, she exclaims, "the least truth of faith must be defended with the same fidelity that we owe to Jesus Christ." And if that means exile, prison, even death, then "let us count ourselves blessed to suffer something for [the sake of] justice." Then she issued her defiant challenge: "Since the bishops are showing the courage of girls, the girls should be showing the courage of bishops . . . .[For] it is not for us to defend the truth; it is for us to die for the truth."[30]

Despite Jacqueline's heroic words, the time for Jansenists to die had not yet come. Indeed, when compared with the sufferings endured by the Huguenots during the Revocation (imprisonment, torture, execution, galleys), the government's treatment of the Jansenists resembles a form of "parlor persecution." Aside from transferring recalcitrant nuns to other convents, sending several men to prison, and exiling a handful of leaders, where is the blood? As R. A. Knox (1950) observed a half century ago, the Jansenists' persecution "has the irresistible atmosphere of make-believe about it all."[31]

But Jansenists loved to suffer, and they insisted that others feel their pain as well. Consequently, they committed their agony to paper. In June 1661 Henri Arnauld, Bishop of Angers, wrote to encourage his sister Angélique Arnauld, depressed at hearing that M. de Sacy had been sent to the Bastille. "[I]t is in the time of combat," he said, "that we have the greatest need of [God's] assistance."[32] Yet because many saw the Jansenists' loyalty to God as disloyalty to their king, Henri tried to explain to Louis XIV a few months later why "the invisible and spiritual chains of conscience" prevented him from signing the Formulary. To disobey that "inner enlightenment" meant "falling into sin" and becoming a "traitor to God." A bishop who "violates God's cause" is "incapable of rendering the most important service to Your Majesty." Henri Arnauld's defense of the right/fact distinction and his refusal to sign the oath angered Louis XIV, the papal nuncio, and the General Assembly of the Clergy.[33]

Seeking a compromise, the vicars-general drew up a new Formulary incorporating the right/fact distinction, but Louis XIV and the General Assembly rejected it. So on Halloween's Day 1661, the vicars-general composed yet another Formulary and demanded that faithful Catholics sign it "pure and simple" without quibbling over the issues of "right" and "fact."[34] This version split the Jansenist camp four ways. Political opportunists close to the Court advocated signing it; Saint-Cyran's group vacillated between submission and refusal; Arnauld and Nicole's camp sought a compromise based on the right/fact distinction; and the *extremistes intramondaine*, led by Jacqueline Pascal and the Port-Royal nuns, refused any compromise measures.[35]

The nuns cited several biblical allusions to support their cause. Jacqueline Pascal opposed Antoine Arnauld's stand because she felt that for the nuns to use their ignorance of theology as an excuse not to sign the Formulary would harm the cause of truth. Fundamentally, she saw the right/fact distinction as an "act of evasion": Christians must uphold truth and avoid dissimulation. Like biblical martyrs, they should be willing to sacrifice their lives for the truth.[36] Angélique de St.-Jean accepted the right/fact distinction; she echoed Pascal's militant call for the nuns to be "heroic women" (like biblical Jael and Deborah) in God's army to "win the battle" for truth.[37] The more pessimistic Agnès Arnauld, on the other hand, predicted that the Port-Royal "vine of God will now be ravaged and trampled upon."[38] Her sister Marie Angélique Arnauld, however, remained optimistic to the last, confident that God would make the nuns "like eagles," flying on "God's wings of charity and grace to His holy mountain" where "He will help us see the light."[39]

Their soldiering brother Robert Arnauld d'Andilly interrupted his forays across Europe to visit Port-Royal for months at a time.[40] Robert employed militant imagery to describe the nuns' conflict over the Formulary. To face "the tempest that has threatened this house for so long a time," he challenges the sisters to be "true Heroes" who will "overcome persecution" and "conquer the heavens." They should be ready "to sacrifice [themselves] if [they] have the courage," for they "will suffer for only a few years."[41] In his essay "Why One Should Prefer His Friend to His Country," he tells the nuns that while personal friendship is natural, useful, and agreeable, patriotism is based on ambition and fear ("the foundation of republics and monarchies"); it leads to domination, violence, feebleness, and "the loss of legitimate liberty." Because friendship is "a holy, divine image," one's friends should be "more dear than the salvation of one's country." They should give their first loyalty to God and stand by their friends who defend the truth.[42]

But what about loyalty to the king? In a glowing letter to Louis XIV in March 1661, he professed "my ardent passion for your service" and described the king as "a living image of God," praising him as "one of the good kings who create the good centuries." If the "arbiter of Europe" will allow "God's will to govern his life" and shape his "generous designs" for Europe, then he will end "the deluge of blood we offered to demons" and bring "peace and justice" to the continent, for "there is nothing of which Your Majesty is incapable." By so doing, he will win "an immortal crown."[43] Yet five months later, he told the marquise de Sablé that the government's "persecution" of Port-Royal would end only "when it pleases God to make the King see to what extent he is abusing his goodness and acting contrary to his piety and justice."[44]

Although in 1661 Louis XIV had made his intention of crushing Jansenism quite clear, it survived for several reasons. First, because its enemies quarreled. Although the monarchy, papacy, General Assembly, and many members in Parlement opposed it, internal jurisdictional issues prevented them from reaching agreement on how to combat this new schism. Many *parlementaires* became "reluctant allies" of Jansenism for its Gallicanism and opposion to papal interference in France's ecclesiastical affairs.[45] Second, because a miracle stiffened the sisters' resistance. As the "Miracle of the Thorn" in 1656 made Mazarin and the Jesuits pause in their harassment of the convent, so in 1662, the perceived miraculous healing of Sister Catherine de Ste.-Suzanne (paralyzed for fourteen months) brought a temporary truce in the battle over the Formulary.[46] Third, because Clement IX feared schism in the Church. This led him to favor the temporary reconciliation known as "The Peace of the Church" (1669–1679) discussed later in this chapter.[47]

Even more importantly, however, several highly placed officials in Louis XIV's government opposed persecuting the Jansenists. Jean-Baptiste Colbert had a pious Jansenist wife (Catherine-Felicité Arnauld de Pomponne), a Jansenist brother (Charles-Joachim Colbert, Bishop of Montpellier), and a militant Jansenist cousin (Honoré d'Albert, *duc* de Chevreuse). This made him sympathetic toward the movement and resonated with his pro-Gallican policies.[48] Equally sympathetic, Chancellor Le Tellier believed that government persecution of Port-Royal was unjust; he worked behind the scenes to establish the "Peace of the Church" in 1669.[49] Although he disliked their secrecy and clandestine publications, Minister of War Louvois sympathized with the Jansenists in the 1660s and welcomed the truce that brought peace in 1669.[50]

If the pro-Jansenist sympathies of Louis XIV's closest advisors made him hesitate to crush Port-Royal, the appointment of a new archbishop of Paris in 1662 provided him with an ally. When the Cardinal de Retz retired in January, Pierre de Marca, the former Archbishop of Toulouse, widely known as "the hammer of Jansenism," took his place, but died four months later. So the king, on the advice of his Jesuit confessor *Père* Annat, chose Hardouin de Beaumont de Péréfixe, Archbishop of Rhodez, to replace him in June.[51] A former protégé of Richelieu, doctor of theology at the Sorbonne, member of the Académie Française, and chief tutor of the boy-king in 1644, Péréfixe intended to carry out his monarch's wishes regarding the Formulary.[52]

In August, the king sent Bishop Henri Arnauld a *lettre de cachet* ordering him to enforce the Formulary in his diocese "for the glory of God and the utility and advantage of His Church."[53] He refused, and his intransigence brought a new storm of persecution to Port-Royal, where Henri's sister Agnès served as abbess. That fall in an encouraging letter to her brother, Agnès compared her nuns to "reeds in the wind," but insisted that "in God's hand we shall become strong palm trees."[54] "All who wish to live in piety," she told Mme. de Foix, coadjutrix of the abbey of Saintes, "must suffer persecution and carry the Cross all their days."[55] The attempt to force the nuns to sign the Formulary, she added, "attacks the truth and charity, which are the two pillars that sustain the Church."[56]

After the truce of 1661–62, the anticipated persecution resumed in the summer of 1663 when Archbishop Péréfixe suggested merging the 67 religious at Port-Royal de Paris with their 22 sisters at Port-Royal des Champs. Immediately, the nuns objected that they "could not in all good conscience assist in the abandonment and destruction of a house so sacred and consecrated to God."[57] On July 2 they staged a protest march around the cloisters, carrying with them the relic of the Holy Thorn—until the archbishop arrived "with much noise" in four carriages and stopped them. Two days later, he came with two carriages and interrupted their prayers. On Sunday, July 5, the civil lieutenant came at 4 a.m. and posted guards in the cloisters and gardens. When the nuns complained, the archbishop removed their domestics and chose new ones. Again they protested that "it is a natural right recognized everywhere that we can choose our own domestics." The exasperated prelate shouted, "It is very strange that no matter what orders you are given, you always find reasons to disobey them."[58]

The archbishop then explained that because of their "revolt and disobedience" to orders given by their "legitimate superiors," their "natural right" of election had been revoked. "I will reduce you to your duty {signing the Formulary}," he told the abbess Marie de Ste.-Madéleine.[59] Two months later, however, the nuns informed the archbishop that "we cannot change our disposition about signing it . . . without wounding our consciences." He asked them if it was a sin to obey their superiors. "Do you prefer your judgment and your wisdom to that of all other authorities?" he queried. "Is it always the same song with you?" "Yes, Monseigneur," they replied.[60]

Despite their objections, by early September, Archbishop Péréfixe had moved 53 stubborn nuns to Port-Royal des Champs, leaving only 14 who agreed to sign the Formulary in Paris.[61] In December, Sister Dorothée sent him a long letter, protesting "this strange captivity." His actions, she declared, undermined "truth and Christian justice." She hoped that the archbishop "will allow yourself to be touched by our sufferings."[62] Hoping that God would change his heart, the nuns added his name to their prayer list, which also included heretics, schismatics, Jews, Turks and other "enemies of the Church."[63]

When prayer failed to change his mind, however, the sisters grabbed their pens and committed their thoughts to paper. During one six-year period alone (1664–1669), these nuns generated sixteen police reports, eleven protests, four appeals, four appositions and refusals, two dispositions and declarations, one disavowal, and one resolution—in short, one negative response every six months.[64] During those same five years, Claude de Sainte-Marthe, their confessor, compiled 176 pages of letters, clarifications, and responses in his *Defense of the Religious of Port-Royal* (1667).[65]

Why this sudden blizzard of propaganda? It arose because the Jansenists saw both Church and state officials collaborating to crush their movement and close Port-Royal. Enforced signing of the Formulary provided a litmus test of orthodoxy to determine who stayed in the Church (and at Port-Royal) and who was expelled. In defense of truth, they felt compelled to respond; when officials ignored their spoken requests, they appealed in writing to public opinion. Unfortunately, their powerful friends who had once defended them at Rome and at Versailles—Antoine Le Maître, Antoine Singlin, Dugué de Bagnols, M. de Bernières—had died, and Arnauld d'Andilly and Antoine Arnauld were aging fast. Also gone were some of Port-Royal's strong female defenders, women like Angélique Arnauld and Jacqueline de Ste.-Euphémie Pascal.[66] Little wonder that Antoine Arnauld complained, "Not one person who could have protected Port-Royal dared to try."[67]

In April 1664, Archbishop Péréfixe tightened the noose around the two convents. He sent spies to Port-Royal des Champs to record the name of every visitor. To fool these spies, Lancelot served as liaison between the sisters and their friends, carrying coded messages to Antoine Arnauld and Le Maître de Sacy. Then the archbishops assigned Port-Royal in Paris a new confessor—Michel Chamillard, a Sorbonne theologian. When Chamillard began pressuring the nuns to sign the Formulary, they refused, saying his advice offended their consciences.[68] When he concocted a new oath—"I submit in heart and mouth to the Pope's Constitutions {bulls}—the submission of the heart being for the *right* and that of the mouth for the *fact*"—they rejected his clever ruse.[69]

Hoping to defuse the situation, Lancelot met with the archbishop of Paris on April 16, assuring him that the sisters at Port-Royal, "the most humble of your daughters," wanted him to be their protector. Péréfixe responded: "Tell them that I admire their virtue, but that they must alter their present views. They must find the means of making the King happy with them." After all, popes, bishops, and doctors of theology had condemned Jansenism, so why would they not submit to those who knew far more than they? To refuse demonstrated "a strange presumption & a dangerous stubbornness." When Lancelot requested that they be left "in repose & silence" out of respect for their feebleness, sex, and "tender consciences," Péréfixe suggested a quid pro quo. "Find me some plank to climb out of this mess," he asked, "and I will be grateful to you for that and you will be obliged to me."[70]

On the very day that Lancelot and the archbishop sought some middle ground, however, *Mère* Agnès was preparing her nuns for resistance. In a letter to Mme. de Foix, the abbess described a "small manual" she had written to help the sisters resist attempts to force them to sign the Formulary. Do not fear the popes' threats in briefs and bulls, she said, or those of bishops in their mandates. These are but "the ceaseless raging of the demon [Satan] against the truth and those who espouse it."[71] To face "the violence of the dragon" would require "the wisdom of the Serpent, the simplicity of the Dove, and the legs of a Lion." To prepare themselves for martyrdom, she advised, the nuns needed prayer, a deeper penitence, and God's infinite mercy.[72]

Parlement provided them an opportunity to practice for martyrdom when two weeks later it registered Louis XIV's Declaration enforcing the signing of the Formulary by "all Ecclesiastics, Secular & Regular." It aimed "to stop the spread of all sorts of new opinions capable of troubling the repose of consciences, the peace of the Church, and the tranquility of the State." By eliminating any compromise based on the right/fact distinction, the king hoped that his Declaration would bring an end to the "deceptions, dissimulations, and manifest rebellions" on the part of the Jansenists and "establish complete uniformity in their thoughts" hereafter.[73]

With the king, *Père* Annat, and the Jesuits breathing down his neck, Péréfixe knew that he had to force Port-Royal's religious to sign the oath "pure and simple" (without reservations) to demonstrate their submission to authority. But when he promised the sisters that he would answer to God for any possible error they might incur in signing, they still refused, calling this subterfuge an assault on their consciences and their spiritual equality with men.[74] So on June 9, the archbishop and his grand vicar once again visited Port-Royal in Paris. After interrogating the women, they gave them three weeks to contemplate signing the Formulary, leaving behind Michel Chamillard and the Oratorian priest *Père* Esprit to guide their reflections.[75]

While the nuns contemplated their next move, their former confessor, Claude de Sainte-Marthe, appealed for the archbishop's compassion:

> What will you have gained, Monseigneur [from forcing the nuns] to sign [theFormulary] against their conscience? . . . You will have destroyed in several souls sincerity, good faith, truth; you will have changed some individuals who had some virtue but were imperfect into hypocrites; you will have filled the Church with dissimulation; you will have crushed the feeble and scandalized the strong; finally . . . you will have destroyed God's temple . . . and created evils that you will not be able to repair and for which you will have everlasting regret.[76]

But these prophetic words fell on deaf ears. Following yet another visit to both convents in early July, during which he interviewed 87 nuns, Péréfixe again rejected their request to sign the Formulary "with reservations."[77] From Agnès Arnauld's perspective, his demand that they sign "pure and simple" would force them to disobey God's ten commandments and place "an insupportable yoke" on the sisters' necks.[78] When he returned on August 21, however, the archbishop was in no mood to compromise. Complaining that "these women are as pure as angels, but as proud as demons," he denied them the sacraments because they were in "rebellion" against Church authority and therefore "unworthy." Then he presented the nuns with copies of the Formulary and demanded that they sign them immediately. Sixteen women at Port-Royal de Paris did so, although nine of those later retracted their signatures (Madéleine de Ste.-Mathilde managed to retract twice). But twelve sisters in Paris and all the nuns at Port-Royal des Champs stubbornly refused to sign.[79]

So on the afternoon of August 26, eight carriages carrying the archbishop, a grand vicar, the civil lieutenant, the captain of the guard, a provost, four commissioners, and two police officers rumbled into the courtyard of the Paris convent. Péréfixe ordered 80 archers and 20 policemen to surround the abbey to prevent anyone from coming or going. Then he summoned the recalcitrant abbess, Madéline de Saint-Agnès, and the nuns who had refused to sign five days earlier, and ordered them into the two vacant carriages. When they shouted, "We protest! We will appeal!" he replied, "Protest, appeal, do what you like, but you will obey me." With the king's approval, Péréfixe sent the disobedient sisters to various orthodox convents (most with ties to the Jesuits) and dispersed the last few students at the *petites écoles* at Le Chenois and The Grange. Those exiled included *Mère* Catherine Agnès de St.-Paul and her three nieces (Angélique de St.-Jean, Marie Charlotte de Ste.-Claire, and Marie Angélique de Ste.-Thérèse), the last remaining members of the Arnauld dynasty at Port-Royal.[80]

After the fifteen nuns[81] had left, the archbishop preached to the remaining sisters for an hour on the importance of submission to Church authority. Before leaving, he appointed *Mère* Eugénie de Fontaine as Port-Royal's new abbess; six Visitation nuns replaced the convent's former officers.[82]

The archbishop soon learned, however, that while he had succeeded in removing a few Jansenist nuns from Port-Royal, he had failed to purge the convent of Jansenism. The remaining sisters, forced to sign the Formulary under duress, refused to keep silent. Abandoning their former defense of "gender ignorance," they now argued that Péréfixe's high-handed treatment violated their right to conduct elections as guaranteed in their constitution. On August 27, Sisters Christine Briquet and Eustoque de Bregy composed a protest document, signed by the remaining nuns, asserting that Henri IV had guaranteed these elections. Then, suiting actions to words, they initiated a lawsuit in September, requesting that their case be transferred from the ecclesiastical courts to Parlement (where Jansenist relatives and supporters could defend them). Péréfixe countered by appealing the case to an even higher court—the Grand Council—presided over by Louis XIV.[83]

Checkmated, the nuns appealed to a court with even broader jurisdiction—public opinion. That fall, Antoine Arnauld, Pierre Nicole, and Claude de Sainte-Marthe wrote their *Apology for the Religious* in the convent's defense. Using highly emotive prose, they described the slanders, "terror & violence," and other "inhumane treatments" being inflicted on the "poor Religious" at Port-Royal by the Archbishop of Paris and the Jesuits. In this biased narrative, Péréfixe embodies all that is evil; he is described as a "dangerous," "violent," "terrible," and "wicked" man whose actions in demanding "blind obedience" are clearly "criminal."[84]

In the same vein, Claude de Sainte-Marthe wrote many letters and penned a short "Request from the Religious of Port-Royal of the Holy Sacrament." By denying the nuns the sacraments, he stated, the archbishop had severed their external, physical ties to the "visible Church," but he could never break their spiritual connection with God which leads to salvation.[85] His "Request" in October asked the procuror-general of Parlement to honor the sisters' *appel comme d'abus* requesting a civil trial, arguing that "never have there been afflictions equal to theirs, neither oppression more foreign than that which they suffer."[86]

To help the magistrates see the justice of this cause, other friends of Port-Royal published written defenses that autumn. Former spiritual advisor Antoine Singlin had recognized that obedience to God could mean disobeying the king. But if one's conscience was being forced, then one was justified in resisting, because the defense of truth and justice outweighed obedience to untruth and injustice. In the end, since "God's will must always be our rule," one should be prepared "to suffer for the Truth" by disobeying a superior who does not understand God's truth.[87]

From the solitude of his estate at Pomponne, Robert Arnauld d'Andilly unleashed a tidal wave of letters defending the sisters at Port-Royal against the "calumnies," "false rumors," and "black malice" levied against them. He appealed to the hearts of their persecutors: "Are you not Christians, Messieurs? Are you not touched with compassion by this extreme violence?"[88] His letters highlight the "suffering," "affliction," and "persecution" endured by "these holy girls" as they face "such a violent and cruel tempest." He hopes that God will deliver them, "if not in this world, then in the next world."[89]

Perhaps seeing herself as God's agent to accomplish that delivery, Catherine Agnès de St.-Paul wrote Péréfixe a bold letter in September 1664. "If I may judge of your intentions by your conduct," she began, then "you have forbidden us to lift up our voices to God [by denying them the sacraments]." But God—not the archbishop —"will be the judge" of "the truth and purity of [our] faith." While the nuns would submit "in matters of faith," they refused to do so regarding tradition and practice. And if this angered Monseigneur, then "I esteem myself happy to have yet more occasions to suffer" and thereby obtain God's mercy.[90]

As if inviting further retaliation, the sisters at Port-Royal des Champs sent three separate requests that December asking for clarification as to whether Péréfixe required "interior belief in the fact of Jansénius" (that the five propositions could in fact be found in the *Augustinus*) before they signed.[91] His Christmas eve reply is almost apoplectic with suppressed anger. Calling them "demi-savants" for "having the presumption to interrogate their Archbishop," he accuses them of pride and disobedience. "You have never learned to pray to God & render your legitimate Superiors submission which is essential for your salvation." Bridling at their "disrespect," he demands compliance "unceasingly & instantly."[92] A week later, responding to their third request, he tells them in measured tones: "I am certain that I have spoken rather clearly up to the present, and if you were not so attached to the defenders of Jansénius . . . you would have long since rendered me the obedience that I requested of you."[93]

Although the archbishop eventually persuaded 76 of the 87 nuns at both convents to sign the Formulary, they had made him the laughing stock of Paris. He resorted to changing carriages in the street to avoid being publicly ridiculed every time he went to Port-Royal to cajole the nuns. For more than six months, they had run circles around him with their finely spun arguments, objections, and appeals. Losing his temper, he sometimes shouted at them. Exasperated at Marguerite de Sainte-Gertrude Dupré's refusal, he yelled, "Get out of here; there is not a drop of reason in you."[94]

But what the nuns lacked in politesse and common sense, they made up for in reason. Their journals, letters, lawsuits, and leaflets (*factums*) show their tremendous wit, literary skill, and clear grasp of the issues. Perhaps using the *Provincial Letters* as their model, they adopted Pascal's tone of wounded innocence, naivete, and deep earnestness. Their writings appeal to conscience and to God's "higher law" as superior to man's laws. They also highlight the disagreements among theologians and bishops regarding the Formulary, asserting that these conflicting views raise "reasonable doubts" about the validity of such an "innovation."[95]

Few did this better than Angélique de St.-Jean, the brilliant daughter of Robert Arnauld d'Andilly and niece of Antoine Arnauld. Mentored by her Aunt Agnès, former abbess of Port-Royal, St.-Jean became the primary chronicler (or "mythographer") who, by documenting the convent's past, shaped its traditions and forged its spirit of resistance at the end of the seventeenth century. A prolific author, she wrote a hagiography of her Aunt Angélique Arnauld, penned her autobiography, and produced numerous devotional works in addition to compiling her speeches, letters, and spiritual lessons as a legacy for her successors.[96]

Her most famous apologetic work, *Relation of the Captivity of Angélique de Saint-Jean Arnauld d'Andilly* (1665), chronicles her experiences at the Annunciades convent in Paris after she had been banished from Port-Royal in 1664. Although her "captivity" lasted barely ten months, Angélique experienced a "crisis of conscience" there and was plagued by doubts. She regales the reader with a detailed record (of 343 handwritten pages) of the "anxieties," "torments," and "privations" that "nearly killed me" in this "very rough prison."[97] Although her primary "torment" was being deprived of the sacraments because she refused to sign the Formulary, Angélique's highly emotional prose evokes readers' sympathies for a woman who had been "deprived of any consolation and all spiritual assistance." Her diary-like reflections, pious prayers, letters, and snippets of dialogue paint a black-and-white picture of Port-Royal's enemies (Louis XIV, Péréfixe, the Jesuits) and friends (the Jansenists). She describes the former as blind, stubborn, ignorant, sinful tyrants who serve the Anti-Christ with their persecution and destruction, and praises the latter as pious, enlightened, virtuous but suffering innocents who remain true to conscience amid unjust persecution. Calling herself "a prisoner of the King," she employs purple prose phrases like "my holocaust," "this great tragedy," "my affliction," "a persecution," and "the oppression of the innocent" to elicit the reader's empathy, declaring that her "persecution was as afflicting as any that exists in the world." Amidst this "persecution," she exclaims, "I placed my confidence in God and in my good angel."[98]

In reality, Angélique enjoyed first-class treatment at the Annunciades. She lived in a clean, comfortable chamber, ate nutritious food, and had the freedom to move about the convent and participate in its worship services (although she strongly objected to the emphasis on the Immaculate Conception). By her own account, this "suffering saint" who "offered to God my tears" spent her "captivity" reading, praying, singing, and worshiping—exactly what she would have done at Port-Royal. Although cut off from her friends, she received (doubtless unwelcome) visits from the archbishop.[99] Despite the alleged "rigors" of her confinement, she refused to sign the Formulary. Péréfixe ordered her to return to Port-Royal des Champs in July 1665, placed her under three months' probation, and when she still refused to sign, prohibited letters and visits from friends and deprived her of the sacraments for four more years.[100]

Clearly exasperated with Port-Royal des Champs and its Jansenist network, the archbishop sent several archers with *lettres de cachet* to arrest its farm manager, gardener, chaplain, sacristan, and confessor in November 1664. Although most had escaped, the archers apprehended the sacristan.[101] For the next four years, the convent experienced a virtual lockdown.[102]

Yet like the hydra in ancient mythology, when Church officials suppressed one of its proponents, others arose to replace him. When Louis XIV issued the Declaration of 1664 ordering all ecclesiastics to sign the Formulary "pure and simple," Nicolas Pavillon, Bishop of Alet, forbade priests in his diocese to do so on penalty of excommunication. Both the king and the General Assembly of the Clergy, he declared, had "exceeded their rights" by imposing this oath. He informed Louis XIV that "[your] declaration, Sire, presupposes that there exists a Jansenist heresy in your kingdom which is making great progress . . . .That is not the truth; it is a pure supposition."[103]

In a letter to his friend Henri Arnauld, Bishop of Angers, Pavillon defended "God's holy daughters" at Port-Royal who "walk the path of justice and truth" despite the "sad extremities" they presently endure.[104] In letters to the nuns, he offered them "consolation and encouragement" amidst their "torment" and urged them to "find God's peace" in nature, in the Gospels, and in meditation while they "make a holy use of their present afflictions."[105] In other epistles, he asserted that "Jesus Christ rests upon the altar of Port-Royal," for they "are the party of truth."[106]

He encouraged them "not to be beaten down by the violence of such rigorous affliction," but to be "happy in your sufferings for [God's] truth."[107]

Pavillon's friend Henri Arnauld also fervently defended Port-Royal. He assured the Archbishop of Paris that, despite the "false accusations & lies" against them, the nuns were "Catholic & orthodox." Yet because "[it is] contrary to the spirit & discipline of the Church" for nuns to engage in theological disputes, they should not be forced to sign the Formulary. Then the bishop made a radical proposal: Because they had been "unjustly mistreated & lied about for twenty years," the nuns deserved compensation for their suffering.[108]

When he replied seven months later, the archbishop first chastised Arnauld for allowing others to use his letters to defend Jansenism. He next made it clear that while he wanted to "extinguish the evil divisions" and bring "peace and unity" to the Church, this could not occur until those hiding behind the "chimera" of Jansenism signed the Formulary. Péréfixe emphasized the need for obedience, order, unity, and peace in the Church—the very goals that the Jansenists, by their disobedience, undermined, with "pernicious consequences for the Church & the State." At the end of his letter, the Archbishop of Paris begged the Bishop of Angers to help him gain Port-Royal's conformity and thus bring "peace in the Church and glory to God."[109]

Henri's brother Antoine Arnauld also boldly defended the convent. In the *Apology for the Religious of Port-Royal* (1664), he asserted that in 1661, after Cardinal Retz's vicar-general M. de Contes had inspected the two convents, his report found them both "in a regular & well-ordered condition, exactly observing their vows, rules & Constitutions . . . with an orthodox faith & legitimate obedience to Our Holy Father the Pope & to all the Decrees of the Church."[110] Therefore, he concluded, in a century "indifferent to truth & justice," Port-Royal provided a model of integrity worth emulating.[111] Far from being "undisciplined rebels," as Jesuit rumors claimed, the sisters were "good Catholics and sincere women," "virgins consecrated to God," and "innocents" being "tormented" for defending the truth.[112]

Seeing Louis XIV as one of their "tormenters," Arnauld composed a "Memoir or Remarks on the Declaration of the King for 29 April 1664" whose bold thesis asserted that "violent means & force are seldom the best way to change men's opinions." "Kings are not prophets," he declared; they do not see the future or understand all truth. Moreover, bad advisors can deceive kings (*Père* Annat and the Jesuits have told Louis XIV lies about Port-Royal).[113] Indeed, before the Archbishop of Paris brought "disorder and corruption" into the convent, the nuns had lived virtuous, self-disciplined lives.[114]

In a not too subtle manner, by praising the neo-Stoic values of the seventeenth century in the lives of the Port-Royal nuns, Arnauld was indirectly criticizing the extravagant, immoral lifestyles of the king and his Court at Versailles. Moreover, by emphasizing the sisters' purity, discipline, and virtues, he showed that the use of force (whether by Louis XIV or Péréfixe) was arbitrary and unjust; in fact, it violated both monastic laws and their individual consciences.[115] In his more direct "Request Presented to the King by the Ecclesiastics Who Have Visited Port-Royal" (1668), Arnauld declared that "those who force others, by whatever means, to embrace their lies" thereby violate "Christian humility & prudence." He believed that the Jesuits and others who "break all the laws to satisfy their vengeance" against the convent perpetrated "abuses in Your Majesty's name."[116]

In a letter to Bishop Nicolas Pavillon, Arnauld asserted that the "cruel and inhumane persecution" unleashed against Port-Royal constituted one of "the two worst misfortunes that God has brought me personally." He called the dispersal of the fifteen recusant nuns "this most unchristian violence . . . a barbarity without precedent in God's house [carried out] without any form of justice." In truth, the act of "destroying" such a convent of "virgins consecrated to God" was "a great crime."[117] Yet because the nuns "suffered for justice's sake," he encouraged them to be "faithful to Christ despite the injustice of men" and to find "joy in persecution, [so] that you suffer . . . without being broken."[118]

The issuing of Alexander VII's new Bull *Regiminis apostolici* brought little joy and much suffering to the Jansenists. After three years of wrangling over its wording, Rome finally released a revised Formulary on 15 February 1665.[119] It closed the door on moderates who would sign only if the right/fact distinction were respected. It stated:

> I [name of signer] submit myself to the apostolic Constitution of Innocent X dated May 31st 1653, and to the Constitution of Alexander VII, dated October 16th 1656, the supreme pontiffs: And I do with a sincere mind reject and condemn the five propositions, taken out of Cornelius Jansen's book, called *Augustinus*, and in the sense intended by the same author, as the apostolic see has by the said Constitution condemned them.[120]

This 1665 Formulary, the first to require signatures by the direct authority of the pope, was carefully worded so as to include a "sincere rejection" of the five propositions in the *Augustinus* without implying that Jansen had misinterpreted St. Augustine's theology. Those who signed it had to appear before the royal judge of their diocese and present evidence of their recent penitence to a bishop as well as written proof that they were reconciled with the Church.[121]

When it reached France in April, the new bull created quite a stir. Parlement refused to register it. Louis XIV had to force the magistrates to declare the new Formulary the law of the land by staging a *lit de justice* on April 29.[122] After the General Assembly of the Clergy endorsed the bull, all but four bishops signed the Formulary. Those four recusants—the bishops of Angers, Beauvais, Pomiers, and Alet—published mandates defending the right/fact distinction. But the Council of State in July issued an *arrêt* breaking these mandates, and Louis XIV asked the pope to form a commission to judge the four bishops.[123] Their courageous example, however, soon inspired others to oppose the bull. Within a year, nineteen bishops refused to sign the Formulary; by 1667, their number had grown to 40. Internal strife and factionalism threatened to destroy Church unity.[124]

Determined to restore unity in the Gallican Church, Louis XIV used the new Formulary to enforce conformity on the Port-Royal religious. Nuns who signed the oath (Gerberon calls them "perjured ones") could remain at Port-Royal de Paris; those who refused were banished to Port-Royal des Champs.[125] During those difficult months, Claude Lancelot, "the most devoted of all the friends of Port-Royal," provided invaluable assistance as an intermediary, carrying dozens of letters and packages from the nuns at both convents to their defenders, particularly Antoine Arnauld, Le Maître de Sacy, and Pierre Nicole. Lancelot himself wrote at least 60 letters, sneaking them past the king's guards in bushels of pears or in laundry baskets.[126] His epistles portray the convent as "a community of saints and martyrs" whose noble example will "edify all the church." He told de Sacy that "the destruction of Port-Royal is its glory. It involves the salvation of souls; it is the edification of the Church in all ages; and it is the protection of all the virgins that God will guarantee to His Church, so no one will dare attack them if they see how unbreakable they remain to the very end." [127]

In their writings, the nuns revealed that their will to survive remained unbreakable. In May 1665, the religious at Port-Royal des Champs signed yet another protest against the new Formulary, objecting not only to its wording but also to the violent way Church officials enforced it. Their objections made Archbishop Péréfixe hesitate to take further action.[128] As the weeks went by and nothing happened, abbess Catherine-Agnès de Saint-Paul rejoiced that the "rigor" and "violence" previously used against them had at last ended.[129]

But she was wrong. Four weeks later on July 26, the archbishop, accompanied by 200 archers armed with muskets and carbines and 20 police officers in eight wagons rumbled into the courtyard of Port-Royal de Paris. Once again, the archbishop gathered the nuns together and threatened them with excommunication if they did not sign the new Formulary immediately. Of the 80 sisters in Paris, only 12 signed, so Péréfixe ordered the 68 recusants into the wagons for the short trip to Port-Royal des Champs. If these sisters expected peace and quiet in their rural retreat, however, they soon had reason to think again. The guards who accompanied them got drunk, marched around the convent singing bawdy songs, organized noisy garden parties at night, threatened their domestics with hanging, and generally made themselves a nuisance. To add insult to injury, the religious had to pay for the soldiers' wood, candles, food, table service, and laundry. Soon the guards forbade the nuns to enter their own garden or send messages to their friends on the outside. Not until 1667, when a new officer and less obnoxious archers replaced the original ones, did the religious have access to their gardens. But when they barricaded the door and put iron bars on the windows, the archers broke down the door and removed the metal bars.[130]

Virtual prisoners, the nuns turned once again to their friends on the outside for support. Antoine Arnauld, praising their "pure spirit" and "fragrance of piety," declared that "there is no convent in France where the religious inmates have less communication with the outside world" than at Port-Royal.[131] In a letter to M. de Sevigné, he condemned "those who are miserably engaged in treating so cruelly one of the holiest institutions of the Church," and predicted that such "deplorable persecution" would "create more apostates than martyrs."[132] Port-Royal's long-time patron the *duchesse* de Longueville agreed, assuring *Mère* Agnès in 1667 that she had "been grieved by the injustice recently done to you in the spoiling of your abbey"; she promised the sisters her support and prayers "more than ever."[133]

Both were needed, especially after M. Chamillard, a doctor of theology at the Sorbonne, accused the nuns of heresy and treason. His lengthy diatribe, published in 1667, charged Port-Royal with forming "a secret party" inside the Church, teaching doctrinal error and unorthodox maxims, slandering popes and bishops, attacking the Jesuits, and seeking to form a "new church" with its own catechism. In addition, he claimed that the convent had grown immensely wealthy by changing its constitution to benefit itself.[134] In his equally long-winded *Defense of the Religious of Port-Royal* (1667), Claude de Saint-Marthe called each of these charges "false slanders." These "innocent" nuns, he asserts, "are being cruelly treated by a priest who had once been their confessor."[135]

The following year, when Archbishop George d'Aubusson de la Feuillade of Embrun attacked Port-Royal, Antoine Arnauld rushed to their defense. The archbishop accused the nuns of forming "an invisible cabal" in rebellion against the Church. Moreover, they had introduced a new heresy "far more dangerous for Church & State than those of centuries past." Furthermore, although they "disguised their malice," they frequently "slandered defenders of truth," employing "false eloquence & lies." Finally, he said, the Jansenists planned to use force to revenge themselves on their enemies and to "establish their sect." All of these accusations, Arnauld asserted, were false. Far from being heretics or schismatics, the religious would gladly suffer for the truth if necessary in order to bring peace to the Church.[136] In an encouraging letter to the sisters themselves, he called them "God's saints" who will be "complete in him through tribulation." He urged them to see their afflictions as "holocausts of [God's] love" that would sanctify them and in the end, bring them golden crowns in glory.[137]

By 1668, Port-Royal's coffers were indeed full of gold. Chamillard was correct: both convents had become immensely rich. The treasury at Port-Royal in Paris contained 14,000 *livres* from nuns' dowries alone, while that at Port-Royal des Champs had 400,000 *livres*—the equivalent of several million U.S. dollars today. In 1669, rental income for the abbey in Paris (with seven religious and three converts) reached 10,000 *livres* a year, about half the rents (19,500 *livres*) taken in every year at Port-Royal des Champs (with 69 religious and 25–30 converts). Persecution had proved highly lucrative; suffering paid big dividends in silver.[138]

Yet just as Agnès Arnauld warned her nuns to take refuge in "our house founded upon a rock so that the winds and tempests cannot shake it,"[139] the storm ended, official persecution ceased, and harmony came to the Church. The "Peace of the Church," which lasted from 1669 to 1679, succeeded thanks to the collaborative effort of many friends and former enemies. Preparing to fight the Dutch in 1668, Louis XIV wanted religious unity at home before he went to war, so he appealed to the new pope, Clement IX, to find some accommodation with the Jansenists.[140] The liberal-spirited Clement, who saw some virtues in Jansenism but feared schism in the Gallican Church, began negotiating with Henri and Antoine Arnauld (among others), seeking a compromise regarding the Formulary. Perhaps, they suggested, the pope could let the Jansenists maintain "a respectful silence" concerning the issue of "fact" or permit them to sign the oath with reservations.[141]

This long-awaited peace owed much to the efforts of some who did not wear clerical garb, including women. Between 1667 and 1669, the marquise de Sablé wrote dozens of letters to archbishops and bishops seeking diplomatic means of bringing about the "Clementine Peace." She assured the pope's nephew, Cardinal de Raspigliosi, that contrary to the rumors he had heard about Port-Royal, the nuns there had "tender consciences" and exhibited "outstanding piety."[142] In July 1667, the *duchesse* de Longueville, one of Port-Royal's most influential patrons, pleaded with the pope and with Cardinal Azzolin, the papal secretary of state, to bring peace to the Church. In her letter, she defended the nuns' orthodoxy, principles, and loyalty despite the slanders of the Jesuits who "for more than 20 years have been tearing them apart."[143]

While preferring peace to persecution, Angélique de St.-Jean shared certain reservations with her Uncle Antoine Arnauld in May 1668. With typical Jansenist pessimism, she feared that

> the result of a settlement . . . would no doubt presuppose the promise to keep silent on the question of fact, from fear of rekindling the debate, and during this silence of the truth, the voice of error would be able to make itself heard throughout the land, and death could take us by surprise before we had the opportunity to acknowledge God and to deliver the truth from its harmful captivity.[144]

Expressing the same idea more colorfully, Angélique's Aunt Agnès Arnauld told her brother Antoine, "We do not fear, by God's grace, the roars of the lion, but we tremble with fear at the deception of the serpent."[145] Perhaps Agnès saw Louis XIV as the lion and the Jesuits (or Archbishop Péréfixe) as the serpent.

The chancellor of France, Michel Le Tellier, also played a key role behind the scenes in bringing about peace in the Church. In his correspondence with Archbishop Gondrin of Sens, Le Tellier urged him to write to Clement IX to find some middle ground with the four recusant bishops. Before the archbishop undertook that delicate mission, however, he conferred with Antoine Arnauld about the wording of his letter to the pope. When their efforts proved successful, Arnauld thanked the archbishop for his role in bringing about the "Peace of the Church," thereby rendering "to our poor persecuted ones [at Port-Royal], the tranquillity they have begun to enjoy."[146]

Meanwhile, Pierre Nicole, another key agent in effecting the peace, tried to persuade the nuns to moderate their "unreasonable" and "stubborn" views concerning the Formulary. "It is essential [that they] be a bit more balanced," he wrote Antoine Arnauld in July.

> I am only thinking of the danger that it seems to me they are facing by engaging [in debates]. It seems to me that there is often as much danger in having too much zeal as in having too little, and as stupidity prevents us from knowing the future, too much light likewise keeps us from discerning it . . . What is

> strange is that virtue and zeal may sometimes be the occasion for deceit and temptation. Because human virtue is never so spiritual nor so pure as our imaginations tell us.[147]

Port-Royal's religious, he declared, should remember that signing the Formulary "is not the frightening monster or beast" that their "violent prose" has claimed. He warned them not to "mix poison with obedience" in their propaganda.[148]

In giving this sage advice, perhaps Nicole had Port-Royal's abbess, Agnès Arnauld, in mind. As peace came to the Church, this die-hard fighter wrote to her brother Antoine expressing "the extreme horror that I have for the Formulary," which she resolved never to sign. She claimed that because she owed her first loyalty to God, and because the pope's bull was not "an indispensable law," refusal to sign the new oath was not a sin.[149]

As Agnès fumed over the Formulary, however, Archbishop Péréfixe, a former enemy, demonstrated his sincere desire to bring peace to the Church. He corresponded at length with Louis XIV and his ministers of state, with the papal nuncio and Cardinal Raspigliosi, and with the French bishops. He urged Raspigliosi to stop requiring signatures to the Formulary "for the good of Religion & the repose of consciences." Then, in an unprecedented move, he secured the release of the Jansenist leaders Fontaine and de Sacy from the Bastille. As a gesture of friendship, he invited them to his palace for a meeting in late July.[150]

Before long, everyone, it seemed, wanted to reach across the table and shake the hand of a Jansenist. On October 13, Cardinal Bargellini, the papal nuncio to France, and the *abbé* Le Tellier, son of the chancellor, dined with Antoine Arnauld and Pierre Nicole. Gushing good will, Bargellini complimented Arnauld: "You have a golden pen, sir!"[151] Eleven days later, Robert Arnauld d'Andilly ushered his Uncle Antoine Arnauld into the king's presence at the palace of Saint-Gemain. As the aging Jansenist bowed, Louis XIV told him how eager he had been to meet the man he so much admired. He only regretted, he said, that Arnauld had not used his God-given talents to defend the Church. Nervously, Arnauld thanked the king "for the greatest happiness that has ever come to me," assured him of his "respect, veneration, and admiration," and praised him for bringing about the "Peace of the Church." The *Gazette de France* broadcast the good news across Europe. In Paris, church bells rang.[152]

As letters of congratulation from Church and government officials poured in to Versailles, Louis XIV, recognizing that this peace had been a collaborative effort, expressed his gratitude to those who had helped him bring it to fruition. In a letter to Cardinal Raspigliosi, he praised Clement IX. "I take this occasion to write to His Holiness to tell him of my joy and my compliments . . . at the glory of the conclusion of this grand work." He assured the pope that "my intention is to support and enforce with all my authority the desires and resolutions of His Holiness."[153] The king told the Bishops of Sens and Châlons, "Messieurs, you will have great fame for arranging this agreement."[154] When Louis XIV complimented the papal nuncio for his part in bringing reconciliation, the nuncio assured the monarch that Clement IX was deeply pleased with him and with the peace.[155]

To show his pleasure, the pope on 1 January 1669 had a medal struck to commemorate this unprecedented event.[156] In letters to the Archbishop of Sens and the Bishops of Châlons and Laon, Clement repeatedly praised them as "mediators of the peace."[157] But he saved his most effusive praise for Antoine Arnauld. In speeches and letters, the pontiff stated that the Church was "greatly indebted" to "the Chrysostom of our century" whose "profound doctrines," eloquence, and "golden pen" had made him "a great hero." "This man must never die," he exclaimed.[158]

It appeared that everyone—Catholic and Jansenist alike—overflowed with compliments and good will. Even *Mère* Agnès Arnauld, the pessimistic worrywart, bubbled with enthusiasm in the thank-you letters she sent those who had played key roles in bringing about the peace. She praised the *duchesse* de Longueville's "zeal and affection" for Port-Royal and commended her "goodness" in bringing this "universal happiness" to the Church. In return, the duchess thanked the abbess "for the role your brother [Antoine Arnauld] contributed to [the peace]."[159] The abbess also thanked the duchess' brother, Louis de Bourbon, prince de Condé, for working with Archbishop Péréfixe to engineer the peace and strengthen Port-Royal. She promised that the sisters would pray for him continually.[160] In a letter to Dominique de Ligny, Bishop of Meaux, Agnès called him "a mediator of the peace" and expressed her gratitude for his using "strong persuasion" with the Archbishop of Paris.[161] Finally, she thanked Archbishop Louis-Henri de Pavillon de Gondrin for his role in effecting reconciliation in the Church. "We [the nuns] think of ourselves as your daughters," she said.[162]

The nuns found much to rejoice about in the "Clementine Peace." According to its terms, Louis XIV, by recognizing the bishops as the highest authority in the Gallican Church, foreswore any future appeals to the pope to settle religious problems in France. Church and state officials adopted the policy of silence regarding the Formulary and forbade all discussion of it in print or public discourse. The terms "Heretics, Jansenists, & Semi-Pelagians" could no longer be used as epithets to refer to any "party." Clement IX and Louis XIV pardoned the four recusant bishops (Alet, Pomiers, Angers, and Beauvais) and reinstated them in their dioceses; they also ended Antoine Arnauld's exile, re-appointed him to the faculty of theology at the Sorbonne, and allowed him to continue as spiritual director of the nuns at Port-Royal. After the nuns at Port-Royal des Champs had assured Archbishop Péréfixe that they "condemned the five propositions with all sincerity, without exception, or any restrictions whatever, in every sense in which the Church has condemned them," he pardoned them "with extreme joy" for their past disobedience. He even dropped his demand that they sign the Formulary. He also removed their armed guards, reinstated the sacraments, restored their right to hold elections, and allowed them to recruit more novices. All restrictions on the movements of the sisters and the solitaires were removed. The archbishop hoped that, in response to these generous terms, the nuns "will increase their efforts in the future to give us more and more proofs of the sincerity of their obedience and their submission to us."[163]

But their obedience and submission was put to the test when they examined the fine print in the "Clementine Peace." A major source of contention concerned the government of the two convents. The nuns at Port-Royal des Champs urged Péréfixe to reunite the two houses so that their combined wealth could accommodate the recruitment of future novices. But the archbishop felt that, given the internal divisions among the sisters concerning the signing of the Formulary, it was better to keep them separate. Furthermore, while Louis XIV agreed to let the nuns at Port-Royal des Champs elect their own abbess, he refused to relinquish his right to nominate the abbesses of Port-Royal in Paris. Therefore, on 12 March 1669, he decided that the two convents would remain separate: Port-Royal in Paris (with ten nuns) would have one-third of the property and its abbess appointed by the king; Port-Royal des Champs (with 72 nuns) would keep two-thirds of the property and elect its abbess. In September 1671, a papal bull confirmed this arrangement. The sisters appealed this decision to Parlement, but the King's Council blocked their appeal.[164]

A closer look at Port-Royal's 1679 Constitution makes it very clear why Louis XIV and the Archbishop of Paris felt so strongly the need to bring the convent under tighter control. This "Explanation of Several Chapters of the Constitutions of the Veneration of the Holy Sacrament" is divided into two parts of 262 pages and 327 pages respectively. The handwritten document contains detailed "chapters" explaining the procedures for elections, assemblies, and conferences, as well as for receiving novices, accepting dowries, instructing students, conducting services, and disbursing alms. It regulates down to the finest detail how the nuns are to sing, worship, labor, write letters, dress, eat and sleep.[165] Yet all these details support one overriding fact: the nuns, accustomed to running their own show, wanted no outside interference. Rejecting the patriarchal hierarchies of Rome, Versailles, and society at large, these women embraced the radical concept of representative democracy. Thanks to the foresight of their founder, Angélique Arnauld, every three years they elected their own abbesses. In business meetings, they deliberated openly and equally. Every sister expressed her opinions; her vote counted as much as that of the abbess. They reached decisions by consensus. The formula read: "We, the Abbess, Prioress, and Religious of Notre Dame de Port-Royal of the Blessed Sacrament, being present in our house and convent in the fields duly assembled in the accustomed manner to deliberate the common affairs of the aforesaid abbey . . . "[166]

Given their penchant for democracy, therefore, it is easy to understand their anger when the king interfered in the election process. In May 1668, as negotiations to establish the "Peace of the Church" continued, Dorothy Perdreau's three-year term as elected abbess at Port-Royal came to an end. The sisters voted to reappoint *Mère* Agnès as their superior. But using the nuns' past refusal to sign the Formulary as his pretext, Louis XIV asked Clement IX for permission to bypass the convent's constitution and appoint Perdreau as the permanent abbess over the convent. The pope consented, and in June, he recognized Perdreau as "perpetual abbess" of Port-Royal de Paris.[167]

The nuns, calling this action "an illegitimate election," appealed the decision to the Archbishop of Paris, but Péréfixe, assuring them that he had had nothing to do with it, advised them to accept it as a *coup d'autorité* (accomplished fact). So they sent the grand vicar a long list of Sister Dorothée's "faults" and "incapacities" that disqualified her for the position of abbess. When this approach failed to get the desired results, they published their objections and distributed them throughout Paris. Leaving no stone unturned, they even sent copies to the procuror-general of the Grand Council of Parlement and to the papal chancellery at Rome.[168]

As doors slammed in their faces, however, they soon recognized that this time, they would have no appeal to any court or jurisdiction. They bewailed the fact that "we have no notary to receive our declarations and acts against the violent injustice and usurpation done against us." Nonetheless, in their 28 June 1669 assembly, the nuns publicly registered their opposition to Louis XIV's action in dividing the two convents and in appointing Dorothée Perdreau as "perpetual abbess"—"an innovation . . . that goes against all the forms of our rules, constitutions, and regular discipline." In a final gesture of defiance, they appealed to Rome, asking Clement IX to overrule the king's decision on the grounds that it "threatens to reverse our reforms and regular discipline."[169]

But their appeals came to naught. In August, Louis XIV directed Cardinal d'Est, French ambassador at Rome, to ask Clement IX to separate the two convents completely on the grounds that Port-Royal de Paris, already split by factions, was deeply in debt. The king would appoint abbesses in Paris while the nuns at Port-Royal des Champs would elect their abbess triennially. Over the loud objections of the rural sisters, the pope agreed with this arrangement.[170]

This dispute over elections and the division of Port-Royal's property rendered the "Peace of the Church" more of a truce or armistice than a genuine, long-lasting peace between the Church, the government, and the Jansenists. And because the parties who drew up the terms of the reconciliation did not consult with the Society of Jesus, the Jesuits continued to oppose the agreement and sought to undermine it.[171] *Père* Annat, Louis XIV's Jesuit confessor, believed it would bring "the ruin of Religion & the State." Miffed, the king replied: "That which concerns Religion is the Pope's Affair; if he is happy with it, then you and I must be content with it."[172]

At Port-Royal des Champs, despite their dissatisfaction with some of the terms of the historic agreement, the nuns continued their lives as before. Yet not everything remained the same. Most of the convent's early historians portray the decade that followed the "Clementine Peace" as "ten years of glory." Aimée Richardt (2002) more accurately depicts that era as a decade of "veiled, embellished decline." On the one hand, these were sweet autumn years. Yet like most Indian summer days, they could not last long. "The solitude flourished once more for a moment, but more troubled than ever."[173]

To all appearances, however, the convent prospered. With clock-like regularity, the rural sisters elected their abbess every three years. Three times in a row (1669, 1672, 1675), they chose Marie de Ste.-Madéleine du Forges, a cousin of their patroness the *duchesse* de Longueville and of the Cardinal de Retz. Appreciating her wisdom and administrative style, they reelected her again in 1684 and 1687 by wide margins of approval.[174] During this Indian summer, the sisters and solitaires also published an amazing array of translations of the scriptures, liturgical books, apologetic treatises, pedagogical works, and moral essays.[175] Perhaps seeking wider recognition of their talents, they asked Minister Colbert in 1666 if they could establish a Department of Theology at the royal Académie des Sciences. After several conferences, negotiations fizzled when Louis XIV let it be known that he wanted the Académie to focus on scientific discoveries; he did not wish its members to become involved in controversial debates about politics and theology.[176]

For this brief moment in its history, Port-Royal des Champs seemed free from controversy. Mme. de Sévigné, a frequent aristocratic visitor, compared it to "a paradise where total devotion to Christianity is the focus." She especially admired the lifestyle of the solitaires, whom she called "angels on earth." She informed her friend Mme. de Grignon that "all is holiness, all is modesty" in this "divine solitude."[177]

But beneath the surface of this "divine solitude," things were changing. Whereas before the "Peace of the Church," Jansenism represented a rigorous penitential discipline that few could fully embrace, after 1669, it began to reflect an ideology of resistance based on established traditions. As it became more politicized, the movement changed its method of attack. As it entered the lists of the world, it eventually lost the spirit and innocence of its origins. Never happy for long with tranquility or anonymity, the religious felt compelled to complain about their glass that was half empty (what they disliked about the Peace) rather than to express thanks that it was half full. Refusing to let muzzled Jesuits lie, they devoted a quarter century to publishing a series of volumes on *The Moral Practice of the Jesuits* (printed at Cologne with help from wealthy supporters). Needless to say, the Jesuits sought ways to get their revenge.[178]

The 1670s also witnessed the loss of many of their powerful Jansenist friends and supporters. Simon Arnauld d'Andilly de Pomponne, arguably one of their most socially prominent friends in government circles, enjoyed Louis XIV's favor for years despite his Jansenists leanings. Rapidly promoted, he became ambassador to Sweden (1666–68) and Holland (1668–71); in 1671 the king chose him to direct the Department of Foreign Affairs and appointed him one of the four Secretaries of State—an honor with a price tag of 450,000 *livres*. Throughout the 1670s he sat on the Council of State. But because Pomponne sent two daughters to Port-Royal, supported it financially, and defended its interests, he gradually lost favor at Court. When in 1679 he expressed reservations concerning the king's new policy of "reunions" (adding territories on France's borders by treaties or military force), Louis XIV demanded his resignation. Disgraced, he could no longer defend the interests of Port-Royal in Court circles. But his sister, abbess Angélique de St.-Jean Arnauld, rejoiced at his demotion, telling a friend that now that he was no longer "in the world," perhaps they could save his soul.[179]

Seven of the convent's greatest defenders and patrons—three of them members of the Arnauld clan—had succumbed to the grim reaper by 1679. Jeanne Catherine Agnès Arnauld, Port-Royal des Champ's courageous but contentious abbess, remained defiant to the end. Her voice and pen fell silent in 1671. In 1678 Sister Marie-Charlotte Arnauld passed to her rest, followed shortly thereafter by Martin de Barcos, the *abbé* de Saint-Cyran.[180]

The charming Madame de Sablé, whose salon near Port-Royal de Paris drew Jansenists, aristocrats, writers, physicians, and Jesuits together to compose *maximes* (witty epigrams), also expired in 1678 and was buried in a pauper's grave. Her Jansenist bon mots, now forgotten, later served as models for La Rouchefoucauld's witticisms. "To be too unhappy with oneself is a weakness," she said; "but to be too happy with oneself is foolishness." "The greatest wisdom of man consists in knowing his follies," she declared. "To know well how to lay bare the inmost nature of others and yet hide one's own soul is a great mark of a superior mind," she opined. Finally, one of her wise sayings that, if heeded, would have saved barrels of ink in the Jansenists' battle with the Jesuits: "The foolishness of others should be more a lesson for us than a subject for our mockery."[181]

The beautiful, intelligent *duchesse* de Longueville, cousin of Louis XIV, who had been "drawn to self-mortification & penitence," wore an iron belt beneath her clothing. From her home near Port-Royal in Paris and at her summer cottage near Port-Royal des Champs, this much-loved "mother in the Church" gave 12,000 *livres* every year to the poor. A major protector of Port-Royal, she sent letters and memoirs to Louis XIV and to popes, cardinals, and bishops refuting slanders against the convent and defending its interests. She died at Paris in 1679, Arnauld wrote, with "a confidence in her Savior's goodness."[182] That same year, the contentious Cardinal de Retz, whose friendship during the Fronde had tainted Jansenism with rebellion, also passed away.[183]

Those not taken by the Grim Reaper often fled the kingdom two steps ahead of the law. Most of the solitaires and many of Port-Royal's long-time defenders chose flight over imprisonment. In the summer of 1679, Le Nain de Tillemont, Ernest Ruth d'Ans, M. Boulanger, Le Maître de Sacy, and Sainte-Marthe all left France and sought refuge in foreign lands.[184] It appeared as though Port-Royal would die a slow death through attrition. Fearing the worst, Abbess Angélique de Saint-Jean moaned in 1680: "Our ruin is too slow for those who wait for our death."[185]

But relief came from an unexpected source. In 1676 the reform-minded Cardinal Odescalchi had ascended the papal throne as Innocent XI. Despising personal comfort, pomp, and nepotism, he adopted an austere lifestyle. Unlike his predecessors, Innocent favored the Jansenists over the Jesuits for their rigorism and asceticism. He soon acquired a reputation as "the champion" of the Jansenist cause. In 1681 he remarked to Cardinal d'Estrées, the French ambassador to the Holy See: "There are no more Jansenists [because] they have been absorbed [within Catholicism]."[186]

Naturally, the Jansenists loved him. In a letter to Cardinal d'Estrées praising the pope's zeal, wisdom, and piety, Antoine Arnauld expressed the hope that Innocent XI, "a man truly apostolic," could find "the remedy for the evils that trouble [the Church]." If the pope could reestablish within it "a holy discipline" and cause "charity & peace to reign," then surely he could restore "unity to the body of Jesus Christ."[187] The Paris Parlement issued an *arrêt* praising the pope for his "strong & sincere piety, his zeal for the faith & for discipline in the Church, the holiness of his manners, his uniform & irreproachable conduct, his disinterested example, [and] his perseverance in renouncing his flesh & blood [nepotism]."[188] Even the Huguenots, Arnauld declared, "esteem him, & believe him capable of reforming the Church, if he was helped & followed."[189] In correspondence both in Latin and French, Innocent XI praised Arnauld for his "piety, erudition, & genius" and assured him of his "esteem & consideration," promising to protect him and his Port-Royal friends from Jesuit slanders.[190] One of Arnauld's eight-page letters (in Latin) highlighting evils in the Church moved the pope to tears.[191]

During the 1670s, this entente inspired a booming tourist trade at Port-Royal des Champs. Sword and robe nobles and wealthy bourgeois sent their daughters there—and insisted on visiting them frequently. M. de Pontchâteau told the *duchesse* d'Epernon in 1677: "I am a little annoyed at all the carriages that I have seen since Easter crowding these quarters."[192] Archbishop of Paris Harlay de Champvallon also felt that Port-Royal "had too much of a reputation." Its many friends "unite with them in making themselves squads [*palotons*] against the State." More ominously, Louis XIV also believed "these unions are dangerous in a State."[193]

One frequent visitor, Mme. de Fontpertuis, became such a close friend with the Arnaulds, Andillys, Pomponnes, and the remaining solitaires (Le Maître de Sacy and Charles-Henri de Luzancy) that she built a chateau near Port-Royal des Champs. Antoine Arnauld and Angélique de St.-Jean Arnauld became her spiritual advisors. A brilliant financier, Fontpertuis served as the financial agent for Arnauld, Quesnel, and Nicole when they were forced to flee in 1679. Her home in Paris became a refuge for Jansenists. Until her death in 1714, she interceded for them with the authorities. When Arnauld and Nicole died, she served as executor of their wills.[194]

Fontpertuis also secretly arranged for the publication and distribution of their books, the number of which grew exponentially in the 1670s and 1680s. As Daniella Kostroun (2000) has emphasized, Jansenist propaganda galvanized support for their cause and helped them resist the encroachment of Church and state authority. By writing letters, lectures, reflections, memoirs, biographies, and historical chronicles, the nuns and solitaires became activists in a well-orchestrated campaign to defend Jansenist truth against the slanders of the Jesuits. Moreover, by reprinting new editions of the convent's constitution, they defended the rights granted them by Henri IV (especially free elections) against Louis XIV's attempts to appoint their abbesses by using the Regale as a political tool.[195] Also, by printing "dictionaries" listing the names of ecclesiastics who had refused to sign the Formulary, the nuns proved that they were not alone in resisting the king's efforts to coerce their submission.[196]

Angélique de St.-Jean, abbess of Port-Royal des Champs in the 1670s, organized this propaganda campaign. She herself wrote over 800 letters and devotional talks emphasizing not only the spiritual themes of faith, poverty, virtue and obedience, but also highlighting the unjust "afflictions" the nuns had suffered by being deprived of the sacraments. Under her direction, the sisters generated a tidal wave of letters and essays testifying of their affection for one another, their genuine happiness in solitude, their diligent pursuit of virtue and piety, and their punctual observation of every holy day and spiritual duty. The sisters consistently asserted that, despite continued "persecution," they had already submitted to the pope, the king, and the archbishop of Paris in 1669.[197]

These hundreds of letters and petitions testify just how well Angélique de St.-Jean learned the lessons her Uncle Antoine Arnauld had taught her. Like him, she knew Latin and Greek, was thoroughly conversant with the Church Fathers, and loved a good argument in defense of truth. Despite her considerable charm and affection for those closest to her, she shared her uncle's doctrinaire spirit and rigid intellectualism, but was even more unbending than he when it came to signing the Formulary.[198] In a 1679 letter seeking Innocent XI's protection for "the infants of the Church," she pulled no punches in asserting that "Authorities of the Church and the State plot our ruin." Despite "following all the rules" of their order, behaving well, obeying their superiors, and "serving God with humility," she explained, they continued to "suffer public defamation and injurious treatment" so terrible that "this final blow will finish us altogether." In conclusion, she begged the pope to defend them because "everyone else in the world has abandoned us."[199]

The nuns' compulsive need to explain themselves, to answer every objection, to justify their actions, and to complain every time someone threatened their rights clearly annoyed Louis XIV. Like many good people whose common failing is not being able to leave well enough alone, they refused to be silent and submissive; their friends in high places defended them so often that the king—who never forgot the Fronde—sensed "an air of conspiracy" about them.[200] "The Jansenists," he told Bishop Vialart of Châlons, "are restless spirits, a bunch of confused people who only seek occasions to stir things up and make a lot of noise." To quiet their noise, he issued another Declaration in 1673 ordering all bishops to command their ecclesiastics to sign the Formulary on pain of losing their positions.[201] Four bishops refused to comply. One of them—Bishop Henri Arnauld—instead released an ordinance in 1676 forbidding the faculty at the University of Angers to sign the Formulary "pure and simple." When they protested, the Council of State issued an *arrêt* canceling the bishop's ordinance.[202]

Yet with a pro-Jansenist pope in Rome, Louis XIV clearly needed someone closer to home to help him suppress the noisy nuns at Port-Royal. Harlay de Champvallon, for 20 years Archbishop of Rouen, became the king's man. Highly intelligent, skillful, clever, and ambitious to become either a cardinal or a chancellor, Champvallon enthusiastically joined with the Jesuits in tightening the noose around Port-Royal after 1676. The Jesuit La Chaise resented Antoine Arnauld's friendship with Clement XI, disliked Henri Arnauld for resisting the Formulary in his diocese, and hated the Port-Royal publications attacking Jesuit moral theology. He convinced Louis XIV that by their refusal to submit, the Jansenists (like the Calvinists) implicitly challenged his divine right sovereignty. By de-sanctifying everything between their consciences and God, they limited divinity to God alone.[203]

Unwilling to tolerate these challenges to his divine authority, Louis XIV counterattacked with two strategies. First, he increasingly invoked his regalian rights to suspend prelates who refused to sign the Formulary. Second, in November 1677 he issued an edict to suppress Jansenism in Paris and especially at Port-Royal. As expected, Clement XI protested these actions, but to no avail. The fact that in 1678, the 106 pacifist nuns, novices, converts, and postulants at Port-Royal des Champs knelt to pray for the success of the king's armies in the War of the Devolution also gained them no reprieve.[204]

Instead, on 16 May 1679, when the archbishop of Paris arrived at the gates of Port-Royal des Champs, he bragged that he "was going to put the axe to the root" of the problem. First, Champvallon ordered Abbess Angélique de St.-Jean to reduce to 50 the number of women there. Then he sent the remainder of the sisters, postulants, and novices to other convents or to their parents' homes. Finally, noting that "there are yet several frogs who croak in the marshes of Port-Royal," the archbishop dispersed the last of the solitaires. The "Peace of the Church" was over; as the Bishop of Châlons told the nuns ten days later, their "troubles" had begun.[205]

Why did the ten-year "Clementine Peace" disintegrate? Antoine Arnauld listed several reasons for its failure, and despite his biases, they remain convincing today. First, because it was a peace between unequal parties: the powerful (pope and king) on the one hand and the powerless (Jansenists) on the other. Second, because these two parties represented disharmonious elements: prestige and authority on the one hand and justice and truth on the other. Third, because many (presumably on both sides) disobeyed the command to remain silent and published attacks on each other. Fourth, because the Jesuits hated the peace and tried to undo it. Fifth, because of continued resistance to the Formulary, which Jansenists saw as an artificial device to define as heretics those who defended St. Augustine's doctrine of efficacious grace and then deny them the sacraments. Finally, because "the King is not satisfied with our conduct."[206]

In fact, Champvallon told Arnauld that Louis XIV considered him Jansenism's "principal heretic chief" for holding "secret assemblies prejudicial to Church and State." When Arnauld's request for a hearing before the king was denied, he (naturally) sent the monarch a letter instead.[207] He argued that because "the name of the alleged party [Jansenists] so odious to Your Majesty . . . signifies nothing very precise and determined," others "apply it to whomever they wish" to demean. Jansenists could be defined as those who hate Jesuits or who read certain pious books or who praise St. Augustine's teachings or who hate casuistry. After disproving "false charges" against them, Arnauld defends the "community" of Port-Royal as orthodox in faith and doctrine and united by "the most profound respect, perfect obedience, and inviolable fidelity" to the king.[208]

Arnauld's words, however, failed to convince Louis XIV of his innocence. Fearing arrest and imprisonment, on 17 June 1679, heavily disguised, he fled Paris in a coach and three days later arrived at Mons in the Spanish Netherlands (Belgium today). For the next fourteen years he found refuge in Holland, Neercassel, Utrecht, Ghent, Courtrai, Tournoi, and Antwerp. Although the damp climate of the Low Countries exacerbated his bronchial asthma, he never returned to France. Instead, his self-imposed exile became his liberation. Despite being constantly watched by agents of the pope, Louis XIV, Spain, and the Jesuits, Arnauld enjoyed freedom to write and speak on matters that concerned him. He also hobnobbed with Gottfried von Leibnitz, Christian Huygens, Nicolas Malebranche, and other famous scientists and philosophers in the "Republic of Letters." Moreover, far from the Court of Louis XIV, he was no longer an embarrassment to his nephew, Minister Pomponne.[209]

Other solitaires, including Pasquier Quesnel and Pierre Nicole, joined him. These French refugees made the University of Louvain the nerve center of their movement; from there they published and shipped books and pamphlets defending the Jansenist cause back into France, much to the annoyance of the king, archbishop, and police who failed to destroy this network.[210] Archbishop Champvallon, venting his frustration to the president of Parlement, M. de Guédreville (whose daughter lived at Port-Royal), complained that Louis XIV strongly disapproved of the convent's popularity and its links to "various foreigners" who defended and supported it.[211]

In letters to Rome, Louis XIV expressed increasing annoyance with the Jansenist nuns at Port-Royal. Referring to the convent as "a hydra [serpent] that has done nothing but sprout too many others for nearly thirty years," he concluded that "cutting off the head of the hydra" was the only way to "uproot such novelties from my kingdom." In another letter, he employed the metaphor of "uprooting" the "seeds of error" from the fields of France. But he found Innocent XI unsympathetic toward his efforts to crush Port-Royal.[212]

Undeterred, the king, with Champvallon's assistance, tried a different strategy. Having already asserted his right to appoint abbesses at Port-Royal in Paris, Louis XIV demanded the restoration of his *commendam* right to nominate abbesses at Port-Royal des Champs. As expected, the nuns objected; defying royal orders, they re-elected Angélique de St.-Jean as their abbess in August 1681, citing St. Benedict's *On the Election of the Abbot* as their justification. When the archbishop of Paris opened a two-front war with the Sorbonne and the Gallican bishops over the Formulary, the distraction enabled the sisters to catch their breath before the next royal onslaught.[213]

When Champvallon tried to impose the *Ratio studiorum* (an abridgment of Catholic doctrines with a Molinist slant) on the Church in Paris, both the Oratorians and the doctors of theology at the Sorbonne girded themselves for battle. Soon Jansenists and Jesuits crossed pens in the inky battle that followed. The controversy inspired Quesnel to write his two-volume *Summary of Apostolic Morality* and eventually, his longer *French New Testament with Moral Reflections on Each Verse* to answer the Jesuits' charges against Port-Royal.[214]

Within months, however, this tempest in the Paris teapot had boiled over into the rest of France when Alexandre Dubois, the pro-Jansenist *curé* of Rumegies in the diocese of Tournai, raised the bloody banner of Gallicanism. Dubois publicly opposed the papacy's new formula for creating bishops ("by the grace of the Holy See, named bishop of ____"). Instead, he recommended returning to the older, apostolic formula ("by the grace of God, bishop of ____").[215] Then in 1681–82, Bishop Bossuet and 52 of his colleagues in the General Assembly of the Clergy drew up four controversial assertions. These famous "Gallican Articles" stated:

1 That the king has absolute sovereignty concerning temporal matters in his kingdom and the pope may not interfere.
2 That the pope's spiritual authority is subject to the superior authority of a general council.
3 That the Gallican Church enjoys special liberties based on custom, tradition, and consent that limit papal authority in France.
4 That the pope's decisions, even in matters of faith, must have the consent of the whole Gallican Church to be effective.[216]

As would be expected, Innocent XI and his successor, Alexander VIII, categorically rejected the Four Articles, recognizing their roots in conciliarism. For the next eleven years, the papacy refused to approve any ecclesiastical appointments in France.[217]

These controversies over the Regale and the "Four Gallican Articles" helped shape the politics of Port-Royal. The Jansenists' political model differed from the nationalistic Gallicanism of the French bishops and from the ultramontanism of clerics in Spain, Portugal, and Italy by limiting the authority of both kings and popes and exalting a form of conciliarism.[218] Antoine Arnauld expressed this new model in *Considerations on Matters in the Church* (1681), which supports a balance between Gallican liberties and papal power. For example, he defends the pope and condemns the king for "usurping" regalian rights. The Regale, he states, belongs to the pope, who grants it to the king as a concession; it is illegal for kings to extend the Regale for the sake of profit. While popes have supreme authority in spiritual matters (something the royalist politiques denied), representative Church councils alone are infallible. Moreover, secular judges should not decide ecclesiastical cases, nor should bishops decide civil suits. In short, Church and State should operate in separate but complementary spheres; they must not compete against or seek to usurp the power of each other.[219]

Arnauld's *Considerations* provides but one example of the critical method that Jansenist writers of the new "historical school" employed to defend their cause in the 1680s. Authors like Le Nain de Tillemont and Pasquier Quesnel, aided by contemporary thinkers such as Richard Simon and Jean Mabillon (themselves the intellectual heirs of Baruch Spinoza and René Descartes) broke with tradition and sought certainty, using the critical method and systematic doubt. They wanted to demystify history, beginning with the Ancient and Medieval roots of Christianity. Aware of the biases in recent sources, they wrote historical critiques based on primary, archival manuscripts. Although their carefully researched tomes, full of uncompromising gravity and moral strictures, appear harmless (and boring) today, Church and government officials, distrusting the historical-critical method, regularly censored and suppressed their works (but not before hiding copies at Versailles and Notre Dame Cathedral).[220]

One by one, the authors of these now-forgotten works passed from the scene in the 1680s. Isaac Louis Le Maître de Sacy, solitaire, spiritual director, teacher in the *petites écoles*, writer of books and more than 300 pious letters, died in January 1684; his friends buried him at Port-Royal des Champs. Two weeks later, his cousin, the assertive abbess Angélique de St.-Jean Arnauld d'Andilly, passed to her rest reciting stimulating passages from the Song of Solomon.[221] In a letter to Mme. de Fontpertuis, Antoine Arnauld mourned her passing as "a cruel blow," yet took comfort in knowing that her death was "so precious in [God's] eyes."[222]

Far less precious—at least to Antoine Arnauld—were the deaths of the stubborn Huguenots who refused to convert to Catholicism when Louis XIV issued the Edict of Fontainebleau in 1685. Three years before, Arnauld had criticized the bishops' use of *lettres de cachet* to force Calvinists to convert, believing that such "unscrupulous persecution" would "render the Catholic Religion odious." In 1682 he attacked the law that forced Huguenot children (seven years old or older) to become Catholics against their parents' wishes.[223]

By 1685, however, as the Calvinists endured torture, imprisonment, the galleys, and execution, Arnauld had changed his tune. Like most Jansenists, he approved of the edict revoking the Huguenots' civil and religious rights, but not of its brutality. Five days after Louis XIV signed the edict, Arnauld told Mme. de Fontpertuis that he "greatly rejoiced" at this "strong measure" against the "schismatic Donatists."[224] Invoking the example of St. Augustine's campaign against this North African sect, he informed Prince Ernest, Landgrave of Hesse-Rhinfels, that "it is good that the king's orders take away their [Calvinists'] temporal rights to force them to return [to Catholicism], which is the same conduct taken against the Donatists with great success."[225] In letters to M. du Vaucel, he heartily approved of banishing their pastors and "completely crushing this sect," wishing only that "less violent" methods had been used.[226] When Queen Christina of Sweden publicly attacked the Revocation's violent methods, however, Arnauld, believing that she had spoken with more "passion" than "reason," objected that her "quarrel with the King's behavior is bad for France's reputation." After all, the Huguenots were "rebels" and "heretics"; the "spirit of Satan" motivated their "abominable calumnies against the King."[227]

By 1687, however, after Louis XIV and Church officials had sent thousands of Huguenots to prison, the galleys, and the scaffold, a terrible truth began to dawn on Arnauld's mind: what goes around may come around. In a letter to Cardinal Paolo Walloni in Rome, he predicted: "It will never satisfy [Louis XIV] to ruin the Calvinist party, but he will certainly ruin this other party of Jansenism [which he believes is] even more dangerous than the first party . . . and equally pernicious to Church and State."[228] Yet the entrepreneur in Arnauld saw the Revocation as a unique opportunity to distribute copies of his book *Apology for the Catholics* to the *nouveaux convertis* (newly converted Catholics) and by so doing, help these Augustinian Protestants understand the Jansenist interpretation of Catholicism. Persecution might, after all, be profitable.[229]

But should persecution be resisted? During the Regale controversy in 1676, the moderate Jansenist Pierre Nicole had agreed with Bishop Pavillon and Bishop Le Camus that it was "useless to resist" the king's will. Like his friend and fellow exile Antoine Arnauld, however, events during the 1680s transformed Nicole into an activist. Returning to France, he criticized bishops who harassed Jansenists in their dioceses, picked debates with theologians, and even wrote a letter to the Archbishop of Paris "to reduce him to silence . . . by reason." While he defended Arnauld against Nicolas Malebranche's charges, he also attacked the exiled Calvinist leader Pierre Jurieu for writing "libels rather than facts." He concluded that his "new vocation" would be to defend "the embattled truths" upheld by Port-Royal.[230]

Always eager to cross swords with any combatant, Antoine Arnauld joined Nicole in defending the convent's interests. In 1680 he opposed Minister Colbert's "unjust and odious" attempt to have his sister appointed abbess of Port-Royal. Declaring that "I do not believe there is any power on earth that can force them to submit to some one whom they have not elected," he urged the 80 nuns to resist like the Maccabees and choose their own mother superior.[231] Resisting Colbert, of course, meant resisting the king himself. But by 1682, in private at least, Arnauld considered Louis XIV to be "a sluggard who sleeps on the throne" and who pursued "the passion of glory, ambition, and folly" in his foreign wars. Believing his Jesuit advisors' lies concerning the Jansenists, the king "mocked those who preached the truth" as "heretics" and believed that crushing them pleased God.[232] He told the Bishop of Castorie: "Kings are not so scrupulous about taking counsel of unjust persons and those without conscience, but they do not like others to think that they place their confidence in persons of bad life who have no sound judgment."[233]

Believing Louis XIV would listen to a good man who had sound judgment, Arnauld sent him two memoirs, hoping that if he read them, he would be convinced. He thought that his 1682 "Remonstrance" would "make [the king] see that all that has been done against the alleged

Jansenists . . . is unjust and unreasonable and that God is offended by it." The first memoir, therefore, focused on the injustices done to Port-Royal and urged Louis XIV not to listen to the "chicanery of the Jesuits" or to the bad advice Archbishop Champvallon and *Père* La Chaise gave him concerning "the phantom of Jansenism." Instead, he should "restore the liberties of the Church" and thereby bring peaceful reform.[234]

Somewhat less optimistic by the summer of 1683, Arnauld told M. de Fontpertuis that he planned to send Louis XIV a second memoir to "disabuse him" concerning the slanders he had heard about the Jansenists, although he doubted the king would read it. Nonetheless, "the cause of truth and justice" demanded that he "persuade His Majesty that he need have no more fear of this specter of Jansenism." Yet with Augustinian foreboding, he admitted "that perhaps it is within God's will that the King never be disabused on the subject of Jansenism."[235]

Despite Arnauld's dislike of Louis XIV's persecution of Port-Royal, however, he deeply respected the person and authority of the king. He assured Prince Ernest of Hesse-Rhinfels that "[I] always have the same affection & veneration for [Louis XIV's] sacred person. I come from a family who has always professed loyalty, in the worst of times, and zealously sustained the cause of Kings & Royalty."[236] Although he worried that if the king believed the rumors concerning the "phantom of Jansenism," his "glory & salvation" would be in jeopardy, he promised the Archbishop of Reims that "nothing will diminish the affection, veneration, & zeal which God has given me for the King."[237] Instead of criticizing the monarch, Arnauld felt Jansenists should pray that God would change his heart and help him stop persecuting Port-Royal.[238]

In addition to praying, Arnauld argued that religious toleration was really the best policy. Given his approval for Louis XIV's rigorous treatment of the Huguenots, it is ironic that he would tell Prince Ernest that tolerance was the most reasonable, equitable approach rulers should take toward schismatics and heretics, for "this is the law of the Gospels." "There are no Jansenists," he opined, "only Jesuits who refuse to observe Christian tolerance."[239] Likewise, the same Arnauld who approved of forcing Calvinists to convert opposed the Jesuits' "introducing the Gospel into the East Indies by force and arms" because "these methods are entirely opposed to the spirit for the Sacred Propagation of the Faith." In his *Moral Practice of the Jesuits* (1683), he declared that Christ and his apostles "established the Gospel without using violence"; Jesuit missionaries should do likewise, for Jesus wants to redeem the world, not by iron, but by the wood of his Cross."[240]

By 1685, Arnauld recognized that Louis XIV and his close advisors, La Chaise and Champvallon, preferred the iron-fisted approach in dealing with the "phantom" of Jansenism. By their abuse of *lettres de cachet*, Arnauld told M. du Vaucel, they "govern the Church [in France] far more despotically than the Popes have dared to do."[241] To end this persecution, answer falsehoods, tell the truth about Jansenism, heal the schism, and bring back the "Peace of the Church," Arnauld published his famous *Phantom of Jansenism* in 1686. In its 20 chapters, he answers Jesuit charges, cites testimonies from leading ecclesiastics, demonstrates that Jansenism is neither a heresy nor a rebellion, and asserts that the Church is fallible when teaching truths not divinely revealed.[242]

Did Arnauld really believe his book could exorcise the king's phobia regarding the specter of Jansenism? Evidently not, for in a letter to M. du Vaucel three years later, he confessed that "this Phantom will yet last a long time [because] everyone is too timid to touch it."[243] Never timid himself, throughout his life Arnauld felt called to pen letters, write books, and send memoirs and petitions clarifying the truth about Jansenism and defending his friends at Port-Royal, whom he saw as "innocents oppressed."[244] "My cause," he boasted to Cardinal Paolo Walloni, "is the cause of Port-Royal." He was proud to be called "one of the great friends of Port-Royal."[245]

During the 1690s, the convent desperately needed its friends, for the political battles surrounding the Formulary, the Regale, and the "Four Gallican Articles" had increased the Jesuits' influence over the ailing king. They took advantage of every opportunity to strengthen his animosity toward the Jansenists and to persuade him to crush Port-Royal. Although successful, the Jesuits overreached themselves, creating a powerful Jansenist-Gallican coalition that would eventually crush them.[246] Similarly, when Alexander VIII in 1690 issued a decree condemning 31 propositions in the works of Jansen and Arnauld as "rigorist and Jansenist," this revived Jansenism rather than suppressing it.[247]

When Alexander VII died in 1691, he was succeeded by Innocent XII. Two years later, when Louis XIV repudiated the "Four Gallican Articles," the new pope expressed his pleasure and agreed to help the king crush Jansenism. The Jansenists feared that this "Compromise of 1693" (pitting the pope, king, Jesuits, and Quietists against the Jansenists) would give birth to more repressive laws.[248] They heard rumors of an impending bull. In a letter to Vaucel, Antoine Arnauld confessed that "this project of the Bull which is going ahead already . . . gives me great uneasiness." He worried that it might compel him to sign another Formulary without the opportunity "to explain oneself." Even more, he feared that a new bull would bring the ruin of Port-Royal.[249]

Sure enough, when Innocent XII's decree appeared on 28 January 1694, it condemned the five propositions *in sensu obvio* ("by their obvious meaning" as determined by the papacy rather than by Jansen himself).[250] Arnauld told his friend Vaucel that if the Jesuits decided to force this Formulary on the Church and thereby "continue to torment the best-intentioned people," then "there will be continual war" between Jansenists and the Society of Jesus.[251]

But once again, fate intervened. As so often happened on the chessboard of Church politics, an anti-Jansenist pope in Rome could be checkmated by a pro-Jansenist Archbishop of Paris, and vice-versa. Thus, when Archbishop Harlay de Champvallon died in 1695 (too quickly to receive Last Rites), Louis XIV chose the Bishop of Châlons-sur-Marne, Louis-Antoine Le Maire de Noailles, to succeed him. The king's wife, Madame de Maintenon, initially preferred Noailles, a model cleric soft on Jansenism and friendly toward Port-Royal, to Bishop Bossuet, who hated Calvinists and Jansenists.[252]

Noailles had praised both of Quesnel's books (*Moral Instructions* and *Reflections on the New Testament*) as "an entire library you may own at home to fill you with the eminent science of Jesus Christ." His 25 June 1695 mandate recommended *Moral Instructions* as "holy reading . . . full of the unction & light of the Holy Spirit" for all priests, *curés*, and vicars to own and read.[253] Still, Louis XIV asked Innocent XII to make him a cardinal. Despite vociferous objections from La Chaise, Le Tellier, and the Jesuits, Louis XIV himself placed the red hat on Noailles' head in July 1700 and appointed him president over the General Assembly of the Clergy.[254]

Although the Jansenists rejoiced at Noailles' elevation, the joy of the nuns at Port-Royal was marred by the passing of several long-time friends and defenders. Henri Arnauld, Bishop of Angers, died in June 1692 after serving the Church for 44 years. The sisters remembered him for his "vigilance, zeal, and assiduity" in supporting the interests of their convent "on all occasions and in the worst of times."[255] In 1695 the last two solitaires from The Grange—Claude Lancelot and Pierre Nicole—passed away in April and November respectively. Teachers in the *petites écoles*, prolific scholars and writers, indefatigable defenders of Port-Royal—their voices and pens were now silent. Then the beautiful and intelligent Mme. de Sevigné, whose name Louis XIV had struck from his guest list at Marly for her support of Port-Royal, died in April 1696.[256]

But Jansenism's greatest loss came in August 1694 when Antoine "the Great" Arnauld expired in Brussels, far from his beloved Port-Royal des Champs retreat. In 1691 he had begged Prince Ernest to intercede for him with Louis XIV and negotiate the terms for his return to France. "I would much prefer to return incognito with the King's consent," he said, "which would spare me from having to make an infinite number of visits to the Archbishop of Paris to beg his permission."[257] To his nephew, Isaac Arnauld d'Andilly de Pomponne, he boasted: "His Majesty has no subject more faithful than I am, nor one more desirous for the glory of his reign, nor more ardent for that which is his true interests."[258] But he never realized his dream of returning home.

Nonetheless, to his dying day, Arnauld continued writing (Jansenists did not take vacations). He penned long letters to Prince Ernest listing the reforms he hoped to see effected in the Church. These included stopping false accusations against Jansenists; abolishing forced signatures to the Formulary; allowing worship services, Bibles, and missals in French; ending book censorship by the Inquisition; and popes refusing to issue bulls when kings requested them. Realistically, however, he recognized that his pipe dreams had little chance of being accepted at Rome or Versailles.[259] Undeterred, he continued writing to combat "the miserable affair of the Formulary [which] always advances." Grieved at the "confusion it will bring into the Church," he hoped to see the matter settled quickly. Those who refused to sign, he said, were being treated as "pariahs" and "rebels against the Church."[260] In "Reflections on the Decree of the Holy Office for 28 January 1694," his final word on the subject, Arnauld advanced five reasons why the faithful should not sign the Formulary. To do so "undermined the foundation of society by perverting the use of [God's] word"; contradicted "the rules of the Gospel"; advanced "the Devil's grand design"; "tarnished the Church's honor"; and precipitated "horrible and pernicious results."[261]

Slandering the Arnauld family name, one of those "pernicious results" he blamed on the Jesuits, led him to call a recent rumor that his parents had been Huguenots "the blackest malice."[262] Perhaps to counter such slander, he made it clear in his last will that "[I] die as a true Christian and a humble son of the Catholic Church, outside of which I recognize there is no salvation."[263]

When he died on 8 August 1694, friends placed Arnauld's body in an oak coffin sheathed in lead and secretly buried it in the crypt beneath the choir of Saint Catherine's Church in Brussels. In accordance with his wishes, however, they placed his heart in a silver container which, after appropriate vigils, a Mass, and public ceremonies, was buried at Port-Royal des Champs. Eulogies (both in Latin and French) praised "this heart which has always been full of tenderness for us" and compared Arnauld to "a brilliant lamp" now extinguished, "a vase which Jesus Christ has broken," and "a fragile monument" now cracked. Dozens of poems and epitaphs added new metaphors honoring him as "This martyr of the truth, Who was banished [and] persecuted, And [who] died on foreign soil, Where his body was content to rest, But his heart, always strong & innocent, Was transported by love . . . Into a peaceful retreat, From which it will never be absent."[264]

Following Arnauld's death, however, that peaceful retreat grew increasingly troubled. In 1697, Agnès de Ste.-Theele, abbess of Port-Royal des Champs, wrote to Archbishop Noailles expressing concern about "the noise of peril of a new flood [of persecution] with which we are threatened." She and her 35 nuns had heard rumors that Louis XIV intended to prevent them from receiving novices. Responding to slanders against the convent, Agnès assures Noailles of "our innocence and the purity of our faith"; "we have given reproach to no one . . . we are guilty of nothing." Boasting that "no one else in the world can surpass us in doing works of charity," she pleads with the archbishop to intercede for them "with pastoral charity" and to tell Louis XIV that "we have done nothing to excite his indignation against us." Sensing "the peril that presses us," the abbess compares the religious to "poor sheep who dare not open our mouths to defend ourselves before the powers of the century." Therefore, they place themselves in the hands of their "pastor, father, and shepherd" (Noailles) to defend them against the "plots" and "oppression" which threaten "to make us die."[265]

Although death was not as imminent as the sisters imagined, a "plot" was brewing that threatened to "oppress" them. Known as the "Case of Conscience,"[266] it began in 1700 when the General Assembly of the Clergy condemned the five propositions in a lackluster manner that offended both the Jansenists and the Jesuits. Then at Clermont, Blaise Pascal's nephew, the Jansenist *abbé* Louis Périer, informed his confessor, the *abbé* Fréhel, that Catholics could remain silent regarding the right/fact distinction in the Formulary. Consequently, Fréhel's confessor, the *abbé* Gay, who required his penitents to show "interior consent" prior to absolution, refused to hear Fréhel's confession. This little "tempest in a chalice" spilled over when Périer's friends published a provocative pamphlet, *The Case of Conscience Proposed by a Provincial Confessor Regarding an Ecclesiastic Who Is Under His Guidance, to Be Resolved by Several Doctors of the Faculty of Theology in Paris*. In it, they posed the following question: Can a priest who for several years has confessed a man without any scruples regarding his beliefs concerning the five propositions suddenly refuse to give him absolution upon discovering he is a quasi-Jansenist?[267]

When Fréhel submitted this case to the theologians at the Sorbonne in January 1701, they debated it vigorously for six months. Theologian Jacques Boileau advanced the debate to a new level by broadening the scope of the case. Could a confessor refuse absolution to a priest who did not attribute the five propositions to Jansen as condemned by the pope in 1653 and who contested the value of attrition in saving the repentant sinner? In July the theologians agreed that, indeed, a confessor could not refuse absolution to a man even after his Jansenist views came to light.[268]

The controversy might still have been contained within the walls of the Sorbonne except that 40 theologians who signed their names to a thesis concerning the "Case of Conscience" decided to publish it. They added what the Jesuits called an "impertinent preface" distinguishing "right" from "fact" and justifying "respectful silence" regarding the five propositions. After two editions of their pamphlet sold out, the "Case of Conscience" became the "Case of Quarrels." Bishop Bossuet in 1703 published his *Reflections on the Case of Conscience*. Pierre Nicole countered in 1704 with his *Apology for the Resolution of the Famous Case of Conscience*, rehashing old arguments and declaring that forced signing of the Formulary brought "much harm & no good" to the Church. Then Pasquier Quesnel (who had recently escaped from prison disguised as a woman and fled to Amsterdam) trumped the opposition with an eight-volume *History of the Case of Conscience*, begun in 1705. When Archbishop Noailles remained neutral, the Jansenists saw him as a traitor to their cause, while the Jesuits accused him of protecting Jansenism.[269]

When word of this quarrel reached Rome, Clement XI released the brief *Cum nuper* on 13 February 1703 condemning the "Case of Conscience" and excommunicating its anonymous author and anyone who read it. The brief declared that "respectful silence" regarding the five propositions "will not suffice to satisfy the obedience due to the Holy See, because it has been evident for a long time that this is the means by which many evade the Church's pronouncements and raise questions that have already been decided." Therefore, he demanded that the 40 theologians retract their statement. All of them did except Nicolas Petitpied; the faculty later expelled him from the Sorbonne. Under increasing pressure from Bossuet, Noailles issued a mandate nine days after the pope's brief condemning the views of the 40 theologians. When Louis XIV sent *lettres de cachet* ordering Parlement to condemn the Case, however, President de Harlay resisted, strengthened by the knowledge that Chancellor Pontchartrain supported him.[270]

Temporarily checkmated but not defeated, the king sent copies of the pope's brief to all the French bishops along with letters from his secretaries of state Chamillart and La Vrillière. These letters condemning the errors contained in the Case of Conscience showed "how the piety of His Majesty agrees with the zeal of His Holiness to maintain the integrity of the faith . . . and to strongly oppose the renewal of troubles which the condemned propositions of Jansénius have brought."[271] To strengthen this impression, Louis XIV wrote to Clement XI, thanking him "for the brief that Your Holiness has written" and assuring him of his "zeal to maintain the peace in the Church . . . and to prevent the dangerous effects of new opinions."[272] This letter thrilled the Holy See; papal nuncio Gualterio praised the king's "zeal for the crushing of novelties."[273]

Port-Royal represented the "nest" of such "novelties," the heart of intransigent Jansenism, the center of what the Society of Jesus called "a vast Jansenist plot." It had become a by-word for resistance, obstinacy, and disobedience to the wishes of Rome and Versailles, a place where (as Mme. de Maintenon put it) "this storm of Jansenism" originated. She told Cardinal Noailles that the only way he could "erase the suspicion of favoring the Jansenist party" would be to "dissipate" the "storm" at its source.[274] While the fence-sitting Noailles pondered her advice, the Council of State issued an *arrêt* mandating silence regarding the Formulary, the five propositions, and the "Case of Conscience." It prohibited the composing, printing, or selling of any works discussing Jansen's doctrines.[275] Shortly thereafter, Noailles told the nuns to sign the Formulary without reservations. They refused.[276]

For the aging, impatient king, this was the last straw. Frustrated by the nuns' endless stream of complaints and petitions and angered by their continual disobedience, he resolved to force them to submit. To accomplish this, he called on Clement XI, a pope widely seen as uncertain, variable, and weak, who, when embarrassed or contradicted, wept.[277] In June 1703, hoping to pave the way for a cooperative effort, the king told Cardinal Janson, the French ambassador to the Holy See: "When we act in concert, His Holiness and I, for the good of religion, we will be able to take measures so just that his good intentions will have their complete effects."[278] The following month, Louis XIV urged Janson to persuade the pope to issue a constitution "renewing the bulls of his predecessors against Jansenism." "I am persuaded," he argued, "that a new constitution on the subject would be useful to the Church." After another month had passed and Clement XI had not responded, the king sent him a rough draft of a bull and asked him to read and revise it.[279]

The request for a new bull put the pope in a bind. On the one hand, he was reluctant to take any action that might strengthen French Gallicanism. On the other, he could hardly issue a bull condemning "respectful silence" on the question of fact and right when Clement IX's bull had sanctioned this right. According to canon law, later pontiffs could not contradict the rulings of earlier ones. Perhaps if he drew up a constitution that merely repeated what Innocent X and Alexander VII had stated in their bulls, accompanied by a "strong objection" to—but not a condemnation of—"respectful silence," Louis XIV would be satisfied.[280] Trapped by this dilemma and uncertain how to respond, the pope dragged his feet for another two years.

Exasperated by Clement's delays, the French monarch told the pope in January 1705 that if he did not have a bull ready to present at the spring session of the General Assembly of the Clergy, he would authorize the Assembly to draw up its own anti-Jansenist resolution. This threat—coupled with a plea from Philip V of Spain for a bull to help him combat Jansenism in the Netherlands—broke the papal logjam. On July 16, after three days of fasting and special Masses, Clement issued the Bull *Vineam Domini Sabaoth* ("The vine of the Lord of Sabaoth"). When the first copies reached Paris and Versailles eleven days later, Cardinal Noailles, who saw "no difficulty in receiving it," described the bull as "very beautiful and good."[281]

Louis XIV was equally pleased. He told Ambassador Janson that the new bull contained all that he desired. Likewise, he assured the papal nuncio that he was "very satisfied" with the bull and expressed the hope that together, Clement XI and he could "vanquish" Jansenism in France. He resolved that since "His Holiness had furnished him with new arms, he would take up the struggle against heresy with greater vigor."[282]

Warmly welcomed in France, *Vineam Domini* received the unanimous approval of the General Assembly of the Clergy on August 21. The bishops voted their congratulations and thanks to Clement XI and Louis XIV, ordered that the bull be accepted "with respect and submission," instructed all bishops to post it in their dioceses, and asked the king to have it registered and published throughout his kingdom. Three days later, the monarch thanked the bishops for "accepting [the constitution] with joy and unanimous consent." A week later, *lettres patentes* gave it the force of law over the Gallican Church. The following week it sailed through Parlement. The magistrates registered it with minimal discussion and much praise for His Holiness.[283]

While *Vineam Domini* pleased many in France, it disturbed others who looked more closely at its content. Basically, the bull repudiated the views of the advocates of the "Case of Conscience" and condemned the position of "respectful silence" concerning the issue of "fact" and "right" in the five propositions. Because the bull marked the end of relative peace in the Church (1669–1705), it could be seen as a kind of "revocation of the Edict of Nantes" for Jansenism, which faced increasing struggles with both Church and state in the years ahead. It also affirmed the pope's infallibility when he spoke on matters of faith and doctrine.[284]

Although they approved the anti-Jansenist features in the bull, the Gallican bishops refused to let the pope's claim to infallibility go unchallenged. Therefore, on the same day they unanimously approved *Vineam Domini*, the bishops also passed three propositions. First, bishops have the right, by divine institution, to judge doctrinal matters. Second, papal constitutions are binding over the Church only after being accepted by the "body of pastors." Third, this acceptance occurs only by the collective judgment of the General Assembly of the Clergy.[285] Clement XI, angered by the bishops' propositions, called their actions "a mark of ingratitude and an injury to the Holy See."[286]

The Gallican bishops, however, were not alone in expressing reservations about the bull. At Port-Royal des Champs, the 25 nuns, led by Abbess Elizabeth de Saint-Anne, braced themselves for the storm they saw coming.[287] When Louis XIV commanded them to sign the Formulary in 1705, they protested that without a "qualifying clause," they could not do so. In March 1706, M. Gilbert, Noailles' grand vicar, again demanded that they adhere to the bull without "respectful silence" and sign the oath "without distinction of fact or right." Once more, after hours of "extraordinary prayer" and "consulting their consciences," they refused. On March 22 the abbess informed the archbishop that "neither passion, interest, or politics" would make them change their minds, for they had "learned in the school of Jesus Christ to love the truth and to suffer for it." Angered by their intransigence, Noailles threatened to scatter the nuns 200 leagues to other convents on bread and water diets. Considering them "criminally disobedient," he promised that unless their submission to his authority "be like that of a child, you will suffer even more for a long time."[288] During the next five years, those ominous words became a self-fulfilling prophecy as Port-Royal des Champs experienced new waves of persecution.

But why should such a tiny, isolated convent with a handful of aging nuns arouse the ire of so many enemies? The reasons are many and complicated. Fundamentally, Church leaders viewed these Jansenist sisters as schismatic at best and heretical at worst; if they refused to submit to Church authority and testify to their orthodoxy by signing the Formulary, they deserved to be excommunicated and suppressed. The issue of submission, of course, raised the specter of female independence from male authority. Although the abbesses chose male confessors and welcomed the solitaires to live nearby, for over a century, the nuns' rejection of appropriate male supervision and their resistance to patriarchal control made their relationship with Church and state authorities contentious. In tune with Archbishop Péréfixe's famous 1664 dictum that they were "pure as angels and proud as Lucifer," by the end of the century some people considered these women witches. Therefore, no matter which negative image one believed—schismatics, heretics, or witches—the conclusion was the same: Port-Royal represented a foyer of dissent and potential subversion against authority.

Furthermore, the endless stream of apologetic literature—books, memoirs, petitions, remonstrances, necrologies, and letters—produced by the religious annoyed those (especially the Jesuits) who disagreed with their viewpoints. Their opponents retaliated by publishing further "lies and calumnies" (as the Jansenists described them) about Port-Royal—leading to an endless tit-for-tat game of poisoned pen publications. Ever eager for combat in defense of "the truth," the convent's defenders engaged in so many quarrels—with the Jesuits, the Huguenots, the pope, the king, Parlement, the General Assembly of the Clergy, various archbishops and bishops—that they eventually depleted their forces. As one by one its wealthy and powerful friends and patrons died, the convent by 1700 had almost no one left to defend it against the onslaughts of state and Church.[289]

From Louis XIV's perspective, Port-Royal represented everything that he, as a divine right absolute monarch, abhorred: novelty, schism, heresy, liberty, independence, and dissent. Because the abbey had supported Cardinal de Retz during the Fronde, to his mind, its nuns and solitaires would never come clean of the taint of being *frondeurs*, rebels against his absolute authority. Therefore, no matter how pious their spiritual devotion to Catholicism or how sanctimonious their writings, Louis XIV saw this community as the center of a religiously deviant and socially disruptive movement that threatened the cohesion of his kingdom.[290]

To some extent, the king's personal experience during the Fronde shaped his image of Jansenism and Port-Royal. But many in whom he trusted and confided—the Jesuits, his confessor Le Tellier, his mistress (and after 1683 his wife) Mme. de Maintenon—also influenced his opinions. In 1706 Quesnel (and Jansenists in general) believed that the Jesuits, who had wanted to suppress the convent for years, played a key role in convincing the king to destroy it.[291] Moreover, the community's moral rigorism contrasted with the Jesuits' casuism and indirectly condemned the Court's pleasure-seeking ways. Furthermore, the Jesuits resented the popularity and success of the *petites écoles*, seeing them as rivals drawing students away from their own colleges. They also hated the solitaires (especially Saint-Cyran, Arnauld, Singlin, and de Sacy) for their relentless attacks on the Society of Jesus, their independence of thought, and their advocacy of liberty of conscience.[292]

Although Louis XIV's Jesuit confessor *Père* La Chaise disliked Jansenism, he did not want to destroy Port-Royal.[293] But his successor, Charles-Maurice Le Tellier, who "had lived his life supporting scholars who wrote against the Jansenists," did want to crush this "nest of heresy."[294] He persuaded the king that the Jansenists were as much heretics as the Huguenots, and just as great a threat to Church unity. Playing on Louis XIV's pride and vanity, he urged him to abolish Port-Royal des Champs before he died. As subsequent events show, Le Tellier himself played a key role in the destruction of the convent.[295]

Near the end of Madame de Maintenon's life, a phobia of heterodoxy made her deeply suspicious of Jansenists. Accusing them of bad faith, party spirit, and intrigues, she called them "political rebels." She disliked hearing courtiers like Mme. de Dangeau praise them as "the most honest people." Because Noailles was soft on Jansenism, Maintenon once referred to him as "the Cardinal who is no longer ours." "I'd shed my blood," she declared, "to hear it said: M. le cardinal has definitely decided against Jansenism." In collaboration with the Jesuits whom she favored, she encouraged the destruction of Port-Royal.[296]

Cardinal Noailles' leniency toward Jansenism and his private opposition to closing Port-Royal, however, did not mean that he approved of the nuns' behavior. "They are not heretics," he declared, "but rebels and disobedient ones. Therefore, I accuse them of criminal disobedience . . . Nothing is worse than half-learned women [*demi-savantes*)."[297] Nonetheless, many accused the cardinal of holding Jansenist views himself, a charge he denied in letters to Louis XIV and his nephew, the *duc* de Noailles. "Yet it is sometimes necessary that I appear to be a Jansenist to certain people," he explained. While he professed a desire to please the king, he also admitted, "I like those girls" at Port-Royal.[298] Consequently, much to the annoyance of Clement XI and Louis XIV, Noailles delayed closing the convent. When his nephew urged him to hasten its demise, the cardinal explained that terminating a religious community was a complex and delicate matter. Secretly, he hoped the sisters could live out their natural lives at Port-Royal des Champs and then, after the last nun had died, he could suppress the convent. He told them that it would greatly help their cause if they agreed to sign the Formulary and stopped writing protest letters and threatening lawsuits at the ecclesiastical court in Lyon.[299] They did neither.

When their insubordination came to Louis XIV's attention, he stopped them from receiving any more novices on the ground that they "hold bad doctrines contrary to the decision of the Church regarding Jansenism, condemned by the judgment of all the Church as capable of troubling the peace." Their refusal to sign the Formulary, he declared, "constitutes disobedience and perpetual scandal."[300] Coming so soon after the deaths of the convent's abbess, sub-prioress, and storeroom supervisor, this restrcition threatened to halt their supply of new recruits to replace the sisters who had died.[301] In their (collectively signed) letter of protest in September 1706, the seventeen sisters declared that "several persons badly disposed toward our convent and acting in the same spirit that caused our former afflictions . . . have formed the design of troubling us again." This "persecution," they opined, "will destroy the Peace of the Church." Although the nuns mentioned no names, their letter alluded to "plots" in Rome and at Versailles to keep the two convents divided, to prevent the rural priory from electing a new abbess, and to cancel many of their traditional rights. They pledged to oppose "so great an injustice by all means possible."[302]

Unfortunately for the nuns, however, while the number of their powerful defenders had diminished to almost nothing, the ranks of those perpetrating "injustices" had grown alarmingly. By 1707 their enemies included Clement XI, Louis XIV, Le Tellier, Mme. de Maintenon, Secretary of State Pontchartrain, Lieutenant-General of Police d'Argenson, and Cardinal de la Trémouille, French ambassador to Rome. At the Holy See, one observer exclaimed, "It will be a miracle . . . if anyone can save Port-Royal des Champs from collapsing under the weight of the authority which these adverse parties bring against it."[303]

Despite having few friends on the outside to protect them from the coming storm, however, these damsels in distress were not helpless. When the Council of State issued an *arrêt* in January 1707 ordering the closure of Port-Royal des Champs, they fought tooth and nail with every means at their disposal.[304] "The people who are making us suffer," declared *Mère* Du Mesnil, "are more to be pitied than we are."[305] Using a strategy they had perfected for more than half a century, these suffering saints generated a tidal wave of letters, petitions, lawsuits, and appeals protesting their mistreatment. Mlle. de Joncoux, a lawyer's daughter with an impressive network of friends, orchestrated their defense through the courts. She directed a team of female paralegals, secretaries, copyists, and couriers in producing so many documents that they clogged the legal system for three years. Her clandestine network connected the sisters at Port-Royal des Champs with exiled Jansenists in the Netherlands and with lawyers and theologians in Paris. By putting pressure on the pope, the king, the Archbishop of Paris, and other officials, the sisters hoped to push them into taking extreme measures and thus bring public opinion on their side.[306]

Almost before the ink on the Council's January 1707 *arrêt* had dried, for example, the nuns responded with a four-page response answering the charges of heresy and disobedience leveled against them. "We are not heretics," they cried, but innocent ones who "for 26 years have endured affliction without protesting." The letter, which defends their honor and proves the purity of their faith and the sincerity of their obedience, asserts "that we have never introduced among us any doctrine contrary to the decisions of the Church or refused to submit to the Constitution of Our Holy Father Pope Clement XI." Far from "troubling the Peace of the Church," their submission has been "genuine and complete," as an affidavit from Archbishop Péréfixe attests. In closing, they praise the king as "a prodigy of patience" for considering their request.[307]

Louis XIV's patience with them, however, had run out. On 9 February 1707, the Council of

State, revoking its *arrêt* of 13 May 1669 (which had divided the properties of the two convents), reunited the two houses and ordered the seventeen nuns and nine converts at Port-Royal des Champs transferred to Port-Royal in Paris.[308] Righteously indignant, the nuns unleashed a blizzard of letters, lawsuits, appeals, and procurations defending their orthodoxy and obedience to the Church, explaining why they could not sign the Formulary, and begging for mercy and understanding. These handwritten documents (which fill several folio volumes in the manuscript room at the Bibliothèque Nationale on the *rue* de Richelieu) reveal that the sisters and their friends could write Latin and French very well and knew how to use history, theology, reason, and past experience to their advantage. No infraction of their constitution, no sleight, however small, escaped their notice. They spilled as much ink protesting the "crime" of uniting their two houses as they did in sharing their "extreme astonishment" at the "crime" of allowing others to sell off their horses and cows. When Vicar-General François Vivant came to inventory their goods in August, they protested. When Archbishop Noailles retaliated by refusing them the sacraments in October, they protested again. When Louis XIV seized their revenues and sent their lawyer, M. de St.-Claude, to the Bastille in November, they protested yet again.[309] Once a pious movement, Jansenism had become a protest movement.

Yet Louis XIV, Clement XI, and even Cardinal Noailles had run out of patience with these geriatric protestors. On November 22, 1707, Noailles forbade the nuns to elect a new abbess "on pain of excommunication." They appealed his decision, not only to the ecclesiastical court in Lyons, but also to Rome. But when the primate in Lyons indicated his desire to reunite the two religious houses ("a wicked conjuncture," they said), these "very submissive, obedient, and afflicted daughters" (as they signed themselves) begged him to reconsider. When he refused, they sent another memoir to Clement XI via Cardinal Sacriponti in Rome, asking for his protection, justice, and grace.[310]

Clement XI, under pressure, decided to support Louis XIV. His bull of 27 March 1708 (which Parlement took eight months to register) suppressed Port-Royal des Champs and united the two convents under one administration at Port-Royal de Paris.[311] In a letter to his friend M. Schort, Quesnel asserted: "This affair, which is of the devil, has been prosecuted with fury." Then he added: "It will take a great miracle to stop [the convent's] complete destruction. I consider the complete union of the two convents to be their ruin."[312]

Despite facing imminent ruin, however, the nuns continued to protest. On 14 December 1708, they sent three nearly identical letters to Louis XIV, Cardinal Noailles, and Cardinal d'Estrées. In the first, they were "convinced that Your Majesty places his highest glory in rendering justice to innocent ones." But since the king was "badly informed" by "false exposés" concerning their heresy and disobedience, they hastened to enlighten him regarding their "innocence" and need for his "justice and goodness" in their behalf.[313] They informed Cardinal Noailles that they would appeal their case "to God's Tribunal, where all is weighed on the scales of the sanctuary [in heaven]." Just in case God refused to hear them, however, they begged Cardinal d'Estrées to intercede for them with his vicar on earth.[314]

In every case, their pleas fell on deaf ears. Even their request for Noailles to offer the sacraments to Sister Catherine le Pavaneu (66), a long-time paralytic who died of a stroke in December 1708, was rejected. The cardinal intended "to make an example of her before all the other sisters" who refused to sign the Formulary.[315] Then came the *annus horribilis* of 1709 when temperatures fell to –20 degrees Celsius. Wine froze in the convent's barrels, glasses, and chalices. Across France men and beasts froze to death in the fields and forests; harvests failed and fruit trees died and were cut down and burned in a desperate attempt to keep warm.[316] But for these women shivering in their cassocks, that terrible winter was an omen of worse things to come. Despite all their protests and appeals, Noailles' decree of 11 July 1709 "suppressed and extinguished forever" the convent of Port-Royal des Champs, "whose goods, rights, and revenues shall [henceforth] be transferred to the abbey and convent of Port-Royal de Paris."[317] Two months later, the Council of State's *arrêt* approved of "this just and natural reunion."[318]

With reunification, of course, came a new abbess—one whom the sisters could not elect. To bring order and discipline to Port-Royal, Louis XIV had personally chosen Mme. de Château-Renaud. But when the new abbess knocked at the gate of Port-Royal des Champs on October 1, the prioress, Louise de Ste.-Anastasie Du Mesnil, refused to let her enter. Angry at being outfoxed, Renaud stormed into Cardinal Noailles' office and told him what the sisters had done to her. When Noailles reported their actions to Louis XIV, the king called the Council of State together and emerged with an *arrêt* ordering the nuns to receive Renaud as their new abbess, give her the keys to the convent, and obey her instructions. Once again, they refused, protesting that since the time of Henri IV they had enjoyed the right of electing their abbesses. That was the last straw. The king decided to teach the nuns a lesson they would never forget.[319]

On October 26, the Council of State issued an *arrêt* authorizing the lieutenant-general of police, Marc-René de Voyer de Paulmy d'Argenson, to arrest and disperse the nuns and postulants at Port-Royal des Champs. Three days later at 7:30 a.m. (as the sisters came from Mass), d'Argenson, accompanied by three police officers and 300 archers, knocked at the gate. In his hand were 23 *lettres de cachet en blanc* (blank warrants) to arrest each of the fifteen nuns and seven postulants (Sister Marguerite de Ste.-Romaine-Lévy had died three months before). When *Mère* Du Mesnil opened only the grate in the door (reminiscent of the "Day of the Wicket Gate" a century earlier), the police chief grew angry at this disrespect to a minister of the king. When he asked the prioress to help him write the sisters' names in the blanks, she refused. When he showed her the *arrêt* from the Council of State, she declined to sign the *procès verbal* unless he gave her a copy of it, but he refused her request.

Gathering the nuns together, d'Argenson gave them three hours to pack their bags and climb aboard one of the twelve carriages waiting in the courtyard. While they ate their last meal and gathered their few belongings, the police officers collected the convent's manuscripts and records, a process that took much longer than d'Argenson had expected. As the hours passed, the archers griped and complained. But at 5 p.m., with all the sisters and postulants on board and the archers shouting commands to the horses, the heavily loaded carriages made their way down the narrow country road.[320] Much later, an anonymous scribe wrote in the *Port-Royal Necrology* that on October 29, 1709, "occurred the general Dispersion of all the Religious from Port-Royal des Champs and the Destruction of this celebrated and holy Convent."[321]

In reality, both the "dispersion" of the nuns and the "destruction" of their convent required more than a year to accomplish. First, separate *lettres de cachet* had to be filled out for each of the fifteen nuns, specifying their name, the convent they were being sent to, and the rules governing their future treatment. One such order, addressed to the abbess of a recipient convent, read as follows:

> BY ORDER OF THE KING
>
> Dear & much beloved, having given our orders to accept into your convent Sister Marie Madéleine de Ste. Gertrude de Valois, religious of the order of Cistercians, We command & order you to receive her & to hold her there until a new order. A payment of her pension will be regularly forwarded to you by the Abbey of Port-Royal at Paris. Make no mistakes in this: for such is our pleasure. Given at Versailles the 26 October 1709. (Signed) Louis Phélypeaux[322]

To wean these sisters from their Jansenist errors, Louis XIV ordered them dispersed to orthodox convents belonging to the Ursulines, Filles de Sainte-Marie, Visitadines, Veronicas, Benedictines, and Saint-Juliens as follows:

Louise de Sainte-Anastasie Du Mesnil—Ursulines at Blois
Françoise de Sainte-Marthe—Veronicas at Blois
Anne-Julie de Sainte-Synclétique de Remicourt—Benedictines at Rouen
Marie de Sainte-Gertrude du Valois—Ursulines at Chartres
Françoise de Sainte-Agathe Le Juge—Visitations at Chartres
Marie de Sainte-Euphrasie Robert—Ursulines at Mantes
Marie de Sainte-Catherine Issoly—Ursulines at Meaux
Marie-Catherine de Sainte-Célinie Benoise—Filles de Sainte-Marie at Meaux
Anne de Sainte-Cécile de Boicervoise—Saint-Juliens at Amiens
Marie-Madéleine de Sainte-Cécile Bertrand—Filles de Sainte-Marie at Amiens
Jeanne de Sainte-Apolline Le Bègue—Filles de Sainte-Marie at Compiègne
Marguerite de Sainte-Lucie Pépin—Filles de la Visitation at Autun
Marie-Madéleine de Sainte-Sophie Flescelles—unknown convent at Moncenis
Madéleine de Sainte-Ide Le Vavasseur—Ursulines at Nevers
Marie de Sainte-Anne Couturier—Ursulines at Nevers[323]

Although the nuns ranged in age from 50 to 86 years of age, nine (60%) were in their fifties, three (20%) in their sixties, one (7%) in her seventies, and two (13%) in their eighties. The oldest—Sister Anne de Sainte-Cécile Boicervoise (86)—who had entered Port-Royal des Champs at 33 in 1656, died of a heart attack only five days after being transferred to the convent of the Cordelières de St.-Julien in Amiens.[324] As convent life tended to promote longevity, however, most of the sisters could hope to live 20 to 30 more years in their new surroundings.

To prevent them from "corrupting" their fellow sisters, Minister Pontchartrain issued seven guidelines to the abbesses of each convent and to the bishops of that diocese. Although the Port-Royal nuns should be treated "with kindness and charity," they must not be allowed to "foment stubbornness" or "spoil the convents" where they resided by discussing controversial doctrines with other sisters. They may not write letters to or receive gifts from those outside the convent without the bishop's permission. The king wants to be informed, Pontchartrain said, if any of the nuns attempts a clandestine correspondence. Such disobedience will be punished by solitary confinement. Every book they read must first receive the bishop's approval. They must follow the schedules and observe all the rules of their host convent "without any resistance." Finally, they must sign the Formulary "purely & simply" as a sign of their submission to Clement XI. All did so except for their prioress, *Mère* Du Mesnil, and Sister Marie Madéleine de Saint-Gertrude du Valois.[325] Following Louis XIV's death in 1715, the *duc* d'Orléans, regent for the young Louis XV, allowed the remaining twelve nuns to return to Paris where the Cardinal de Noailles could impose "good discipline" on them. As they (still) refused to go to Port-Royal de Paris, Noailles placed them in other convents in the capital, where they lived out their natural lives, the last one dying in 1738.[326] The Jesuits, hoping to establish another seminary in the Saint Jacques district, asked Noailles if they could occupy Port-Royal, but he denied their request.[327]

Meanwhile, back in the Chevreuse Valley, the *abbé* Madot and several archers, at Le Tellier's orders, rifled through the convent's books, manuscripts, and pictures. Seeing heresy everywhere, Madot tore up pictures of Saint-Cyran and Antoine Arnauld, but gave Mlle. Joncoux many of the most valuable manuscripts, records, and books (which, at her death in 1715, went to the Bibliothèque de Saint-Germain-des-Près and now reside at the Bibliothèque Nationale on the rue de Richelieu). When *Mère* Château-Renaud arrived (this time without being rebuffed), she commandeered the archers to load the convent's goods into 150 wagons for the trip back to Port-Royal de Paris. From the larder, they hauled potted butter, hogsheads of prunes, barrels of grain, boxes of eggs, pitchers of olive and nut oil, bags of salt, and candle wax. From the laundry's shelves they packed linens, coverlets, mattresses, robes, stockings, and thread, in addition to a tapestry from the royal Gobelins factory.[328]

Moving on to the chapel, library, and storerooms, they gathered 500 years' worth of gold, silver, and gem-incrusted relics donated by kings, dukes, duchesses, bishops, and wealthy friends since 1204. These priceless treasures included silver crosses, crimson reliquaries, gilded paintings of saints, crystal vases, pearl-studded tableaux, gold-covered shrines, paintings matted with expensive satin and embroidered with flowers. Like wide-eyed explorers in a pharaoh's tomb, everywhere they turned they saw gold, silver, lapis lazuli, gilded leather, black and crimson velvet, white silk, crystal, and enamel. Despite the abbess's watchfulness, a few relics disappeared into the archers' pockets.[329]

Having removed the convent's inhabitants in one day and confiscated its treasures over several weeks, the archers next proceeded to tear down its buildings, a task that took nearly a year. Louis XIV's Jesuit advisor, *Père* Le Tellier, had convinced him that, to save maintenance expenses and prevent pilgrims and tourists from flocking to the site, all physical traces of the convent should be obliterated. The Council of State, in its *arrêt* of 22 January 1710, ordered all but the chapel (used as a warehouse) to be torn down. Not until June, however, did the wrecking crew begin carrying out these orders, demolishing the convent, guest house, barns, and outbuildings, including the pavilions where the *duchesse* de Longueville and Mlle. de Vertus had once lived. During 1711, they also tore down the chaplain's lodgings and the tenant farmer's house. When Jansenist pilgrims crowded the grounds in 1712 to worship in the old chapel, the king ordered that destroyed as well. When the dust finally settled, only one barn, the solitaires' dwelling known as The Grange, the wall, and the huge dovecote remained standing.[330]

But underneath the ground, possibly 3000 skeletons[331]—few of which had belonged to Jansenist bodies—remained. In his effort to eradicate all traces of this "nest of heresy," Louis XIV ordered the cadavers dug up and moved to the cemeteries of Saint-Lambert-des-Bois and Magny-les-Hameaux in Paris. Warned in advance about the king's intentions, several prominent families exhumed their relatives' bodies and reburied them in family plots. Thanks to the intervention of Minister of State Pomponne, six members of the Arnauld family (including former abbesses Angélique Arnauld and Angélique de St.-Jean), and the bodies of the *duchesse* de Longueville, the *princesse* de Conti, Le Maître de Sacy, and Jean Racine, were exhumed and moved elsewhere. The rest, however, suffered a ghoulish fate. To make the corpses fit into the boxes, the workmen sometimes chopped off their heads, arms, or legs before loading them onto the wagons. The stench must have been horrible. Once in Paris, the gravediggers buried the bodies in unmarked graves.[332]

But what to do with the cemetery markers left behind? According to long-standing legends, some tombstones became paving stones in nearby roads; others appeared as tables at inns. After workers blew up the old chapel with gunpowder, they sold its timbers to the highest bidder, while the Archbishop of Beaumont used its foundation stones to build a new aqueduct. Where the fruit orchard had once stood, farmers plowed up the soil and sowed wheat. To all appearances, Port-royal des Champs had disappeared.[333]

By destroying the physical reminders of Port-Royal des Champs and scattering its nuns, Louis XIV demonstrated that he had won the battle against the convent in the short run. But over the long run, neither the king nor Clement XI nor Cardinal Noailles could win the war to erase the memory of Port-Royal. By their courageous but hopeless resistance, the sisters, too, had won a short-term victory by preventing officials from forcing them to participate in the reunification of the two convents. During the seventeenth century, they had ably played the role of suffering saints as the drama of Jansenism unfolded. Throughout the eighteenth century and beyond, as martyrs for the truth, their cause would endure in the hearts and minds of Jansenists everywhere.[334]

Long before 1709, the religious insured that they would be remembered by carefully preparing their legacy for posterity. To vindicate their beliefs and defend their resistance to persecution, they carefully preserved their memoirs, relations, letters, biographies, and legal documents.[335] Their meticulous necrologies, handwritten in fading brown ink, lauded the virtues and deeds of their abbesses, solitaires, and Jansenist benefactors. Decades before Diderot's and d'Alembert's *Encyclopédie* popularized alphabetical organization, the nuns wrote biographical entries in these sacred almanacs according to the day that person died. As one would expect, they wrote longer entries for famous Jansenists like Antoine Arnauld (seventeen pages), Angélique Arnauld (eleven pages), Antoine Le Maître (nine pages), and Blaise Pascal (eight pages). Key figures like the *abbé* de Saint-Cyran, Robert Arnauld d'Andilly, Pierre Nicole, Edmond Richer, and the Bishop of Alet got three or four pages each, while many friends (like Cardinal de Retz) and even former abbesses (like Catherine de Ste.-Agnès Arnauld) garnered only a page. Significantly, the nuns summarized Louis XIV's reign in *one single line.* Even non-Jansenist figures like Alphonse IX of Spain, Queen Berengaria of Jerusalem, and Bishop Palafax in New Spain (Mexico) received more attention.[336]

Almost before the dust had settled at Port-Royal des Champs, Jansenist apologists began writing militant histories portraying the nuns as "a community of holy examples destined for the faith" and "instruments of the divine plan" defending truth in the midst of persecution.[337] Jacques Fouillou (1709), who called the convent's destruction "the abomination of desolation," provided the nuns with heroic lines like "We will obey even to the death" and "Today is the day of man; soon the day of God will come" as they stumbled, defiant to the end, toward the carriages.[338] He imagined that someone posted the following verse on the wall at Versailles:

Let us weep, alas! The fatal dispersal
Of these Saints of Port-Royal
Without any form of justice
This convent devoted to God
By the Magistrate of Police
Is treated as a wicked place.[339]

Other poems, odes, and epitaphs praised the memory of Port-Royal des Champs as a "Temple of pure faith, obedience, charity, and penitence" set amidst a "peaceful solitude so full of charms." Its destruction came about because of the Jesuits' "devouring hatred" and the "fury of hundreds of criminal ministers," all of them "traitors and models of iniquity" whose "infernal design" made them commit "this horrible crime."[340]

Until her death in 1715, Mlle. de Joncoux assisted in the publication of several apologetic works defending the memory of Port-Royal, including that of Jacques Fouilou. Others who benefited from her assistance included Michel Tronchay (1710) and Pasquier Quesnel (1711). Both men wrote emotional treatises describing the destruction of the convent and praising the nuns as Christian heroes who resisted evil persecutors. Tronchay (1710), who saw the convent as a symbol of faith, vigilance, virtue, godly conduct, and the disciplined life, portrayed the nuns as "innocent Victims of man's passion" and the closing of the abbey as "pillaging this holy House." Its ruins, he exclaimed, "are worthy of veneration."[341] Even that perpetual curmudgeon, the *duc* de Saint-Simon, waxed superlative in his praise of Port-Royal. "That which in recent centuries has produced all that is most holy, pure, wise, instructive, practical, exalted, brilliant and clear has come from that school which we know under the name of Port-Royal," he said.[342]

When Louis XIV tried to ram the Bull *Unigenitus* (1713) down the throats of the ecclesiastics and *parlementaires*, (see chapter 5) Jansenists and *appelants* resisted in the name of Port-Royal. To the *abbé* Etemare, leader of the *Figuristes*, "the cause of appeal and the cause of Port-Royal are one." Louis-Adrien le Paige, another *Figuriste*, wrote voluminously to prove that the Parlement of Paris represented "a second Port-Royal" charged with conserving fundamental laws. Many Jansenist magistrates invoked the image of the "luminous utopia" in their battles against the Jesuits. The nuns' courageous stand against government persecution likewise inspired the followers of the Deacon Pâris, known in the 1730s as *convulsionnaires* (discussed in chapter 7).[343]

Between 1730 and the expulsion of the Jesuits in 1764, many memoirs about Port-Royal as well as collections of letters written by the religious were published.[344] One author, Nicolas Fontaine (1736), focused on the positive, praising the convent as "the most precious source of the purest light & most solid virtue in the Church today."[345] Others, like Olivier Pinault (1750) and Charles Clémencet (1757), explained how defeats in battle, famine, expulsion from France, and sudden death represented "the finger of God" raised against those (Louis XIV, Cardinal Noailles, and the Abbess Château-Ranaud) who had dared to destroy such a holy place.[346] In addition, authors and editors like Pierre Leclerc (1753), Charles Clémencet (1757), and René Cerveau (1760) collected and published previously unknown hagiographies, letters, speeches, biographies, and book excerpts written by the sisters and solitaires, bringing them to the attention of a wider (and often sympathetic) public.[347] After reading this material, many wanted to visit the two convents. So in the 1770s "manuals for pilgrims" appeared to guide tourists to the locations of the two convents and provide them with a brief (and biased) history.[348]

Finally, just two years before the French Revolution, the underground Jansenist paper *Les Nouvelles Ecclésiastiques* ("The Ecclesiastical News") praised the memory of Port-Royal as "this Holy House," "the glory & ornament of the Church," "that illustrious solitide" where the "solid & enlightened piety" of its nuns and solitaires had produced such "immortal works."[349]

When the government nationalized Church property after 1789, Mme. Desprez purchased Port-Royal des Champs. However, she permitted the Society of Christian Philosophy, a small group of writers, to hold their meetings at The Grange and discuss science, medicine, philosophy, and literature. Port-Royal de Paris, on the other hand, became Port-Libre Prison where aristocrats awaiting their turn at the guillotine formed a literary salon and played games to while away the time.[350] Nineteenth-century writers portrayed Port-Royal as part of "the moral world that has perished" where faith, excellence, austerity, genius, and joy resided.[351]

For the most part, twentieth century historians have preserved the halo around Port-Royal. In addition to praising the austere, rigorist lifestyles of its religious, H. Bremond (1923) lauded the "spirit of reflection" and "depth of analysis" of their "devout humanism."[352] Louis Cognet (1952) surmised that for most of its visitors, Port-Royal des Champs represented "an austerity, a rigor, a resistance to authority, the refuge of noble souls and the crossroads of passions."[353]

Today, in a far different sense of the word, Port-Royal in Paris still represents "the crossroads of passions" to the hundreds of expectant mothers who come to its maternity hospital for assistance in giving birth. A hospice for orphans and bastards after 1795, the former convent was renamed *Maternité Baudelocque* in 1895. But in 1966 it became *La Maternité de Port-Royal*. Here at 169, *rue* Saint-Jacques, where aging celibate nuns once sang in the chapel and walked in the gardens, young mothers today enjoy that same experience, as the gardens and many of the interior buildings have been restored. At Port-Royal des Champs, on the other hand, only the pigeon house, one barn, The Grange, and part of the outer wall survive today. But in the Louis XIII-style building where boys once studied their lessons in the *petites écoles*, the National Museum of the Grange of Port-Royal, opened in 1962, preserves many of the precious manuscripts and artifacts of Port-Royal's glory days three centuries ago.[354]

CHAPTER 5

Jansenism Enters the Political Arena, 1713–1750

"[The Bull] *Unigenitus* will be the Cross not only of theologians but also of the highest magistrates of the realm."—*Henri-François d'Aguesseau*[1]

Louis XIV considered the demolition of Port-Royal des Champs a major victory in his war against Jansenism. No doubt he thought that without a visible headquarters such as the convent had provided, the Jansenists would scatter and soon their heresy would cease to trouble the Church. Government officials had used the same reasoning when in the 1680s they demolished Huguenot temples, believing that without places to worship, the Calvinists would soon convert to Catholicism.[2] Officials had failed to realize, however, that heart-felt convictions could endure—indeed, could grow stronger in the minds of their adherents—without physical structures to contain them.

Just as the persecution that followed the Edict of Fontainebleau in 1685 (which revoked the civil and religious rights of the Huguenots) had strengthened French Calvinism, so the papal Bull *Unigenitus* in 1713 gave Jansenism its second wind and transformed a religious controversy into a major affair of state.[3] As Catherine Maire (1998) so aptly stated: "The shock wave [of *Unigenitus*] reverberated across the century. The history of France and, to a certain degree, the history of Christianity in the eighteenth century revolved around it."[4]

This controversial new bull marked the passing of the first or spiritual phase (seventeenth century) of Jansenism, with its Augustinian emphasis on sin, grace, penitence, and self-denial in the devotional and polemical works of Jansen, Saint-Cyran, and members of the Arnauld family. It gave birth to a second, political phase (eighteenth century) in which prominent Jansenists battled popes, kings, and bishops in Parlement, at the Bastille, and in the pages of clandestine publications like the underground paper *Les Nouvelles Ecclésiastiques (The Ecclesiastical News).*

In a sense, Pasquier Quesnel inadvertently inaugurated the political phase of Jansenism when in 1692 he published his *Moral Reflections on the New Testament* with comments on each verse in French. Shortly after the Archbishop of Paris banished him from Paris, Parlement condemned the work and had it publicly burned in 1699. In a typical case of overkill, the Church placed it on the *Index* in 1700, Louis XIV issued an ordinance against it in 1703, and in 1708 Clement XI condemned the book.[5]

But Louis XIV wanted to crush Jansenism, not merely ban books. Unfortunately, Clement XI's Bull *Vineam domini* (1705) had proved disappointing in eliminating the Jansenist scourge in France. So in November 1711, the king told La Trémoille, his ambassador to the Holy See, to ask the pope for permission to convene a national council of bishops to solve the problem. But Clement, afraid of conciliarism, refused. So Louis suggested a compromise: convene an assembly of Church leaders and theologians to draft a new constitution condemning Quesnel's *Moral*

Reflections and Jansenism.[6] While this request flattered the pope's pride, it also presented him with a dilemma. In the early eighteenth century, when many Church officials opposed the pope's claim of infallibility, papal documents often met with hostile receptions across Europe, engendering contentious debates among theologians, professors, and magistrates. Given the highly charged atmosphere in France, it was more than likely that Parlement would oppose making any bull the law of the land. Moreover, many bishops who supported the "Four Gallican Articles" of 1682 would argue that they had as much right as the pope to judge doctrinal matters. In addition, the bull might raise the hackles of the General Assembly of the Clergy, who, as the "body of French pastors," steadfastly defended its right to accept or reject papal pronouncements. Finally, by issuing such a bull, Clement risked alienating Jansenist sympathizers in Europe as he had done in 1705.[7]

Consequently, the pope stalled for time. Months passed with no action taken as Louis XIV became increasingly impatient and letters flew back and forth. In 1710 and 1711, Louis offended the pope during the Regale controversy and Clement angered the king by refusing to support his grandson Philip for the vacant Spanish throne. Yet king and pope genuinely wanted reconciliation. Certain individuals began pressuring the pope for a new bull: Cardinal Fabroni (secretary of the Congregation of Propaganda), Cardinal Paolucci (papal secretary of state), *Père* La Chaise and his successor, *Père* Le Tellier (Louis XIV's Jesuit confessors), and of course, the king himself.[8]

Finally, Clement XI formed a committee (called a "congregation") composed of two cardinals, two members of the Holy Office, and nine theologians. Between early June and late December 1712, this committee met 20 times by itself, followed by another 23 sessions with the pope from early February to late August 1713. During those fourteen months of deliberations, its members reduced the original 155 condemned propositions they found in Quesnel's *Moral Reflections* to 101. Then they scrutinized the writings of Catholic theologians to decide in what sense each proposition was susceptible to condemnation (heresy, blasphemy, offensive, error, etc.).[9]

Chafing at their slow deliberations, Louis XIV shared with La Trémoille "the impatience that I have that he [Clement XI] remedy it [the problem of Jansenism] as soon as possible by this constitution." He told the ambassador in June to "renew my insistence for the constitution that I have requested for such a long time . . . I order you to press this affair." When two months passed without progress, the king commanded La Trémoille to "push the matter to a short conclusion."[10] Finally, at the end of August, the committee completed its work. On September 8, Clement XI signed the Constitution *Unigenitus Dei Filius* ("The Only Son of God").[11]

In it, the pope expressed (in French, not Latin this time) his "profound grief" at the "pernicious enterprises" of "false prophets" and "wolves" like Quesnel and Nicole who attacked the Catholic "flock" and spread their "venom of errors" (even papal documents could mix metaphors). Among other epithets, the preamble calls Quesnel a "master of falsehood," an "inventor of seditious sects," a "falsifier of Scriptures," a "poisoner of souls," and a "child of the devil." His *Moral Reflections* is packed with "novelties," "pernicious maxims," and "seductive & wicked insinuations." Yet "the venom of this book is well hidden, like an abscess that must be cut out." Mingled with its "pious appearances and smooth style," the committee discovered 101 "detailed errors." They therefore forbade the faithful to possess, read, print, or distribute this book on pain of excommunication by the Church and further punishment by the state. After "ardently imploring the help of Heaven" in personal and public prayers, the pope released the bull on September 10, hoping that it would protect his flock across Europe.[12]

Yet many members of that flock found portions of the bull deeply disturbing. In its buckshot attack on Jansenism, Augustinians asserted that it condemned several orthodox theses on grace in order to support Molinist positions held by the Jesuits. Its rejection of liturgical innovations and opposition to granting the laity access to the Bible in their own language offended progressives. Gallicans naturally objected to certain clauses implying the pre-eminence of Rome over the French Church and the Holy See's right to control kings. Still others pointed out that in order to condemn Quesnel, the committee had taken some of his phrases out of context, twisted many of his innocent biblical citations, and misinterpreted most of his references to St. Augustine and a few to the other Church Fathers. The magistrates in Parlement took offense at Article 91 asserting the pope's right to excommunicate kings and absolve subjects of their natural allegiance. Overall, the bull attacked 43 propositions on grace and predestination, 28 on charity and faith, seven on Church organization and hierarchy, and 23 on penitence, morality, and the Holy Scriptures. However, unlike earlier bulls condemning the five propositions ascribed to Jansen's *Augustinus* (only some of which could actually be found therein), the 101 propositions condemned by *Unigenitus* were authentically in Quesnel's book.[13]

While some theologians debated what the bull asserted, however, others quibbled over what it did not say. Its carefully nuanced, ambiguous prose applied none of its 22 condemnatory qualifications specifically to any of the 101 propositions allegedly taken from Quesnel's book. Therefore, it did not clarify which propositions were merely "shocking" or "offensive to pious ears" and which "outright heresy." Those with legalistic minds (and all Jansenists had such minds) could argue, therefore, that the bull did not constitute a rule of faith and that those who opposed it were not heretics.[14]

Unigenitus received a warm welcome in Italy, Germany, Hungary, Poland, Dalmatia, and among Catholics in England. Savoy, Spain, and Poland welcomed it also, but allowed individual bishops to accept or reject it. Only in France did the bull create controversy.[15] Hoping perhaps to smooth the way for the its acceptance there, Clement flattered Louis XIV. "We cannot applaud enough the zeal of our most dear son in Jesus Christ, Louis, the Most Christian King of France . . . for the defense and preservation of the purity of the Catholic faith, and for the extirpation of heresy."[16]

A courier from Rome reached Fontainebleau on September 25 and presented the king with his personal copy of the bull; other copies went to Cardinal Noailles and First President of Parlement De Mesmes. Quickly backpedaling, Noailles issued a (rather unconvincing) mandate disavowing his previous praise for *Moral Reflections* as a bishop ("We do not want to lose a moment in revoking the approval that we gave it in another diocese," he declared).[17] Thrilled with *Unigenitus*, Louis issued *lettres patentes* on 14 February 1714 to enforce the bull in the Gallican Church. He hoped, no doubt sincerely, that the bull would stop all disputes disturbing the "peace of the Church and the purity of the Faith"; halt publication and distribution of Quesnel's book; and destroy "errors against the faith."[18] Ironically, however, by enforcing the bull to crush Jansenism, Louis instead gave the movement a shot in the arm that invigorated it, because his vision of a unified French Church clashed with the Jansenists' call for independence regarding "fact" and "right."[19]

The bull required three separate "registrations"—by the Gallican bishops, by Parlement, and by the Sorbonne—before it could be effectively enforced in France. Louis XIV promised the pope that, after a cursory examination "to verify that it contained nothing contrary to Gallican liberties," the bishops would accept it quickly.[20] But Cardinal Noailles hesitated to accept a bull condemning a work he had once approved, and the clergy were reluctant to accept the authority of a committee of eight bishops (chaired by Armand Gaston, Cardinal de Rohan and handpicked by the king) to enforce the bull in France. Therefore, in October, 29 bishops (and eventually 49) meeting in Paris formed an ad hoc committee that deliberated over the bull for five months. This committee took three months to determine the authenticity of the French and Latin texts, to examine the bull's theology (Was each of the 101 propositions really in Quesnel's work?), and to decide if they agreed with the pope's level of condemnation on each point. Not all did. Nonetheless, the bishops signed a congratulatory letter thanking Clement XI for "the zeal he has shown in condemning a work so dangerous" and thanked him for his "excellent and solemn bull." They also thanked Louis XIV "for his continual protection over the Church and the zeal he has always shown to crush errors." On December 21, 29 bishops issued a circular letter urging French bishops to accept, post, and enforce the bull. Most of them did, eagerly condemning Quesnel's ideas as "venom," "the most dangerous artifice," and an "abuse of Holy Scripture."[21]

But by January 1714, the Assembly as a whole had still not voted in favor of the bull. As Louis XIV and Clement XI grew increasingly impatient, a subcommittee of six clerics suggested six proposals for the group to approve. They should receive the bull with "respectful submission," express their joy at finding consistent Catholic doctrines within it, agree to censure the *Moral Reflections*, send letters of pastoral instruction to all French bishops, and letters of thanks to the pope and king. When put to a vote on January 23, 40 bishops approved and nine (including the chair Noailles) rejected this motion. The nine recusants, believing that the bull would do great harm to Catholic doctrine, Church discipline, and Christian piety, declared that "their consciences forbade them from receiving this document."[22] Many saw Article 91 giving the pope authority to excommunicate kings and absolve subjects of their allegiance as "contrary to royal maxims" and Gallican liberties.[23]

Therefore, despite Cardinal Rohan's pleas that they all unite and accept the bull, the recusants, led by Cardinal Noailles, sent Louis XIV a letter begging him to allow them to accept *Unigenitus* "with some explications." When deliberating about papal constitutions, they said, bishops are "judges of the faith," so their consciences should never be coerced.[24] Gaston de Noailles, Bishop of Châlons-sur-Marne, told his brother, the Cardinal de Noailles: "I am your brother and would love to do anything for you, but my conscience will not permit it. There are times when Christian prudence demands that one resist openly . . . The authority of the pope and the King is being carried too far."[25]

The eight intransigent bishops soon learned just how far their monarch could carry his authority. In February he signed *lettres de cachet* sending each of them back to their dioceses and ordering them not to move without his permission.[26] After Cardinal Noailles issued mandates forbidding the Paris clergy to read the bull to their parishioners on penalty of being removed from office, Louis XIV, calling him a heretic, removed him as president of the General Assembly and banned him from appearing at Court. Mme. de Maintenon, who accused Noailles of trying to "undermine the King," reminded him that "you have the pope and most of the bishops against you." In fact, Cardinal Paolucci, the papal secretary of state, sent him a blistering letter informing him of the pope's "astonishment" at this "scandal." Clement XI threatened to summon Noailles to Rome to answer charges against him unless he at once prepared a pastoral letter of instruction supporting the bull. After waiting six months, the pope set October 18 as the deadline to receive Noailles' letter of submission. It arrived the day before the deadline.[27]

Although Noailles complied with the pope's demand for a pastoral letter, he still did not accept the bull. He told his friend M. de Mirepoix in June 1714: "I have the misfortune of being out of the King's good graces. But I cannot desire his favor at the expense of my conscience."[28] Recognizing that he could not coerce Noailles' conscience, the king sought some other way of gaining episcopal support for the bull. In October, he once again asked Clement to authorize a national council of French bishops to decide matters of discipline and dogma in the French Church. As before, however, the pope rejected this plan, fearing schism in the Church if the bishops developed a spirit of independence from Rome's control. "I do not want to deliver myself to a hundred bears who would eat me alive," he quipped.[29] Cardinal Fabroni gently reminded Louis XIV that "It is to St. Peter and his successors that Jesus Christ has confided the government of the Church . . . One reads nowhere in the Gospels 'exceptis Gallis' [except in France]."[30]

To increase pressure on the Archbishop of Paris, Clement sent the king two briefs: the first urged Noailles to write another pastoral letter accepting the bull and citing this brief; the second threatened to summon him to Rome and strip him of his cardinal's hat. The pope also suggested that Louis revoke the cardinal's French citizenship.[31]

Despite being persona non grata at Court and in Rome, Noailles stood by his convictions. In March 1715 he informed Chancellor Voysin:

> Blind obedience, submission pure and simple, degradation of the episcopate so clearly established cannot be separated from threats and reproofs . . . I have done nothing except to uphold the purity of the faith, the authority of the bishops, the service of the King, and the maxims of the State . . . If this is a crime in Rome, it must not be so for you, Monsieur, since you are charged with defending our liberties and the rights of the Crown.[32]

Although fifteen bishops attempted to find some compromise formula that would satisfy the pope, the king, and Noailles, negotiations disintegrated when the group split over the wording. Thirteen bishops drew up the "Body of Doctrine" highlighting the truths and errors in *Unigenitus*. Although Louis XIV approved this document, Parlement refused to register it.[33] Bishop Broglie, secretary of the General Assembly of the Clergy, worried "that the spark they had lighted would one day cause a great conflagration if it were not quickly extinguished."[34]

To prevent the bull from sparking lengthy debates in Parlement, Le Tellier and Mme. de Maintenon urged the king to pressure procurer-general D'Aguesseau and advocate-general Joly de Fleury to register it quickly. Unlike the bishops, the magistrates needed only a week (September 26–October 2) to examine *Unigenitus*.[35] From their initial reading, they concluded that "Rome has never sent into France a bull more innocent and less contrary to the traditions of the kingdom and to the liberties of the Gallican Church." Although they cautioned Louis XIV that Article 91 could "cause trouble in the State," they recommended registering it, but with "a measured reserve on that point."[36]

But some of the leading *gens du roi*—among them 16 Jansenist barristers—felt that Article 91 merited closer examination. Could it subvert Parlement's jurisdictional authority to hear appeals from Church courts? Might it allow the pope to excommunicate the king and absolve his subjects from their natural allegiance to him?[37] Like Antoine Arnauld before them, these Jansenist lawyers envisioned Parlement playing a leading role in the on-going struggle between the papacy, the Gallican Church, and the king. As judges, they had the right to police the external affairs of the Church when ecclesiastical cases were referred to them and, if necessary, to censure or punish offending clerics, including bishops, cardinals, and even the papal nuncio to France. Parlement had the power, they asserted, to refuse to recognize papal bulls, decrees, and briefs, and the pope should not excommunicate them for carrying out their legal duty.[38] Nor should the king curtail their freedom to express their opinions about the bull in legal arguments printed and distributed among the public (such "judicial memoirs" ran to hundreds of pages).[39]

Procurer-general D'Aguesseau, himself a Jansenist, expressed his Gallican concerns for parliamentary liberties when he told Louis XIV: "No Constitution of the popes in matters of doctrine . . . may be invested with the king's authority without a legitimate and sufficient acceptance by the Gallican Church. To do otherwise would be to recognize the pope as infallible and sole judge of faith against the fundamental maxims of our liberties."[40] D'Aguesseau confided in his private journal that this bull "would be a cross, not only to the theologians, but also to the first magistrates of the realm."[41]

Angered by their debates and delays, Louis XIV seemed ready to nail his magistrates to a cross. On 8 February 1714 he summoned First President De Mesmes and Advocate-General Joly de Fleury to Versailles and ordered them to have Parlement register the bull quickly. During this brief but heated encounter, the king reminded the two men that he was the master and wished to be obeyed; if they caused him "the least trouble, he would stomp on [their] stomachs with both feet." As a parting shot, Louis reminded them that "it was not very far from his office to the Bastille."[42] Five days later, he warned them to cease writing their memoirs and commentaries and simply register the bull because "I wish it."[43]

Two days later in a speech on February 15, Joly de Fleury told his colleagues in Parlement that the king wanted *Unigenitus* registered to restore peace in the Church, crush Jansenist errors, and condemn Quesnel's book. Then the advocate-general expressed his personal reservations. The bishops, he said, are divided in their opinions regarding the bull, especially regarding Articles 90, 91, and 92 which "are dangerous to the liberties of the Gallican Church, the maxims of the Realm, the authority of kings, the independence of the Crown, and the loyalty due him by his subjects." He urged his colleagues to consider these points carefully before voting.[44]

The magistrates did so. After further deliberations, they voted 150:9 to register the bull and the king's *lettres patentes*, but provided the following generous loophole regarding Article 91:

> [The bull and the king's *lettres patentes*] are to be executed according to their form and function without approving the decrees not received in this Kingdom, enunciated in the said Constitution, and also without prejudice to the liberties of the Gallican Church, the rights and preeminence of the Crown, the power and jurisdiction of the bishops in the kingdom; and so long as the condemnation of the Propositions which concern the matter of excommunication bring no attack to the Maxims and customs of this Realm . . . nor to the fidelity & obedience owed to the King, and the observation of the laws of the State.[45]

Dissatisfied with his magistrates' half-hearted compliance, Louis XIV told De Mesmes and Joly de Fleury in July 1715 to have Parlement reregister the bull without any qualifying remarks. They refused, telling the monarch that they would rather resign ("turn in our robes") than to "dishonor the Crown." Angered, Louis shouted: "When I say 'I wish it,' it is necessary that [you] obey me." To force the magistrates to bend to his will, the king planned a *lit de justice* (a personal appearance in Parlement), but his deteriorating health prevented it.[46]

Finally, it was the Sorbonne's turn to register the bull. Considered the premier theological faculty in Catholic Europe, the 200 doctors of theology at the University of Paris met monthly to determine policy, set the standards for academic degrees, and deliberate on theological issues. The fact that Jansenists comprised a higher percentage of its faculty than among the French clergy at large helps explain why these professors valued their independence and frequently clashed with popes, kings, and Parlement.[47] Wishing to avoid such contention, Louis XIV instructed the Sorbonne on 28 February 1714 to receive the bull "with respect and submission" and to register it promptly, "because such is our pleasure." When the doctors gathered on March 1, half (15) of those who spoke (28) favored the bull; one suggested the compromise of registering the bull (to please the king) without accepting or approving it (to salve their consciences). Believing their debate had gone on long enough, the king ordered them to register the bull "without any delays or modifications" on March 3, threatening to fire them if they did not comply. At their third meeting on March 5, after lengthy deliberations (theologians, like magistrates, loved debating), a bare majority (68 out of 128 present) voted to register the bull "purely and simply." When the King received them on March 14, he expressed his satisfaction with their dispatch.[48] As for the 28 doctors of theology brave enough to register protests against the bull, Louis threatened them with loss of their positions and exile from Paris if they did not comply. By the time of his death, however, only three members of the faculty had been exiled.[49]

Realizing the contentiousness that *Unigenitus* left in its wake—a badly divided General

Assembly, Parlement, and Sorbonne—helps one understand the long-term consequences of Louis XIV's policy of enforcing it over the objections of the bishops, magistrates, and theologians simply "because such is my pleasure." As Cardinal de Trémoille said in July 1714: "The affair of the bull does not seem to me to be finishing up soon; on the contrary, it seems that it has only begun."[50] The Archbishop of Tours called the crisis "the most important affair since the Apostle's time."[51]

Exaggerated as that claim may sound, recent historians agree that *Unigenitus* cast a long, baleful shadow over France throughout the eighteenth century. Grès-Gayer (1988) asserted that the bull precipitated a crisis on four levels: It challenged papal authority, redefined Church doctrine, gave birth to "ecclesiastical Gallicanism," and sharpened the lines between orthodox Catholics and Jansenists.[52] Jeffrey Merrick (1990) believed that the conflicts surrounding the bull "accentuated the subversive nature of Jansenism" and played an even more significant role than the Enlightenment in undermining "the judicial fictions that bound the *ancien régime* together." These judicial fictions included the identification of the corporate kingdom with the divinely ordained kingship and the conjunction of citizenship and Catholicity.[53] David Bell (1994) concurred, declaring that "Jansenism was probably the most divisive political issue of Louis XV's reign" because it sparked debate in Parlement and in the press about political sovereignty and royal despotism.[54] Pierre Chaunu, Madeleine Foisil, and Françoise de Noirfontaine (1998) described *Unigenitus* as "that machine to crush unity" because it "established the battle lines in France" by "drawing circles around fields of truth" and demarcating the limits of orthodoxy and heresy.[55]

Debate over the bull often created coalitions of strange bedfellows. Gallicans, Jansenists, Richerists, and *parlementaires* made common cause against the papacy, the monarchy, and the Jesuits. The former group, who rejected the bull, took the names *opposants* (because they opposed the bull) and *appelants* (because they wished to appeal it to a Church council), while the latter coalition, who welcomed the bull, were called *constitutionnaires* or *acceptants.*[56] But one could add three other groups. The *accommodants* neither accepted nor rejected the bull; instead, they sought a compromise satisfactory to both sides. The *politiques*, who wanted to maintain stability in the state and Church, avoided debating the issues raised by the bull. The moderate "episcopal party" tried to maintain equilibrium between the *constitutionnaires* and the *appelants.*[57]

In effect, instead of uniting the Gallican Church, Louis XIV's bulldogged enforcement of *Unigenitus* badly divided it. It forced Cardinal Noailles, fifteen bishops, dozens of Sorbonne professors, and hundreds of parish priests to openly declare their allegiance to the Jansenist cause. *Unigenitus* became the catalyst that merged several elements within Jansenism (ecclesiastical, parliamentary, Gallican, and constitutional) in opposition to the "despotism and blind authority" of popes and kings. McManners (1998) estimates that while perhaps 3000 ecclesiastics across France (3% of the total) registered their appeal to a General Council, in Paris, 385 out of 450 *curés* (86%) did so. This potent opposition would cause controversy to the era of the French Revolution.[58]

One such controversy occurred in 1715 when Louis XIV ordered all French clerics to publish the bull in their dioceses, parishes, and religious houses. While 112 bishops (88%) agreed to do so, 15 (12%) refused. Of the approximately 100,000 clergy across France, roughly 97,000 (97%) supported the bull while a mere 3000 (3%) opposed it. Yet those few *appelants*, united by their refusal to compromise and vocal in their intransigence, exerted an influence far out of proportion to their numbers.[59]

Naturally, they looked to the Archbishop of Paris for leadership. Recognizing that by his opposition to Clement XI and Louis XIV, Cardinal Noailles had placed himself firmly in the *appelant* camp, these bishops wrote hundreds of letters asking for his advice. In these letters, they seek clarity on such doctrines as efficacious grace, contrition, predestination, interior holiness, confession, and absolutism. They express their concerns about schism ("the spirit of cabal") in the Church, the pope's real authority in France and the extent of his infallibility, and whether the bull, by pitting Parlement against the papacy, could "imperil the health of the Church." The bishops complain that their parishioners are being "seduced" by the Jesuits and forced to become "traitors to their consciences." They share their sincere anxiety and pain that *Unigenitus* has ruined the "Peace of the Church," disturbed the relationship of bishops to the pope and king, eroded Gallican liberties, brought bad publicity to their beloved Church, and besmirched the honor of the episcopate. Finally, their letters echo the fear that the bull will create even greater difficulties for the Church and the state after Louis XIV dies.[60]

Parlement's involvement in the *appels comme d'abus* (appeals by writ of error in lower courts) also concerned the bishops. After 1713, growing numbers of laity with complaints against ecclesiastical authority appealed their cases to the *parlements* to block decisions they considered contrary to canon law and recognized precedents, especially when such ecclesiastical judgments threatened their Gallican liberties. Most often this occurred when *appelants* considered the Church courts biased, incompetent, or too ultramontane. They then had the right to appeal their cases to a temporal jurisdiction—such as the Council of State or the Grand Chamber of Parlement. In the wake of *Unigenitus*, more and more laity (and clerics) took advantage of the *appel comme d'abus* to appeal bishops' mandates, ordinances, and pastoral instructions enforcing the bull. The magistrates, considering this practice "the finest jewel in the parlementary crown," were just as determined to safeguard their right to hear these appeals from Church courts as the bishops were to stop them.[61]

Since the sixteenth century, Parlement had invoked this right against infractions of royal ordinances dealing with ecclesiastical affairs and violations of the Pragmatic Sanction of Bourges (1438) and of the Concordat of Bologna (1516)—in short, against any infringement on their Gallican liberties. In the past, priests, monks, and nuns had invoked the *appel comme d'abus* to challenge their superiors, contest convent elections or the acceptance of novices, and occasionally to annul their vows. But now, everybody, it seemed, was using it to escape censure by Church courts, counter charges of Jansenism, and haul their superiors into secular courts. Naturally, the bishops saw this practice as an attack on their ancient judicial prerogatives to decide, unhindered by the king or Parlement, what was best for the spiritual health of the Church.[62]

As his own health deteriorated in August 1715, Louis XIV, deeply worried about the future of the Gallican Church, pondered his options. He considered asking Clement XI once again for permission to summon a national council of Church officials to depose Cardinal Noailles and to register their acceptance of *Unigenitus* once and for all. Believing the pope would never consent to that, he thought about issuing a declaration "exhorting and enjoining all cardinals, archbishops, and bishops in France" who had not published the bull in their dioceses to do so immediately "without distinction or restrictions." As late as August 13, the king urged the chancellor, the procurer-general, and the first president to push the registration of this declaration through Parlement. If the magistrates refused to register it, he planned a *lit de justice* to force their hand.[63]

But the Grim Reaper spared these officials from having to ram yet another unwelcome declaration down the throats of the magistrates. On September 1, as Louis XIV lay dying, he shared with Cardinal de Rohan and Cardinal de Bissy his regrets at not solving "the troubles of the Church":

> But God has not permitted it. It was all done for his glory. The public has perhaps believed that I acted through suspicion and to show my authority. But God knows the truth. Since I have failed in the attempt to reunite the bishops, perhaps things would have progressed more advantageously by someone else's hand more agreeable to God. But I die Catholic, Apostolic, and Roman.[64]

The king also regretted his estrangement from the Archbishop of Paris. "Truthfully," he said, "I would like to see him [Cardinal Noailles] and I am upset to be dying while in disagreement with him."[65] But time had run out for Louis XIV. He died at 8:15 a.m. with the words, "O my God, come to my aid, hasten to give me help" on his lips.[66] An anonymous Jansenist scribe devoted one single line to this important event in the *Necrology of Port-Royal*: "On this day [1 September] died Louis XIV, King of France, when he was still trying to force Parlement to register the Constitution [*Unigenitus*]."[67]

On the day he died, Louis XIV left behind a deeply divided Church and kingdom. In 1715, 385 (86%) of the 450 priests in Paris and 97 (87%) of the 110 doctors of theology at the Sorbonne opposed the bull. Throughout France, 17 bishops and over 3000 parish priests likewise remained hostile to *Unigenitus*.[68] They resented attempts by the *constitutionnaires* to force their compliance. Sometimes bishops made unannounced visits to inspect the libraries of priests and religious houses, looking for Jansenist works to confiscate and condemn. Suddenly, even private libraries had become potential spaces of subversion to orthodox beliefs.[69]

Attempts to enforce the bull unleashed a tidal wave of pro-Jansenist publications. Between 1713 and 1731, over 1000 books, pamphlets, and articles appeared hostile to *Unigenitus*—180 of them in 1714 alone—or about one every single week for nearly two decades. From 1713 to 1760, almost 70 per cent of the individuals arrested for Jansenism were charged with printing offenses (see chapter 6).[70]

As she had helped the religious of Port-Royal des Champs publish their works before 1709, so now Mlle. Françoise-Marguerite de Joncoux spearheaded a publications blitz against the bull until her death at 47 in 1715. As general-in-chief, she invested her time, talents, and wealth in finding clandestine publishers for Saint-Cyran's *Abridged History of Jansenism*, Pascal's *Provincial Letters*, the eight-volume *History of the Case of Conscience* set, and various other printed attacks on the Bull *Unigenitus*. The content and tone of these works differed greatly from the majestic erudition of the debates on grace that had characterized the seventeenth-century Jansenist works of Saint-Cyran, the Arnaulds, and Nicole. Hostility toward the bull inspired a new generation of lawyers and ecclesiastics to adopt a more combative tone as they waged a guerilla war in print against the evils of *Unigenitus*.[71] One anonymous cleric in 1714 predicted: "What a noise will be raised everywhere as soon as [the bull] is available in French."[72]

Yet not everyone made a noise. Given the fact that *Unigenitus* specifically targeted Pasquier Quesnel and his book *Moral Reflections on the New Testament*, it is interesting to note his own reaction. He received a copy of the bull one evening while dining with three friends. He read it in silence, tears streaming down his face. While his friends remained at the table arguing about the bull, Quesnel went to the chapel and spent four hours praying. Then, emboldened by prayer, he took up his pen and attacked the bull as "a wolf in sheep's clothing," a "false prophet," an "artful seducer," and a "master of lies." Since *Moral Reflections* propounded Augustinian theology, he declared, then if it contained false doctrines, "it will be necessary to burn St. Augustine." He had regained his cutting Jansenist edge.[73]

He would need it, for all across France, bishops attacked his book in mandates and letters of pastoral instruction that grew increasingly more vitriolic. In 1710 the bishops of Luçon and La Rochelle jointly released one mammoth 542-page "Ordinance and Pastoral Letter" attacking *Moral Reflections* for containing Jansen's five condemned propositions and for contradicting Catholic teachings on grace, free will, sin, God's law, and human merit.[74]

Such lengthy "pastoral letters" inspired wits and pundits to write humorous poems and satires attacking the pope, king, bishops, and especially the bull. One amusing "Mandate from Monseigneur the Bishop of Bethlehem on the Affairs of the Time" parodied the style and content of these letters. No doubt the following lines entertained many listeners at wayside inns:

Mandates are all the rage today.
Paris is crammed full of their [bishops'] bulletins.
Pascal and St.-Cyran's books are all from Satan and deserve equal anathema.
Jansenism is an abyss without a bottom.
Jansenists who spread this venom are guiltier than damnable poisoners.
Quesnel the revolutionary is a famous and impious monster.
The King [Louis XIV] is a Caligula, a true Nero.[75]

Another 21-stanza satire on "Innocent XI," blasphemously sung to the tune of the *Pater Noster* ("Our Father"), makes fun of the pope and his purported infallibility. In harsher tones it attacks *Unigenitus* as "an injustice before God" for "enslaving the French to a sovereign pope," "spilling our blood . . . and violating our laws," and bringing "a thousand anguishes" upon France.[76]

Jansenists, however, lacking both wit and humor, took the bull more seriously. One group of 30 theologians, militant young students at the Collège de Sainte-Barbe and the Seminary de Saint-Magloire, hatched a "Jansenist plot" to overthrow *Unigenitus*. Deeply influenced by the theology and eschatology of Jacques-Joseph Duguet, their mentor, they spearheaded a movement to appeal the bull to a national council. Adopting the conciliarist position that it had never been accepted by the "universal Church" (which meant, of course, that the Jansenists had had no say in its development), they argued the necessity of calling together representatives from the entire Church to approve it. Recognizing (as Louis XIV had been forced to do) that Clement XI would never call such a council, they felt certain that the bull would never gain universal approval, so they could continue with clear consciences to attack it.[77]

But one did not have to be a Jansenist to oppose the bull. The *duc* de Saint-Simon, for example, who sided neither with the Jesuits nor with the Jansenists, strongly criticized *Unigenitus*. He saw it as "fatal to the Church and to the State, shameful to Rome, harmful to religion, advantageous to the Jesuits, Sulpicians, Ultramontanists, and the ignorant" who thrived on disorder, falsehood, confusion, and violence.[78] "Everything shines in it," he quipped, "except the truth." Only one year after the bull appeared in France, Saint-Simon declared: "We are now living . . . in a time of persecution, which has depopulated the schools, introduced ignorance, fanaticism and disorder, crowned vice, thrown every community into the utmost confusion, with disorder everywhere, and established the most arbitrary and barbarous inquisition."[79] More laconically, the *princesse* Palatine confessed, "I am overcome with boredom every time I hear someone speak of it, and have decided that it will not stop me from sleeping well at night."[80]

The spread of Jansenism in Paris and across France, however, gave many Church leaders sleepless nights. Although popes' bulls and bishops' mandates had suppressed its theological and religious vitality and Louis XIV had destroyed its heart at Port-Royal des Champs, like the legendary phoenix, it arose from the ashes rejuvenated and transformed as a political and judicial phenomenon after the king's death. Thanks largely to the controversy over *Unigenitus*, by the 1720s the majority of the clergy in Paris embraced Jansenist ideas, with the exception of the Jesuits, Capuchins, and Sulpicians. Across France, some 6500 to 7000 religious—regular and secular—in 45 dioceses (one-third of them in Paris) sided with the *appelants*.[81]

Although it possessed regional peculiarities, eighteenth-century Jansenism also reflected certain common geographic, social, and cultural traits. It was, for the most part, a northern movement. About 83 percent of Jansenists lived north of the Loire River in Paris, Châlons-sur-Marne, Tours, Montpellier, Boulogne-sur-Mer, and Rouen. It was also largely an urban phenomenon. At least 65–70 percent of the *appelants* lived in Paris and its suburbs or in other large cities. It attracted well-educated men and women who enjoyed high social status. At least 75 percent of the men, for example, had degrees in law or theology; many women, privately tutored, could read and write French (and sometimes Latin) very well. They came from comfortable, even wealthy backgrounds: 38 percent were robe nobles, 35 percent came from the bourgeoisie. Nonetheless, they adopted ascetic lifestyles, spending hours in prayer and devotional reading, eating little, writing much, and helping the poor. Naturally, they all refused to sign the Formulary, sometimes engaged in violent debates, and hoped that the new Regent would be favorable to reforming the Church.[82]

Although Philippe, *duc* d'Orléans' daughter Louise-Adélaide, *abbesse* de Chelles, was an ardent Jansenist, he himself held notoriously irreligious views. Far more tolerant than his predecessor ever thought of being, the Duke placated the Jansenists and welcomed many of them (including D'Aguesseau, Joly de Fleury, and the *abbé* Pucelle) to his Court; but he sent Mme. de Maintenon and Jesuit confessor Le Tellier into exile. Just hours after Louis XIV's death, Orléans summoned Cardinal Noailles to Versailles and appointed him president of the Council of Conscience, which dealt with appointments to Church offices, ecclesiastical finances, and disputes over Jansenism. Overnight, Noailles had become the most powerful prelate in the realm.[83]

But the Regent went further, seeking to undo some of the harm his grandfather had done. Guided by his new confessor, the *abbé* de Fleury, he revoked the *lettres de cachet* that had sent some bishops into exile for opposing *Unigenitus*, released scores of imprisoned Jansenists (and 68 Huguenot galley slaves), and invited hundreds of fugitive *appelants* to return to France. He welcomed the remaining sisters of Port-Royal des Champs, scattered in 1709, to dwell at the Abbey of Malnoue, where the last one died in 1738. "[Paris] is Jansenist from head to toe," one contemporary quipped.[84]

The Regent's tolerant attitude, however, displeased Clement XI. In April 1716, when the Duke asked the pope to invest several new bishops he had chosen, Clement declined to do so unless the Regent agreed to accept *Unigenitus*. When Orléans, after consulting 32 bishops in 1717, asked the pope to revise his recent bull to make its wording less offensive, Clement refused, claiming that the Holy Spirit had guided him in writing *Unigenitus*.[85]

Blocked by the pope, the Regent shifted his position late in 1716, aligning himself with the ultramontanists and the Jesuits. Delegating to his Council of State all matters relating to *Unigenitus*, Orléans created a chamber to examine heretical writings. In December, Parlement issued an *arrêt* forbidding publication, printing, selling, or distributing anything relating to the bull without royal approval (by *lettres patentes*).[86] The Duke's Declaration of 7 October 1717 imposing silence on partisans and adversaries of the bull raised cries of protest around the kingdom. His exiling of Jansenist Chancellor D'Aguesseau and replacing him with the anti-Jansenist marquis d'Argenson proved equally unpopular with the *appelants*.[87]

As a handful of clerics in 1717 began denying communion to those who had rejected *Unigenitus* (this practice of "refusing the sacraments" would dominate the 1750s), four bishops stepped into the national limelight to protest this practice and register their opposition to the bull. But when the bishops of Montpellier, Boulogne, Mirepoix, and Senez asked the pope to call a general council, the Regent banished them to their dioceses and sent the notary who had received their act of appeal to the Bastille. But the Duke's heavy-handed approach inspired 26 more bishops to join the *appelant* cause. By 1718, those 30 bishops, joined by most of the theology faculty at Reims, Nantes, Poitiers, and Caen, a growing number of cathedral chapters, and thousands of *curés*, vicars, and regular clergy (especially among the Oratorians, Benedictines, Dominicans, and Génovésains) had also joined the *opposant* camp. With a reputation for free-thinking, the Oratorians opposed the bull because (as Cartesians), its ideas were not "clear and distinct" and because (as *appelants*), they demanded a General Council to decide its legitimacy.[88]

As the climate in France grew colder toward Jansenism, many *appelants* fled to countries where they could continue waging war on the bull in relative security. Quesnel, now 83, escaped to

Amsterdam and published his *Two Acts of Appeal* in 1717, a defense of the four recusant bishops and a ringing call for a general Church council. The book articulates the platform set forth by the four bishops and the faculty of theology at Paris, Reims, and Nantes. *Unigenitus*, he states, is a flawed document that divides and "wounds" the Church. Therefore, the pope should call a general council of ecclesiastics to rewrite it and to examine all papal decrees "prejudicial to the faith, manners, or discipline of the Church." Popes are not infallible; only general Church councils are "sovereign and infallible." To allay Clement XI's fears concerning his orthodoxy, Quesnel assures His Holiness that "I always have had and always will have, to my dying breath, an unbreakable attachment to the Faith of the Roman Catholic Church, to Catholic Unity, and to the Authority & the Primacy of the Holy See."[89]

Clement XI, however, remained unmoved by such assurances. Instead, he believed that the only way to solve the "Jansenist problem" in France was to issue yet another bull. Drawn up by Cardinal Fabroni and released in 1718, *Pastoralis Officii* ("The Pastoral Office") condemned those who refused to accept *Unigenitus* and forbade everyone to agitate the issue by voice or pen. The bull would have excommunicated some 3000 *appelant* bishops, but it offended the Regent and many Jansenist sympathizers in Parlement; the magistrates refused to register it and as a consequence, it never officially became law in France.[90]

Despite Clement XI's call for silence and submission, however, the new bull (like its predecessors) engendered a noisy response in France. Jean-Joseph Languet de Gergy, Bishop of Soissons (and later Archbishop of Sens) strongly supported and loudly defended the bull. In his lengthy mandates, he not only attacked Jansenists as "the party of error," but also criticized bishops he felt were "soft" on Jansenism. At the end of his 655-page "Advertisement" in 1718, the bishop remained convinced that "these wicked appeals create a scandal in the Church, cause the triumph of the Protestants, and bring desolation to all true believers."[91]

The magistrates in many provincial *parlements*, of course, felt the same way about the pope's bulls. Although they devoted weeks to debating the merits and demerits of the 1713 and 1718 bulls, they refused to register them, finding them "contrary to the rights of the bishops, to canon laws, to Gallican liberties, and to the principles of natural right." In addition, many *parlements* issued *arrêts* forbidding anyone to print or distribute copies of the bulls without royal permission. Those who did would be punished as "disturbers of the public peace."[92] This new emphasis on "natural right" and disturbing the "public [not Church] peace" marks a significant shift in thinking away from the spiritual ideals of the seventeenth century and toward the more secular goals of the nascent Enlightenment.

Refusing to keep silent himself, the disgraced Cardinal Noailles released a lengthy pastoral letter in January 1719. In it he justified the 101 propositions condemned by *Unigenitus*, stated that papal bulls were not "unchangeable judgments of the Church," and condemned the "pretended doctrine of the infallibility of popes." Shocked, Clement XI immediately placed Noailles' letter on the *Index*.[93] Five months later, when the Regent issued the Declaration of 5 June 1719 seeking a new "Peace in the Church" by again imposing silence on everyone, the bishops were not impressed. Nor did they like the Regent's heavy-handed *lettre de cachet* of 28 June 1720 ordering the censure and exclusion of all clerics who refused to sign the Formulary. This order also upset the theology faculty at the Sorbonne and caused a ruckus at the General Assembly of the Clergy in August.[94]

Bragging that "I have bridled my asses," the *duc* d'Orléans, now supported by Chancellor D'Aguesseau, issued the Declaration of 4 August 1720 to enforce "order & tranquility in our Estates . . . choke out the old seeds of discord . . . stop the party spirit . . . and bring a much-desired peace" into Church affairs. This declaration enforced all previous laws regarding *Unigenitus*, commanded Parlement to register the 1713 Bull, suppressed all appeals to a general council, and forbade anyone to write against it. Furthermore, it required all prelates to sign the Formulary "purely and simply." Among the Gallican bishops, 97 signed (twelve with reservations), but 19 (five *constitutionnaires* and fourteen *appelants*) refused to sign. After weeks of negotiation, however, Cardinal d'Estrée and Cardinal de Polignac engineered the famous "accommodation" by which 40 bishops (including both *acceptants* and *opposants*) agreed to accept *Unigenitus* as "a rule of faith" only. In the end, they persuaded 98 prelates to sign.[95]

The fact that the bishops had agreed on their compromise (known as "the Body of Doctrine") provided a basis for their negotiations with Parlement. For their refusal to register the pope's bull, several magistrates had been banned from Paris. With the help of Archbishop Dubois of Cambrai, they now cut a deal with the Regent. If he agreed to let them return to the capital and dismissed John Law (a Scottish speculator hated for the failure of the Mississippi Company), they would register *Unigenitus*. When Orléans kept his part of the bargain, the magistrates registered the bull on 4 December 1720. Five days later, Law resigned and fled to Venice.[96]

But as many began to hope that peace had finally returned to the Church, four bishops in Paris (led by Jean Soanen, Bishop of Senez) published the "Maxims on the Duties of Ecclesiastics" in September 1720. This call to arms, laced with Richerism ("a *curé* . . . is one of the depositories and interpreters of Truth"), urged clerics to reject any compromise concerning the bull. Nine months later, seven bishops asked the new pope, Innocent XIII, to annul *Unigenitus*, calling it "harmful and calamitous" to the French Church. Instead, Innocent issued two briefs defending the bull and calling the seven bishops "audacious and insolent." Adding fuel to the flame, a royal declaration in July 1722 ordered bishops and university officials to require all those seeking admission to holy orders, benefices, or academic degrees to sign the Formulary. Those who refused—as well as those who had appealed against *Unigenitus*—were to be refused. Then at the 1723 Assembly of the Clergy, Archbishop Vintimille of Aix suggested convoking provincial councils to force recalcitrant bishops to submit to the bull.[97]

Suddenly, however, the cast of characters changed, leaving the outcome very much in doubt. First, Philippe, *duc* d'Orléans died in 1723 and the *duc* de Bourbon became Principal Minister of France. Second, Innocent XIII passed away in 1724 and Benedict XIII became the new pope. Bourbon, who took a laissez-faire attitude toward *Unigenitus*, wanted to permit the bishops to issue "new explications" regarding it, but Cardinal Fleury (as head of the Council of Conscience) opposed it. Therefore, in June 1725, the Council of State issued an *arrêt* suppressing any new explanations of the bull. Likewise the new pope, who favored restoring "Peace in the Church," issued the brief *Demissas preces* in November 1723 declaring that the 1713 Bull had not attacked the doctrines of St. Augustine and St. Thomas regarding grace and predestination. But only three years later, Benedict denied the grace of the Jubilee Year (1726) to any diocese whose bishop had refused to accept *Unigenitus*.[98]

By the late 1720s, therefore, the attitude of Church and government officials toward the *appelants* had hardened. Under increased pressure, Bishop Soanen accepted the bull in 1727; Cardinal Noailles did likewise in 1728. That same year, Minister Fleury launched an offensive against Jansenism that resulted in the interdiction of 300 French clergy and the dismissal of almost that number by 1730.[99] Placards threatening Louis XV, Fleury, and Vintimille appeared in Paris; seditious talk filled the streets.[100] Monsieur Barbier exclaimed: "It is a known fact . . . that the greater part of Parisians . . . are Jansenists, that is to say, in the main [they are] against the court of Rome and the Jesuits."[101] From this climate of conflicting opinions and emotions arose the longest-running underground religious newspaper in European history—*Les Nouvelles Ecclésiastiques* (*Ecclesiastical News*). First printed in 1728, it lasted until 1803, a phenomenal run of 75 years.

This printed newspaper, however, owed its inspiration to the *gazettes à la main* (handwritten news sheets) begun 50 years earlier by Louis Foucquet, Bishop of Agde. Protégé of Saint-Vincent de Paul, friend of Archbishop Harlay de Champvallon, and member of the Company of the Most Holy Sacrament, Foucquet espoused Gallicanism, conciliarism, and strict morality. Although he had signed the Formulary in 1660, he later repudiated his signature and in 1664 openly declared himself for the Jansenist cause. For his attacks on the Jesuits, his strong defense of Port-Royal, and his alleged complicity with his relative Nicolas Foucquet's embezzlement of state funds, Bishop Foucquet was exiled to Villefranche in 1675. Fifteen years later, when he opposed the revenue schemes of Paul Pellisson (whose "conscience fund" bribed Calvinists to convert to Catholicism) to enrich his heirs, another *lettre de cachet* banished him to his diocese at Issoudun.[102]

Because of his two exiles (1675 and 1690) and Louis XIV's orders that he could not leave his diocese even after his release, Foucquet's personal freedoms were curtailed for 30 years. Little wonder that he considered liberty "the essential thing in life"; to lose it meant "shameful servitude." From his perspective, the government, working hand in glove with the Jesuits, had reduced the Gallican Church to "servitude" by enforcing papal bulls and using *lettres de cachet*, which constituted an "Inquisition." Consequently, during his first exile in Villefranche, Foucquet began writing pastoral letters attacking Jesuit casuistry and praising the example of the early Christian martyrs that "suffered for the truth." These handwritten letters became *gazettes à la main* which he called *Mémoires ecclésiastiques* (1675–1680) and later *Les Nouvelles ecclésiastiques* (1680–1698).[103]

In these gazettes, he provided clerics and laity information about ecclesiastical matters relevant to the "liberties of the Church." "To help others love the truth is the best means of defending it," he declared. Authors of articles (who were assigned numbers) remained anonymous; as editor and compiler, Foucquet kept their identities a secret from Minister of War Louvois' spies for nearly a quarter of a century. He took circuitous routes in contacting writers; he burned written messages after reading them; and he relied on members of the Oratoire to hand copy and distribute these gazettes. Between 1657 and 1688, the two- to ten-page *Ecclesiastical News* appeared weekly; from 1689 to 1698, it filled 50 pages and appeared once a month.[104]

In many ways, Bishop Foucquet's small (28 cm. x 18 cm.), handwritten (in brown or black ink) gazettes provided a model for the printed *Nouvelles Ecclésiastiques* that first appeared in 1728. Each issue summarizes the highpoints of a year and how its events impact Port-Royal and Jansenism in general, giving special attention to the actions taken by popes, Louis XIV, the Council of State, the General Assembly of the Clergy, the *parlements*, and the Sorbonne faculty. In its pages, one reads reviews of books, the text of bishops' mandates, funeral orations, precis of articles and dissertations, and extracts from letters and sermons supporting or attacking Jansenism. Its authors gloat over Jesuit defeats and bemoan the mistreatment of Jansenists in court trials and in print. They share the gossip about leading individuals at Court, in the Church, and in society, protecting their sources by using the tagline "It is said" or "We have heard." In its pages, Jansenists *always* receive positive remarks; Jesuits *always* emerge as the villains.[105]

Although the last issues of Bishop Foucquet's *Ecclesiastical News* appeared in 1698, he stated in a mandate written in 1700 that he would devote his remaining days "to banishing all error and making the truth triumph." When he died in 1702 after serving as Bishop of Agde for 46 years, others took up the challenge to keep the torch of truth burning brightly.[106]

After 1708, the wealthy Desessarts brothers financed and produced handwritten bulletins or broadsides (known as *nouvelles à la main*) concerning events related to the Bull *Unigenitus*. Issues appeared irregularly for the first dozen years, but by 1721, became quite numerous (if rather illegibly written).[107] Known collectively as the *Histoire Ecclésiastique* (*Ecclesiastical History*), the issues from 1708 to 1721 fill 930 handwritten pages. While most articles focus on news concerning the Gallican Church, others provide excerpts from Dutch newspapers like the *Gazette d'Hollande* and the *Gazette d'Amsterdam*. Like its printed successor the *Nouvelles Ecclésiastiques*, the *Histoire*

Ecclésiastique also summarizes news notes from Rome, Vienna, Madrid, Cologne, Hamburg and other European centers. Its authors praise Cardinal Noailles, Pasquier Quesnel, the *duc* d'Orléans, and a host of Jansenist bishops, but excoriate the actions and writings of Clement XI, *Père* La Chaise, *Père* Le Tellier, the Archbishop of Embrun, the Jesuits, and anyone enforcing the Bull *Unigenitus*. Between 1708 and 1713, authors discuss a variety of issues relating to the *Régale*, papal infallibility, Jesuit missions, the Inquisition, the growth of Quietism and Protestantism, and the mistreatment of Jansenists. From 1713 to 1721, however, the major focus of every article is on how *Unigenitus* affects the Church, Gallicanism, the Sorbonne, the *parlements*, bishops' mandates, provincial synods, or police actions (the use of *lettres de cachet* against *appelants*).[108]

In addition to the impact of Clement XI's 1713 Bull, the actions of a provincial assembly called the Council of Embrun gave the faltering *Ecclesiastical News* a shot in the arm that guaranteed its continued health for 75 years. In February 1727, Church and state officials conspired to condemn the outspoken *appelant* Bishop Jean Soanen. His rigged trial, presided over by the corrupt Archbishop Tencin, began in August. Within a month, Soanen was reduced to a lay communion and banished to the abbey of the Chaise-Dieu, where he survived thirteen more years as a martyr of the *appelant* cause. The council also condemned one-fourth of France's bishops to imprisonment or exile as *appelants*, thereby doing incalculable harm to the cause of religion in France. The *News,* decrying this "brigandage of Embrun," embraced their cause.[109]

By a remarkable coincidence, both the *Nouvelles Ecclésiastiques* and the Masonic Society began in Paris in 1728. Both formed clandestine organizations, founded on secrecy, and proclaimed hidden truths. Like the secret rituals of masonry shared only with the elite, the *Ecclesiastical News* served as the cement holding Jansenism together like a secret lodge of Christian Masons preaching "the truth" in a hostile environment. During the eighteenth century, both Masons and Jansenists would face persecution from Church and state officials.[110]

Financed by Jean-Baptiste and Marc-Antoine Desessart, wealthy brothers with close ties to the Jansenist convent of Saint-Magloire, the *Gazette ecclésiastique* began (like its predecessors) as a handwritten paper edited by the *abbé* Vaillant in 1725. When the first printed issue came from the press on 23 February 1728, however, its name had been changed to *Les Nouvelles Ecclésiastiques, ou mémoires pour servir à l'histoire de la Constitution Unigenitus* (*Ecclesiastical News, or Memoirs to Serve as a History of the Bull Unigenitus*). It succeeded largely because of the cooperation of a host of anonymous individuals. Its editorial board (who met at secret locations on the *rue* des Bourguignons and the *rue* de la Parcheminerie in Paris) included the *abbés* Boucher, Troya, Duguet, and D'Etemare and the *curé* Jean Fontaine de la Roche. During nearly eight decades, the paper had only three editors: Jean Fontaine de la Roche (1728–1761), who died in office; Marc-Claude Guénin (1761–1793), forced to flee to Holland; and the *abbé* Mouton (1793–1803), who published the paper in Utrecht during its last decade.[111]

From 1728 to 1791, this weekly paper appeared clandestinely in Paris, with occasional issues printed in Senlis, Mantes, Nantes, La Puisaye, Geneva or The Hague when police surveillance made it impossible to publish it in the capital. Beginning in 1791 during the French Revolution, however, the *Nouvelles* was distributed openly. Colporteurs brought handwritten manuscripts, gathered from writers in Champagne and Auxerrois, to Paris to be set in type at one of 20 presses.[112]

Like its contemporary institution the Masonic Order, the process for printing and distributing the *Nouvelles* remained highly secret and complex. Around 1730, Mme. de Joncoux created her famous organizational chart showing the precise relationship of a vast network of authors, correspondents, printers, and colporteurs that Mme. Françoise Elizabeth Jourdain Théodon had helped establish in and around Paris.[113] This chart depicts a five-tiered hierarchy with the author at the top; correspondants A, B, and C below him; sub-correspondants D, E, F, G, and H beneath them; printers J, K, L, M, N, O, and P in the fourth tier; and colporteur-distributors Q, R, S, T, U, V, X, Y, and Z at the base of the pyramid. A note at the bottom explains:

> Each one of the 24 persons designated by letters of the alphabet knows only the person to whom he must report and those who report directly to him. The author is known only to the three correspondents. When one of these persons fails to report within a half hour to the person he must report to, the latter goes immediately to a designated house as a place of refuge [one of twelve such houses] and gives the news to one of the correspondents.[114]

As this chart demonstrates, one author might know three correspondents (A, B, C) and two sub-correspondents (G and H), but G and H did not know each other or the identity of B or C. Thus, if H proved to be a traitor, he could only betray A whom he knew, but no one else in the chain of command. After writing an article, an author also burned his notes and gave his manuscript to a correspondent, who edited, polished, and copied it, again throwing the original manuscript into the fire. A sub-correspondent took this polished copy to a printer, after which 20 or more individuals distributed 100 issues each to different offices around Paris. If the police arrested one office manager, the other nineteen managers, upon hearing about it, redirected their copies to yet another secret office. In all, this secret web included 160 regular distributors and 32 professional colporteurs. Of the former, 80 (50%) were laymen, 45 (29%) laywomen, and 35 (21%) clerics. For over six decades, they successfully smuggled copies in and out of Paris in the luggage of bishops and nobles whose lackeys had been bribed.[115]

The scope of their achievement is absolutely staggering. For three-quarters of a century, under the watchful but unseeing eyes of government officials, these secret Jansenist presses churned out 4000 (and sometimes 5000–6000) four-page issues of the *Ecclesiastical News* every single week—and not a single issue ever failed to come out on schedule! Its national readership included tens of thousands of eager bourgeoisie, clerics, robe nobles, merchants, shopkeepers, and artisans. Not until the rise of the cheap secular newspapers of the 1770s did any medium surpass the circulation of the *Nouvelles*.[116] As D. A. Coward (1981) correctly stated: "In a century adept at propaganda, the *Nouvelles Ecclésiastiques*, an underground journal published by a secret army on a perpetual war footing, was a propaganda machine which had no equal."[117] Although wildly popular among students in the parishes of Saint-Jacques, Saint-André-des-Arts, Saint-Séverin, and Saint-Etienne-du-Mont where many colleges and seminaries were located, the *Nouvelles* also attracted dukes, bishops, and many women. Much to police chief d'Argenson's annoyance, a copy even appeared in his carriage![118]

The paper literally created its own readership not only because of its content, but even more due to its competitive price. From 1728 to the mid-1740s, it sold for three *sous* an issue; after 1744 each issue cost four *sous*; during the 1770s and 1780s, the price rose to six *sous* per issue. This compared favorably with other newspapers of the time. For example, in the 1760s, when the *Journal Ecclésiastique* sold for 9 *livres* 2 *sous* per year, the *Nouvelles Ecclésiastiques* cost 7 *livres* 16 *sous* annually. By the French Revolution, when a subscription to the *Journal de Paris* cost 30 *livres* a year and the *Année Littéraire* cost 24 *livres*, the *Nouvelles Ecclésiastiques* sold for 26 *livres* a year. While not exactly cheap, those who wanted to subscribe to the *Nouvelles* could do so for the price of a couple loaves of bread each day.[119]

While bread nourished readers' bodies, the newspaper strengthened their opposition to *Unigenitus*. Every page contains two columns of 56 lines each featuring articles and news notes highlighting "the great evils that exist in the Church" because of "that wicked decree." Every issue features a dramatic frontispiece. The 1728 edition includes black-and-white scenes depicting the destruction of Port-Royal des Champs, the Council of Embrun, *lettres de cachet*, torture, the Bastille, the destruction of the convent of Sainte-Barbe, and a meeting of the

Sorbonne. Each issue also contains a dramatic scripture text as a rallying cry to readers. One favorite—Isaiah 58:1—proclaims: "Cry without ceasing, make your voice sound as the trumpet, announce to my people the crimes they have committed & to the house of Jacob the sins they have committed." In their articles, writers praise "defenders of the truth," attack the Jesuits, warn of persecution against specific Jansenists, and critique bishops' mandates.[120]

During the eighteenth century, of course, all those who wrote for the paper remained anonymous, not only to the public but also to one another. That way, if the police arrested one of them, he could not betray any of his colleagues even under torture. But thanks to the publication of three indexes for the *Ecclesiastical News* (the 1760 index covers 1728–1760; the 1790 one covers 1761–1790; and the 1803 one covers 1791–1803) and the efforts of recent historians, a handful of these authors are now known.[121] The *abbé* Louis de Troya d'Asigny, who worked among the poor at the prisons of Bicêtre and La Salpêtrière, wrote many of the articles in the earlier issues, while the *abbés* Guenin and Mouton wrote (and edited) articles after 1760. Authors Philippe Boucher and the *abbé* d'Etemare lived on the *rue* Judas in Paris. Editor Jacques Fontaine, always ready for a quick getaway, used a boat on the Seine River as his floating office. Other ardent contributors included Bishop Le Camus of Grenoble and the *abbé* François Genet, professor at the Grand Seminaire. Amazingly, although the police arrested several printers and colporteurs over the newspaper's 75-year history, not once did they apprehend a single author or editor.[122]

The popular chroniclers of the century (including Marios, Buvot, and Barbier) frequently quoted from its pages. They treated the *Nouvelles* with malicious admiration for its continual defiance, unfailing subversiveness, and cat-and-mouse elusiveness with police. In an era of harsh censorship, this underground newspaper became the tribunal of the public and the linchpin in the Jansenist propaganda effort to galvanize popular opposition to *Unigenitus.* As such, it chronicled the after effects of the Bull, spearheaded a popular resistance movement to Clement XI's authority, and by focusing attention on the "persecution" of *appelants* (by the police and bishops), helped develop a Jansenist mindset among the lower classes.[123]

By combining serious prose, narrative, satire, name-calling, gossip, and innuendo, the *Ecclesiastical News* created a kind of pious yellow journalism designed to recruit readers to the Jansenist cause. In its columns, writers focused attention on every repressive act by bishops (decrees, mandates) and the police (raids, *lettre de cachet* arrests, imprisonment) and every vexatious act perpetrated by anyone anywhere against the *appelant* cause. A sufficient number of racy rumors—like quarter proofs in French criminal justice—added conviction to the truth editors sought to propagate. Articles beginning with "It is said," "People are saying," "We have heard," or "We have received word" gave credence to the opinions of ordinary people. The use of the familiar "we" (*on*) united all kinds of Jansenist sympathizers (Gallicans, conciliarists, Richerists, Jesuit haters) against "them" (Louis XV, Clement XI, Minister Fleury, the Society of Jesus), creating a community of thought. Safely hidden behind their anonymity, authors could, for example, call Fleury a "heretic" and an "imbecile" and Archbishop Beaumont a "firebrand"—epithets that under normal circumstances would have earned them an all expenses paid chamber in the Bastille.[124]

One must, therefore, read *Les Nouvelles Ecclésiastiques* with great care, because its bias is clearly ultra-Jansenist: In its pages, "*appelants* are the persecuted innocents and *constitutionnaires* are their unjust persecutors."[125] For three-quarters of a century, its target list of evils and enemies remained remarkably consistent: the Bull *Unigenitus*, Molinist theologians, the Jesuits, popes opposed to Jansenism, bishops who made life difficult for Jansenists, and the philosophes of the Enlightenment.[126]

Employing a strident tone and an aggressive, biting vocabulary, the editors and authors of the *Nouvelles* combated "error and vice," denounced "public scandals," and defended their version of "truth and justice." The newspaper provided information regarding Jansenist struggles primarily in Paris and in the provinces and to a lesser extent, in foreign countries. By the use of anecdotes, reports, dialogs, and scandals, it instructed the faithful and shaped public opinion. A masterly vehicle of modern propaganda, the paper employed the techniques of persuasion, repetition, rhetorical questions, and didactic prose somewhat like the Jehovah's Witness *Watchtower* magazine does today. But unlike the *Watchtower*, the *Ecclesiastical News* revealed scandals in solemn style, recounted pious cliches with relish, expounded theological debates with clarity, and throughout, flattered readers' intellectual self-esteem.[127]

Consistently, editors and authors repeated several well-chosen arguments. *Unigenitus*, which has not been passed unanimously by a representative Church council, does not constitute a canonical judgment; those who excommunicate opponents of the Bull are persecuting true Christians. Church reform is progressive and should lead to the teaching of a common doctrine, better training for the clergy, stricter rules in seminaries, tighter control of convents and monasteries, manual training in schools, frequent conferences and councils for clerics, and the elimination of pluralism. Church officials should place increased emphasis on penitence and true contrition, celebrate communion less often, revive the liturgy, show greater devotion to the Virgin Mary, and place limits on privileged altars (a source of great profit to the local church). Articles regularly attack "the tyranny of the Jesuits," the interference of secular powers (king, Parlement, and police) in ecclesiastical affairs, the Regale controversy, Quietism, Islam, and Calvinism (while opposing dragoon violence during the Revocation). On the other hand, authors consistently uphold the memory of Port-Royal des Champs, praise the Oratorians, trumpet the triumphs of Jansenists everywhere, encourage charitable deeds, and promote mission work (in Siam, Tonkin, and China)—as long as it is not being done by the Society of Jesus.[128]

As might be expected, however, over the 75-year life span of the newspaper, subtle differences emerged in format, content, emphasis, and style. These will be examined by decades. At its inception in 1728–29, most news reports focused on events in Paris, Rouen, Castellanne, Reims, Nancy, and Tours, with minor references to eight other provincial centers, and only a handful of news notes drawn from sources in Rome, Brussels, Utrecht, and Savoy. In short, the *Nouvelles* had a very provincial focus on Gallican Church affairs. Issues featured articles describing papal briefs, excerpting bishops' letters and mandates concerning *Unigenitus*, reviewing books for and against the Bull, giving reactions to the Council of Embrun (1727), calling for a national council, highlighting actions by the king and Parlement, and bemoaning the persecution of Jansenists. The paper's strident tone is reflected in the choice of Habakkuk 2:2 as the key Bible text for the 1729 edition: "The Lord spoke to me and told me: 'Write what you see & mark it down clearly on tablets so that he that runs may read it.'"[129]

Such bold declarations, however, offended a growing roster of enemies, which by 1730 included Louis XV, the police, the Jesuits, the philosophes, and most Gallican bishops. To the editors' rhetorical question—"If the *Ecclesiastical News* is contrary to the Constitution [*Unigenitus*], is it necessarily opposed to the State and Church?"— government officials and ecclesiastics gave a resounding "Yes!" In fact, by attacking hierarchies, reviving the sixteenth-century Calvinist *monarchomach* arguments (under the guise of Richerism), and encouraging open criticism (something it denounced in the philosophes), the newspaper radicalized society and undermined absolute monarchy.[130]

Recognizing this threat, the police tried to uproot this propaganda weed before it spread too far. In September 1728, the Council of State ordered Lieutenant-General René Hérault to stop the *abbés* Petitpied and Blondel from printing the *Nouvelles*, describing it as "contrary to the authority of the Church and to the laws of the State and to public tranquility." When the police found in these clerics' lodgings "packages . . . full of pernicious maxims tending to foment division and trouble," they decided to arrest them and bring them to trial, but both abbots had fled the kingdom.[131]

Hérault, however, was soft on Jansenism himself; on occasion, he interceded with the government to ease the punishment of *appelants*. Indeed, a *lettre de cachet* once sent his domestic to the Bastille charged with aiding and abetting Jansenists by sharing with them secret reports about what happened inside the police bureau. Unlike his successor, Feydeau de Marville, Hérault made only half-hearted attempts to ferret out the editors and writers of the *Ecclesiastical News*.[132] In 1728 he declared: "In the provinces and even more so in Paris, there have always been printers whose greed for gain leads them to overcome the most rigorous prohibitions" to unlicensed publication.[133] Even if the police chief had been disposed to arrest *appelants*, three-fourths of his officers, inspectors, and spies sympathized with the Jansenist cause, accepted bribes to look the other way, and sometimes—as in the case of the *abbé* Guilbert in 1736—let suspects escape.[134]

But the *Nouvelles'* most unrelenting enemy proved to be the Jesuits, who, despite their casuism, could not be bribed to look the other way. A closer examination of its pages helps one understand why they hated the newspaper so much. In the "A-J" index to the *Nouvelles Ecclésiastiques*, the entry for "Jésuites" fills 209 pages—23 percent of the entire first volume. By contrast, the entry for "Jansénisme" fills only 1.5 pages. Separate entries for "Louis XIV" (5 lines) and "Louis XV" (20 lines) are miniscule by comparison.[135] Not surprisingly, the Society of Jesus garners only negative comments. They are repeatedly called "morally perverse," "criminals," "profaners," "monstrous," "idolators," "the true enemies of religion," as well as "detestable doctors," "public poisoners," "false and odious," "dangerous for the State," and "the shame of the Church."[136] In addition to name-calling, the newspaper lambastes the Society's theology, morality, mission work, and pedagogical methods, particularly attacking Jesuit colleges for banning dances and ballets while sponsoring comedies and tragedies.[137] Despairing of police efforts to squelch the paper, the Jesuits, led by *Père* Patouillet, counterattacked by publishing a clever counterfeit—*The Supplement to the Ecclesiastical News*—from 1734 to 1748.[138]

Frustrated by its failures to suppress this underground paper, the government reacted with increasingly harsh laws punishing editors, authors, printers, distributors, and subscribers the police managed to catch. Louis XV's Declarations of 29 May 1728 and 24 March 1730 condemned first-time offenders to be chained to the *carcan* (stocks) in prison; recidivists rowed the king's galley ships around the Mediterranean Sea for several years. A successful police sting in Mantes, Champagne, and Burgundy sent the following individuals to the Bastille: the editors Vaillant and Troya (1728), the *abbés* Ferlant and Failly (1729), financier Marc Desessarts (1730), and the *abbé* Nivelle (1730). Police sent the *abbé* de Rougemont to the Conciergerie prison in 1731 while a printer named Lefebvre and a colporteur named Mozart went to Bicêtre in 1740. Throughout the kingdom, executioners publicly burned confiscated copies of the *Nouvelles*. As chapter 6 shows, 70 percent of Jansenists arrested after 1713 were charged with printing, engraving, or selling works promoting Jansenism (including the *Ecclesiastical News*)—and the vast majority of them went to the Bastille.[139]

Paradoxically, efforts by Church and government officials to suppress the *Nouvelles Ecclésiastiques* provided free publicity for the paper and increased the demand for *appelant* publications in Paris and the provinces. In short, far from suppressing Jansenism, persecution spread it like a virus that soon infected a major portion of the Gallican clergy. During the 1720s, when Jansenism reached its maximum extent, between 66 and 75 percent of the *curés*, 69 percent of the nuns, 54 percent of the priests, 50 percent of the canons, and 42 percent of the monks in Paris embraced the *appelant* cause. Its teachings permeated the Benedictines, Jacobins, and Oratorians.[140] In the 1720s, Jansenism had taken firm root in nine Paris parishes: St.-Germain-des-Près, St.-Roch, St.-Séverin, St.-André-des-Arts, St.-Gervais, St.-Jacques-du-Haut-Pas,

St.-Etienne-du-Mont, St.-Médard, and St.-Méry. But by 1739, when Monseigneur Nicolo Lercori, interim nuncio to France, sent Benedict XIV a list of "Jansenist" and "suspected Jansenist" parishes in Paris, their number had doubled. Lercori labeled 13 out of 44 parishes (30 percent) as "bad" and 4 parishes (9 percent) as "suspect." These 17 infected parishes included St.-Germaine-l'Auxerrois, St.-Eustache, St.-Jean-en-Grève, St.-Leu, St.-Séverin, St.-Gervais, St.-Landry, La Magdalaine de la Ville l'Evêque, St.-Pierre aux Boeufs, St.-Geneviève, Ste.-Marine, St.-Germain le Vieux, St.-Josse, St.-Paul, St.-Etienne-du-Mont, St.-Jacques de la Bouderie, and St.-Martin.[141]

Beyond Paris, strongholds of the *appelant* cause could be found in eastern France, especially in the southeastern Paris Basin, Lorraine, and Verdun. In northwestern France (possibly 40 percent Jansenist), its centers included Rouen, Pontoise, and Le Vexin. In the west and southwest, Senez, Cotignac, Pignons, Nantes, the Loire Valley, and Bayonne (Saint-Cyran's home) were Jansenist bastions. Contrary to the normal pattern of urban strength in northern France, in the south—and especially in Provence—Jansenism had a rural base of support. At Marseilles, the College of the Oratorians espoused it with support from the Parlement of Aix. Nevertheless, in three-fourths of the kingdom, the impact of Jansenism could be described as "fleeting."[142]

Once *appelants* gained the upper hand in a parish, however, a power struggle ensued, because they frequently raised questions other Catholics found uncomfortable. Who would run the parish administration? What kind of liturgy should be followed? Which saints' days should be observed? Would *curés* and clerics (the Catholic position) or local notables (the Jansenist view) have the final word in theological, ecclesiastic, and political disputes in the parish? Dozens of *placets* (petitions) sent by bishops, priests, canons, and *curés* to Cardinal Noailles and police chief Hérault mirror the pain and horror Catholics felt at the "disorders" and "violent & scandalous conduct" *appelants* had brought to their dioceses. These prelates beg Noailles to demonstrate his "compassion," "justice," and "equity" by protecting them and their flock from Jansenist "libels and gazettes." Repress these Jansenist upstarts, they plead; arrest and imprison them.[143]

But no one loved a dispute like the *appelants*. Protesting the harassment of Bishop Soanen of Senez by Cardinal Fleury and the Council of Embrun, 800 priests and 32 *curés* in Paris (and 500–600 priests in Troyes, Auxerres, and Châlons) signed a petition to Cardinal Noailles in March 1728. Dozens of clerics also penned memoirs defending Bishop Soanen—documents whose language would reappear during the 1730s in the remonstrances and consultations issued by Parlement.[144] Others, waxing poetic, wrote allegories and satires. One clever fifteen-page poem, allegedly "discovered" by a Chinese Mandarin and published "by permission of the Chinese Emperor," portrays the division within the Church as a "war" between "wolves" (Jansenists) and "dogs" (orthodox Catholics). Its anonymous author pleads with the "Good Shepherd" (the pope? the king?) to mediate a peace between them. Following several stanzas (in which the Jansenists, Church officials, advocates in Parlement, and even the devil play roles), the "dogs" and "wolves" sign a "concordat of peace," agree to jointly "guard the sheep," and celebrate a *Te Deum* (Mass) together.[145]

In real life, however, things could get more beastly. Although 707 (87 percent) doctors of theology at the Sorbonne finally accepted *Unigenitus* in September 1729, 104 (13 percent) of their colleagues refused to sign the Formulary.[146] Across France, the bishops were also divided following the Council of Embrun's exile of Bishop Soanen. Although the majority supported the Bull, a vocal minority opposed it during the late 1720s and 1730s. These recusants (including the bishops of Nîmes, Gap, Senez, Laon, Auxerre, Mirepoix, Montpellier, Boulogne, and Soissons) formed a "correspondence league" to support one another in resisting efforts to force their compliance. By means of letters, pastoral instructions, remonstrances, responses, and petitions, these bishops banded together to defend themselves and the larger cause of truth.[147]

Despite the old adage that "sticks and stones may break my bones, but words can never hurt me," these sources show the power of words—sharp, unorthodox, accusing words—doing great harm both at the personal and parish level. The emotional prose in these documents reveals the spiritual and psychological shock these Church officials endured as they desperately searched for a compromise between the two parties.[148] Some—like the Bishops of Senez, Mirepoix, Montpellier, and Boulogne—call for a national council to address the issues dividing them.[149] Others—like the Bishops of Vannes, Montpellier, and Soissons—wield the club of excommunication against "restless spirits" who "trouble consciences" with their speeches and writings against the Bull.[150]

The Jansenist bishops express concerns about their rights within the Gallican Church. They fear that the recent Council of Embrun's actions will threaten their authority as judges and blur the line between secular and religious power. They see the "liberties of the Church" under attack when a provincial council or parlement can put a bishop on trial, something they consider irregular, unprecedented, unjust, uncharitable, and "contrary to the faith, to tradition, and to the fundamental maxims of the realm." Every bishop, they assert, should be allowed to impose discipline in his diocese by means of decrees, synods, and ecclesiastical courts without the interference of parlements or police.[151] As Bishop Jean Colbert of Montpellier told Minister Maurepas: "All good Frenchmen must be enemies of the Bull because it contradicts those principles dear to the national [Gallican] Church."[152]

In an even bolder letter to Louis XV, Bishop Caylus of Auxerre warned the king in 1729 that the current debate over *Unigenitus* "foments a fanaticism which may soon ignite a war throughout the kingdom."[153] In his July 24 mandate, Caylus stated that just because the laws of the Church and the *arrêts* of Parlement have established *Unigenitus* in France, this "does not mean that the Bull must be regarded as a decision of the universal Church" or as "a law of Church and State." In fact, because the bishops (and not Parlement) are the true judges of doctrine, they have the right to revise the Bull before publishing it in their dioceses. For the pope or the king to force them to accept the Bull goes against canon law and disturbs the peace of the Church. To counter such attempts, the bishops had the right of appeal.[154]

While the Archbishop of Cambrai agrees with Bishop Caylus that "the power of the Keys" belongs to bishops and not to Parlement or secular authorities, he completely disagrees with the bishop's pro-Jansenist stance. In his 6 March 1731 mandate, he calls on the bishops to "raise their voices" against the "latest insolence" and "pernicious designs" of Jansenism. Jansenists, he asserts, "corrupt the faith of the Church" and "attack its authority"; moreover, they seek "to ruin this flourishing Monarchy" with their "scandalous excesses" (propaganda). Therefore, he calls on the Gallican bishops to "[take up] spiritual arms" to "repulse" the insults of "these enterprises of Heresy." Furthermore, he accuses 40 advocates in the Parlement of Paris (Jansenist sympathizers) of promoting Protestant reforms, because Richerism is the same as Protestantism in principle. These magistrates, he asserts, are trying to establish "a monstrous Republic" to the "horror of all good Frenchmen."[155]

This "republican spirit" had also infected the lower clergy, inspiring insubordination on a massive scale. Beginning in the 1720s, literally thousands of priests, canons, curates, nuns and monks used the *actes d'appel comme d'abus* to block attempts by their superiors (bishops, abbots, abbesses) to force them to accept the Bull. The dossiers at the Bibliothèque de l'Arsenal show that widespread disobedience had permeated the ranks of more than two dozen monastic orders in and around Paris. These included the Carmelites, Ursulines, Franciscans, Bernardins, Augustinians, Dominicans, Oratorians, Grandmontains, Feuillants, Mathurins, Theatins, Recollects, Cordeliers, Pratorians, Lazaristes, Minimes, Missionaires, Premonstratines, Annonciades, and Visitandines.[156]

Church and government leaders, who described this tidal wave of insubordination as "rebellion," "revolt," "scandal," "the spirit of intrigue," and "sedition," took it very seriously indeed. In fact, as the dossiers reveal, cases involving a single monk or nun could elicit the personal attention of Louis XV, the Council of State, government ministers (La Vrillière, Fleury, Maurepas, Phélyppeaux, Florentin), Parlement, police chiefs (Hérault, Marville), cardinals (Noailles, Polignac, Tencin), the Assembly of the Clergy, and the Sorbonne. But each case first passed through the bureau of Inspector Duval, who specialized in cases of religious dissidence. He and his staff assembled complete dossiers concerning the particulars of each individual's disobedience.[157]

Those who, after lengthy interrogations and intimidation, agreed to submit to *Unigenitus*, signed "Acts of Retraction." These oaths, with blank spaces for the recipient's name, date, and the place of signing, read as follows:

> I the undersigned____ submit to the Church; I respect all of its decisions relating to the faith and good manners; I accept all that it accepts and condemn all that it condemns. I receive as a decision of the Church the Constitution [*Unigenitus*] . . . and I ask pardon of God and of the Church for my error in signing this letter [of protest], and of my sisters [or brothers] for the scandal that I have caused them on this occasion.[158]

After signing an "Act of Retraction," the penitent had to perform an "act of restitution" (such as the renewal of their vows or some penitential act) before being reinstated into the fellowship of their order.

But these dossiers reveal that most of the clerics who signed "Acts of Protest" (*Actes d'appels*) stuck by their convictions. Phrases like "To put my conscience at ease," "I must decide my eternal destiny," and "We declare for the Truth" indicate that the vast majority believed that the Bull transgressed the principles of justice, right, and truth and cancelled their God-given freedom to choose. Yet protesting Church authority exacted a tremendous emotional price. The anguish many priests, monks, and nuns felt is revealed in such statements as "We are in tears," "We are in a desolate condition," "We are destroyed and ruined," and in the frequent use of words like "embarrassed," "sadness," "anxiety," and "just regrets" to describe their inner turmoil. Almost without exception, they agree on three points: *Unigenitus*, introduced by force, lacks universal approval and canonical justification; the Council of Embrun's (1727) condemnation of the Bishop of Senez should be nullified; and Jansenists are loyal, orthodox Roman Catholics.

Among the hundreds of cases studied, probably none defended herself more articulately than Sister Marie Margaritte Fleury de Saint-Jean Baptiste at the Ursuline convent in Beauvais. In her three-page protest of 10 May 1734, Sister Marie spoke eloquently for herself and for scores of her *appelant* colleagues when she penned the following "Appeal":

> In the name of the Father, Son, and Holy Spirit, Amen. In the uncertainty I feel at this moment when I must decide my eternal destiny, and not wishing death to hinder me from leaving behind certain proofs of my last sentiments, I declare of my own will and with full knowledge:
>
> 1 That having always lived in the fold of the Catholic Apostolic and Roman Church, I wish to die in the protection of that Church, from which no one can separate me.
> 2 I believe firmly with all my heart all the truths taught by the Holy Church, and I condemn with all my heart all the errors it condemns.
> 3 Among the decisions of the Church which are the object of my faith, I do not understand in any way the Constitution *Unigenitus*, which was introduced into the Church without any canonical form and without unanimity, and which was enforced by all kinds of violence and methods opposed to the spirit of Jesus Christ and of the Church, and very prejudicial to the salvation of the Faithful.

4 I renew with all my heart the Appeal that I made on this subject with all our Community [the Ursuline Order] to adhere to the appeal that Our Lords Bishops have interjected against the Constitution, to which appeal several Chapters, Communities, Companies, and Universities, and a great number of ecclesiastics have also adhered.
5 I accept with all my heart all the motives and reasons mentioned in the appeal and in the Memoir of Our Lords the Bishops, and in all the other appeals and writings made to oppose the Constitution, and I am in agreement today with all that will yet be done to oppose that Bull.
6 I regard the Council of Embrun as most unjust, as well as all actions taken against Monseigneur the Bishop of Senez, and I unite myself with this Prelate and with Monseigneur de Montpellier regarding the Constitution and the Formulary.
7 That God may only be pleased if I never consent to anything but what is written by P[asquier] Quesnel in his Preamble to the Constitution.
8 I will live inviolably attached to the Holy See, the center of unity of all the Church, and I remain closely tied to the Communion of Our Father the Pope who is seated on Saint Peter's Throne to whom Jesus Christ gave the primacy among the apostles.
9 I will always have the respect I must for Monseigneur Our Bishop and will, under God, render him all honor and all obedience that I must to a legitimate Superior.
10 I am also in agreement with all the First Pastors, with all the Second Order, and with all the Church Universal. I detest all revolt and Schism, and I wish to die in the unity and the charity of the Church.

These are the sentiments of my heart that I wish to appeal to the Tribunal of a just Judge. I swear by all that [God] has done for me in His great mercy, to increase my faith and make me persevere in the Truth with a confidence full of love until His second coming. Finally, I protest against everything that may be found in me contrary to the above, which cannot be taken from me except by violence or by the enfeebling of my reason. Amen.

[Signed] Soeur Marie Margaritte Fleury called Saint-Jean Baptiste, unworthy Religious, 10 May 1734. Done at the Convent of Ursulines at Beauvais.[159]

Jansenist clerics and nuns who stood firm for the "truths" espoused by Sister Marie did so fully realizing that the personal cost could be high. The police dossiers reveal that the punishments meted out to *appelants* ranged from mild to severe. Some, for example, were confined to their cells, placed on bread and water diets, denied the right to attend divine services or vote in chapter assemblies, sent back to college for refresher courses in Catholic theology, or transferred to other, presumably more orthodox, religious institutions. Their original convents or monasteries were forbidden to receive more novices and pensioners (a chief source of wealth) until given permission to do so. Others were put on trial and coerced into signing the Formulary. Frequently, still others received *lettres de cachet* exiling them far from Paris. Occasionally, as in the case of the Abbey of Orval in 1726, *appelant* brothers fled to Holland to enjoy religious liberty among the Dutch. On rare occasions Louis XV ordered a chapter closed if too many of its members had been infected with Jansenism. However, the most severe penalty was imprisonment, usually to Bicêtre or the Bastille, as chapter 6 shows.[160] Frustrated by one group's resistance, Archbishop Languet de Gergy of Sens exploded: "These women are so opinionated that one could burn them alive without changing their minds."[161]

Such widespread resistance to the Bull placed Cardinal Noailles in a tough position. Clement XI and Louis XV expected the Archbishop of Paris to exterminate Jansenism wherever he found it, yet he himself remained sympathetic to the *appelant* cause, as we have seen. His letters and mandates from 1725 to 1729, therefore, show him wringing his hands and longing for peace in the Church. In January 1725, Rome urged him to issue a mandate to counter "the artifices of the enemies of peace" and restore order before the pope died.[162]

A month later, however, Noailles shifted that responsibility back to the Holy See by assuring the pope that the 20 recusant bishops would all submit to *Unigenitus* as soon as Clement XI sent them his "explanations," for "kindness and charity," he declared, would win the day.[163] Ever the optimist, Noailles told Cardinal de Polignac in March of his "supreme joy" at news of the "approaching peace." "I am so full of happiness with His Holiness," he exclaimed, "that I can refuse him nothing . . . [This is] the happiest I have ever been in my life."[164] When Sister Desclaire, a paralyzed nun from the St. Antoine district of Paris, experienced healing while watching a procession of the relics of Ste.-Genevieve, the Archbishop saw this miracle as "new proof" that God would "hasten the peace that the Church desires" by bringing *appelants* back into the fold.[165]

Yet while he tried to convince Rome of his orthodoxy, Noailles kept one foot in the Jansenist camp. In the autumn of 1725 he sent the pope a "Project for a Mandate" suggesting ways to force recalcitrant clerics to sign the Formulary. At the same time, however, he issued "Secret Instructions" asserting that since the Bull of 1713 "was never put forward in Council as a rule of faith," it should not be held as such now.[166] In the meantime, Noailles—or someone acting with his permission—sent a "Memoir" to Cardinal Graveson denying charges that the Archbishop of Paris favored Jansenism and assuring him of his "irreproachable behavior . . . and orthodox doctrine." Noailles had in fact "absolutely submitted to all the papal bulls," the *Memoir* asserted.[167]

Everyone knew, of course, that Noailles had *not* fully submitted to *Unigenitus*, and his attempts to walk the fence between heresy and orthodoxy took a toll on his health. In a Declaration sent to the Gallican bishops in October 1727, he confessed that "the troubles that afflict the Church" had been for him "a continual source of sadness, so much so that our health succumbs under the weight of this affliction." He admitted to his colleagues that he was torn between "a desire to preserve the doctrines and rules of the Church" and the need to uphold "the peace of the Church." He found it "difficult to reconcile one with the other."[168]

Noailles finally resolved his dilemma a few months later when in July 1728 he agreed to sign the Formulary. Under pressure from Procurer-General Joly de Fleury, Chancellor d'Aguesseau, and members of his own family, he had copies of *Unigenitus* printed and publicly displayed all over Paris along with his letter of acceptance. In an October mandate, he told the new pope, "I have fulfilled my promise; I have done what I must do and what you expected of me."[169] On November 9, Benedict XIII, expressing his "extreme joy," assured Noailles, "I have great confidence in you . . . I have not seen your inner heart, but I have heard your words which are assuredly a testimony of your sincerity."[170]

Although the pope believed Noailles' submission to be sincere, when the Archbishop of Paris died on 4 May 1729 in a state of semi-consciousness, he could not express his true state of mind at the end.[171] Others, however, thinking themselves omniscient, presumed to do so. One anonymous author (possibly a Jansenist), in "Complaints that Religion Addresses to Your Eminence," accused the departed Archbishop of Paris of being "pious without strong zeal," for "beneath his perfect love beat an unfaithful heart." Because of Noailles' "indolence" and "infidelity," he had proved a "wolf most cruel." To prevent his "dangerous" friendship from causing one to "lose one's conscience," the author recommended "fleeing from this false peace which will only cause your eternal ruin."[172]

Noailles' successor, however, suffered no inner tensions concerning his attitude toward Jansenism. Charles Gaspard Guillaume de Vintimille, *comte* de Marseille du Luc and Archbishop of Aix from 1708 to 1729, became Archbishop of Paris at age 74 when he was 100,000 *écus* in debt. He had accepted *Unigenitus* without reservations in 1714, condemned the *appelant* cause in 1718, placed 300 Jansenist priests under interdict in the 1720s, and in his new position, resolved to crush the *Nouvelles Ecclésiastiques.*[173]

Since in their youth, Vintimille and Cardinal Fleury had studied theology together at the

Sorbonne, Louis XV's minister of state felt confident that the Archbishop of Paris would cooperate fully in the war on Jansenism. Vintimille did not disappoint him. In September 1729 he invited the *appelant* canons of Notre Dame Cathedral to a feast; the next day they all signed the Formulary. Others found his pastoral instruction letters demonstrating that *Unigenitus* did not contradict Catholic dogma or morality more convincing. Prior to 1730, out of 1,100 clerical applications to preach and hear confessions, Vintimille refused only 30 (3%). But after 1730, under pressure from Fleury, the Archbishop abandoned his easygoing policies. When Fleury exiled 48 Sorbonne theologians who had refused to sign the Formulary, Vintimille followed by publishing an ordinance revoking recusant priests' rights to confess and preach. During his tenure, he suppressed the rights of regular and secular clergy on 200 different occasions.[174] He urged Fleury to "stand firm" regarding Jansenism. "In the name of God," he exclaimed, "let the King show his anger."[175]

Louis XV did indeed "show his anger." When Parlement issued a "Consultation" trying to block Vintimille's efforts to prevent bishops from administering last rites to those lacking "Approval for Confession" documents, the king had the Council of State annul their action. When the magistrates remonstrated against Vintimille and drew up an *appel comme d'abus* in March 1731, the king imposed silence upon them. When they retaliated by going on strike, he sent ten of them into exile. His message was clear: He would support the Archbishop of Paris in his campaign to crush Jansenism no matter what the cost.[176]

The cost to Vintimille's personal reputation would be high. Even his bending of Catholic dietary rules to allow the faithful to eat eggs during Lent in the 1730s (due to food shortages in wartime) did not enhance his popularity, especially among his Jansenist critics.[177] Instead, some anonymous wit composed a "New Song to the Tune of There You Have It, My Cousin" with a stanza devoted to Vintimille:

> Vintimille sleeps, my cousin,
> To the point of indolence,
> He opens his eyes only half way, my cousin,
> And gives himself to license, my cousin.[178]

If the Archbishop of Paris occasionally slept at the switch, however, his old Sorbonne friend, Cardinal Fleury, remained a rabid anti-Jansenist. Cardinal Noailles, with good reason, had once described the minister of state as "a twenty-four carat Molinist."[179] In a 1734 letter to Bishop Souillac of Montpellier, Fleury warned him of the need to "take necessary precautions to oppose the progress of a fanaticism that is so contagious, especially in a place so filled with Huguenots as Saint-André." During the peak of the convulsionist controversy (discussed in chapter 7), Fleury feared that the Jansenist *convulsionnaires* would conspire with local Protestants. "There are too many connections in several respects between the Jansenists and the Protestants," he explained, "and it is essential to avoid everything that would contribute to their acting in unity to their mutual advantage."[180]

Seeing quarrels and conspiracies over *Unigenitus* as more dangerous than the Bull itself, Fleury expected Parlement, the Sorbonne, and the General Assembly of the Clergy to support Louis XV's anti-Jansenist policy. When 100 doctors of theology refused to fall into line, the minister took away their right to attend assemblies. This government purge effectively left control of the Sorbonne in the hands of the Ultramontanists. He also expelled nearly 300 *appelant* clergy from their parishes and had 300 more clerics arrested and placed under interdict.[181] Fleury assured the pope that with the king's "zeal for the faith" and the government's plan to extinguish Jansenism, the Gallican Church would soon be "reestablished to its former glory."[182]

But the first minister placed too much faith in the long-term effectiveness of his "plan." First, he dismissed Jansenist sympathizers in seminaries, colleges, and universities; required all degree candidates in theology to sign the Formulary; and closed schools "where [Jansenist] error is taught." Second, as a member of the Council of Conscience and the Ecclesiastical Chamber, he controlled all appointments to Church offices. With Louis XV's full support, he nominated only orthodox bishops, abbots, and canons "who favored good doctrine" and promoted only those candidates who graduated from "good seminaries." Third, he purged "corrupted" convents and monasteries. Fourth, emulating the Council of Embrun's handling of Bishop Soanen of Senez's case, he asked the Archbishop of Narbonne to preside over a provincial council to try Bishop Colbert de Croissy of Montpellier. This, he hoped, would send shock waves through the episcopate and bring positive reforms in the Church. Fifth, he imposed severe censorship on all printing establishments in Paris. Finally, he resolved to curb Jansenist influence in the Parlement of Paris—although he recognized that "nothing is more difficult than to find the means of doing this."[183]

Unfazed by the overwhelming challenges he faced, the first minister resolved to use every means at his disposal to punish those who opposed him, including strong reprimands, stiff fines (up to 3000 *livres*), the stocks, confiscation of property, exile, and imprisonment. Together, he and police chief Hérault dispersed religious communities tainted with Jansenism. The *maréchaussée* (rural mounted police) arrested *appelants* in tiny villages and tracked them through the woods. Returning from such a foray, Hérault discovered in his carriage a fresh copy of *Les Nouvelles Ecclésiastiques* criticizing him for attempting to root out Jansenism! *Appelants* apprehended by the police usually went to Vincennes or the Bastille for several weeks or months (see chapter 6).[184]

By following this repressive program, Fleury nearly succeeded in destroying the second wave of Jansenism as a popular movement. By the time he died in 1743, *appelant* clergy in Paris were as rare as hen's teeth in Provence. Yet his "victory" came at a high price, for in his efforts to crush Jansenism, Fleury compromised the monarchy's prestige in the public eye. Eventually, Louis XV would become as unpopular in the eighteenth century as Henri III had been in the sixteenth century.[185] As one police spy told Hérault in 1728: "The mind of the Public . . . is just about universally infected with Jansenism."[186] During the outbreak of convulsionist miracles at St.-Médard in the 1730s, many felt that if Louis XV refused to side with the Jansenists, he could no longer be their king "by the grace of God."[187]

Paradoxically, as Louis XV's popular approval ratings fell, his efforts to enforce *Unigenitus* only grew more determined. On 24 March 1730, he issued a seven-page Declaration making the Bull for the first time the law of the land. Despite the "divisions" and "troubles" that had followed its issuance in 1713, he said, "we had hoped that by 1720 . . . unity, peace, charity, and concord" would have been restored within the Church. Since such harmony had not occurred, the Declaration of 4 August 1720 had demanded that all clerics in France submit to the Bull. As the past decade had made abundantly clear, hundreds of cardinals, bishops, priests, monks and nuns had refused to do so. Therefore, confident that yet another Declaration would solve the problem, the king ordered all prelates to sign the Formulary "pure and simple without distinctions [of fact or right]"—or risk losing their benefices.[188]

If Louis XV expected Parlement to pass this Declaration without debate, he was sadly disappointed. For ten days, the magistrates refused to register it, so on April 3 the king entered the Grand Chamber and held a *lit de justice* to force them to do so. After they had registered the new law, Louis forbade them to hear any more appeals concerning *Unigenitus*. On 10 March and again on 5 September 1731, the Council of State issued *arrêts* imposing silence "general and absolute" on any matter related to the Bull. Henceforth, "all disputes & debates on the subject of the Constitution *Unigenitus* shall cease."[189]

But imposing the "law of silence" only added fuel to the fire of debates raging across France. As the archives make abundantly clear, it required hundreds of *lettres de cachet* to enforce the new law among the Benedictines, Oratorians, Dominicans, Doctrinarians, and Feuillants in Paris. Fleury and Hérault purged scores of *appelant* monks and nuns in these orders. They also expelled Jansenist students from the seminaries of Saint-Magloire and Trente-Trois and closed the colleges of Saint-Barbe, Harcourt, Plessis, and Navarre. By 1731, the *Ecclesiastical News* estimated that Minister Fleury had issued some 600 *lettres de cachet* to send 879 *appelants* to prison or exile.[190]

Although the General Assembly of the Clergy supported the Declaration of 1730, hoping that it would annihilate the Jansenist "conspiracy" that threatened "to destroy the very foundations of the Faith,"[191] the doctors of theology at the Sorbonne opposed it. So in November 1729, the king issued *lettres de cachet* expelling all *appelants* at the University of Paris. The orthodox remnant then dutifully ratified the Bull "with heart and mind" on December 15. When the *abbé* René Pucelle led the expelled theologians in protesting before Parlement the irregularity of their expulsion, Louis XV countered by placing the Faculty of Theology directly under the jurisdiction of his Council of State. When 100 doctors opposed this action and called for a national Church council, he banished them from the Sorbonne in 1732.[192]

When magistrates at the Parlement of Paris, ignoring the law of silence, continued debating issues related to *Unigenitus*, Louis XV issued more *lettres de cachet* forbidding them to do so. Like pouring gasoline on a fire, this action only spread the conflagration. Soon protests poured in from the parlements of Rouen, Rennes, Dijon, Bordeaux, and Metz. When the king sent *lettres de jussion* ordering these parlements to register and publish the 1730 law, they balked. In Paris, where 150 of the 180 *parlementaires* (83 percent) opposed the new law, a clique of 25 to 30 magistrates started a writing campaign against it. They issued *appels comme d'abus* in favor of accused clerics and published the incendiary *Cause of the State Abandoned by the French Clergy* blaming the Jesuits for disrupting the "Peace of the Church" by persecuting Jansenists.[193] They also republished Louis Machon's *Memoir Touching the Origin of Parlement's Authority in France Called Judicium Francorum* (1652), a pamphlet written during the Fronde. This work asserts that the Parlement of Paris, like its ancient predecessors the gatherings of the Gauls and the assemblies of the Franks, represents the entire nation. Its magistrates, therefore, have the right to deliberate over the king's declarations and *arrêts* and to remonstrate when they disapprove of them. Indeed, Jansenist literature in the 1730s considered Parlement to be "the Senate of the nation" charged with upholding the "rights, liberties, and franchises" of the French people.[194]

Angered by Parlement's never-ending remonstrances, Louis XV exiled 140 magistrates (15 presidents and 125 councilors) to the four corners of France in September 1732. An anonymous engraver prepared a humorous black-and-white sketch showing "The Parlement of Paris Oppressed, Exiled, and Placed in Irons" with a sign over the Palace of Justice that read "Palace for Rent." Only after lengthy negotiations by the King of Sardinia did Louis XV agree to recall his disobedient magistrates.[195]

They returned submissive but not silent. In their remonstrance for 6 April 1737, the councilors assured the king that because of their "zeal to maintain peace in the Church and State," they could not ignore the current "troubles" in the kingdom. They reminded their sovereign that Parlement "represents your immediate person and exercises in your name the sovereign authority in the administration of justice." Therefore, during the present "crisis," the magistrates must protect the king's sovereignty and the "liberties of the Gallican Church" against popes whose false claims of infallibility could lead them to pass bulls harmful to Gallican independence.[196] In his reply, Louis XV thanked the magistrates for their careful scrutiny of papal documents, but assured them that he *first* reviewed Church decisions and *then* passed them along to Parlement to enact into law. Magistrates, he reminded them, received their authority from the king; therefore, they should unite with him in promoting "the common and indivisible good of religion and the state." On matters of doctrine, he added, both Parlement and the Gallican Church must submit to Rome.[197]

One such challenge came the following year when Clement XII attempted to canonize the popular French cleric Vincent de Paul "for his noble and pious life." When Parlement passed an *arrêt* suppressing his canonization, the angry pope issued a brief attacking the magistrates. "Who are they," he asked, "to oppose the Apostolic authority of the Vicar of Christ?" With typical papal overkill, the brief declared the magistrates' *arrêt* "vain, reproved, broken, null, annulled, abolished, and without effect or force whatsoever." The pope threatened to excommunicate those who read or distributed the *arrêt*.[198]

As the magistrates explained to Louis XV in an "Address" on 28 June 1738, however, the real issue did not concern Vincent de Paul's worthiness for sainthood, but the pope's bypassing Parlement's traditional right to issue letters patents approving his canonization in order for it to be effective in France. By ignoring their customary and historic rights, the councilors told the king, Clement XII trampled on "our ancient canon laws and on our holy and precious liberties." Such actions could lead to "scandalous tocsins . . . and schisms in the Church and trouble and desolation in the State," they warned.[199] In a reply two months later, Louis XV assured his councilors that he would maintain the laws and uphold repose, order, and tranquility in his realm.[200]

To assist the monarch in maintaining that tranquility, the Council of State had previously issued the *arrêt* of 5 September 1731 forbidding the printing, selling, and distribution of any work dealing with the Bull which used the terms "injurious and innovative, heretical, schismatic, Jansenist, semi-Pelagian, and any other names of parties."[201] But this *arrêt* proved useless in stopping the circulation of over 1000 Jansenist books, articles, and pamphlets already in print.[202] Nonetheless, after 1737, the *comte* d'Argenson, newly appointed Inspector of the Publishing Trade, with the help of *Dom* La Taste and the police, began enforcing strict surveillance of Parisian printers and booksellers. In a short time he had put 180 out of 200 (90 percent) Jansenist printers out of business; only 20 remained active by 1740.[203]

D'Argenson failed, however, to find and suppress the underground presses that produced the *Nouvelles Ecclésiastiques*, Jansenism's premiere propaganda paper. Its continued success in the 1730s owed more to the talents of its clandestine editors, authors, and distributors than to the lack of effort by Church and government institutions to suppress it. Parlement issued *arrêts* against the newspaper on 9 February 1731 and 13 June 1732, ordering copies of it to be "torn & burned by the Executioner of High Justice." The magistrates felt that its "audacious satires," full of slander and libel, "show a lack of respect for secular & ecclesiastical authority." Even worse, it creates scandals, profanes "the mysteries of religion," and "arouses the public voice" (public opinion), something that should remain quiet and submissive.[204]

Archbishop Vintimille, who on this subject at least agreed completely with Parlement, condemned the *Nouvelles* in his mandate of 25 April 1732, labeling it "a great scandal throughout the kingdom." Finding its "wicked, libelous prose" full of lies and calumnies "most dark and artificial," he called it "an enemy of the truth and a damnable slave to politics . . . without manners, probity, or conscience." Its "venom" insults Church authorities, "turns the faithful from obedience," "favors schism & heresy," and "violates all the rights of truth, charity, & justice." Therefore, he warned, all those who print, distribute, or read it will be excommunicated.[205] Scores of *appelant* priests and abbots, however, refused to read the Archbishop's mandate from their pulpits. When he threatened them, they defended the newspaper's attacks on the Holy See and the Jesuits while rejecting their superior's assertion that they were "disobedient" clerics. At wit's end, Vintimille confessed to Minister Fleury: "It is a question of knowing whether the Paris *curés* are leading me or if I am leading them as their Archbishop."[206]

Following Vintimille's lead, the Bishop of Marseilles issued a mandate two months later condemning the *Nouvelles* for its libels and lies. The newspaper is full of "wicked profanities & sacrilege," he declares. It promotes "disrespect for legitimate authority," "increases the spirit of independence & rebellion," and "inspires revolt & sedition." Employing a style "like a comedian," it purports to amuse the reader with its "odious portraits," "astonishing scandals," and "Molinist errors." Although he did not threaten excommunication, the bishop forbade the faithful to read the paper.[207]

Not to be outdone, the Council of State on 3 May and again on 16 June 1732 condemned the *Ecclesiastical News* as a rag that "troubles the tranquility of Church & State." They ordered its authors and editors "to cease all disputes & debates" related to *Unigenitus* and forbade anyone to read, sell, or distribute the paper. The Council told the courts to "take convenient measures" to enforce this law.[208] Yet as the newspaper proudly declared in 1732: "The public is a judge which they [Crown and Church] have been unable to corrupt."[209] And the public hungered for copies of the *Nouvelles* like street urchins begging bread.

During the 1730s, the Church news reported in the paper came from all over Europe. Although 90 percent of the articles focused on Gallican affairs, more often now, writers also described ecclesiastical events in Naples, Rhodes, Utrecht, Brussels, and Flanders. As in the 1720s, the paper carried two columns per page and four pages per issue, but it came off the press more regularly now, usually every five to ten days (from 1730 to 1735) and once every week (after 1735). Like the 1720s, issues in the 1730s contained reports and commentary on Louis XV's declarations, Council of State *arrêts*, Parlement's new laws, bishops' mandates, university decrees, and civil and criminal trials involving *appelants* in France.

Authors wrote hagiographies on and obituaries for Jansenist worthies (nearly always men), penned virulent attacks on Jesuits and Quietists, reviewed books favorable and unfavorable to Jansenism, reprinted extracts from foreign papers, and followed the controversy between Louis XV and the Sorbonne. As before, reporters sniffed out examples of persecution wherever they could find them and blamed the Jesuits, police, or the bishops for the exile and imprisonment of their *appelant* colleagues. Accurate reports in the 1738 issue concerning police chief Hérault's plans and movements and the treatment of ecclesiastics inside the highly secure Bastille raise the question as to whether the editors had planted a mole inside the police force.

What was new in the 1730s was the increased, favorable attention given to the more than 200 people healed at Deacon Pâris' grave in the Cemetery of St.-Médard (see chapter 7). The *Nouvelles* argued that these "genuine miracles" proved that "God has spoken against that Bull [*Unigenitus*]." The masthead of the 1733 issue quoted Ecclesiastes 36:6–7, 10: "Do miracles that have not been seen." Articles strongly defended these healing incidents as Jansenist "weapons" in the battle for truth against the Jesuits (whose "weapons" included exile, prison, torture, and book burning). As one title page in 1732 illustrated, God's miraculous intervention empowered *appelant* doves to drive Molinist hawks from the Gallican skies. Beginning in 1737, the newspaper also favorably reviewed the speeches and writings of Carré de Montgeron, a *parlementaire* defender of Jansenist miracles (discussed in chapter 7).[210]

One friendly critic—the "*abbé* D.G." (probably a Jansenist)—suggested several improvements to make the paper more effective. In a letter to an anonymous professor of literature in 1732, he said: "I think . . . that the *Nouvelles Ecclésiastiques* would be more useful and more widely approved if the facts were simply reported without comment, without emotion, without any design of prejudicing the judgment of the reader, in the style of novels." Because authors did not sign their names, "their authority for what they write is unknown. This leads them to think and write as authorities on every subject . . . which is a very dangerous job." He regretted the paper's penchant for name-calling and making "impertinent and unreasonable" assertions, believing that such yellow journalism biased readers' minds and injured "the good cause & those who defend it."[211]

But many of those who defended the *appelant* cause disagreed with "*abbé* D.G." and believed that the use of satirical songs, poems, and engravings promoted the Jansenist cause, especially among the illiterate lower classes. The Fonds Sainte-Beuve at the Bibliothèque de l'Histoire du Protestantisme Français in Paris contains dozens of these humorous works.[212] One black-and-white engraving, printed in Amsterdam, shows the papal nuncio to France surrounded by cardinals and Jesuits, all plucking chickens in a courtyard. The accompanying verse states:

> You came, imprudent nuncio, to pluck the French:
> You want to deprive them of their ancient rights
> By dangerous views of a dark cabal
> Of priests always ready to serve Papal ambition;
> But remember, Parlement's wise integrity
> Can regain Italy with all diligence;
> So soon you will receive in France
> The just chastisement that Malta deserves.[213]

Offended by such impertinent propaganda, Louis XV pleaded for religious unity in the realm. In a circular letter to the Gallican bishops in July 1731, he asserted that further disputes over *Unigenitus* would not only be "dangerous and useless," but would also represent an "attack upon the King." Since the Bull was now law in France, he urged the bishops to enforce it in their dioceses so that "uniformity in doctrine" and "subordination to the hierarchy" might prevail. Optimistically, he declared that "the end of all disputes" would soon bring "calm and peace to all minds."[214]

But during the 1730s, the Church experienced very little "calm and peace." Priests who refused to sign the Formulary had their revenues frozen or sequestered, lost their benefices, and suffered exile or imprisonment.[215] Meanwhile, bishops from every corner of the kingdom debated the issues surrounding the Bull in their mandates, pastoral instructions, personal letters, and responses.[216] Those who favored *Unigenitus* found "sentiments of rebellion and republicanism and seditious maxims" in the writings of those who opposed it.[217] Such *appelants*, the Archbishop of Aix exclaimed, "commit a grievous mortal sin" and face "a life of damnation without hope of salvation." To save as many souls as he could, the Archbishop composed his own Formulary for all the ecclesiastics in his archdiocese to sign—but Parlement, finding this oath a "novelty without approval," annulled it.[218]

When the Archbishop of Sens issued a similarly stern pastoral letter defending Catholic truth and condemning Jansenism in 1734, the courageous *abbé* Languet reminded his superior that truth was not always easily discerned. "Truth should be distinguished from authority," he asserted. "Pilate and the High Priest had authority, but not the truth; on the contrary, they condemned Jesus Christ, who was the truth."[219]

Perhaps the only way to reconcile the tension between truth and authority, one radical but anonymous author suggested in 1734, was to tolerate one another's beliefs. His "System of Tolerance for This Time" asserted that ecclesiastical unity "is not essential to the Church, nor a divine law," but a man-made rule that can be changed. The author recommended talking with heretics and schismatics rather than condemning them. Let *all* Catholics (except "notorious sinners") receive the sacraments without distinction regarding *appelants* and *constitutionnaires*. Stop priests and bishops from punishing *refusants*, for "prudence and charity" dictate showing "love and communication" toward all sincere Catholics. The author then outlined a 22–step plan showing how Church officials at all levels could implement this policy of tolerance. Among these suggestions, he recommended all-inclusive worship services, no refusals of sacraments, continuous communication, no name-calling, kindness and charity toward all, and recognizing that the spectrum of beliefs within Catholicism, Jansenism, and Quesnelism enriched the Church. Diversity and freedom of belief need not threaten Church unity, he said, for not everyone will be unified in the search for truth, but all can be charitable. In the final analysis, the Gallican Church does not have to follow the drumbeat of Rome's bulls.[220]

But in issues related to *Unigenitus*, tolerance was a scarce commodity. Across France, bishops took sides and vigorously defended their positions in mandates and pastoral letters. One prelate, however, chose a different path. Wanting no part in enforcing "this wicked decree," Jean Charles de Segur, Bishop of St. Papoul, resigned his office in 1735 and joined the Oratorians, seeking "instruction and contemplation." In a mandate addressed to his clergy and parishioners, he explained that "inquietude and alarms in our conscience" concerning the Bull and weariness with the "avarice of the world" had dictated his decision. Although most of his fellow bishops attacked his "scandalous" action ("a bishop does not simply resign," they said), a handful, praising his "public humiliation" at accepting "the Cross of Jesus Christ," believed that he had "the finger of God" upon him.[221] Two months later, however, Segur felt the disapproving finger of his monarch when the Council of State suppressed his mandate.[222]

Yet even those who supported the Bull risked reprisals for defending it in print and breaking the "law of silence" imposed by the king in 1730. François Ilharat de la Chambre, for example, went to Utrecht to have his *Treatise on the Formulary* published in 1736. In it, he vigorously defended the "moral and supernatural right" of Church and state officials to condemn and punish *appelants*, force them to sign the Formulary, and censor their works full of "fantastic heresies and bad doctrines."[223] In a similar vein, Chabaille d'Anvigny (possibly a police spy), called Jansenists "odious hypocrites" and accused them of being Augustinians secretly in league with the Calvinists and the *convulsionnaires* to "deceive an entire people."[224]

Two years later, in his *History of the Constitution Unigenitus* (1738), Pierre-François Lafiteau, Bishop of Sisteron, told his fellow bishops that Jansenism's "venomous" deception presented just as much danger to the Church as Protestantism had in the sixteenth century. He predicted that it would bring "one of the most violent tempests [the Church] has ever suffered." Because the Jansenists' "animosities are so active & bold, their writings so multiplied & licentious . . . there is much to fear in France for Religion & for the State" from their divisive, independent spirit.[225]

Given this divisive climate, even *constitutionnaire* clerics judged it prudent to leave behind written testimonies of their orthodoxy and of their opposition to Jansenism. As he lay dying in 1738, Bishop Daubrière of Soissons penned the following "profession of faith":

> I am and always have been submissive to all the decisions of the Catholic Church and to all the bulls against Jansenism and notably the Bull *Unigenitus*. If I have shown kindness toward the Jansenists, it was to win their hearts and lead them to do their duty, and not because of affection for them, because I have always detested and abhorred them in my heart.[226]

Significantly, the year 1738 also marked the passing of Agnès de Sainte-Blaindine Forget, the last sister exiled from Port-Royal des Champs. She died at Amiens, far from the Chevreuse Valley she had once called home.[227] To keep the memory of Agnès and her deceased sisters alive, Jansenist authors wrote multi-volume hagiographies. One example, *abbé* Claude-Pierre Goujet's *Memoirs to Serve as a History of Port-Royal* (1734–37), is a three-volume supplement to the earlier Port-Royal histories by Fontaine, Lancelot, and du Fossé. In it, Goujet gathered together the letters, testimonies, and tributes penned by the convent's nuns concerning the pious lives and noble deaths of sixteen abbesses and nuns.[228]

But the *abbé* Gaspard Terrasson, a priest at Treigny in the diocese of Auxerre, wanted to do more than revere the memories of the past: he wanted to revive Port-Royal des Champs itself. Expelled from his order and tracked by police, he fled Paris in 1732 to escape imprisonment in the Bastille. At Treigny, he created a rural refuge for persecuted *appelants*. With support from Charles de Caylus, Bishop of Auxerre, Terrasson built two houses for solitaires, a hospital offering free charity to the poor, and two schools (one for boys, one for girls) with three teachers and 60 pupils. Over the next three years, dozens of outcast Jansenists flocked to his rural retreat, proclaiming him "the patriarch of the new Church." But in 1735, when procurer Le Pelletier des Forts learned of the scheme, he informed police chief Hérault, who in turn informed Cardinal Fleury, who told Archbishop Vintimille to investigate the matter. As a result, Louis XV issued *lettres de cachet* dispersing the solitaires, closing the hospital and schools, and imprisoning Terrasson at Vincennes. Nine years later, after the *abbé* had signed the Formulary in 1744, the king allowed him to retire to Nogent-sous-Coucy, where he died in 1752. The phantom of Port-Royal des Champs had once again been exorcised.[229]

Yet its ghost returned to haunt Church and government officials during the growing controversy over the refusal of sacraments to dying Catholics suspected of Jansenism. This practice, more frequent in Paris than elsewhere, deeply disturbed *appelants* (who saw it as virtual excommunication) and annoyed *parlementaires* (who considered it "disturbing to the public order"). Several times—in 1733, 1737, and 1738—Parlement issued remonstrances condemning the practice.[230]

But the bishops argued that they must "follow their consciences" in denying the sacraments to those who opposed *Unigenitus*. "I do not think one should pray for a man who dies an *appelant* any more than one would pray for someone killed in a duel," the Bishop of Amiens asserted. The Bishop of Châlon concurred, declaring that to be an *appelant* was "the most enormous and scandalous crime" of being a schismatic who deserved excommunication. Because *refusants* "are in revolt and schism" against the Church, the Bishop of Marseilles added, "good principles" dictated that they should not receive last rites. Those who died refusing to sign the Formulary, the Bishop of Laon thundered, "become the heritage of demons." The Bishop of Nantes went further: Those who stubbornly resisted Church decisions should be "deprived of Ecclesiastical Sepulcher" (burial in holy ground) after death. The Bishop of Boulogne agreed that such a stand promoted "good discipline" in the Church.[231]

Probably no Church prelate articulated this hard-nosed stance better than Etienne Joseph Delafare, the prolific and controversial Bishop of Laon. During the 1730s, he penned 71 documents (seven per year) defending his apostolic authority, declaring *Unigenitus* a rule of faith, and condemning Jansenism as "an abomination before God" worthy of excommunication.[232] In 1732 he bragged to Minister Fleury that he had "combated and nearly dissipated the heresy which previously dominated" his diocese.[233]

Yet every time he issued a mandate against the *appelants*, a group of lawyers, magistrates in Parlement, or the Council of State struck it down for "troubling the public tranquility" and breaking the 1730 law of silence. Deeply hurt, the bishop would then defend himself and his apostolic prerogatives in writing—only to have that document suppressed as well. Over a period of ten years, the bishop relentlessly upheld the rights of the Gallican Church, defended the authority of the bishops, and denied the power of king and Parlement to intervene in religious affairs. In return, Parlement and the Council of State issued twelve *arrêts* to restrain him. When he appealed his case to the Holy See, the Council of State revoked his printing privilege—but the determined bishop went right on issuing mandates and pastoral letters anyway![234] Carrying his hatred of Jansenists beyond the grave, in 1738 he asked police chief Hérault for a *billet d'exhumation* (a "ticket to exhume") to unearth a corpse buried four weeks before (and subsequently found to be an *appelant*) and rebury it in a distant place. Days later, when Archbishop Vintimille gave his permission, the Bishop of Laon held "a solemn service of exhumation" for the body of Jean Gay, priest and doctor of theology at the Sorbonne.[235]

The Jansenists, of course, expressed horror at the bishop's action. In a short "Memoir Concerning the Public Refusal of the Sacraments on the Deathbed," one anonymous *appelant* argued that only flagrant sinners (those living in "constant crime," "open scandal," or "open revolt") should be refused last rites at death. Denying the sacraments to anyone else is "defamatory & injurious to that person," "prejudicial to the spiritual welfare of the faithful," "contrary to the peace & public tranquility," and "opposed to the letter & spirit of holy canon law." Therefore, those who privately opposed the Bull created no public scandal and should receive the last rites.[236]

Perhaps because the marquis d'Argenson's own brother had espoused the *constitutionnaire* cause in 1739 and feared financial ruin as a result, the minister himself tried to straddle the fence between the two contending camps.[237] In his "Profession of Faith," the Minister of State admitted that concerning Jansenism and *Unigenitus*, "[I] have always been very balanced and worthy of good will." But regarding dogma and ecclesiastical authority, "[I have been] very heretical and worthy of disgrace." Although he agreed that the laity should submit to the pope, to the bishops, and to the Bull "as a guaranteed preservative against abuse," as a politician and magistrate who valued "repose" in the State, he believed "it is wrong to pressure the Jansenists as we do." If government and Church officials could learn one lesson from their failure to convert the Huguenots, he said, it would be that toleration often succeeded where persecution failed.[238] Continued persecution of the Jansenists will plunge France into war, he warned. "The only way to abolish heresy," he asserted, "is by ignoring it."[239]

But nearly everyone agreed that the exponential growth of Jansenism in Paris made it impossible to ignore. In 1733, an anonymous doctor of theology at the Sorbonne had asserted that "Paris is truly possessed by a spirit of vertigo; error and fanaticism dominate it almost completely." He feared that the capital would "carry the entire kingdom over the precipice" into the *appelant* camp.[240] To all appearances, this had occurred, for in 1745, the marquis d'Argenson called Jansenism "the universal religion of the realm."[241] "All Paris is Jansenist!" Barbier exclaimed in 1752.[242]

Perhaps nowhere was this more obvious than among the robe nobility. Lawyers, magistrates, and judges who trained at the colleges and served on the law faculties imbibed instruction reinforced with Jansenist and Oratorian ethics. They studied the *Art of Thinking*, written by a Cartesian, and sharpened their reasoning and syllogistic logic skills by reading the works of Antoine Arnauld and Pierre Nicole.[243] Yet with perhaps a half dozen exceptions, these eighteenth-century jurists did not share the pious, devout, ascetic religious outlook of their seventeenth-century predecessors on the bench. Instead, they had replaced their ancestors' theological mindset with a Gallican outlook that was strongly anti-papal and anti-despotic in nature. Therefore, although these lawyers opposed the 1713 Bull, they did so as Gallican patriots and not as *appelants*. In their minds, Parlement served as a crucial counterweight to the arbitrary actions of the Crown and the bishops. Consequently, the 1730s witnessed frequent conflicts between the *parlementaires* on the one hand and Louis XV and the bishops on the other.[244]

Beginning around 1740, however, the king tried a different tactic. Following the marquis d'Argenson's advice, he decided "to punish those who elevated themselves by imprudence and false zeal" by preventing their advancement to high offices in the Church and state. The children of these "celebrated Jansenist fanatics," he reasoned, being ambitious to rise, would be "the first converters of their fathers."[245]

For those already in high positions, Louis XV required loyalty oaths. In 1741, for example, the Faculty of Theology at the Sorbonne swore the following oath: "I [name] declare, in the presence of the Sacred Faculty, that I acknowledge the *Unigenitus* Constitution as the dogmatic judgment of the Universal Church, following the meaning of the decree of the Sacred Faculty passed on 15 December 1729, to which I adhere, and I request the document to show my adherence."[246]

During the 1740s, at convents and monasteries in Paris and beyond, Archbishop Vintimille and police chief Marville required nuns and monks to sign similar oaths attesting to their orthodoxy. Those who refused were transferred to other convents or sent into exile. Also, when vacancies occurred in dioceses where opposition to *Unigenitus* was centered (Paris, Boulogne, Tours, Orléans, Meaux, Nantes, Montpellier, Aix, and Senez), Church officials appointed strictly orthodox prelates. By the end of the decade, there were virtually no Jansenist bishops left. In addition, police reports show that "peace," "good order," and "tranquility" had returned to many religious houses.[247]

But here and there, individual *appelants* continued to protest. At the Benedictine Monastery of Mortagne, for example, Brother Jean Le Suer, who had signed the Formulary as a novice in 1718 and again as a sub-deacon in 1721, declared on 1 April 1744 that he repudiated "with my blood" those earlier oaths taken "in ignorance." Now that he "knows the Truth" and can "distinguish fact and right," his Declaration asserts, he denounces the Bull of 1713 as "an anti-Christian doctrine." Le Suer defends "the cause of the Holy Bishop [Jean Soanen] of Senez unjustly condemned in the Council of Embrun," the miracles at Deacon Pâris' grave, and the convulsions then raging in Paris. Yet in the same breath, he also acknowledges the pope as the vicar of Christ, professes his adherence to Roman Catholic teachings, and "abhors schism and division" in the Church. The Bishop of Auxerre and Minister St. Florentin, however, saw Le Suer's declaration differently; soon a *lettre de cachet* removed him from the monastery.[248]

Appelant nuns as well—especially among the Benedictines, Carmelites, Ursulines, and Franciscans—occasionally defied officials' efforts to enforce uniformity. In 1747, Sister Saint-Basile, a nun at the Benedictine convent of Notre-Dame du Val-de-Gif, penned a similar declaration. "Today silence is no longer permitted," she said. "The Constitution wishes to reign over all and makes itself adored. No asylum, no solitude, no convent is protected from its violent pursuits. It [*Unigenitus*] troubles all, ravages all, scatters all. One must of necessity opt for one or the other of the two parties."[249]

By the mid-1740s, however, Archbishop Vintimille and Minister Fleury—who both died in office in 1746 at 91 and 93 years of age respectively[250]—had put in place measures to insure that only one party—the *constitutionnaires*—won. With the help of the Council of Conscience and the support of the General Assembly of the Clergy, they rapidly replaced *appelant* clerics with orthodox ones. They also pressured Parlement to censure libels, satirical songs, and pro-Jansenist publications more severely. The *arrêt* of 18 May 1745 sentenced those caught distributing gazettes or newspapers (like the *Nouvelles Ecclésiastiques*) to exile or several years' detention at Bicêtre or the Bastille. Supplying the vigilant police chief Feydeau de Marville with a generous number of *lettres de cachet*, they helped the police arrest and detain dozens of *curés, abbés*, and vicars hiding in Jansenist parishes like St.-Josse and St.-Germaine-des-Près.[251] In 1747, for example, an escort of musketeers removed the last *appelant* nuns from the convent of La Fidelité at Saumur and sent them to Angers.[252]

The government's attempts to purge the University of Paris and the Hôpital-Général of Jansenist influence, on the other hand, met with stiff resistance. In 1745, Louis XV issued an edict permitting bishops to place *curés* in their dioceses without having to consult the university professors who had taught them (as the Concordat of 1516 required). Angered by this attack on their customary prerogatives, the Faculty of Theology protested loudly and often, but their remonstrances fell on deaf ears.[253]

After purging the Sorbonne and most of the capital's parishes of Jansenist priests, authorities set out to do the same at the Hôtel-Dieu, Bicêtre, and La Salpêtrière, all part of a vast complex of eight buildings and 5000 employees known as the Hôpital-Général. Part hospital, part prison, the Hôpital-Général was administered by a council dominated by Jansenists. Since about 1700, half of its bourgeois administrators had been sympathetic to the *appelant* cause.[254]

But in 1747, the new Archbishop of Paris, Christophe de Beaumont, resolved to sweep the place clean of Jansenism. He removed unorthodox books from its library, fired *appelant* employees, and replaced several administrators. But when he appointed the widow Louise-Urbine de Moysan—a non-Jansenist—as the new director, he initiated a "tempest in a teapot" that pitted Jansenists and *parlementaires* against the king, the Jesuits, and himself. Immediately, 19 of the 22 administrators resigned in protest.[255] Secretary of State D'Argenson declared that the Archbishop had "seized for himself the administration of the Hôpital-Général with a despotism that revolts everyone."[256] The philosophe Voltaire quipped: "Never has a smaller affair caused such grand emotion in people's minds."[257]

During the 1740s, the clandestine Jansenist press both mirrored and ignited this emotional state of mind. The *Nouvelles Ecclésiastiques*—whose four-page issues now appeared regularly every seven days—continued to report primarily on news in Paris and around France. But it also closely followed ecclesiastical events in Rome, Utrecht, Turin, Holland, and Spain, and frequently printed excerpts from the *Gazette of Amsterdam*. More often now, it also chronicled the passing of "the defenders of the Truth" (many of them women). Its articles—longer than in the 1730s—tended to ignore happenings at the Holy See. Instead, they repeatedly attacked the Jesuits and Voltaire and focused public attention on the *grands secours* (convulsionist healing and tortures, discussed in chapters 7 and 8). At the end of the decade, authors devoted even more attention to the controversy surrounding the purging of Jansenists at the Hôpital-Général and the fight over the refusal of sacraments, a battle that, thanks to Archbishop Christophe de Beaumont's intransigence, would grow into an all-out war in the 1750s.[258]

The prose employed by *Nouvelles* writers became even harsher than during the previous decade. News reports often repeat the phrase "One will be astonished to hear," "As everyone knows," or "It has been some time since we have warned the Faithful about . . . " Comments concerning the Society of Jesus are especially biting. They are attacked for the "venom of their pernicious doctrines," their "scandalous missions," the "excess of their lies," and their persecution of *appelants*. In context, even references to "the genius of their Society" and acting "with a Jesuit's zeal" are disparaging compliments. The Jesuits are blamed for causing "terrible schisms" in the realm, supporting "false Prophets and false Doctors," "poisoning the roots" of Catholicism, and "plotting to substitute their own doctrines for the old doctrine of the Church."[259]

In addition, authors repeatedly attack the Bishop of Laon as "the Prelate who has made himself famous by the solemn attacks he attracts to himself." They poke fun at his inability (or unwillingness) to distinguish between Jansenists, Quesnellists, *appelants*, and *opposants*. They label his numerous pastoral instructions attempting "to purge [his] diocese of Jansenists" as "scandalous, outrageous, and dangerous," informing readers that no fewer than nine *arrêts* from the Council of State and three *arrêts* from Parlement have condemned his writings.[260] Such satirical prose and embarrassing disclosures alarmed police chief Marville, who told Secretary of State Maurepas that the authors deserved "a severe punishment." Chuckling, the minister of state thanked Marville for "giving me the pleasure" of reading copies of the *Nouvelles*, which he had found amusing. But Maurepas stopped chuckling when, between 1745 and 1747, its writers began mocking police and government efforts to shut it down.[261]

By the end of the decade, therefore, thanks largely to the propaganda success of the *Nouvelles Ecclésiastiques* and increased efforts by a new group of young *appelant* lawyers and magistrates, Jansenism began to win widespread public support. In a series of *causes célèbres* surrounding

Unigenitus, their writings and frequent use of the *appel comme d'abus* (which the Declaration of 1730 had forbidden) helped undermine the authority of the Catholic clergy and the integrity of the Crown.[262] In this highly charged political atmosphere, religious freedom increasingly became the watchword of the Jansenist cause. In February 1749, the *Nouvelles* complained that "the poisoned roots" of *Unigenitus* had "defeated liberty in the Ecclesiastical & Religious Assemblies. This evil perpetuates itself. In nearly all the religious chapters, there are no longer any elections in the Religious Orders of men & women in which the Secular Authority does not intervene to force the vote." Instead, royal commissioners, armed with *lettres de cachet*, "determine the choice of nominees [which is] an abuse of Royal Authority."[263]

Despite such abuses, by the end of the decade, Jansenist advocates began to win small but significant victories for the *appelant* cause. In March 1748, the *abbé* Charles Arnauld de Pomponne, doctor of theology at the Sorbonne, brought a case before Parlement protesting Jesuit Jean Pichon's slander of his uncle Antoine Arnauld in his book *The Spirit of Jesus Christ and the Church in the Book Frequent Communion*. Parlement forced Pichon to retract his libelous comments.[264] While this victory represented a small step for the Arnauld family, in the years ahead, Jansenists would gain more ground against government and Church restrictions.

In conclusion, *Unigenitus* (1713) transformed Jansenism from a spiritual into a political movement, but proved dangerously divisive in the long term. Parlement, recusant bishops, and the Sorbonne battled Louis XIV, Louis XV, popes, the Archbishop of Paris, Minister Fleury, and the police amidst crises ranging from enforced signing of the Formulary to firing Jansenist administrators at the Hôpital-Général in Paris. During the 1720s, '30s, and '40s, proponents of these two opposing camps published incendiary books and pamphlets and successfully distributed the underground newspaper the *Nouvelles Ecclésiastiques*. But as Jansenism became more contentious and politicized, Church and state officials sent more *appelants* (especially printers and colporteurs) to the Bastille and other prisons. And worse battles lay ahead, as chapter 6 shows.

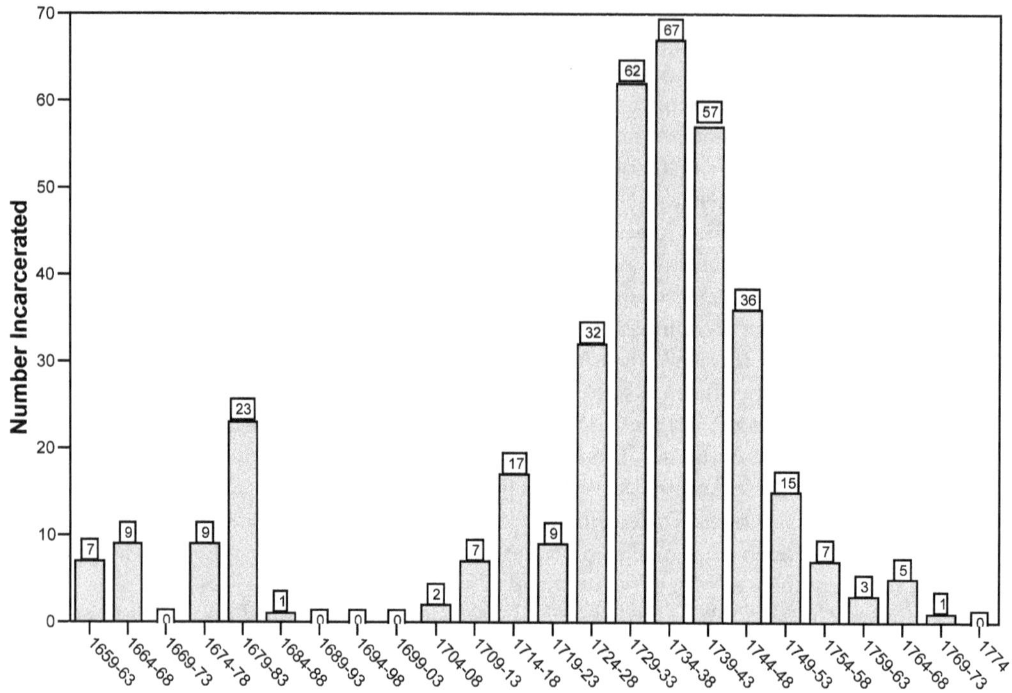

Graph 1 Number of Jansenists at the Bastille under Louis XIV and Louis XV, 1659–1774

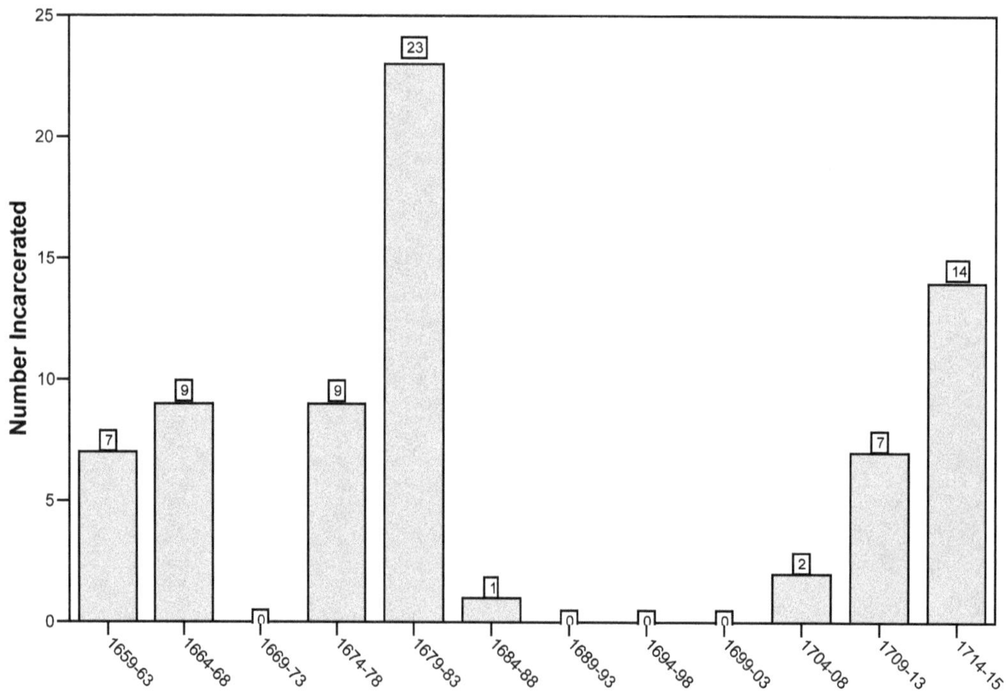

Graph 2 Number of Jansenists at the Bastille under Louis XIV, 1659–1715

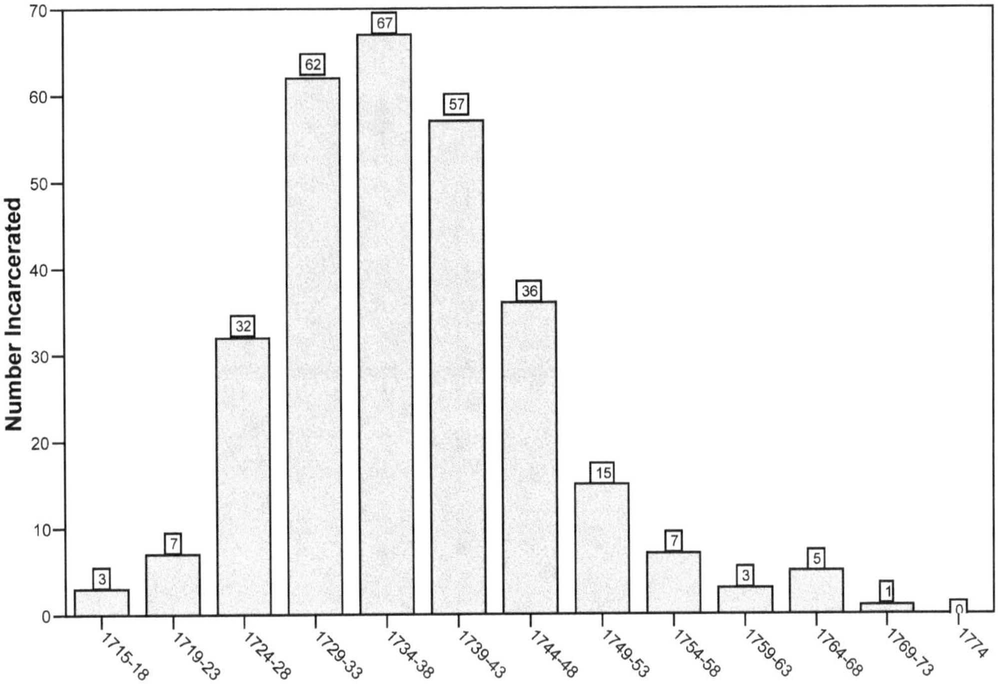

Graph 3 Number of Jansenists at the Bastille under Louis XV, 1715–1774

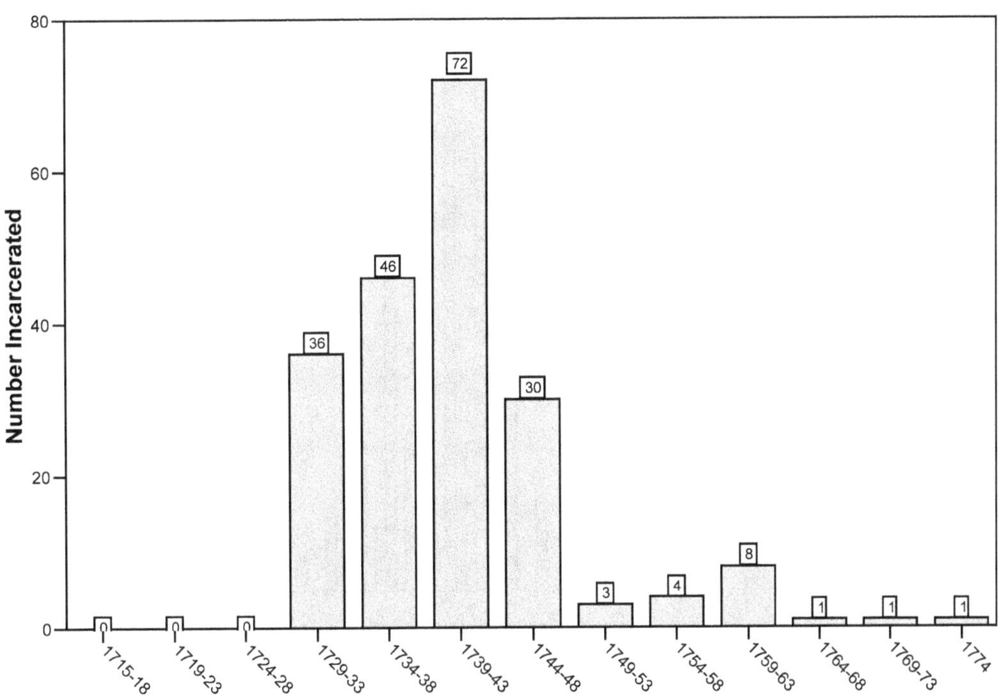

Graph 4 Number of *Convulsionnaires* at the Bastille under Louis XV, 1715–1774

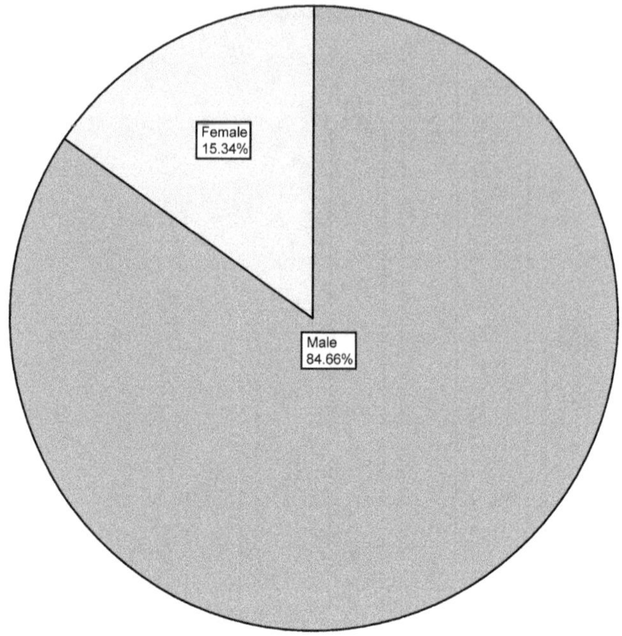

Graph 5 Gender Ratio for Jansenists at the Bastille under Louis XIV and Louis XV, 1659–1774

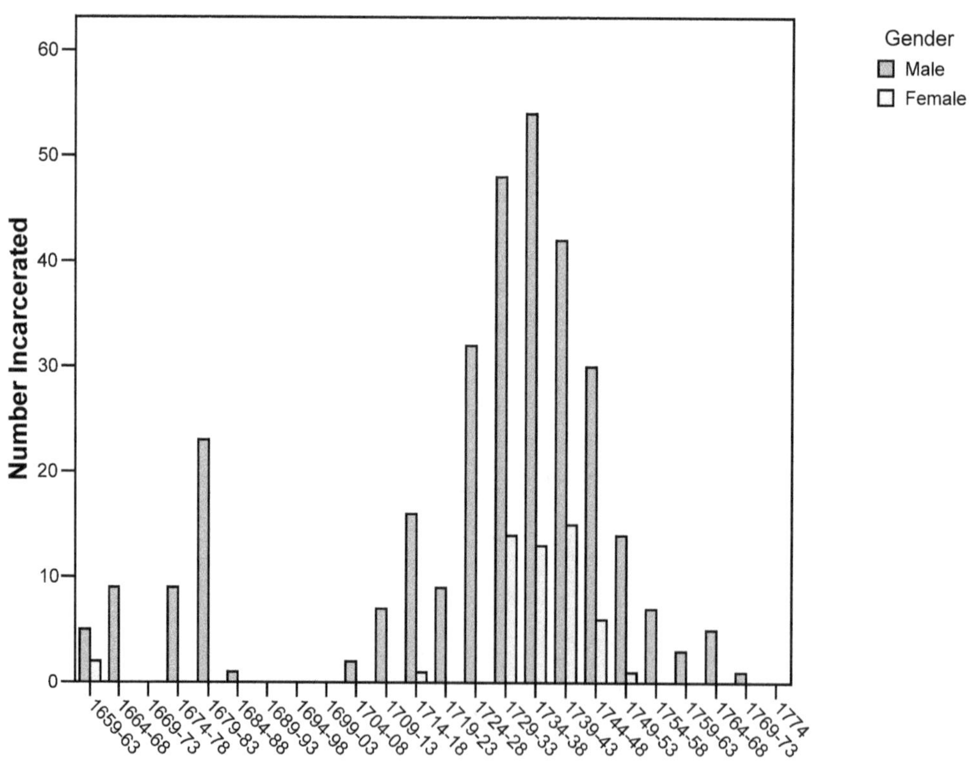

Graph 6 Number of Jansenist Men and Women at the Bastille under Louis XIV and Louis XV, 1659–1774

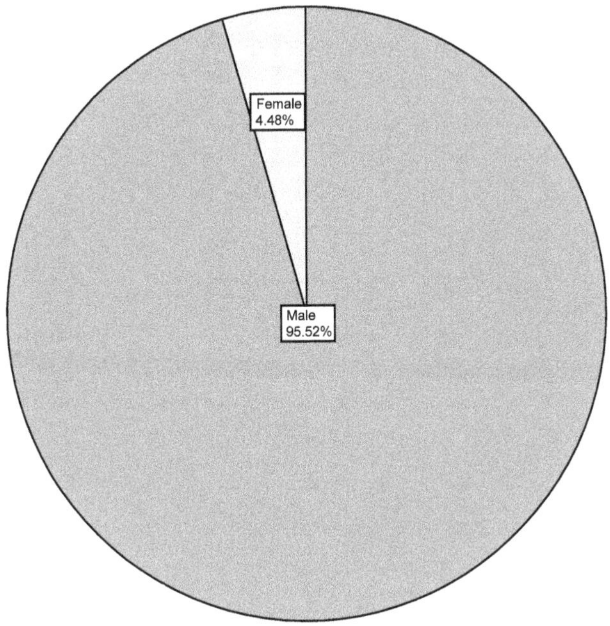

Graph 7 Gender Ratio for Jansenists at the Bastille under Louis XIV, 1659–1715

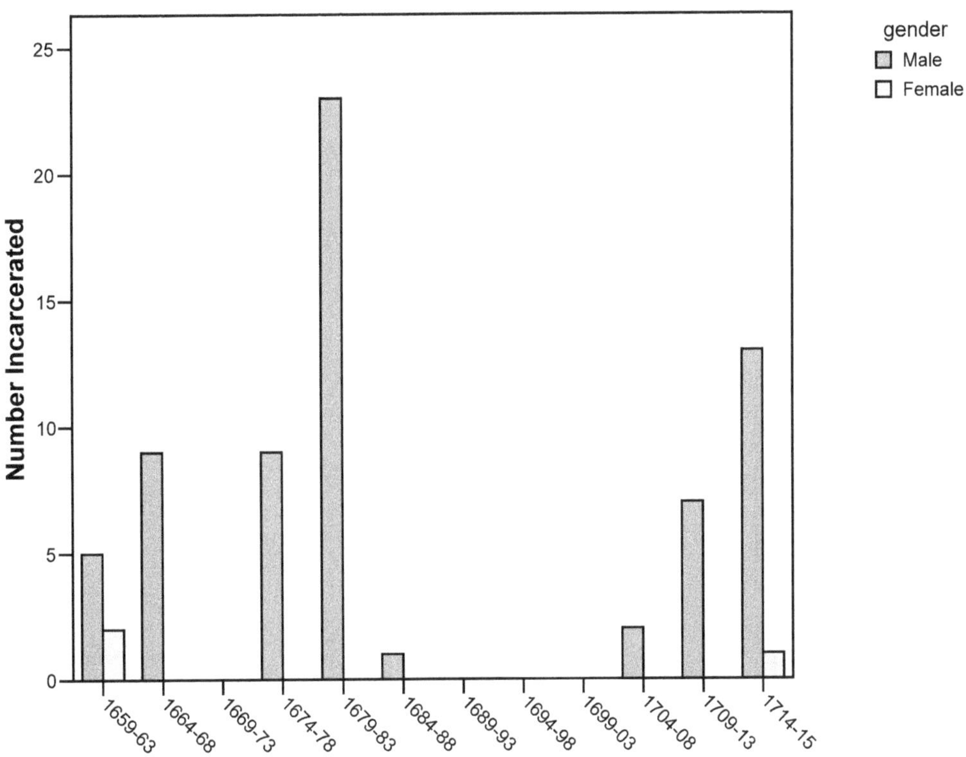

Graph 8 Number of Jansenist Men and Women at the Bastille under Louis XIV, 1659–1715

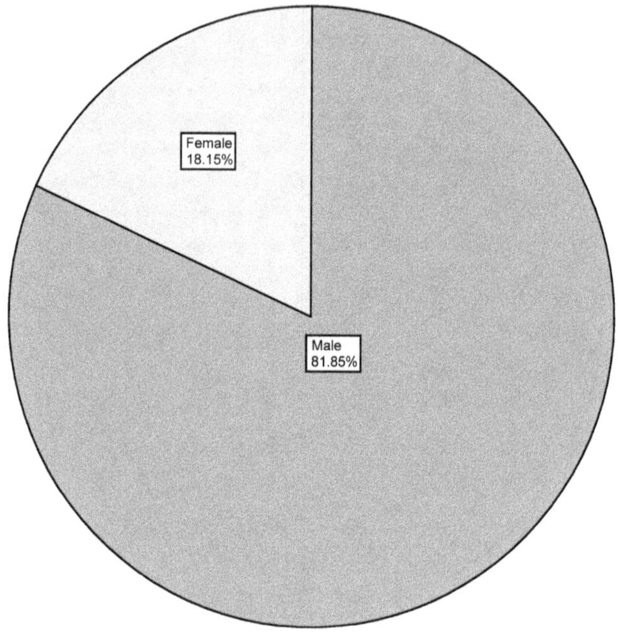

Graph 9 Gender Ratio for Jansenists at the Bastille under Louis XV, 1715–1774

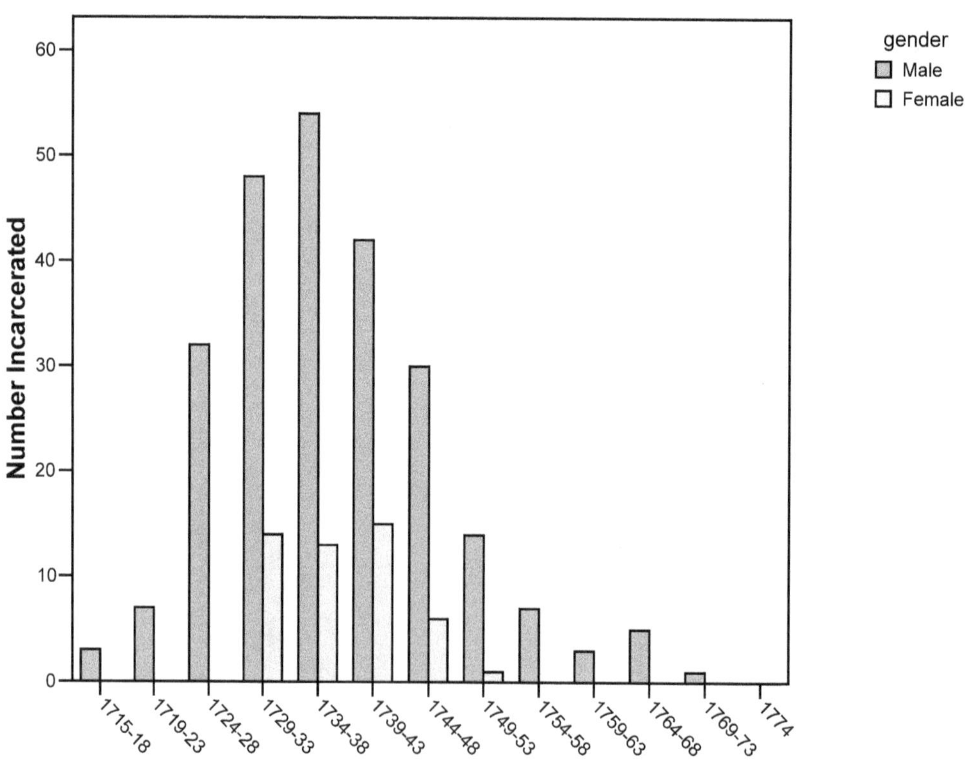

Graph 10 Number of Jansenist Men and Women at the Bastille under Louis XV, 1715–1774

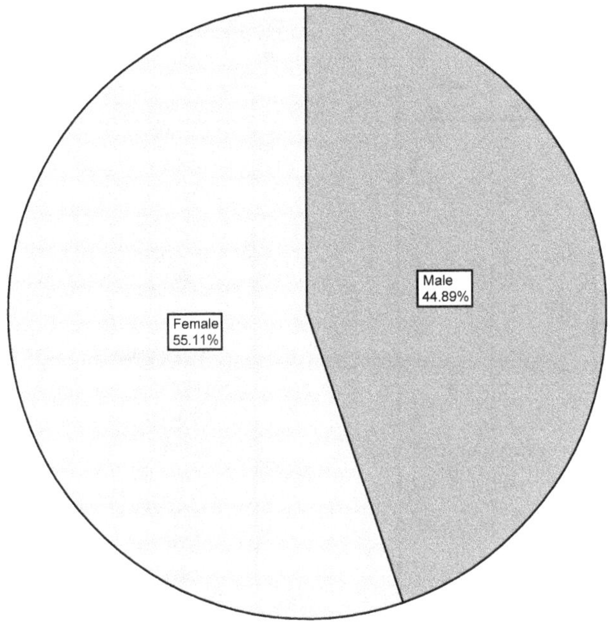

Graph 11 Gender Ratio for *Convulsionnaires* at the Bastille under Louis XV, 1715–1774

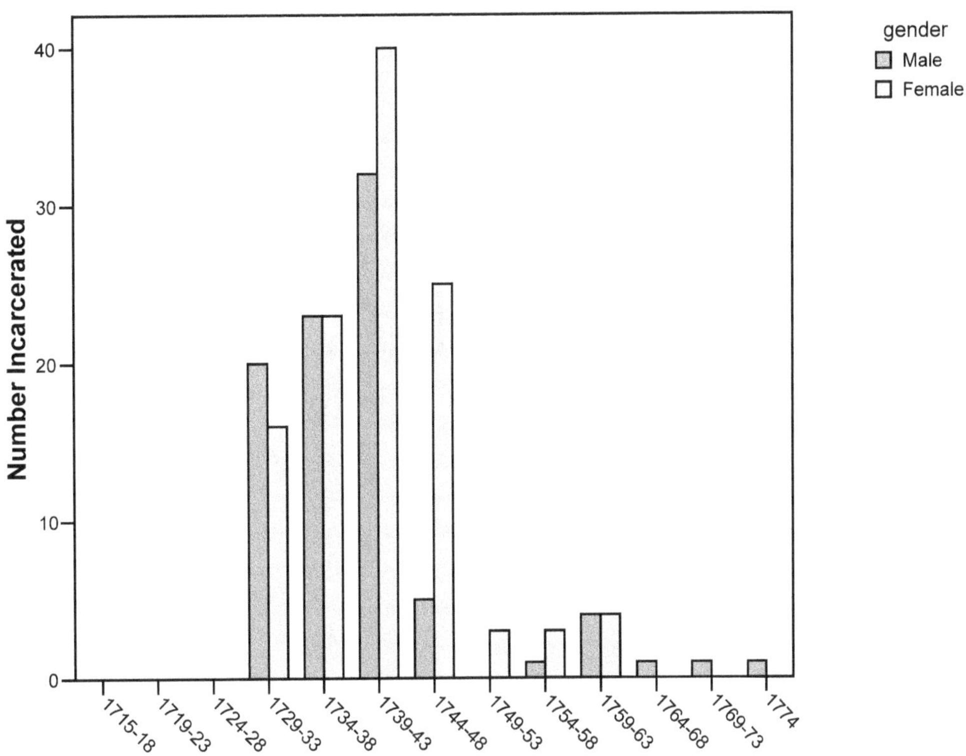

Graph 12 Number of *Convulsionnaire* Men and Women at the Bastille under Louis XV, 1715–1774

	Frequency	Percent
Abbot	58	17.8
Agent	1	.3
Dyers apprentice	2	.6
Archer	1	.3
Architect	1	.3
Colporteur	8	2.5
Bourgeois	1	.3
Canon	2	.6
Military	1	.3
Chevalier	2	.6
Family LC	7	2.1
Legal clerk	4	1.2
Commissioner	1	.3
Cook	1	.3
Copper engraver	4	1.2
Servant	18	5.5
Doorkeeper	2	.6
Engraver	3	.9
Foreigner	1	.3
Friar	1	.3
Fruitseller	1	.3
Gardener	1	.3
Gentleman	2	.6
Glass merchant	1	.3
Goldsmith	1	.3
Haberdasher	2	.6
Hatmaker	2	.6
False hermit	1	.3
Hosiery merchant	1	.3
Master at the hunt	1	.3
Intendant	1	.3
Laborer	1	.3
Lawyer	6	1.8
Librarian	19	5.8
Physician	1	.3
Merchant	2	.6
Lace dealer	3	.9
Messenger	1	.3
Sword cutler	2	.6
Monk	6	1.8
Musician	1	.3
Notary	1	.3
Sergeant	2	.6
Paper maker	1	.3
Practician	1	.3
Priest	7	2.1
Printer	40	12.3
Prior	1	.3
Procureur	1	.3
Teacher	4	1.2
Mistress	1	.3
Protestant	1	.3
Regent	1	.3
Ambassador's secretary	1	.3
Shop worker	1	.3
Servant	1	.3
Student	1	.3
Tax collector	3	.9
Vicar	1	.3
Waggoner	1	.3
Wife	4	1.2
Unknown	77	23.6
Total	326	100.0

Table 1 Status and Occupations of Jansenists at the Bastille under Louis XIV and Louis XV, 1659–1774

	Frequency	Percent
Abbot	9	13.4
Dyers apprentice	1	1.5
Archer	1	1.5
Colporteur	1	1.5
Family LC	2	3.0
Foreigner	1	1.5
Friar	1	1.5
Haberdasher	1	1.5
False hermit	1	1.5
Lawyer	3	4.5
Librarian	15	22.4
Physician	1	1.5
Merchant	1	1.5
Monk	5	7.5
Musician	1	1.5
Sergeant	1	1.5
Printer	4	6.0
Procureur	1	1.5
Teacher	2	3.0
Regent	1	1.5
Ambassador's secretary	1	1.5
Vicar	1	1.5
Unknown	12	17.9
Total	67	100.0

Table 2 Status and Occupations of Jansenists at the Bastille under Louis XIV, 1659–1715

	Frequency	Percent
Abbot	49	18.9
Agent	1	.4
Dyers apprentice	1	.4
Architect	1	.4
Colporteur	7	2.7
Bourgeois	1	.4
Canon	2	.8
Military	1	.4
Chevalier	2	.8
Family LC	5	1.9
Legal clerk	4	1.5
Commissioner	1	.4
Cook	1	.4
Copper engraver	4	1.5
Servant	18	6.9
Doorkeeper	2	.8
Engraver	3	1.2
Fruitseller	1	.4
Gardener	1	.4
Gentleman	2	.8
Glass merchant	1	.4
Goldsmith	1	.4
Haberdasher	1	.4
Hatmaker	2	.8
Hosiery merchant	1	.4
Master at the hunt	1	.4
Intendant	1	.4
Laborer	1	.4
Lawyer	3	1.2
Librarian	4	1.5
Merchant	1	.4
Lace dealer	3	1.2
Messenger	1	.4
Sword cutler	2	.8
Monk	1	.4
Notary	1	.4
Sergeant	1	.4
Paper maker	1	.4
Practician	1	.4
Priest	7	2.7
Printer	36	13.9
Prior	1	.4
Teacher	2	.8
Mistress	1	.4
Protestant	1	.4
Shop worker	1	.4
Servant	1	.4
Student	1	.4
Tax collector	3	1.2
Waggoner	1	.4
Wife	4	1.5
Unknown	65	25.1
Total	259	100.0

Table 3 Status and Occupations of Jansenists at the Bastille under Louis XV, 1715–1774

	Frequency	Percent
Abbot	13	7.4
Butcher	1	.6
Candlemaker	1	.6
Family LC	11	6.3
Legal clerk	1	.6
Colonel in cavalry	1	.6
Cook	1	.6
Parlementary councilor	1	.6
Count	1	.6
Deputy	1	.6
Servant	7	4.0
Muslin embroiderer	1	.6
Foreigner	1	.6
Cutler	1	.6
Furrier	1	.6
Gentleman	3	1.7
Gilder	1	.6
Tapestry worker	1	.6
Guard	1	.6
Harness maker	1	.6
Hosiery merchant	1	.6
Iron merchant	1	.6
Clockmaker	1	.6
Laborer	1	.6
Lace merchant	3	1.7

	Frequency	Percent
Lawyer	2	1.1
Linen worker	2	1.1
Marechal	1	.6
Lace dealer	1	.6
Sword cutler	3	1.7
Monk	4	2.3
Musician	1	.6
Paper maker	1	.6
Perfumer	1	.6
Priest	1	.6
Silk merchant	1	.6
Smelter	1	.6
Squire	1	.6
Servant	1	.6
Surveyor	1	.6
Tailer	5	2.8
Tax collector	1	.6
Pension master	1	.6
Viscount	1	.6
Widow	1	.6
Wife	6	3.4
Wig maker	1	.6
Woodworker	1	.6
Writer	3	1.7
Unknown	77	43.8
Total	176	100.0

Table 4 Status and Occupations of *Convulsionnaires* at the Bastille under Louis XV, 1715–1774

	Frequency	Percent
1 week	18	5.5
2 weeks	14	4.3
3 weeks	11	3.4
1 month	35	10.7
3 months	45	13.8
6 months	70	21.5
9 months	50	15.3
1 year	21	6.4
2 years	33	10.1
3 years	12	3.7
4 years	4	1.2
>4 years	13	4.0
Total	326	100.0

Table 5 Length of Detention for Jansenists at the Bastille under Louis XIV and Louis XV, 1659–1774

	Frequency	Percent
1 week	3	4.5
3 weeks	3	4.5
1 month	7	10.4
3 months	2	3.0
6 months	20	29.9
9 months	10	14.9
1 year	4	6.0
2 years	7	10.4
3 years	6	9.0
4 years	1	1.5
>4 years	4	6.0
Total	67	100.0

Table 6 Length of Detention for Jansenists at the Bastille under Louis XIV, 1659–1715

	Frequency	Percent
1 week	15	5.8
2 weeks	14	5.4
3 weeks	8	3.1
1 month	28	10.8
3 months	43	16.6
6 months	50	19.3
9 months	40	15.4
1 year	17	6.6
2 years	26	10.0
3 years	6	2.3
4 years	3	1.2
>4 years	9	3.5
Total	259	100.0

Table 7 Length of Detention for Jansenists at the Bastille under Louis XV, 1715–1774

	Frequency	Percent
1 week	22	12.5
2 weeks	16	9.1
3 weeks	12	6.8
1 month	14	8.0
3 months	38	21.6
6 months	28	15.9
9 months	11	6.3
1 year	6	3.4
2 years	19	10.8
3 years	4	2.3
4 years	1	.6
>4 years	5	2.8
Total	176	100.0

Table 8 Length of Detention for Convulsionnaires at the Bastille under Louis XV, 1715–1774

	Frequency	Percent
Released	257	78.8
Transferred	18	5.5
Exiled	46	14.1
Galleys	4	1.2
Escaped	1	.3
Total	326	100.0

Table 9 What Happened to Jansenists at the Bastille under Louis XIV and Louis XV, 1659–1774

	Frequency	Percent
1 week	22	12.5
2 weeks	16	9.1
3 weeks	12	6.8
1 month	14	8.0
3 months	38	21.6
6 months	28	15.9
9 months	11	6.3
1 year	6	3.4
2 years	19	10.8
3 years	4	2.3
4 years	1	.6
>4 years	5	2.8
Total	176	100.0

Table 10 What Happened to Jansenists at the Bastille under Louis XIV, 1659–1715

	Frequency	Percent
Released	216	83.4
Transferred	8	3.1
Exiled	32	12.4
Galleys	3	1.2
Total	259	100.0

Table 11 What Happened to Jansenists at the Bastille under Louis XV, 1715–1774

	Frequency	Percent
Released	131	74.4
Transferred	31	17.6
Exiled	13	7.4
Galleys	1	.6
Total	176	100.0

Table 12 What Happened to Convulsionnaires at the Bastille under Louis XV, 1715–1774

CHAPTER 6

Jansenism Loses Its *Raison d'être*, 1751–1799

"The Jansenists, ordinarily the persecuted ones, become persecutors in their turn as soon as they find the occasion, especially against their enemies [the Jesuits]."—*Marquis d'Argenson*[1]

When Minister of State D'Argenson made the above observation in 1752, he also quipped that "Jansenism has become the universal religion and dominates the kingdom," not because everyone had fallen into heresy, but because nearly everyone had become allies of the Jansenists against the Jesuits.[2] Although the Church, as reflected in *Père* Colonia's *Dictionary of Jansenist Books* (1752), continued to define Jansenism as an "innovation" full of "pernicious doctrines,"[3] in the popular mind, Jansenists had become "the party of opposition" to the Society of Jesus. As a vocal minority in Parlement, they had also gained a reputation for being "fomenters of troubles" and leaders in resisting royal policies. Their political enemies considered them "republicans" in principle, worthy of being "humbled and punished" as "the abettors of all the maxims contrary to the monarchy."[4]

In July 1752, Secretary of State for Foreign Affairs Antoine-Louis Rouillé expressed the government's frustration with this vocal lobby group in a confidential letter to retired Attorney General Joly de Fleury. Rouillé admitted that "it would be pointless to try to satisfy both sides and dangerous to give total satisfaction to either one. We can therefore only try to formulate a policy which wins the approval of the reasonable members of both parties."[5]

Rouillé's middle-of-the-road approach might have prevailed had it not faced stiff opposition from several highly placed Church officials who did not want it to succeed. One of those individuals was Christophe de Beaumont, Archbishop of Paris for 35 years. The son of a gendarme in Périgord, Beaumont had studied at Toulouse and Paris before becoming a priest in 1734. Over the next twelve years, he rose from vicar-general at Blois, Bishop of Bayonne in 1741, and Bishop of Vienne in 1744 to become Archbishop of Paris in 1746. He had a reputation as a mediocre but orthodox prelate who gave one-third of his income to the poor (the other two-thirds filled his closets and furnished his lavish homes). Honest, pious, kind, wise, and well-mannered, Beaumont could also be obstinate and confrontational when his conscience dictated.[6] And that conscience, as Cardinal de Bernis quipped, "was a lamp which enlightened none but himself."[7]

The motto on Beaumont's coat of arms—*Impavidum ferient ruinae* ("Catastrophes destroy the fearless")[8]—provides some insight into his character and helps one understand his controversial career as archbishop. As an administrator, he preferred refusing requests to granting them. He could hesitate when faced with insurmountable challenges (such as crushing Jansenism), yet move precipitously on minor issues (like granting last rites to *appelants*). Julian Swann (1995), with good reason, described Beaumont's elevation as "one of the most unwise appointments in the history of the *ancien régime*."[9] When he precipitated the "refusal of sacraments" controversy in the

1750s, his initial popularity plummeted; his enemies thereafter considered him opinionated, foolish, insolent, and "a stubborn sinner . . . incapable of compromising."[10]

Although the Dauphin and Chancellor Lamoignon de Blancmesnil supported Beaumont's uncompromising stand on refusing the sacraments to Jansenist sympathizers, Louis XV and the Parlement of Paris staunchly opposed him.[11] This set the stage for what the marquis d'Argenson called a "noisy standoff" that would precipitate a growing schism within the Church.[12]

This tempest in a teapot concerned a short document, called a *billet de confession* (ticket of confession), that Catholics had to present to their priest to prove their orthodoxy before being allowed to partake of the sacraments (especially communion, confession, and last rites). To be valid, a *billet* had to be signed by a priest or bishop who favored the Bull *Unigenitus* and had signed the Formulary "without reservations." One tiny "ticket" (about 4.5" × 3") stated: "I have heard the confession of Denys de la Fosse this 11th day of January 1755. [Signed] De la Ville, priest of the Company of Jesus." In a society where dying and preparation for death played a vitally important role, where everyone fell to their knees when funeral processions approached, and where cemeteries were located at the center of every parish, refusing confession or last rites struck terror into the hearts of Catholics and Jansenists alike. To answer "No" to the priest's question "Do you have a *billet*?" could damn one eternally in hell, deprived forever of the Church's final blessing and forgiveness.[13]

Appelants, with good reason, argued that denying them the sacraments simply because they refused to sign the Formulary defied charity, represented sinister coercion, and constituted a tacit excommunication because it stripped them of their Catholicity. Moreover, this practice contradicted Roman Catholic handbooks for priests in the confessional advising them that only habitual sinners should be denied Last Rites. As one lay dying, a brief confession in general terms covering one's life was generally thought to be sufficient. Furthermore, the confessor should be praying for the dying person, not judging him or her. Although some claimed that being deprived of the sacraments did not cause Catholics to lose their rights as citizens, the majority of bishops countered that being citizens did not guarantee their right to partake of the sacraments: Catholic citizens must first prove their orthodoxy by presenting a *billet*. In a very real sense, Church officials in the 1750s imposed a higher standard on Jansenists (conformity to *Unigenitus* or excommunication) than they did on Protestants (who now worshiped secretly and performed civil weddings as prelates looked the other way).[14]

The consequences for not possessing a "ticket of orthodoxy" could be severe. A dying *appelant,* denied last rites and excommunicated, was deprived of sepulcher in holy ground. Instead, the body was buried in common ground (a field, yard, or ditch) next to heretics, atheists, actors, comedians, and notorious libertines.[15] Sometimes this led to ludicrous results. In 1754 a priest in Boulogne buried an elderly Jansenist with his feet in sacred ground and his head and body under the street, declaring that "since he had made an appeal against the Bull *Unigenitus*, it was his head and heart that sinned and not his feet."[16] As the "tickets of confession" controversy heated up, however, many priests and bishops who refused the sacraments to *opposants* found themselves prohibited from exercising their ecclesiastical functions, suspended from office, or arrested and imprisoned. Those who fled their dioceses were hanged in effigy.[17]

The use of these *billets de confession* had begun, as we have seen, a century before Archbishop Beaumont came to Paris. Cardinal Charles Borromeo had sanctioned their use at the Councils of Milan from 1565 to 1582. In France, Archbishop Vintimille had used them occasionally in the 1730s. In 1746, the year Beaumont came to Paris, Bishop de La Force had ordered priests in Amiens to deny the sacraments to all persons who could not present a "ticket of confession" signed by a *constitutionnaire* priest. In June 1749, the *curé* of St.-Etienne du Mont in Paris, *Père* Bouettin, had denied last rites to Charles Coffin, the dying rector of the University of Paris and an outspoken opponent of *Unigenitus*. When the family asked the First President of Parlement to intercede with the Archbishop of Paris, Beaumont responded that the *curé* had merely been following his orders. By March 1750, six cases of refusals had come to Parlement's attention.[18]

But the simmering controversy boiled over in December 1750 when Bouettin denied the sacraments to Charles Coffin's nephew, Daniel Coffin, a councilor at the Châtelet Court—again on Beaumont's orders. When the magistrates summoned Bouettin to answer for his actions before Parlement, he declared that " he did not have to answer to them." The *parlementaires* had him arrested and sent to a dungeon in the Conciergerie. A day later, however, following the Archbishop's intervention, the king ordered Bouettin released. Before long, this zealous curate had denied the sacraments to a dozen *appelants* in his parish (including yet a third member of the Coffin family)—half the total number (24) of refusals for the entire city of Paris between 1749 and 1755. Louis XV, annoyed at Parlement's interference with Church affairs, begged the magistrates to "moderate" their actions in the interest of "public tranquility."[19]

The *parlementaires*, however, esteemed their customary rights more important than keeping the public peace. When the Archbishop of Paris personally denied the last rites to the *duc* d'Orléans (son of the former Regent) on his deathbed in February 1751, the Duke appealed "this improper and illegal" behavior to Parlement. Then in March 1752, when Bouettin defied the magistrates by refusing the sacraments to the priest Lemère (former chaplain of the *abbesse* de Chelles), they arrested him, fined him three *livres*, and ordered him imprisoned. But Louis XV remanded the case to his Council of State and imposed silence concerning the affair. Ignoring the king's command, the *parlementaires* ordered all clerics to administer the sacraments to everyone without requiring *billets of confession*—or face punishment for being "disturbers of the public peace." Despite that order, during the 1750s, at least 60 Parisians (45 clerics and 15 laity) suspected of Jansenism were denied the sacraments.[20]

This "refusal of sacraments" controversy ignited a firestorm of debate and reactivated the quarrel over *Unigenitus* that had nearly burned itself out in the 1740s. It precipitated a war of words during which Benedict XIV, Louis XV, Parlement, the Archbishop of Paris, and numerous clerics penned scores of remonstrances, appeals, letters, encyclicals, and *arrêts* to defend their positions. Examining some of these dusty documents opens windows of understanding into the deeper issues involved.[21]

In their 4 March 1751 remonstrance, the magistrates inform the king that by refusing to recognize Parlement's right to regulate the "public domain," Church officials show disrespect for the authority of the king and Parlement, disrupt the public order, and therefore must be punished "with the greatest rigor." They find the refusal of sacraments a "reprehensible" practice that will cause "dangerous consequences." It should be used "to correct" wayward Catholics, not "to damn" them to hell.[22]

Despite this warning, however, the practice of denying the sacraments to *appelants* spread from Paris to Troyes, Orléans, Chartres, and other cities in 1752 and 1753. In 22 instances, Parlement tried to stop clerics from denying last rites to those without tickets, but in every case, Archbishop Beaumont overruled the magistrates.[23] "This is serious," the advocate Barbier exclaimed in 1752. "The greatest part of Paris is Jansenist . . . Liberty is precious to all men and no one likes the constraint of these tickets of confession."[24]

For disobeying Parlement's order and ignoring the king's imposition of silence, the Archbishop of Paris and several bishops lost their own freedom. In May 1752, the Bishop of Amiens and the Bishop of Marseilles were stripped of their sources of income and exiled. On December 3, a *lettre de cachet* banished Archbishop Beaumont to his estate at Conflans. But when Parlement attempted to seize his temporal property in Paris two weeks later, the Council of State blocked their action.[25]

Although separated from his see, Beaumont remained defiant. He told the magistrates that "regarding the administration of the sacraments, it is a purely spiritual matter, so I am accountable only to God for the exercise of an authority He has confided to me. There is no other person than the King to whom I owe the duty to give an account."[26] Considering this "impertinent" response a sign that Beaumont refused to submit to the king's authority (of which Parlement was the depository), the magistrates issued an *arrêt* commanding the Archbishop to administer the sacraments to everyone. They also imprisoned two of his vicars for refusing to do so.[27] Although an ostensibly repentant Archbishop assured the magistrates of his desire for peace and silence, continued insubordination soon brought him an even more distant exile at Brie in Lagny-sur-Marne in February 1753. "I am more and more discontented with the Archbishop of Paris," Louis XV told the First President of Parlement.[28]

After Beaumont's second exile, 29 bishops, led by Bishop La Rochefoucauld, attempted to find some common ground on which the king, Parlement, and the Archbishop of Paris could stand. Calling themselves "The Tolerant Ones," they searched for a compromise concerning the denial of sacraments impasse.[29] But Beaumont was not the compromising type. For refusing to comply with Louis XV's Declaration of 2 September 1754 ordering clerics to administer the sacraments to all "to keep peace in my kingdom," he once again found himself banished to Conflans—this time for over three years (March 1754–October 1757). For his sharp tongue and uncompromising pen, he would be exiled twice more in 1758 and 1764.[30]

Even in isolation, however, the Archbishop had faithful spies keeping him informed of events in Paris.[31] When pro-Jansenist books appeared, he exercised his ecclesiastical right to ban them. Even though Lamoignon de Malesherbes, Louis XV's official censor, thought some of these books deserved tacit permission, Beaumont disapproved. "Your prudence" and "your love for Religion will lead you to order this work suppressed," he repeatedly told Malesherbes.[32] Police chief Berryer's letters to Malesherbes echo the frequent refrain that the Archbishop has decided yet another book "is contrary to Religion and should not be published." In fact, this historian has not found a single instance between 1746 and 1781 in which Beaumont *approved* of a new book![33] Perhaps that explains why in 1754 one press began printing *Les Sarcelades*, a series of wickedly funny satires attacking the Archbishop of Paris.[34]

But Beaumont and his *constitutionnaire* colleagues failed to appreciate such humor. For them, the difference between orthodoxy and heresy was a matter of eternal life or everlasting damnation. At one session of the 1755 General Assembly of the Clergy, 33 bishops voted on whether refusing to accept *Unigenitus* constituted "a mortal sin" (sixteen bishops) or merely "a sin concerning a grave matter" (seventeen bishops).[35]

As the frequency of refusals of sacraments grew, the marquis d'Argenson became increasingly alarmed at "this ridiculous quarrel of the priests." While the number of bishops "who cry out against this foolish Archbishop [Beaumont] is great," at least twelve bishops and 60 priests had joined his "schismatic order." "The Archbishop of Paris is more stubborn than ever," he confided to his diary. "Certainly this Archbishop is as much of a fool as the Bishop of Troyes" for disobeying the king's order for silence. Perhaps, he hoped, Parlement will put him on trial.[36]

In reality, the magistrates did everything in their power to bring to trial not only the Archbishop of Paris but also every other cleric who refused the sacraments, but Louis XV checkmated their every move throughout the decade. Here, for example, is a typical pattern of tit-for-tat actions between the king and Parlement for six months in 1750–51:

December 1750—*Pére* Bouettin denies the sacraments to Councilor Coffin; Parlement sends Bouettin to prison.
2 January 1751—Louis XV rebukes Parlement for its mistreatment of Bouettin.
4 March—Parlement sends the king a remonstrance concerning his rebuke.

23 March—Parlement orders Bouettin to appear for trial.
26 March—The Council of State's *arrêt* suppresses Parlement's decision.
28 March—Parlement orders the arrest of Bouettin.
4 April—Louis XV forbids Parlement to proceed with Bouettin's trial.
15 April—Parlement sends another remonstrance to the king.
5 May—Parlement's *arrêt* protests royal interference with their judicial proceedings.
14 May—Louis XV replies, forbidding the magistrates to proceed with Bouettin's trial.[37]

Extending this pattern over eight years gives some idea just how contentious relations became between Church and judicial officials regarding the refusal of sacraments to *appelants*. When Parlement issued registrations, investigations, decrees and arrests, Louis XV countered with *lettres de cachet*, *Declarations du Roi*, and *arrêts* from his Council of State. An examination of a few of these documents will elucidate the deeper issues involved from the perspective of Louis XV, Parlement, and Church officials.[38]

Above all else, Louis XV wanted obedience, order, and peace in the realm. In his 17 April 1752 response to Parlement's April 15 remonstrance, the king listed his key concerns as "the good of Religion and the tranquility of the State" in order to avoid "schism and scandal." To achieve these goals, he forbade the magistrates to debate any issues concerning *Unigenitus*. "My Parlement, being fully instructed and obedient to my orders, will cease all pursuits and procedures that it has begun . . . and it will return to its ordinary functions of rendering justice to my people."[39] Five months later, he instructed the *parlementaires* to "maintain the laws of the realm without deviating from the respect due to religion." While he allowed them to handle cases involving priests, he alone would deal with the bishops.[40]

When the magistrates continued remonstrating, the king's Declaration of 2 September 1754 demanded their "absolute silence" on the *billets* controversy. "I will have no one speak again on this matter," he thundered; "rest assured, I expect to be obeyed." He told Archbishop Beaumont to "be more circumspect; that's the best advice I can give you."[41] But magistrates and Church officials continued debating. So two weeks later, Louis signed the Declaration of September 16 imposing the "Law of Silence" on the kingdom. Whereas the 1730 "Law of Silence" had exempted the clergy, the 1754 Declaration subjected them to parlementary prosecution if they broke the law. Copies went to the parlements of Dijon, Grenoble, Pau, Douai, and Metz, for they had been the most active in the refusal of sacraments controversy.[42] A month later, the Declaration of October 8 quashed debates in the Parlement of Brittany. Recognizing that "silence is the best method of arresting the course of an evil so dangerous" that "troubles the repose & happiness of our Subjects," Louis hoped these two laws would reestablish "order & public tranquility."[43]

When they did not, the king pondered more radical options to restore peace in his kingdom. According to the marquis d'Argenson, in January 1756 Louis XV even considered offering a general amnesty to Jansenists in prison and recalling the exiled bishops, nearly all of whom (according to D'Argenson) "disapproved of the tickets of confession."[44] A month later, in a conciliatory gesture, he promised the magistrates that he would "listen to the views" of princes, peers, great nobles, and Parlement if they felt that "the fundamental Laws of the Monarchy are being openly attacked."[45]

But in August, exasperated with Parlement's endless debating and disobedience, the king held a *lit de justice* lasting nearly two hours, during which he offered his *parlementaires* neither food nor drink. At its conclusion, he demanded the magistrates' silence: the five-year debate over the *billets de confession* would end—now![46] When the magistrates continued remonstrating, Louis issued the Declaration of December 10 and three days later, held another *lit de justice* forcing them to register it. This Declaration (and a subsequent edict) "for the discipline of Parlement" suppressed the two Chambers of Inquest, abolished 65 offices, and again imposed silence on clerics and magistrates concerning the issues surrounding *Unigenitus*.[47] Many of the magistrates, objecting to its clauses allowing ecclesiastical courts to handle cases concerning refusal of sacraments that they felt should be under civil litigation, resigned their offices. The king dismissed several other troublemakers in the *parti janséniste* and exiled them.[48]

This "Jansenist Party," a highly organized cadre of 20 to 60 *parlementaires* led by their chief spokesman Louis-Adrien Le Paige ("the oracle of Parlement"), dominated religious debates in the high court during the 1750s and '60s. Although a minority, their persuasive arguments, organization, and persistence gave them a disproportionate influence over their peers. As the most effective party within the high court, they organized their colleagues to protest the Church's refusal of sacraments to those without tickets of confession and thus counterbalance the influence of the *parti dévot* who supported such actions. By issuing *arrêts,* remonstrances, pamphlets, and books, and by refusing to do their official duties, they made it clear to the king that they disapproved of the bishops' actions. Le Paige alone wrote 70 volumes on Parlement's disputes with government and Church officials, 30 volumes dealing with the convulsions (see chapters 7 and 8), and twelve more focusing on the Jesuits' expulsion in 1764. Adopting a tone of "respectful inflexibility," he built the platform of truth that his colleagues in Parlement defended in their 40 remonstrances during the 1750s and '60s.[49]

That platform, hammered together during the course of some 65 cases relating to *Unigenitus* that came before Parlement from 1750 to 1756,[50] emphasized protecting the independent authority of the Crown and the customary rights of Parlement. In their 15 April 1752 remonstrance, the magistrates told Louis XV: "Sire, never has such an important matter been deliberated by your Parlement at the foot of Your throne. Religion, the State, the laws, & the rights of Your Crown—all are equally threatened by a fatal, bold schism." This "inhumane" refusal of sacraments, they declared, has caused impiety, public scandals, animosity, persecution, and the denial of inheritances to legitimate heirs. Then, melodramatically, they warned the king that the *billets* controversy also undermined the fundamental laws of France and even threatened the monarchy. "What a strange calamity for a Christian Kingdom," they exclaimed. At the end of the document, the *parlementaires* expressed another concern: the fear that enforcing *Unigenitus* would "extinguish our voice."[51]

Those fears became a reality when in May 1753, Louis XV, exasperated by their never-ending debates and refusal to register his *lettres patentes*, exiled 176 magistrates to Pontoise and half a dozen other places and sent four councilors to provincial prisons for over a year. But the high court's prestige had never been so great. Public opinion saw the king's actions in dissolving Parlement as an attack on national liberty. When the *parlementaires* left the Grand Chamber, the crowd shouted, "Hurrah for Parlement! Death to the King and to the bishops!"[52]

The marquis d'Argenson, concerned that "all the other parlements in the kingdom will follow the Parlement of Paris' lead," feared that this might cause "a revolution in the ministry."[53] Those fears came to fruition in 1753 as one after another, the parlements of Provence, Toulouse, Pontoise, Rouen, Normandy, and Aix issued *arrêts* ordering priests to stop requiring tickets of confession. These new laws called the *billets* "a foreign innovation" and "an inhumane practice."[54]

When in 1755, thanks to the efforts of the prince de Conti and others, Louis XV recalled the Parlement of Paris, the councilors returned older and wiser but not silent and submissive.[55] Their *arrêt* of 18 March 1755, declaring the 1713 Bull "not a rule of faith," ordered the bishops to obey the 1754 "Law of Silence." When Archbishop Beaumont told priests to ask the dying if they submitted to the Bull, Parlement called him "a disturber of the public peace" and ordered clerics not to obey him.[56] In May, they ordered the Sorbonne faculty to censor "suspect opinions" and screen masters' theses for "indiscreet" references to *Unigenitus* so that "order and tranquility may one day be reestablished" at the University of Paris. This mandate to maintain "purity of doctrine" while pursuing "peace & moderation" proved impossible, given the contradictory nature of those two goals.[57]

As tensions grew, D'Argenson confided in his *Journal*: "The fermentation is great in Parlement."[58] On 13 December 1756, the magisterial bottles blew their corks when eleven presidents and councilors in the Grand Chamber resigned their posts, claiming that the king's *lits de justice* "degraded or deprived them of their functions." Feeling "disappointed," "disgraced," and "useless," they asked Louis XV "to take back the titles and offices and functions to which he has appointed us." A week later, to their surprise, he accepted their resignations and declared their positions vacant.[59]

But if the king had won the battle with his magistrates in the controversy over the *billets de confession*, Parlement, in the long run, won the war. As recent historians have emphasized, this debate over the refusal of sacraments shifted the political initiative in the 1750s from the Crown and the Church to Parlement. It likewise opened a serious rift between the monarchy and the magistrates that boded ill for revolutionary developments in the 1780s.[60]

If the king valued order and tranquility and Parlement sought to protect its jurisdictional rights, Church officials wanted to uphold doctrinal orthodoxy and maintain their independence amidst the tickets of confession controversy. When Parlement in 1752 ordered priests to administer the sacraments to everyone regardless of whether they had a "ticket" or not, the Archbishop of Paris objected that this action contradicted Louis XIV's Edict of 1695 granting ecclesiastical courts exclusive jurisdiction over cases concerning the sacraments.[61] "I am accountable only to God for the authority He has given me," Beaumont told Parlement. "The priests who have refused the sacraments . . . have acted by my orders and followed the light of their consciences."[62]

By mid-1753, as such refusals multiplied, the number of parishioners celebrating the Eucharist at Catholic churches in Paris had dropped 50 percent—and "for several past years," the marquis d'Argenson noted, "this has dropped below half."[63] In short, the Church faced a *cris de conscience*: It badly needed someone with a "Half-Way Covenant" to bring the contending parties together. D'Argenson hoped that "a good pope . . . can alleviate the rigor of this foolishness [refusing the sacraments to *appelants*]."[64] But in Rome, Benedict XIV approved of Louis XV's 1754 "Law of Silence," hoping that it would finally end the quarrels over the tickets of confession and bring peace to the Gallican Church.[65]

It had exactly the opposite effect. By mid-decade, dozens of priests and curates in Paris, Orléans, Troyes, Montigny, Toulouse, Montpellier, and Auvergne were being arrested, tried, and imprisoned or exiled for denying the sacraments to Jansenists. Hauled into civil (not Church) courts, they were charged with being "disturbers of the public peace" for their refusal to treat all Catholics equally. In February 1755, the Parlement of Paris wanted to place Archbishop Beaumont on trial for undermining their authority to rule on ecclesiastical matters, but Louis XV blocked this move. Instead, he exiled Beaumont to Champeaux (near Melun) and forbade him to speak or write on religious matters. When the Archbishop of Aix-en-Provence issued his own Formulary and the Parlement of Aix fined him 10,000 *livres* and confiscated his property, the king let the judgment stand.[66] Some priests (rumors said) had declared that "it will require bloodshed [the decapitation of several magistrates] to extinguish this controversy."[67]

Before any magistrates lost their heads, Rome found a solution to the problem. Benedict XIV, with a reputation for strict probity and sympathy for the Jansenists, did not share Archbishop Beaumont's exalted view of *Unigenitus*. A moderate Augustinian in his theology, he surrounded himself with prelates who in many ways were more Gallican than the French clergy.[68] On 16 October 1756, Benedict issued the encyclical *Ex omnibus christiani orbis regionibus* ("To All Christians Around the World") as his solution to France's crisis.

By calling the 1713 Bull a "judgment" (rather than a "rule of faith and doctrine"), the encyclical (or brief) sought to appease both the *constitutionnaires* and the *appelants*. Priests, it stated, must no longer require *billets de confession* nor deny the sacraments to anyone except "public & notorious refractory persons" found guilty in secular courts and "public sinners" charged in ecclesiastical courts. Those admitted to Holy Communion during their lives must not be refused the last rites at death, for denying them the Church's final blessing "prejudges" their state of mind and motives and creates "public scandals."[69]

Ex omnibus so circumscribed the case for refusing sacraments that it reduced the issue more or less from a doctrinal necessity to a metaphysical possibility. Two months later, Louis XV's Declaration of 10 December 1756 supported the pope's brief. The new law, which declared that *Unigenitus* did not have "the denomination, the character, or the effects of a rule of faith," limited the refusal of sacraments to judicially convicted opponents of the Bull.[70]

However, if Benedict XIV and Louis XV saw this encyclical as a permanent solution to France's religious crisis, they were soon disappointed, for it pleased almost no one. When the king tried to censor theological theses at the Sorbonne and impose the "Law of Silence" on its doctors of theology, they reacted as explosively as had the magistrates in Parlement. In their February 1758 reply to the king, 83 (of the 133) theologians declared "that Religion, conscience, and honor did not permit them to obey the orders of His Majesty," for silence will only "open the door to heresy . . . and give rise to even greater troubles." They remind the king that "the essence of the faculty [of theology] is to teach the truths of Religion." Therefore, maintaining silence will "go contrary to their statutes and the oath they have taken." Displeased with this response, Louis and Minister of State St.-Florentin banished several professors to their estates and told the rest to maintain "absolute silence" regarding the Bull. Instead, the faculty went on strike, suspending all classes for bachelors' students.[71] Once again Crown, Parlement, and Church officials faced off, hopelessly divided over seemingly incompatible goals.

But on 5 January 1757, an event occurred that temporarily, at least, brought them together. While returning from his daughter's apartment, Louis XV felt a stab to his chest. "I am wounded," he cried, "and it is that man who has struck me." Robert Damiens, the would-be assassin, was immediately arrested, detained, tortured, and interrogated six times in five sessions. Although he denied the existence of any plot or accomplices, Damiens confessed that he hated the king and detested the Archbishop of Paris for denying sacraments to "honest people" whom they then "buried like dogs" in common ground.[72]

Since Damiens had once worked as a domestic for the Society of Jesus, many people blamed the Jesuits as the instigators of his crime. Others, however, pointed their fingers at the Archbishop of Paris, whose sharp disagreements with his sovereign allegedly gave him reason to conspire against the throne. Despite these differences, however, Archbishop Beaumont immediately ordered Church officials in Paris to pray for the king and celebrate special masses (*Te Deums*) for his recovery. Publicly, he called Damiens "a monstrous murderer," "the agent of Satan," and "a man of blood."[73]

The Jansenists reacted with equal shock and horror. The *Nouvelles Ecclésiastiques* called the attempted murder "a horrible attack on the sacred person" of the king by "a fanatic" who deserved to be spitted like a pig over the fire. Naturally, Jansenists everywhere suspected the Jesuits of being Damiens' accomplices in this "execrable parricide." They conveniently ignored the fact that he had also worked for Jansenist employers.[74]

The judges, after pondering Damiens' responses to their 539 questions, reached equally contradictory opinions. Some tried to implicate him in a "Jansenist plot" against the king because of his brother Antoine-Joseph Damiens' association with the *appelant* Fenes brothers of Saint-Omer. When the police arrested him, Antoine had 140 bound volumes of (mostly) Jansenist literature stashed in his house. But Robert protested that he detested Jansenist priests and had never attended meetings at his brother's house. A police attempt to connect him with a "Convulsionist plot" fell through for lack of evidence. Efforts to prove that he had the backing of the "Devot Party" collapsed when the court learned that he had not gone to confession for over three years. Regarding the "Jesuit plot" (popular with the Jansenists and the philosophes), although Robert admitted that he had once worked for the Society, he asserted that if he had the power, he would expel them from France within 24 hours. Under torture (which was legal in French trials until 1788), he claimed that he had acted alone, not to kill Louis XV, but to warn him to listen to Parlement's remonstrances.[75]

Apparently the king got the point, because after Damiens' execution, he recalled the exiled magistrates without imposing any conditions. All sides thereafter basically ignored the 1754 "Law of Silence." Meanwhile, as public opinion, inflamed by the philosophes and Jansenist propaganda, grew more hostile toward the Society of Jesus in France and across Europe, Louis XV and the Council of Conscience began choosing moderate bishops to replace Jesuit ones.[76]

With the increasing popularity of salons, clubs, societies, cafés, taverns, public gardens, and other centers of public discussion in Paris, the 1750s refusal of sacraments controversy (and other divisive issues like free trade and parliamentary reforms) whetted the common people's love of debate. As a result, public opinion became a key force to be reckoned with—a "Fourth Estate" in many ways more sovereign than the king.[77] Printing presses (with moderate censorship in the 1750s and '60s under Malesherbes' administration) made primary documents (circular letters, relations, memoirs, mandates, and remonstrances) as well as secondary ones (books, tracts, pamphlets) more widely available to the public. These publications both reflected what the public thought and shaped popular opinion, inspiring new authors to publish still more writings.[78]

Perhaps one noticeable difference in the 1750s was that people from varied backgrounds took up their pens to address the refusal of sacraments issue. Jansenist writers abhorred the practice of denying communion and the last rites to Catholics. A century earlier, Antoine Arnauld had argued that according to St. Augustine, no one (except the "wicked & schismatic") should be denied the sacraments so long as they acknowledged their sins. To do otherwise would bring "confusion & disorder" into the Church.[79] Pasquier Quesnel had concurred, asserting that "to use violent means to extort the sacraments is enough to render them worthless."[80]

In the 1750s even more than in the 1740s, a growing number of satirical verses attacked the 1713 Bull and the practice of refusing the last rites to the dying. On the streets of Paris, people sang songs calling the Jesuits enemies of the king.[81] On every hand, the marquis d'Argenson wrote, "we are assured that all is prepared in France for a great reform in religion." One sign of the anticipated reform was the "decided fermentation against the priests" in respectable Paris circles. Many proudly took the name "Deist," meaning one who "has the true religion in his heart and who has given up superstition." Public opinion held that "with this religious reform will come government reform." The *billets*' controversy had occurred because "secular tyranny is married to ecclesiastical tyranny" in France, but when both are destroyed, democratic government and religious freedom will result.[82] In his *Letters from a Man of the World on the Subject of Confession and the Bull Unigenitus* (1753), the *abbé* Bon declared that all Catholics, regardless of their political views, "have the right to the sacraments."[83]

During this controversial decade, numerous writers looked back with nostalgic feelings to a "golden age" when Port-Royal championed the Jansenist cause. In his seven-volume *Historical Memories and Chronologies on the Abbey of Port-Royal des Champs* (1755–56), the *abbé* Pierre Guilbert portrayed the convent as an oasis where holiness, charity, and love of the truth reigned. In the "violence and injustice of our time," he said, the "praiseworthy lives" of those Port-Royal sisters and solitaires offers "great examples" of "virtue" to "respect and imitate" today. Such noble "defenders" are needed now to counter the Jesuits' "false rumors" and end the "abuse of authority" and "oppression of the truth" so prevalent in France.[84]

As it had for two decades already, the *Nouvelles Ecclésiastiques* during the 1750s defended Jansenist truth and attacked the Jesuits. Appearing regularly every week, its two-column, four-page issues provided between 204 and 212 pages of scintillating information drawn from international sources as far afield as Brussels, Amsterdam, Rome, Flanders, Vienna, Luxembourg, Italy, Syria and Turkey. As before, the editors often reprinted news from the *Gazette de Hollande* and the *Gazette d'Utrecht*.[85]

Its articles, which for two decades had focused primarily on religious debates related to *Unigenitus*, now featured social and political issues as well. Authors devoted entire issues to the controversies surrounding the Hôpital-Général (1750, 1751, 1757), the refusal of sacraments (1751–1756), the use of *lettres de cachet* against clerics (1753), censorship of Jansenist works (1754–55), and the struggle of Parlement against Louis XV and the Council of State (1754–56). The editors' "list of enemies" grew longer still; it now included Mme. Guyon and the Quietists (1750), Montesquieu (1750), Buffon (1754), Diderot (1758–59), and Voltaire (1759).

Above all else, the *Nouvelles* loved to attack the Society of Jesus and the philosophes. Authors closely followed "the Affair of the Jesuits" in Paraguay and Portugal; they gloated when the Portuguese king expelled the Society in 1759. Articles described "the horrors" revealed in the Jesuits' "insolent writings."[86] But writers saw the growing influence of the philosophes as even more dangerous to Catholic truth and Christian morality. They panned Montesquieu's *Spirit of the Laws* for its irreligious tone, called Buffon's *Natural History* "that pernicious Book," and attacked the materialistic atheism in Diderot's *Of the Mind*. The editors warned subscribers not to read the *Encyclopédie* because of "its dangerous maxims," "seductive poison," "philosophical jargon," and the "irreligious spirit" that filled its pages. In a word, the *Nouvelles* found the *Encyclopédie*—and by extension, the entire Enlightenment—"disgusting."[87]

But *appelants* and Jansenist sympathizers, as before, received glowing reviews. When they died, eulogies routinely praised them for their "humility," "attachment to the truth," "charity to the poor," "love of penitence," and (spiritual) "enlightenment." Their passing nearly always constituted "an irreparable loss," and if they had published anything, those writings were remembered as "extremely useful and precious." In short, obituaries became fill-in-the-blank encomiums to departed saints.[88]

Authors continued to cover controversial issues using satirical, often biting language. A few examples will suffice. Describing one hard-shelled *constitutionnaire* cleric who demanded *billets de confession*: "There are few bishops in France who carry despotic domination further than the Archbishop of Aix."[89] Writers loved to use emotive words like "horror" ("the horrors we have just heard" and "that horrible treason"[90]), "sad" ("the sad affair" of the Abbey of Chatrice[91]), "pernicious" ("the pernicious custom of enjoying the Comedy"[92]), and "despotic" ("the despotism of the bishops"[93]). The refusal of sacraments to *appelants* was "so horrible," the editor opined, "that among the scandals of this type, we have seen none worse than this."[94]

Naturally, such biased prose offended the *constitutionnaires* and invited equally passionate attacks on the *Nouvelles Ecclésiastiques*. In his *Dictionary of Jansenist Books* (1752), Dominique de Colonia called the newspaper "a treasury of lies" and "fearful blasphemies against God," a collection of "mad declarations against the decisions of the Church," and "seditious expressions against the King, his Ministers, & all the Authorities established by God." Colonia took 20 pages to warn readers against the paper's "atrocious impostures against the Faithful," its "tangible errors 100 times condemned," and its many "falsifications," "contradictions," "blasphemies," and "libels." Because of its "bizarre and revolting partiality," "horrible impiety," and "despicable platitudes," the *Nouvelles* was "an infernal gazette," "the shame of our century." He called its editors and writers "rabid rebels" who, by insulting the king and his ministers and bishops, did the devil's work on earth.[95]

In attacking the *Ecclesiastical News* as a radical, rebellious newspaper, Colonia expressed more prescience than he realized at the time, for modern historians have seen in the popular press' reaction to the refusal of sacraments controversy a precursor of the French Revolution. F. Rocquain (1877), for example, asserted that the popular debate from 1751 to 1754 sowed the "seeds" of the Revolution of 1789. Discussions about limiting the king's power, taxing the clergy, and granting civil and religious rights to Protestants, Jews, and Jansenists reveal that the "spirit of revolution" existed already in France more than three decades before the Revolution. During the denial of sacraments controversy, many called for a "national senate" to examine Louis XV's conduct and the bishops' actions. New labels like "national" and "sacerdotal" replaced older terms like "Jansenists" and "Molinists" in what the marquis d'Argenson called a "revolution in thought."[96]

A century later, Dale Van Kley, in *The Damiens Affair* (1984), agreed. Everything about the refusal of sacraments controversy, he asserted, demonstrates the growing tension between the sacred and secular, between the Church and society, that fed this revolutionary spirit. In the 1750s, debates focused on distinctions between *for intérieur* (conscience) and *for extérieur* (outside authority), opposing considerations regarding the holiness of the sacraments, and a growing interest in one's reputation as a citizen.[97]

But as the 1760s dawned, the nature and reputation of Jansenism itself changed. The denial of sacraments controversy from 1751 to 1756 and Damiens' attack on the king in 1757 represented a decisive turning point for the movement. The former larva of ecclesiastical Jansenism was reborn as the butterfly of parlementary Jansenism. With their enemies discredited and public opinion now on their side, the *parlementaires* emerged from the controversy more popular than ever. Seen as the representative institution of the nation, the depository of the laws, and the guardian of the throne, Parlement's reputation had grown stronger as a result of its combat with the king.[98]

In a realistic sense, however, Jansenism was both retreating and advancing. Thanks in part to the Council of Conscience's judicious appointments, by 1760, only one in twenty (five percent) Gallican bishops sympathized with the *appelant* cause. Yet among the lower clergy and lay orders (who favored Richerism and defended their independence from episcopal control), Jansenism was more popular than ever.[99] And if one defined a Jansenist as anyone who hated the Jesuits, then the number of adherents increased exponentially and could even be said to include the king's mistress, Mme. de Pompadour, a "Jansenist of circumstances."[100]

At mid-century, the Society of Jesus had 26,000 religious throughout the world. In France, it boasted 3300 male and female religious (one-third of them in or near Paris), 111 *collèges* (high schools for boys), 21 seminaries, 25 residences, eight missions, and four professional houses. As confessors of kings, directors of conscience for the nobility, and educators of youth for nearly two centuries, the Order permeated society and appeared invincible. But it was not. Long before the 1760s, cracks had begun to appear in its foundation. Many associated the Jesuits with the worst horrors inflicted by the sixteenth-century "Catholic League" whose pro-Spanish leanings and fanatical persecution had brought so much bloodshed during the Religious Wars. Writers presented colorful tales about "Jesuit plots" to assassinate kings. They portrayed the Society as the enemy of Gallican liberties and national freedoms, the incarnation of servility and despotism. After all, did Jesuits not swear "blind obedience" to a superior general who acted without constitutional restraints? Throughout history, the Jesuits had been court intriguers and enemies of constitutional legalities—in short, "foreigners" to French religious and patriotic ideals.[101]

The Dominicans, jealous of the Jesuits' wealth and power, had carried on a long-running feud with them. Many Paris *curés* remained suspicious and critical of their intentions. *Appelants*, seeing them as old enemies, remembered the Society's polemical attacks on Saint-Cyran, Antoine Arnauld, and other Jansenist stalwarts of the previous century; they also blamed the Jesuits for the destruction of Port-Royal des Champs. The *encyclopédistes* (especially Voltaire) hated them for "plotting" to censure the *Encyclopédie* in 1752 and 1758. The Parlement of Paris had a strong anti-Jesuit bias, for many of its Gallican magistrates had imbibed a hatred for the Order in the course of their legal studies.[102]

Ironically, the Jesuits themselves provided their enemies with the proverbial last straw that destroyed their power in France. In 1761 *Père* Antoine Lavalette, director of the Society's headquarters in Martinique (where the Jesuits made huge profits off the backs of Negro slaves on coffee, cocoa, sugar, and vinegar), was caught red-handed engaging in risky speculation and went bankrupt. An epidemic that killed many slaves and English privateers who captured his cargoes exacerbated the disaster, driving the Society some 6,200,000 *livres* in debt. One of Lavalette's creditors was a large firm in Marseilles to whom he owed over 1,500,000 *livres*. The Parlement of Paris took an interest in the case when the procurer-general of Jesuit missions, *Père* de Sacy, asked the magistrates for help. The trial began in April and lasted four months. At its conclusion, the high court issued *arrêts* stopping Jesuit recruitment, dissolving their congregations, and closing their colleges in the capital. By March 1762, the parlements in Rouen, Rennes, Toulouse, Metz, Aix, and Bordeaux had followed suit. A month later, after reading a 542-page list of "dangerous and pernicious assertions" compiled for him by the Parlement of Paris, Louis XV ordered all Jesuit colleges in France closed.[103]

Immediately, the press went into high gear to undermine the Jesuits' credibility from every conceivable angle. This "cabal" (involving magistrates and philosophes as well as Jansenists) unleashed a veritable campaign of hatred and disinformation through the underground press. Authors blamed the Jesuits for the assassination of Henri III and Henri IV and for attempts on the lives of Louis XV (1757) and Joseph I (1758), saying these proved "a visible conspiracy against all authority." They unearthed scandals concerning the Society's mission work, including robbing Peru's silver mines, stealing the wealth of India and the West Indies, and despoiling the plains of Paraguay. The Jesuits, so rumors said, had embezzled the riches of France, Germany, and Spain; by hoarding grain, they had perpetrated the "famine plot" in France. Throughout history, they had corrupted the youth in their schools, given kings bad counsel, monopolized wealth, and (like Renaissance Italians), had poisoned those who opposed them. In short, the Jesuits, full of vices, played the role of "monsters" in this propaganda farce; Parlement, a cornucopia of virtues, became the people's hero to deliver them from the Molinist dragon.[104]

In their official court documents, the *parlementaires* promoted this image of the Jesuits as wicked casuists, regicides, plotters, anarchists, and assassins. They rejoiced when Joseph I expelled them from Portugal.[105] Led by Louis-Adrien Le Paige, a key Jansenist spokesman, the magistrates voted on 6 August 1761 to close all Jesuit colleges, associations, and seminaries in France.[106] Parlement considered their doctrines "perverse, destructive to all religious principles, injurious to Christian morality, pernicious to civil society, seditious, harmful to the rights of nature and royal power, tending to cause great troubles in States and to form and nurture the most profound corruption in the hearts of men."[107]

Two years later, Louis XV's Edict of 18 November 1764 suppressed the Society in France. The king told Secretary of State Choiseul:

> I do not cordially love the Jesuits, but have always detested heresies, which is their triumph. I will say no more about them. For the peace of the realm, if I banish them against my wishes, at least I do not want people to think that I have agreed with all that the Parlements have done and said against them.[108]

However, although this edict proscribed the Society as a body, it permitted individual Jesuits to remain in France if they submitted to the authority of the bishops or joined other religious orders (as Le Paige had suggested). As late as 1790, at least 515 Jesuits still received state pensions.[109] But their days were numbered across Europe. Expelled from Portugal in 1759, from Spain, Naples, and Parma in 1767, and finally from Rome itself, they awaited the final blow. It came in 1773 in the form of Clement XIV's Bull *Dominis ac Redemptor* ("God the Redeemer"), which abolished the 200-year-old Society of Jesus.[110]

The Jansenists were not the only ones savoring victory after the expulsion of the Jesuits. In truth, Parlement was the greatest victor, for by 1764 it had won the refusal of sacraments crisis, crushed the Jesuits, earned the support of Versailles, buried *Unigenitus* as the law of the land, and sent the Archbishop of Paris on his third exile.[111]

After each exile, however, the Archbishop returned to Paris as stubborn as before. During the 1760s, he continued to assert that only *constitutionnaire* priests and bishops could officiate at baptisms, confirmations, marriages, masses, and ordinations—and no secular power (king or Parlement) could intervene in their spiritual duties.[112] In one 320-page letter to the Gallican bishops in 1763, he defended the Jesuits against all the charges Parlement had brought against them. Incensed, the magistrates condemned his *Pastoral Instruction* as "insidious, slanderous, and tending toward fanaticism, troubling the public peace and encouraging minds to deny the respect and obedience due to the authority of the king and his court [Parlement]." The councilors then ordered Beaumont's letter to be burned by the public executioner.[113]

With Archbishop Beaumont cooling his heels far from Paris, the refusal of sacraments debate lost momentum. In 1765, the General Assembly of the Clergy redefined *Unigenitus* as "a dogmatic judgment of the Universal Church" and "an unchangeable judgment . . . in matters of doctrine"—but not (as previously) "a rule of faith." The faithful, it said, should give the Bull "sincere submission of heart and mind"; anything less would be "revolt."[114] This mollified the *appelants*. Yet the controversy did not entirely disappear in the capital. Documents show, for example, that the Archbishop kept very well informed concerning such refusals in Paris. So did Louis XV and his ministers (St.-Florentin, Bertin), Procurer-General Joly de Fleury, members of Parlement, the police (Berryer and Sartine), and a host of bishops, vicars, priests, deacons, and lawyers (who probably profited most from the controversy). Clerics of all types were hauled into the Châtelet courts and, if found guilty, transferred to other religious houses, sent to the Bastille, or banished from Paris.[115]

Naturally, these *causes célèbres* made those being punished heroes throughout France, thanks largely to the growing influence of the press and especially of the *Nouvelles Ecclésiastiques*. To curtail that influence, the General Assembly of the Clergy asked Louis XV in 1760 to crush "this atrocious libel." Its "outrageous praise of the Church's enemies, exalting the abominable work of the convulsions, [and] declaiming outrageously against papal decisions and authority," they declared, "[destroys] . . . all that is most respectable on the earth."[116]

During the 1760s, however, that "atrocious libel" appeared regularly every week. Over a year's time, its two-column, four-page issues added up to between 208 and 228 pages. As its network spread across Europe, news reports poured in from Italy, Sicily, Spain, Portugal, the United Provinces, Luxembourg, Austria, Bavaria and other German states. Occasionally, the *Nouvelles* also carried reports from as far away as Santo Domingo, Martinique, and China. More often now, the editors excerpted articles from secular papers like the *Gazette de France*, the *Gazette de Leyden*, the *Gazette de Madrid*, and the *Bibliothèque des Sciences & des Beaux Arts*.[117]

While articles in the *Nouvelles* followed Archbishop Beaumont's struggles with Parlement and the king (1764), actions taken by the General Assembly of the Clergy (1765), and the controversy surrounding the Hôtel Dieu Hospital (1769), coverage of the refusal of sacraments cases declined markedly. Authors continued to decry the immoral influence of the Enlightenment, attacking Jean-Jacque Rousseau's *Emile* (1763) and all of Voltaire's works (1763) because their "chicaneries destroy the authority of [divine] Revelation."[118]

But nearly every four-page issue throughout the decade carried news concerning the demise of the Society of Jesus. With euphoric prose, authors traced the steps in the Jesuits' downfall. They rejoiced at their condemnation by Louis XV and Parlement (1761–64) and their expulsion from Portugal, Naples, China, France, Spain, the New World, Italy, and Malta (1760–61, 1764–68). With pens dipped in gall, writers traced the long history of Jesuit "evils" in the sixteenth, seventeenth, and eighteenth centuries, pausing to highlight every law, *arrêt,* and bull by kings, parliaments, and popes that condemned their teachings. Articles entitled "The End of Jesuit Affairs at ____" appeared regularly in the pages of the *Nouvelles*, as did articles carrying positive and negative reactions to the Jesuits' expulsion by Church and government officials. Between the 1764 and 1765 editions, the editor inserted the *pièce de victoire*: the complete text of Louis XV's Edict of 18 November 1764 expelling the Jesuits from France.

In truth, the normally biased prose employed by the newspaper's contributors turned a darker purple in the 1760s. Writers attacked the Jesuits' "cupidity," "cruel persecution," and "the despotism that [they] have always exercised in every state to which they have been admitted."[119] Their downfall, one author declared in 1761, "proves that there is a God in heaven."[120] Hoping for the same result in France, another writer in 1762 suggested: "We can crush the Jesuits . . . by using their own Constitutions against them."[121] One reporter worried in 1763 that although "the Society of Jesus has been destroyed in France, their doctrines . . . did not die with them."[122] Another expressed the concern that the Holy See's "blind devotion to the interests of the former Jesuits" could resurrect the Order in the future.[123]

Voltaire, Diderot, and D'Alembert had no such illusions. Ironically, these three men, universally condemned in the pages of the *Nouvelles*, credited the Jansenists with destroying the Jesuits in France. Members of a loose "cabal" consisting of philosophes, *parlementaires*, and *appelants*, they had made the Society so odious in the pages of the *Nouvelles Ecclésiastiques* that the Jesuits had become "victims of public hatred." Not "universal reason," but "purple prose" had defeated the Society of Jesus.[124]

The *Nouvelles* employed that same biased prose to burnish the halos of its supporters. The passing of the *appelant* Bishop of Soissons, for example, was "a loss to the French Church and even more, to the Church Universal."[125] The editors occasionally devoted entire issues to eulogizing the pious lives and noble deaths of the suffering saints, whose demise always constituted "an irreparable loss."[126]

During the bitter religio-political battles waged between the Crown, Parlement, and the Jansenists for more than a century, at least 326 of these suffering saints were imprisoned during the reigns of Louis XIII, Louis XIV and Louis XV. It is important to understand the nature of their offenses, the qualitative differences in the conditions of their detentions, and the statistical trends in their punishment. Therefore, this portion of the chapter will provide a comprehensive overview—both quantitatively through the use of previously unavailable statistics and qualitatively by the inclusion of brief anecdotes—of the treatment of Jansenists sent to Vincennes and the Bastille between 1638 and 1774.

Jansenists in the Bastille: A Quantitative and Qualitative Analysis

Between 1659 and 1774, of the 772 individuals sent to the Bastille for religious offenses, at least 326 (42%) of them were charged with Jansenism [Graph 1]—roughly 30% more than the number of Protestants (250) incarcerated during the same time period. Similarly, male Jansenists

(276 or 84.7%) outnumbered female Jansenists (50 or 15.3%) by more than five to one.[Graphs 5 and 6] Yet despite his hatred for Jansenism, Louis XIV was responsible for only 67 (20.5%) of these arrests between 1659 and 1715. Among these, men (64 or 95.5%) outnumbered women (3 of 4.5%) by more than twenty to one.[Graphs 7 and 8]

As might be expected, the incarceration of Jansenists at the Bastille followed a cyclical pattern roughly coterminous with the peaks and valleys of Port-Royal's fortune at the hands of government and Church officials.[Graph 2] From 1659 to 1669, a decade of tension between the state and the solitaires, the Bastille held 16 Jansenists, an average of 1.6 per year. During the "Peace of the Church" from 1669 to 1679, however, this number dropped to only nine, or fewer than one per year. But during the 1680s, as Louis XIV increased pressure on both Huguenots and Jansenists to conform, arrests for the latter jumped to 24 (about 2.4 per year). Then, as Church and state officials united their efforts to crush Jansenism and close Port-Royal des Champs after 1704, at least nine Jansenists went to the chateau (about one per year). In the last two years of Louis XIV's reign, however, as the *Unigenitus* controversy heated up, the number of Jansenists sent to the Bastille jumped to 14, or about seven per year in 1714 and 1715. The average stay for Jansenists at the Bastille was 370 days, or about one year [Table 6], but their median stay was only 156 days (about five months).

The fates of only 67 Jansenist detainees under Louis XIV are known: 41 (61.2%) of them were released outright, fourteen (20.9%) were exiled, ten (14.9%) were transferred to other penal institutions, one (1.5%) went to the galleys and one (1.5%) succeeded in escaping.[Table 10] But who were these imprisoned Jansenists? What status groups and occupations did they represent? The largest group came from the Third Estate—printers, booksellers, and librarians (20 or 30%). Close behind and representing the First Estate came the clergy, with abbots, monks, and friars (fifteen) making up another 22.4% of the total. The occupations of twelve (18%) are not known. Among the remaining 29% (20 individuals), all but one (an ambassador's secretary) came from the Third Estate. Adding their numbers to those of the first group above shows that at least 40 (59%) of those Louis XIV sent to the Bastille came from the Third Estate.[Table 2][127]

Comparing statistics on the treatment of Jansenists by Louis XIV and Louis XV demonstrates that in many ways, the latter treated them more harshly. Of the 326 Jansenists sent to the Bastille from 1659 to 1774 [Table 1], Louis XV incarcerated 259 (roughly 80%) of them.[Graph 10] Whereas Louis XIV sent only 67 Jansenists to the Bastille over a 55-year period (1659–1715), Louis XV incarcerated 259 over a 59-year period (1715–1774). Under Louis XV, the 212 men sent to the chateau constituted a lower percentage (81.9%) of males than under Louis XIV (95.5%), while the 47 women sent there by Louis XV represented a percentage (18.2%) exactly four times higher than that for women under Louis XIV (4.5%). [Graph 9]

As during the Sun King's reign, imprisonment under Louis XV came in cycles. [Graph 3] The harshest periods (peaks) occurred from 1724 to 1748 (254 or about eleven at the Bastille each year) during the crackdowns led by Cardinal Fleury and police chiefs René Hérault and Feydeau de Marville. Far fewer detentions at the Bastille occurred during the Regency from 1715 to 1724 (ten or one each year) and at the end of Louis XV's reign from 1749 to 1774 (31 or about one each year). The "Refusal of the Sacraments" controversy during the 1750s sent only 24 Jansenists to the Bastille, about 2.4 each year.

But if Louis XV sent more Jansenists there than his predecessor, he did not detain them nearly as long [Table 7]. Whereas Jansenists under Louis XIV had spent an average of 370 days (about one year) at the Bastille, those under Louis XV stayed about 312 days (about 10.5 months). Their median stay, which under Louis XIV had been 156 days (roughly five months), likewise fell to 123 days (four months) under Louis XV [Table 5]. Whereas Louis XIV had released outright only 61.2% of his Jansenists, Louis XV released 83.4% of his, transferring only eight of them (3%) to other prisons (as opposed to 15% for Louis XIV). Louis XV also exiled only half as many Jansenists (12.4%) as Louis XIV had done (21%) once they were released from the Bastille. While Louis XIV sent one prisoner to the galley ships, Louis XV sent three Jansenists there. No Jansenists escaped from the chateau during Louis XV's reign [Tables 9, 10 and 11].

As for their status and occupations under Louis XV, 60 (23.2%) Jansenist inmates came from the First Estate (abbots, canons, priests, etc.), only six (2.4%) from the Second Estate (two chevaliers, one *intendant*, and three tax collectors from the Court of Aids), and at least 138 (49.3%) from the Third Estate [Table 3]. At least 47 from this last group (34%) were colporteurs, printers, book binders, librarians, and engravers, the occupations most directly connected with producing and distributing the *Nouvelles Ecclésiastiques*. The occupations of 65 Jansenists (25.1%) are unknown, but it is likely that they, too, came primarily from the lower class trades (servants, colporteurs, hat-makers, cutlers, apprentices, etc.) In the 20 cases where other charges were recorded against these Jansenists,five (25%) had assisted other prisoners, five (25%) had attended illicit assemblies, two (10%) had attacked religion, and one each had been charged with writing *nouvelles à la main* (handwritten sheets), debauchery, attempting to escape, intrigues, and one (ironically) with Calvinism. The accusations for two others are unknown.

While computer-generated statistics contribute precise quantitative information about Jansenist inmates over long periods of time, personal anecdotes provide human interest details and insights into the qualitative differences in their treatment during the reigns of Louis XIII, Louis XIV, and Louis XV. Pro-Jansenist writers like Augustin Gazier (1924) have asserted that the vast majority of Jansenists sent to Vincennes and the Bastille endured "very hard" treatment, being denied the right to exercise, write, and receive the sacraments.[128] Such generalizations, although accurate for the early seventeenth century, do not fit the reality for late-seventeenth and eighteenth century treatment of Jansenists according to the sources cited below.

Abbé de Saint-Cyran (1638–1643)

When Saint-Cyran was arrested by 22 archers and sent to Vincennes in May 1638, Chancellor Séguier actually wanted him executed. Because the *abbé* was an outspoken proponent of Spain, a close friend of Jansen, and an enemy of the Jesuits (who suspected him of Calvinism), Richelieu considered him "more dangerous than six armies."[129] The first minister initially had him placed in chains and incarcerated in a dungeon chamber, then moved him to a more healthful room, and finally placed him in a commodious chamber of twenty square meters with a garden view and a servant to assist him.[130] Despite Saint-Cyran's exclamation that "I am astonished that I did not die from all the evils I have endured [at Vincennes],"[131] he was, in fact, treated fairly well. Although tightly guarded, he wrote more than 50 letters, promenaded in the courtyard gardens, and entertained a long line of visitors (including scholars from the *petites écoles*, who each received three sugared almonds). He prayed often, sang loudly, and ate a daily diet costing eight *livres*—more than the average French subject spent on food. Nonetheless, he was not released until 6 February 1643, two months after Richelieu's death; his detention (four years and eight months) was almost five times longer than the mean for Jansenists sent to the Bastille in Louis XIV's reign.[132]

Cardinal de Retz (1652–1653)

Cardinal de Retz, the scion of an old Italian family famous for its intrigues, had a reputation for being rich, clever, crafty, and immoral, which made many distrust him. Cardinal Mazarin had him arrested in 1652 and sent to Vincennes under suspicion of plotting against Louis XIII and Queen Anne. Although Retz spent only a few months in its chambers, his noble status and high position as Archbishop of Paris entitled him to receive the best care available. In a letter to a friend, Mazarin declared: "Never has any prisoner of State been so favorably treated." Nonetheless, the first minister refused to release Retz, choosing instead to transfer him to another chateau in Nantes.[133]

Pères Terrasson and Creigny

By contrast, two curates sent to Vincennes in November 1735 experienced far less comfortable incarcerations. *Père* Terrasson, arrested for distributing Jansenist literature, became somewhat "delirious in his mind" during several months at the chateau and was exiled first to Troyes and then to Turin. Only after he signed the Formulary did Louis XV permit him to reenter France. *Père* Creigny, a pistol-packing priest accused of convulsionism, sexual improprieties, and bilking his followers of 14,000 *livres* (and many pounds of chocolate), certainly did not fit the conventional Jansenist mold. Yet his hellfire and brimstone sermons enjoyed the support of the Bishop of Auxerre, the Congregation of the Oratory, and several local *curés*. Nevertheless, in November 1735, he too found himself incarcerated at Vincennes—and there is no record of when he was released.[134] Most likely, the serious nature of both men's offenses and their low social status earned them long detentions.

Both priests also had the misfortune of being arrested during a peak period when Louis XV, the Church, and the police were cracking down on fanatical Jansenists known as the *Convulsionnaires* (see chapters 7 and 8). Between 1732 and 1760, at least 250 of them were sent to the Bastille or the Châtelet prisons—nearly 80% of all Jansenists detained during Louis XV's reign. Police chiefs Hérault, Marville, and Berryer also ferreted out clandestine Jansenist presses in the capital; Hérault alone closed down 30 of them, earning him the nickname of "the Grand French Inquisitor." Minister Fleury extended the prison terms for Jansenists from earlier sentences of eight to ten months to lengthier stays of one to three years—and often banished those he released.[135]

The social makeup of those being arrested changed as well. By the 1720s and '30s, only about one-third of the detainees were clerics; the other two-thirds comprised printers, colporteurs, merchants, and artisans. In fact, from 1713 to 1765, the police charged nearly three-fourths (72%) of those they arrested with being involved in the clandestine printing trade (as booksellers, partners, laborers, colporteurs, or hack writers). This becomes understandable when viewed in the context of another trend. From 1640 to 1713 (73 years), French presses (never more than 40) printed around 500 Jansenist works (7 per year), but from 1713 to 1765 (52 years), these presses (an estimated 200 by 1739) churned out 2,600 Jansenist publications (50 per year).[136] Not all of those involved in this underground publishing trade came from the lower classes either. Presidents from the Chamber of Inquests, councilors in Parlement, masters of requests, and numerous lawyers and advocates funded these clandestine presses.[137]

Pouiray (1659) and Pierre Baudelot (1661)

Pouiray (also spelled "Preveray") may have been the first French printer in Paris arrested for publishing Jansenist works and selling them from Port-Royal. A humble bookseller, he spent only thirteen weeks at the Bastille. Another bookseller, Pierre Baudelot, charged with peddling tracts dedicated to Saint-Cyran, entered the chateau in May 1661, but was shortly transferred to an unknown prison outside Paris.[138]

Isaac le Maître de Sacy and Pierre du Fossé (1666–1668)

Isaac de Sacy entered the Bastille in 1666 for his French translation of the New Testament. Although he had taken no prominent part in the Jansenist-Jesuit disputes of the period, he was, nonetheless, a prominent solitaire at Port-Royal des Champs. Contrary to Augustin Gazier's

(1924) claim that he endured "a very hard captivity"[139] (due to prison Governor Besmaus' reputation for being "unfeeling and disagreeable)," Sacy entered the chateau with his servant Hérissant and received visits from friends and relatives. During his stay at "the retreat" (as he called the Bastille), he read numerous books, took walks on the outer walls, wrote many coded letters, and completed his translation of the Old Testament (later published in Amsterdam). Being deprived of the sacraments, he and Hérissant prayed, studied, and consoled each other during what he later called "the sweetest years" of his life. Just after completing his biblical translation, he was released (to mark the "Peace of the Church") on 1 November 1668 after two and a half years at the Bastille. This was still twice as long as the average stay for a Jansenist detainee, but only half the length of Saint-Cyran's detention at Vincennes a generation earlier.[140]

Arrested at the same time as his housemate de Sacy, Pierre du Fossé was lodged in a separate chamber of the Bastille. Suffering from palpitations of the heart, he found the nights especially painful. But like Sacy, he obtained paper, ink, pens, and books and spent his detention praying, reading, writing, singing, and exercising in his room. Thanks to family ties with Minister Le Tellier, du Fossé left after a month, but was banished to Normandy until the "Peace of the Church" freed him to return to Paris in 1668.[141]

Le Noir de Saint-Claude and Germain Vuillart (1707–1715)

A councilor in the Parlement of Paris, Saint-Claude served as the defense attorney for the religious at Port-Royal des Champs. As such, he urged them to resist Louis XIV's attempts to merge the two convents. With the help of his friend Germain Vuillart, the two prepared legal briefs defending the rural convent's cause in court. This so annoyed the king that he sent both men to the Bastille for one of the longest detentions any Jansenist ever endured. During their eight years at the chateau, Saint-Claude became gravely ill and Vuillart went blind. Only the death of the king and Mlle. de Joncoux's intervention with the *duc* d'Orléans secured their release on 12 September 1715. Saint-Claude died a month later, but Vuillart lived until 1742.[142]

Dom François Louvard and Julien Mellinet (1728–1734)

For his vocal opposition to *Unigenitus* and his peddling of 5000 *livres* worth of Jansenist literature in Maine, Louis XV sent Doctor of Theology Dom Louvard to the Bastille in December 1728. A recidivist who had previously been detained in Nantes for raising "revolts" in Benedictine monasteries, Louvard denounced the pope and the Jesuits (whom he blamed for crafting the 1713 Bull) and planned an insurrection against it. Although Hérault denied him the sacraments, he gave him paper, pens, and ink to write letters defending himself, books to read, and the privilege of exercising in the prison gardens and receiving visitors. In addition, Hérault sent him clothing, medicines, and a physician to bandage his hernia. Because Louvard wrote strongly worded letters to Hérault and refused to sign the Formulary, however, his stay stretched into five years. His friend Mellinet, on the other hand, signed the Formulary and was released after eight months. Finally released in January 1734, Louvard went to a monastery in Meaux. His continued disruption of monastic life led Louis XV to order his arrest in March—but Louvard fled to Utrecht and died there in 1739 at age 78.[143]

Jansenist Printers and Colporteurs (1730s–1740s)

Most of those involved in the clandestine printing trade in the 1730s and '40s, however, spent only a few weeks or months at the Bastille. For distributing Jansenist materials, the *abbé* Angevin went there for six months in 1736.[144] The Jansenist Ladourny de Caseau spent fourteen months at the Bastille in 1736–37, but in addition to possessing Jansenist literature, he had counterfeited false contracts and allegedly plotted to murder Cardinal de Fleury.[145] In some instances, the same minister of state ordered widely varying periods of detention for the same offense. For example, in the mid-1730s, Minister Phélyppeaux sent François Cadet Noel to the chateau for 20 months, Guillaume Bachelier for three months, and the wife of Edme Michel Briard for only sixteen days—all for operating clandestine Jansenist presses.[146] At the same time, Phélyppeaux sent the printer Michel Rivier—who had no Jansenist connections—to the Bastille for six months.[147]

In 1742, the *abbé* Roquette, who had already been exiled several times for his opposition to *Unigenitus*, entered the chateau. As a recidivist, he received a six-month term, but that was sufficient to insure his fame once the *Nouvelles Ecclésiastiques* printed his *Relation* in its pages. The paper informed readers that the poor, suffering Roquette had been isolated in a tower chamber without exercise, writing implements, adequate food, or visitors. In reality, police chief Marville allowed him to exercise an hour each day in the courtyard, offered him two meals a day (soup, entrée, bread, roast, vegetables, and wine), permitted his brother to visit him, and provided him books. Because he refused to sign the Formulary, however, it required the intercession of three princesses and the death of Minister Fleury in 1743 to release him from the chateau.[148]

The *abbé* Jean Boullemois, one of several "dangerous composers of the *Nouvelles Ecclésiastiques*," spent several months at the Bastille in 1747–48 when the police found articles for the newspaper in his home. During his interrogation, police chief Berryer asked him if he knew the authors who wrote for the newspaper. Boullemois replied that no one person knew all their names or where they lived, and that "his conscience would not permit" him to reveal those he did know. Because of his poor health, Minister Fleury released Boullemois after six months on condition that he leave Paris and go to a health resort at Bourg-la-Reine, which he did in June 1748. Three other men arrested with him (and also connected with the *Nouvelles*) spent six to ten months at the chateau before being exiled to Lyon and Alsace.[149]

But the *abbé* de St.-Jean Lamoureux earned the prize for the longest stay of any Jansenist at the Bastille. His persistent activities in the underground Jansenist press landed him there in 1747—and he did not emerge until 1757.[150]

Although Louis XIV condemned 3500 Huguenot men to the galleys,[151] he sent no Jansenists to row in his Mediterranean fleet. Louis XV, however, sent two *appelant* priests to the galleys in May 1755. One of them (whose name is unknown) had been accused of fanaticism and denying the king's authority to legislate regarding *Unigenitus* and the refusal of sacraments. The other, an *abbé* Dubois, was part of a group suspected of plotting to kill the king. One of its members had been overheard saying, "There are still some Ravaillacs [the assassin of Henri IV in 1610] around." The records do not reveal how long these priests served in the royal galleys.[152]

As one would expect, the *Nouvelles* kept its readers well informed about the arrests, trials, and imprisonment of Jansenist adherents. In fact, its articles reflect such detailed, accurate knowledge of police intentions, the time, place, and reason for arrests, and the place of detention that one can only conclude that the *Nouvelles* must have had one or more *mouches* (spies) working inside the police force in the 1730s and '40s.[153] Consistently throughout its pages, the paper spread the myth that the Bastille was a horrible prison in which Jansenists suffered terrible fates deprived of adequate food, water, companionship, books, and spiritual consolation. One poem attacked the chateau as "an infernal catacomb" where "abbots [were] fed like dogs in the courtyard. For having nourished many Christians, you will suffer at the Bastille."[154]

A comparison of the quantitative and qualitative evidence regarding the treatment of Jansenists during the reigns of Louis XIII, Louis XIV, and Louis XV, however, leads one to draw several conclusions. First, that Jansenists' (and others') myths concerning the suffering endured by imprisoned *appelants* were greatly exaggerated; the legends do not usually square with the evidence provided by government, police, Church, and private documents found in the Parisian archives.[155] Second, that the Jansenists, who enjoyed writing about their sufferings, did not in reality endure the degree of pain and punishment that Louis XIV and Louis XV inflicted on the Huguenots: longer prison terms, more frequent exiles, galley servitude, torture, and execution.[156] Third, that the treatment of Jansenists followed "peaks" and "valleys" determined by such factors as papal bulls, external wars, the Gallican Church's demands, royal and parlementary laws, and the willingness (or resistance) of police to enforce those laws. Finally, the treatment of specific Jansenists—their care, privileges, and the length of their detention—differed according to their social status, the seriousness of their offenses, their degree of cooperation while in prison (for example, whether they signed the Formulary), and the intervention of powerful friends to secure their release. In the main, however, the statistical evidence demonstrates that while more Jansenists went to prison in the eighteenth century than in the seventeenth century, they experienced shorter sentences and better treatment during Louis XV's reign than they had under Louis XIV.

However, as the 1770s dawned, Jansenists ceased to suffer at all. Their old enemies the Jesuits had left and Louis XVI sent no *appelants* to prison. Paradoxically, however, with its old nemesis suppressed, Jansenism suffered a kind of identity crisis. For decades, *appelants* had so exclusively defined themselves by what they opposed—the Society of Jesus—that once that force disappeared, they lacked doctrinal specificity and political momentum. So Jansenism ceased to be a movement and became a legacy, and a fragmented one at that. Its various groups—*appelants, convulsionnaires, figuristes*, to name a few—constituted the flotsam and jetsam of a much larger stream that now included the *philosophes*, the *physiocrates*, the *parti janséniste* and the *parti patriote*.[157]

Through their opposition to *billets de confession*, episcopal mandates, and the Society of Jesus during the 1750s and '60s, the members of this "Jansenist Party," with roots in Gallicanism and Richerism, had helped to develop opposition thought in France. Their propaganda and political strategies, in the final analysis, shaped the course of French politics and Church decisions during the reign of Louis XVI.[158] In 1772, the *Historical Journal of the Revolution Operating under the Constitution of the French Monarchy* stated:

> Jansenism . . . having lost its true focus after the expulsion of the Jesuits from France, has been transformed into the party of patriotism . . . It has always had a great attraction to independence: it fought against papal despotism with invincible courage: political despotism is a hydra no less terrible to fight, and it is necessary today to direct against this enemy all the forces henceforth rendered useless in the former genre of combat.[159]

With the Jesuits gone, the members of this "Jansenist Party" sought new enemies to fight. Seeing the bishops, those "tools of the popes" and "natural despots," as their continued persecutors, Jansenist lawyers penned briefs attacking their arbitrary power. Inspired by Jansenism's Richerist core, they sued bishops for under-representing the lower clergy on diocesan panels. Priests and abbots demanded more ecclesiastical assemblies, more efficient diocesan organization, better record keeping and financial accounting, precise scheduling of sacred services, the establishment of charity schools, and the rejection of all ostentation. In this secular, materialistic age, Jansenism, which for over a century had rejected the world and its values, now embraced the pragmatism and utilitarianism of the Enlightenment.[160]

But if the Jansenists (despite their protests) were adopting many of the values of the Enlightenment, Archbishop of Paris Christophe de Beaumont, their old nemesis, refused to change with the times. Although old and feeble, he continued defending the Jesuits, despite the fact that Clement XIV had suppressed the Society in 1773. This stance earned him the animosity of *appelants* everywhere.[161] Nor did it endear him to the new king. Shortly after taking the throne, Louis XVI told the Archbishop: "I will not exile you, but I will make you suffer the full severity of the laws. I give you my royal word that I will not arrest you for your activity . . . [but] you may retire."[162] Forced out after 35 years as Archbishop of Paris, Beaumont died in 1781 at 78 years. Although he had greatly harmed religion by his intolerance, before his death, he gave away two-thirds of his vast income to 1000 ecclesiastics and 500 nuns, and 500,000 *livres* (won in a lawsuit) to the Protestant Madame Necker for her hospital charities. While the *Gazette de France*, praising him for his frankness and loyalty, asserted that he had "practiced just severity like [the biblical prophet] Samuel," in reality, the inflexible septuagenarian was out of step with the spirit of the times.[163]

So was René Nicolas de Maupeau, former First President of Parlement whom Louis XV had chosen as his chancellor in 1768. Beginning in 1770, Maupeau's determination to introduce certain administrative reforms in Parlement precipitated a constitutional crisis that brought the exile of the magistrates from Paris. Although the "Jansenist Party" did not take the lead in this anti-Maupeau campaign, they did participate in it, joining with old enemies (including the philosophes) who understood that the chancellor's reform program would undermine Parlement's authority. Led by *abbé* Claude Mey and *parlementaire* Louis-Adrien Le Paige, these "Jansenist patriots" published 80 pamphlets comparing Maupeou's "despotism" to past papal "despotism," calling it "Molinism of the State" and "a Jesuit coup." These tracts (many carrying ideas plagiarized from Montesquieu) contrast Henri IV (the patriot-king) and Louis XV (the despot-king), and assert that all true patriots must unite to check the "despotism" of Maupeou. The "Patriots" picture themselves as defenders of the laws of the realm and the rights of the nation, and demand genuinely representative institutions (an "Assembly of Notables") and elected assemblies.[164]

When Louis XVI asked for Maupeou's resignation in 1774 and restored Parlement's authority, the Jansenists rejoiced. The fact that defeating the chancellor had required them to cooperate with some very strange bedfellows—princes of the blood, courtiers, clients of Minister Choiseul, robe nobles, and philosophes—shows just how much Jansenism had been changed by its involvement in the political battles of the century. By nature, Jansenism had always been "revolutionary," given its emphasis on conscience, love of truth, individualism, anti-establishmentarianism, and representative democracy, as well as its conscientious opposition to any form of arbitrary power. The nuns at Port-Royal des Champs had espoused these values in the seventeenth century, and in the eighteenth century, their female heirs played a key role in spreading anti-Maupeou propaganda around Paris. By the 1770s, these "Jansenist Patriots" shared several traits in common with their secular colleagues: youthfulness, bourgeois origins, an ambition to rise in society, and an inveterate hatred of all forms of despotism. As Shanti-Marie Singham (1990) so aptly declared, the "Maupeou Revolution" of 1770–74 had brought about "the secularization of Jansenism and the sanctification of the political."[165]

As the Jansenists embraced social and political causes, society became more tolerant of them as well. Their campaigns to expel the Jesuits, abolish the Inquisition, soften the penal codes against heresy, and revive the spirit of tolerance that Christ had taught won them many friends. As the debate over granting French Protestants religious and civil rights heated up after 1775, the authors of the *Nouvelles Ecclésiastiques* championed the cause of civil toleration. Paradoxically, ever since the Revocation in 1685, Calvinists had been forced to receive the sacraments they did not want while *appelants* had been denied the sacraments they very much desired.[166]

Therefore, in 1775 a magistrate in Parlement asked Louis XVI for some "solid indication" that he would soon grant the Jansenists religious toleration.[167] Minister of the King's Household Lamoignon de Malesherbes believed the time had come to do this. Seeing the Jansenists as one of the three great causes of France's past "troubles" (the Jesuits and Calvinists were the other two), he told Louis XVI that it was hardly right for clerics to grant *appelants* the sacraments all their lives and then deny them at death. Some bishops, he said, had even employed *lettres de cachet* to punish those who refused to conform—but Malesherbes had intervened to stop those arrests. Now he pleaded with the king to release imprisoned Jansenists and restore their rights.[168]

Since restoring human rights was one of the goals of the Enlightenment, this should have placed the Jansenists and the philosophes on the same side of the fence. But for over a century, the two groups had been sworn enemies. In his *Necessity of the Faith* (1641), Antoine Arnauld had written that philosophy must be the servant of faith, for only faith could save humanity from sin.[169] "Outside the Christian Religion," he had declared in *Of the True Religion* (1656), "one can never find true philosophy or true wisdom."[170] Throughout his writings, Arnauld attacked philosophers as "pagans" and "infidels," motivated by vanity and vice, whose science was "useless for salvation."[171]

Arnauld's hatred of Jesuits and philosophers cast a long shadow over his spiritual descendants. Therefore, after the Jesuits were expelled from France, the Jansenists "adopted" the philosophes as their new enemies. Their books, pamphlets, and newspapers considered them irreligious, materialistic, secular, immoral pagans. Writers criticized the philosophes' emphasis on pleasure-seeking, free-thinking, Deism, human reason, and natural law (rather than God's laws). As we have seen, the *Nouvelles Ecclésiastiques* panned the works of Montesquieu, Buffon, Diderot, Voltaire, and D'Alembert.[172]

Yet despite their aversion for the philosophes, the Jansenists admired some aspects of the Enlightenment, such as its emphasis on individual freedom. In 1754, for example, a Jansenist translated John Locke's *Two Treatises on Government* (1688) into French—which Minister of State D'Argenson considered "a delicate matter" that would "annoy royalty."[173] During the 1760s, *appelants* and philosophes had cooperated in undermining the Society of Jesus and securing its expulsion from France. In the early 1770s, they worked hand in glove to defeat Maupeou's reforms and restore the old Parlement; by the end of the decade, they found themselves on the same platform reclaiming the civil and religious rights of French Protestants. Involvement in these reform movements had made them—in spite of themselves—more tolerant.[174]

Although historically, Jansenists had always been aristocratic in ethics and elitist on grace, their bourgeois, utilitarian emphasis on hard work, sobriety, success, ambition, and taking personal responsibility drew them closer to the Enlightenment. Like the philosophes they loved to hate, the *appelants* opposed Molinism, the Jesuits, Maupeou, and persecution of any kind. Also like the philosophes, they defended the rights of conscience and Christian liberty. In the pages of the *Nouvelles*, authors praised Joseph II for his tolerant laws toward Lutherans and Calvinists in Austria, Bohemia, Hungary, and the Austrian Netherlands (Belgium). However, the Jansenists supported civil toleration (granting all religious groups civil rights, something the Jesuits opposed) rather than "theological tolerance" (saving everyone regardless of their state of grace, a position the Jesuits favored). Nonetheless, they saw toleration as preferable to the alternatives: hypocrisy, persecution, forced emigration, and sedition.[175]

For their part, the philosophes experienced a love/hate relationship with the Jansenists as well, finding in their theology, lifestyles, and actions much to condemn and little to admire. Probably none had felt the lash of *appelants'* criticism as much as François Arouet de Voltaire. They condemned him as a fool, devil, imposter, and *débauchée* and attacked his "foolish arrogance," "diabolic letters," and "irreligious prose." Jansenist opposition to his tragedy *Mahomet* in 1739 persuaded procurer-general Joly de Fleury to ban that drama in France.[176]

Little wonder then that Voltaire, in his war against "the infamous thing," made his famous suggestion that the police "should hang the last Jesuit with the entrails of the last Jansenist."[177] He considered their religious quarrels puerile and their "chimerical ideas" unintelligible and useless for human progress.[178] Nonetheless, when Minister Fleury and police chief Hérault pressured him to use his pen against the Jansenists, he refused. Although he tried to write a satire on

Pascal's *Provincial Letters*, he threw his efforts into the fire, refusing to "dishonor" himself by becoming the state's "mercenary penman."[179]

Although Voltaire called Pascal "that misanthrope" and made critical remarks about him in his *English Letters* and *Philosophical Letters*, he praised his *Provincial Letters* as "the first work of genius in prose to be seen in France."[180] As a playwright, he could also appreciate Jean Racine's dramatic efforts, but rejected his religious views. In his "Poem on Grace" (1720), Voltaire asserted: "Your God is not mine, You have made Him a tyrant, I want Him to be my father. Your homage is forced, mine is voluntary."[181] He felt that the *appelants*' "false ideas" dishonored the Christian religion.[182] Regarding Pasquier Quesnel's imprisonment, however, Voltaire wrote: "Your persecutors are abominable . . . I pity you for being oppressed, but I also pity you for being a Jansenist. All sects appear to me as the joining together of error. Tell me if there are sects in geometry."[183]

While he considered the Jansenists valuable allies in expelling the Jesuits from France, Voltaire decried their "theological quarrels and pen wars." In his writings, he lampoons them as "atrocious wild men," "wicked wolves far worse than the Jesuit foxes," and "Presbyterians more dangerous than those in England."[184] The legacy these "virtuous but stubborn savants" have left France, he declares in his *Century of Louis XIV* (1751), includes abstract theological quarrels, intrigues, cabals, and a century of persecution.[185]

Jansenists also attacked the Baron de Montesquieu's *Spirit of the Laws* (1748) as "unchristian" because it spoke favorably of suicide, polygamy, and celibacy. In its pages, they found "Spinozism," "Atheism," the "Natural Religion," and human free will emphasized. They also accused Montesquieu of asserting that religion should accommodate itself to the manners and customs of the different countries it enters.[186]

Montesquieu was a moderate Gallican who opposed *Unigenitus* (calling it "a great evil" and "a gigantic political error") and favored the Jesuits. He disagreed with priests' refusing the sacraments to the dying. Although not as publicly hostile toward the *appelants* as Voltaire, Montesquieu privately disapproved of their theology. In the 33rd letter in his *Persian Letters*, he mocked a Tartuffe-like Molinist bishop as "a fat man with a rosy complexion." He ridiculed Pascal's famous argument that one gains more by believing in God than by not believing as "very good for Atheists. But it does not establish one religion over another." "If God predestines," he said, "those He predestines are saved. But it does not follow that all those He does not predestine are lost." Despite his description of Quesnel's *Moral Reflections* as "so many shallow thoughts and puerile ideas," he believed that neither *appelants* nor *constitutionnaires* should be excluded from the Church for conscience's sake.[187]

The Jansenists joined the pope and the Sorbonne in condemning Denis Diderot's *Of the Mind* for attacking "all religions and all morality, and establishing systematically the most alarming libertinage"; it also promoted "the natural religion." Behind the author's "infernal doctrines," Jansenists smelled "the doctrine of the Jesuits."[188]

Yet of all the philosophes, Diderot expressed the most sympathy toward the *appelant* cause. Between 1732 and 1736, he had studied theology at the Sorbonne, then dominated by Jansenists. He considered the Jesuits a "pest inseparable from cholera." In his political works, Diderot borrowed much of his imagery from the chronicles of the religious of Port-Royal des Champs, including phrases like "the depository of truth," "God's absolute power," and "the time of troubles." He showed less antagonism toward Pascal than Voltaire and Diderot, describing him as "an elegant writer and profound thinker [who was] honest, but also timid and credulous." Persecuting the Jansenists, he told Catherine II of Russia, had cost France dearly; tolerating them would render them harmless.[189]

When the government banned Diderot's and D'Alembert's *Encyclopédie* in 1759, writers in the *Nouvelles Ecclésiastiques* rejoiced. But the editors of the *Encyclopédie* had the last word. In its pages, D'Alembert called the *Nouvelles* "a vagabond gazette," "an insipid and scandalous collection of obscenities and falsehoods," and "a libelous periodical without intelligence, truth, charity, or approval" that circulated "blind and sterile commentaries" and attacked the Society of Jesus.[190]

Although D'Alembert himself called the Jesuits "the grand grenadiers of intolerance," he preferred a Jesuit "tyranny" to a Jansenist one. In his book *On the Destruction of the Jesuits* (1765), he rejoiced that "Jansenist intolerance" had not replaced the "Jesuit intolerance" crushed in 1764. While he found the beliefs of both groups "wicked and pernicious," the Jesuits were "less tyrannous" because their theology was "more accommodating " of diverse thought.[191] "If the wretched posterity of Port-Royal" had prevailed in France, he declared, they would have "exercised over books, minds, discourses, and morals the most virulent kind of inquisition."[192]

Jean-Jacques Rousseau agreed, predicting in *The New Heloise* (1763) that "as soon as the Jansenists are the masters, they will be more intolerant and cruel than their enemies [the Jesuits]."[193] Like the other philosophes, he, too, had good reason to dislike them, for the *Nouvelles Ecclésiastiques* had criticized him for his "lax morality" and Molinism and had attacked *Emile* (1762) for its "atheism" and advocacy of the "natural religion."[194] Yet their dislike for his lifestyle and writings did not prevent them from plagiarizing phrases like "the social contract," "the general will," and "essential unanimity" from his *Social Contract* (1762) to defend the rights of minority groups.[195]

For his part, Rousseau treated the Jansenists with a mixture of humor, sarcasm, and hostility. Although he called them "detestable insects" in his *Letter to Christophe de Beaumont*, he modeled the Savoyard vicar in *Emile* (1762) after Jean-Claude Gaime, a quasi-Jansenist prelate at Turin whom he knew personally. In fact, Rousseau read *appelant* writings more frequently than he would admit. His *Verger of Mme. de Warens* (1735–37) has a distinctly Jansenist tone to it. And shortly after he re-converted to Protestantism in 1754, he criticized the arts and the theater in his *Letter to D'Alembert* (1756) every bit as harshly as any Jansenist would have done.[196]

In actuality, Rousseau and the Jansenists shared many values in common. They both valorized the past and used its heroes to condemn leaders in the present. They loved primitivism, and especially the simple Christianity of the apostolic era. Both Rousseau and the Jansenists condemned usury, profit, and luxury and opposed capitalism and progress. In their place, they exalted the simple virtues of rural living and criticized urban excess and immorality. They shared an attraction for the solitary life devoted to duty, truth, right, obedience, and temperance. Likewise, they both championed the separation of Church and state.[197]

But the similarities they shared failed to unite the Jansenists and the philosophes as much as their differences and mutual distrust divided them. The Jansenist writer, orator, and *parlementaire* Louis-Adrien Le Paige, equating the moral laxity of Molinism with the free thought of the Enlightenment, summarized it this way: "What is a true Jesuit if not a disguised philosophe, and what is a philosophe if not a disguised Jesuit?"[198]

In the 1770s, this seemed to be the prevailing view of the *Nouvelles Ecclésiastiques*, whose two-column, four-page issues appeared like clockwork every week and totaled exactly 208 pages every year. Reports about the progress of the Enlightenment "in this licentious century" poured in from all over Europe. Regularly, the *Nouvelles* carried excerpts from Portugal, Spain, Italy, Belgium, the German states, the Netherlands, Poland, Switzerland, Austria, Ireland, England, Hungary and Moravia. But occasionally, the editors reported on events (even wars) in distant India, Siam, and China. They frequently reprinted articles from secular papers like the *Mercure de France*, the *Journal Politique de Bouillon*, the *Gazette de Florence*, and the *Journal des Savants*.[199]

The newspaper continued as before criticizing the works of Voltaire, although his passing blunted those attacks. In August 1778, the paper informed its readers that Voltaire, "this famous chief of miscreants in our time," had died.[200] Of all the philosophes, only Rousseau earned favorable reviews for his contempt of worldly luxury and his hostility to despotic power.[201]

But the Society of Jesus never garnered favorable remarks. Although the Jesuits had been suppressed in France since 1764, writers continued attacking their old nemesis (now referred to as "former Jesuits") as if their very identity depended on it. The *Nouvelles* reviewed prominent anti-Jesuit publications, highlighted national laws against them, and gloated over their expulsion from Austria, Hungary, Poland, Germany, Belgium, Milan, and China. Authors expressed unrestrained joy at Clement XIV's brief suppressing the Society in 1773 (although they worried about the Jesuits still occupying faculty positions in Florence, Sienna, and Tuscany).[202]

"The Jesuits are no more," one writer proclaimed. "That Society, once so powerful & so formidable, is extinguished; its reign and empire . . . remain only a memory."[203] Yet writers continued beating the dead horse of Jesuitism as if, phoenix-like, it might resurrect itself. They repeated the familiar litany about its "perverse nature," "animosity," "lies," "frauds," "fanaticism," and "plots."[204]

Naturally, the actions and writings of *appelants* received glowing reviews, as they always had in the pages of the *Nouvelles*. Indeed, throughout the decade, the paper devoted far more pages to printing excerpts of Jansenist prelates' letters and reviewing their books than to covering the news in France and Europe. For example, regular notices appeared concerning the assembling and publishing of the works of Antoine Arnauld and Blaise Pascal.[205] Yet in an article announcing Louis XV's death in 1774, the author criticized the funeral sermon given by the Bishop of Langres, but wrote not a single kind word about the former king.[206] By contrast, the paper filled several columns on the life and death of Clement XIV and the good deeds of his successor, Pius VI.[207]

From the philosophes' point of view, however, the *Nouvelles'* emphasis on such "foolishness" while failing to crush fanaticism and intolerance proved its misguided nature. "We laugh at the death of Jansenism and Molinism," Condorcet stated in his *Eulogy to Pascal*, "at concomitant grace and medicinal grace, and at sufficient and efficacious grace."[208] As a whole, the proponents of the Enlightenment laughed along with him. Seeing the *Nouvelles* as virulent, corrosive, and contemptible, they felt that it had "infected" France with its "obscure religious fanaticism" and "deplorable teachings" (which they had hoped to destroy) for half a century. Its "base thoughts" and "puerile ideas" appeared "unintelligible" to them and offered no benefit to humanity.[209]

Far more serious, however, was the fact that some Jansenists questioned the value of these ideals as well, for Jansenism had become "a creed for nostalgic older men and younger troublemakers." In most dioceses, its controversies had lost their former asperity because the public no longer cared about theological issues. After 1775, Jansenism ceased being a movement and became a legacy—and a very fragmented one at that. During this "era of decomposition" when political Gallicanism replaced ecclesiastical Gallicanism, Jansenism became merely flotsam and jetsam in a swift-flowing stream. Discussions on human sin and God's efficacious grace seemed totally irrelevant in the face of crises such as the Diamond Necklace Affair (1785), the *lits de justice* to enforce registration of fiscal edicts (1786), and the debates over granting civil rights to Protestants and convoking the Estates-General (1787–88).[210]

Despite the skepticism, rationalism, and materialism of the late Enlightenment, the Benedictines of Saint-Maur and the Genovesains and Dominicans in Paris experienced revivals. Never had so many Catholic churches and sanctuaries been built in France as were erected between the 1750s and the 1780s. On the eve of the French Revolution, over 63 percent of all books published dealt with religious topics. Over 2,000,000 copies of liturgical works, offices of the saints, books of prayers, and songbooks came from the presses in Paris during the 1780s—including Thomas à Kempis' *Imitation of Christ*, still a best seller after 300 years. Never had devotion to the Sacred Heart of Jesus been so strong as on the eve of the Revolution. French

Catholicism would enter the nineteenth century quantitatively diminished but qualitatively purified. As Pius IX later said: "There were fewer Christians, but they were better Christians."[211]

Doubtless Pius IX would not have considered the Jansenists "better Christians," yet by 1781, 62 percent of the parishes in Paris had *appelant* priests and *curés* at their head. To replace the Jansenist-hating Christophe de Beaumont (who died in 1781), Louis XVI chose Antoine Le Clerc de Juigné as the new Archbishop of Paris. Praised for his conciliatory and benevolent nature, de Juigné steered a middle course, seeking to placate both the *constitutionnaires* and the *appelants.*[212]

By the 1780s, the Jansenists themselves had passed from the camp of the *devôts* to that of the *politiques*, becoming "apostles of tolerance" willing to champion religious freedom even for French Protestants and Jews. If Antoine Arnauld had applauded the Revocation of Calvinists' rights in 1685, a century later, the *appelants* regretted Louis XIV's persecuting policies and denounced forced worship. Seeing the Huguenots as their "separated brothers," Jansenist writers took up their pens to advocate granting them civil rights. Following Maultrot and Tailhe's *Essay on Christian Tolerance* (published in Geneva in 1758), Clément de Boissy, Robert de Saint-Vincent, Charles Adrien Le Paige and others argued that Louis XVI should follow the example of Emperor Joseph II of Austria in granting French Protestants their full legal rights.[213]

Saint-Vincent, exclaiming that "those who destroyed Port-Royal are the same ones who persecuted the Protestants," directed the campaign to persuade the king to issue the Declaration of 1787 restoring the Reformed to full French citizenship.[214] Not all of his Jansenist colleagues agreed with him, however. For the opposition, *parlementaires* A.-A. Clément de Boissy and J.-J. Bonnaud argued that such an edict would harm the Church and be useless to the state. Granting Protestants (and Jews and Muslims) civil toleration would "unleash a deluge of errors" on France because these religious groups were "seditious, republican, and anti-Roman Catholic." Both asserted that the current de facto toleration (recognizing Protestants' marriages, protecting their property, abolishing penal laws against them) was sufficient; anything more would "allow the camel's nose to enter the tent."[215]

At least one writer in the *Nouvelles Ecclésiastiques* argued that the camel deserved to enter the tent. Granting equality to Protestants demonstrated "zeal for the public good, good faith, and good sense," he declared. Civil toleration, which "follows reason & justice," would bring positive benefits not only to the Reformed but also to France. Furthermore, such civil toleration should be extended to the Jews as well.[216]

The *abbé* Grégoire wholeheartedly agreed. A nominal Jansenist, post-millennialist, and political activist, Grégoire opposed Negro slavery and championed civil equality for Jews. He belonged to a group whose millennial beliefs assigned a key role to the Jews at the end of time. Based on their interpretation of certain Old Testament prophecies, these neo-Jansenists tried to reconcile God's old covenant promises to Israel with Christian belief in a Messiah. They concluded that the True Church would include not only Catholics but also Jews, who, once they converted to Christianity, would reorganize this new church to focus on preaching, prayer, and charitable acts. Although Grégoire did not totally agree with this group's eschatology, he prayed regularly for the Jews' conversion and worked diligently to improve their legal conditions.[217]

During the 1780s, the *Nouvelles Ecclésiastiques* also demonstrated its more tolerant stance by championing the cause of Jews, Protestants, and other persecuted groups and individuals. Appearing regularly each week in French, and after 1784, in German as well (from Vienna), the newspaper's double column, four-page issues comprised 208 pages in each annual edition. For the first time in its history, reports from across Europe nearly equaled the space devoted to French religious news. Of its 1,175 news notes, 613 (52%) came from France and 562 (48%) from Europe and around the world, including new venues like St. Petersburg, Prague, Harlem, and Bonn. The editors also reprinted excerpts from an enormous array of French and foreign journals. These included the *Gazette Française de Cologne*, the *Journal de Paris*, the *Journal de Luxembourg*, the *Journal de Monsieur*, the *Journal des Savants*, the *Journal Historique et Littéraire*, *L'Année Littéraire*, the *Gazette Universelle*, the *Gazette Française de Vienne*, and the *Annales Ecclésiastiques de Florence*, to mention a few.[218]

Its authors also devoted considerable attention to several new issues. They rejoiced whenever Jews converted to Christianity (1780, 1781), approved European countries passing laws tolerating Protestants (1784), and supported the Edict of 1787 for the Non-Catholics (1788). They immediately informed subscribers whenever new volumes containing the works of Antoine Arnauld, Bishop Bossuet, and Biship Fénelon (1780–1784) became available. In fact, the pages of the *Nouvelles* contained more notices of recently published articles, theses, and books on Jansenism and other religious issues (46 percent) than it did on news events (45.5 percent).[219]

By the 1780s, the embers of Jansenist hatred for the Jesuits and the philosophes were also beginning to cool as the number of news notes referring to these two groups diminished. Articles occasionally warned of Jesuit "plots, intrigues, & strategies" (the Order had been "resurrected" in Russia) and rejoiced at their "defeats" (1781) while placing the entire blame for the past persecution of the Protestants firmly in their lap (1788). As the number of column inches devoted to the Society diminished, so did the biased rhetoric, although authors occasionally attacked the Jesuits for their "obstinacy" and their "spirit of error and opposition to all solid reform and useful projects." The paper even labeled De Juigné a "Casuist" and feared that during his term as Archbishop of Paris the "Molinist innovators [would] proudly raise their heads in France."[220]

Regarding the philosophes, the *Nouvelles* condemned "the false principles" and "excesses" of Bouffon, the "anti-Christian Works" of the *abbé* Raynal, and Voltaire's "criminal efforts to overthrow Altar, Throne, Manners, Virtue & Religion." While emphasizing "the danger of their pernicious writings," the newspaper frequently referred to Voltaire, Rousseau, Raynal, and Buffon as "pretended Philosophes" much as the government had once referred to Calvinists as the "pretended reformed religion."[221]

The editorial policy of the 1780s seemed determined to transform even Jansenism itself into a pretended hoax perpetrated by its enemies. Mirroring the very words of Antoine Arnauld a century earlier, authors called it "a chimerical heresy without reality," "the pretended Jansenism," "this alleged Jansenism," and "a phantom." "All sensible people have recognized that the pretended Jansenism is only a phantom created by an ambitious and vindictive Society [of Jesus]," one author wrote in 1788.[222] Consequently, people had nothing to fear from this ghost of the past.

The *Nouvelle's* almost nonexistent coverage of the rapidly changing political scene in France could lull its readers into thinking that they had nothing to worry about. The newspaper showed little or no interest in social, political, economic, or intellectual developments during the last decade of the *ancien régime*. The convoking of the Estates-General to solve the fiscal crisis in France, for example, received only brief mention in four articles in 1789—and the editors were interested only in how the debate related to Church issues.[223] Instead, to the very end of its existence, the "mission statement" of the *Ecclesiastical News* remained "to portray the actual condition of the Church, its evils & its resources, the abuses that disfigure it, the superstitions some seek to introduce into it, & the continual efforts of good Christians to rebuff these."[224]

Nonetheless, if the *Nouvelles* ignored events leading to the French Revolution, individual Jansenists could not, because the political upheaval in France would eventually have an impact on *appelants* not only in France, but also in Spain, Italy, Belgium, and Holland.[225] Yet the nature of that impact has been a matter of dispute among historians for two centuries. The *abbé* Grégoire (1809) claimed that the solitaires, emphasizing the "principles of patriotism" and republicanism in their writings, had been "precursors" of the French Revolution.[226] Nineteenth-century writers such as the historian Jules Michelet and the socialist Jean Jaurès agreed, claiming that a "Jansenist conspiracy" precipitated the Revolution.[227]

Joseph Dedieu (1936) concurred, suggesting that by its attacks on Rome, royal authority, and the bishops, its appeals to a national council, and its alliance with Parlement and the philosophes, Jansenism "undermined throne and altar which had held in check the revolutionary spirit."[228] René Taveneux (1965), who questioned the direct causal link between Jansenism and the Revolution, nonetheless admitted that its political theory could easily take on a "revolutionary character."[229] But Ruth Necheles (1971) argued that the *abbé* Grégoire and the *appelants* were not good "party men" at the time of the Revolution because their rigid adherence to truth forced them to evaluate each political issue on its own merits; therefore, they could never accept any program dictated by others.[230]

Yet Jansenism had nevertheless become a "symbol of resistance," Françoise Hildesheimer (1992) opined, because everyone recognized Port-Royal's historic role in fighting the arbitrary power of popes and kings.[231] Catherine Maire (1998) agreed, adding that one needs to understand this attitude of "passive" or "negative resistance" in order to explain Jansenist actions from 1640 to 1789. But the Richerism within the movement "proved incapable of making a place for a superior echelon in a hierarchy" in order to maintain an equilibrium between the contradictory claims of divine right (pope and king) and those of the Gallican episcopacy. After the Jansenist-led Parlement desacralized the state of its absolutism, it served the nobility, not the *appelant* cause. Consequently, "Jansenism died in the French Revolution" because it "dissolved in its own contradictions."[232]

The Jansenists, William Doyle (2000) asserted, had always been "republicans and heretics." Therefore, they saw the Revolution's break with Rome and the overthrow of Louis XVI as "the revenge of Port-Royal" on the papacy and the Bourbon dynasty.[233] By helping to overthrow the king, David Bell (2001) added, Jansenists assisted in the rise of French nationalism by encouraging "radically new ways of imagining the relationship between the heavenly and terrestrial cities . . . and new ways of imagining the nation."[234] David Garrioch (2002) suggested that because the Jansenists spread anticlericalism, encouraged independence of mind, and made politics relevant to ordinary people's lives, they prepared the stage for the Revolution.[235] Most recently, Jotham Parsons (2004) has stated that the seventeenth-century debate over Gallican liberties pitted Jansenist magistrates against bishops and boosted royal power and each group's reliance on the king's support. But like Humpty-Dumpty in the children's fairy tale, when the king fell, so did all his bishops and the Jansenists.[236]

Realistically, however, it is difficult to claim that the Jansenists "caused" the French Revolution when in fact they did not approve of much that it accomplished. Although the Figurist writer Claude Guénin de Saint-Marc professed to see in the Revolution "the finger of God in a marked and striking manner," others disagreed.[237] The *appelant abbés* Claude Mey and Gabriel-Nicolas Maultrot, for example, denounced the "despotism" of the Constituent Assembly in stripping the Gallican clergy of its property and then attempting to reform it through the Civil Constitution of the Clergy in 1790 (a document some Jansenists helped to write).[238]

Despite these differences, between 30 and 40 Jansenist clergy, jurists, nobles, judges, and lawyers served as deputies in the National Assembly, usually siding with the political left (including the Protestants). Far from being silent observers, Timothy Tacket (1996) has shown that they were some of the most outspoken members of the Assembly. In fact, eight Jansenist deputies gave 95 of the 261 speeches (36 percent) during the debate over the Civil Constitution of the Clergy in 1790.[239] John McManners (1998) agreed, pointing out that the Oratorians (who pioneered the ideas that all men are equal in a state of nature and that kingly power is delegated from the people rather than directly from God) welcomed the collapse of royal absolutism in 1789 and strongly supported the Civil Constitution in 1790.[240] This Constitution implicitly condemned *Unigenitus* and rehabilitated Richerism. It supported several historic *appelant* attitudes and ideals: a hostility toward the papacy, a desire to see the bishops subjected to election, hatred of formularies, the demand for a national representative Church council, and a commitment to the laity's playing an active role in Church governance.[241]

But many Jansenist deputies (and their Protestant allies) feared that the Constituent Assembly might settle for religious toleration rather than religious liberty. In a bold speech reminding his colleagues that toleration had often led to persecution, Rabaut de Saint-Etienne declared:

> But, Sirs, it is not the old tolerance that I wish to reclaim; it is liberty. Tolerance! Support! Pardon! These ideas are supremely unjust to dissidents, to the extent that it will be true that differences of religion and opinions is not a crime. Tolerance! I demand that it be proscribed among us; and it must be, for this unjust word presents to us citizens worthy of pity, as guilty ones whom we pardon.[242]

Saint-Etienne's moving speech helped carry the day. When the Assembly voted in favor of religious liberty, the *Nouvelles Ecclésiastiques* printed its resolution in its pages, including the phrase that "no one must be disturbed for his religious beliefs."[243]

However, the Revolution *did* disturb the Jansenists. Nearly a century after Louis XIV had closed Port-Royal des Champs, the Constituent Assembly suppressed Port-Royal de Paris in 1790 along with all the other convents and monasteries. In an ironic twist of fate, it became for a few months in 1791 the Prison of Port-Libre. After the government abandoned it, vandals looted it in 1792, doing considerable damage.[244] But many Jansenists did some looting of their own. Joining the mob that desecrated the Bourbon tombs at St.-Denis Cathedral, they scattered the royal bones of the kings who had once made life so difficult for them.[245] But the pope, it seemed, would have the final word. While the Terror reigned in France, Pius VI issued the Bull *Auctorem Fidei* (1794), a kind of smorgasbord *Unigenitus* that condemned conciliarism, Erastianism, iconoclasm, vernacular worship, and several Jansenist works. This time, however, there were no appeals to his bull. Instead, the absolutely unthinkable happened: On the orders of Napoleon Bonaparte, First Consul of France, General Berthier invaded Rome and took the pope hostage in 1798. Pius VI died in captivity the following year. Thanks to his bull and those of his predecessors over the previous century and a half, few Jansenists remained to mourn his passing.[246]

Despite Jansenism's comatose state, however, its propaganda machine continued producing issues of the *Nouvelles Ecclésiastiques* every week during the 1790s. But now, for the first time in its history, the newspaper enjoyed legal protection and could operate openly in Paris (at the print shop of M. Le Clère at 254, *rue* St. Martin near the sign of the Bear from 1790 to 1794) and Utrecht (at P. Muntendam's shop on the Place Sainte-Marie from 1794 onward). An annual subscription now cost 12 *livres* (15 *livres* in the provinces), and beginning in 1791, subscribers could purchase a two-volume index for all the back issues from 1728 to 1790.[247]

Its writers reported on ecclesiastical news from every country in Europe, including Protestant England, with special attention given to news from Rome, Italy, the Netherlands, Belgium, and, of course, France. Authors discussed the pontificate of Pius VI (1790), public education (1790), Joseph II's reforms (1791), and commented on the debates in the National and Legislative Assemblies and the Convention (1790–1794). To a greater degree than ever before, writers in the *Nouvelles* debated issues like the abuses discussed in the *cahiers de doléance* (1790), the Civil Constitution of the Clergy (1791–1792), and the religious issues before the Convention (1793).

Although the Jesuits were long gone and the philosophes nearly all dead, a few writers criticized them. Authors alerted readers to Jesuit "plots" across Europe, but their tired warnings lacked the passionate prose of previous years.[248] They attacked the philosophy of Voltaire, Mably, and Rousseau and disapproved of the "honors" that the Assembly heaped on Voltaire.[249]

They had mixed reactions to the reforms of the Revolution. Initially, writers were cautiously optimistic that the delegates to the National Assembly would promote just reforms in the Church and state. In the lead issue for 2 January 1790, the editor remarked: "The events in Paris & all of France over the past eight months are a theatre holding Europe's attention & presenting to the eyes of reason & faith a spectacle worthy of serious reflections." Finding the changes already effected in government "astonishing," he believed that all of this was "God's plan to hold in his hand men and their passions and make them serve . . . his eternal designs." These "eternal designs" included the overthrow of "arbitrary power," the downfall of "blind Ministers," and the "restoration of our Liberties."[250]

But as deputies' words outstripped their actions, one author quipped: "The Revolution in France has transformed our mute prelates, at one blow, into Ambroses and Chrysostoms."[251] Somewhat more optimistic, another writer gushed: "The French Revolution has been achieved; the signal for reunion is given; & the Empire of the Law begins. Thinking is now free."[252] The paper favored the confiscation of ecclesiastical benefices and the suppression of temporal jurisdiction by the Church, seeing in these reforms the promise of religious renewal. Then, beginning in 1793, it carried as its banner headline Article 7 of the Declaration of the Rights of Man and the Citizen and Article 122 of the Constitution concerning freedom of the press, assembly, and worship. From 1796 onward, it used the revolutionary names for the dates on its masthead—although it decried the use of the *decadi* (ten-day week) because "it abolishes Sunday, which is the Lord's day."[253]

Yet as the Revolution turned bloody during the "Reign of Terror," the *Nouvelles* expressed pessimism about its legacy, regretting the Convention's "oppression" of Catholics, bemoaning its attack on Sunday, and predicting a "violent crisis" in the Church if such radical reforms continued.[254] One author exclaimed: "One of the most singular phenomena of our time is that the Roman Catholic religion, which formerly was the only recognized and respected religion in France, seems today to be the least tolerated."[255] When editor Guénin attacked the Convention in 1793, however, he was forced to flee to Holland for safety.[256] The loss of editorial anonymity certainly had its drawbacks.

In conclusion, as Jansenism spread out after 1750, Jansenists became more strident as a "party of opposition." Jansenist *parlementaires* opposed Archbishop de Beaumont during the refusal of the sacraments controversy and remonstrated against Louis XV's challenges to their judicial sovereignty. They played a leading role in the suppression of the Jesuits in the 1760s and in the Maupeou crisis of the early 1770s. Paradoxically, despite their hostility toward the Enlightenment, by the 1780s, they advocated equal rights for Protestants, Jews, and Negroes. Some of them (Maultrot, Saint-Vincent, Le Paige, Grégoire), as elected delegates to the National Assembly, taking the side of Protestant members their ancestors would have considered heretics, became outspoken advocates of civil and religious liberty during the French Revolution.

CHAPTER 7

The Shaking of Jansenism: Miracle Cures and the *Convulsionnaires*, 1727–1740

> "[There is] something supernatural in the invincible obstinacy of all these sorts of people [*convulsionnaires*], including those who are the dregs of the populace, from whom we cannot extract the least confession nor the smallest clarification."—*Minister of State Fleury*[1]

As Philippe Loupès (1993) has pointed out, Jansenism was riddled with paradoxes. While on one hand Jansenists preached efficacious grace, practiced asceticism, and promoted charitable works, on the other, their belief that divine healing validated their movement spawned incredulity with its bizarre eighteenth-century offspring of miracles, convulsions, and self-torture.[2] These violent phenomena, arising in the late-1720s, split the Jansenist movement into antagonistic factions. While nearly all *convulsionnaires* were Jansenists theologically (at least initially), few Jansenists embraced the bizarre behavior of the *convulsionnaires*. Because of this huge divide between the two camps, I have chosen to discuss the eighteenth-century *convulsionnaire* movement in two separate chapters.[3]

Because convulsionism emerged from the Jansenist movement, however, that division took some time to develop. Jansenism first had to establish a foothold in Paris. But as we have seen in chapters 5 and 6, the *appelants* gradually began taking over leadership positions in many parishes. Between 1653 and 1662, at least 38 of the 68 *curés* (56 %) in the city were either Jansenists or sympathetic to Jansenism.[4] From 1669 to 1730, the parishes with the highest concentration of *appelant* priests included St.-Merry (100%), St.-Séverin (84%), St.-Roch (77%), St.-André-des-Arts (74%), St.-Germain-l'Auxerrois (73%), St.-Etienne-du-Mont (72%), St.-Laurent (71.5%), St.-Gervais (71%), St.-Médard (61.5%), and St.-Jacques-du-Haut-Pas (46%). These ten parishes clustered around the Ile-de-la-Cité and the Ile-St.-Louis district along the left and right banks of the Seine.[5]

Other parishes with significant concentrations of Jansenist priests (but under 50%) included St.-Benoît, Ste.-Marguerite, St.-Germain-le-Vieux, Ste.-Marine, St.-Landry, St.-Leu, and St.-Jean-en-Grève. In addition, the faculties at the colleges of Ste.-Barbe and Harcourt and the staff at the convents of Ste.-Agathe and Ste.-Pélagie contained many Jansenists.[6] According to a 1739 list sent by Nicolo Lercari, intermediary to the papal nuncio to France, to Cardinal Firrao, secretary of state at the Holy See, 13 (31%) of the 42 parishes in Paris were *cattovo* ("bad" or Jansenist), another 4 (9%) were *equivoci* (suspected of Jansenism), while 25 (60%) were rated as *buoni* ("good" or orthodox). In addition, 4 (9%) of the 36 colleges in Paris—Boissy, Ecossois, Cambrai, and Ave Maria—had Jansenist directors or faculty suspected of Jansenism. Finally, Lercari reported that 26 of the city's 200 printing establishments (13%) were operated by known Jansenists, primarily in the parishes of St.-Séverin and St.-Benoît.[7]

Collectively, Church leaders in these Jansenist parishes exhibited many similar characteristics. They came from similar social backgrounds (38% from the robe nobility, 35% from the upper bourgeoisie); most (75%) had graduated with theology or law degrees. They shared a conservative organizational philosophy, made serious attempts to systematize record keeping, and enforced strict financial accounting procedures. As would be expected, these clerics lived ascetic lifestyles, gave liberally to charities, and promoted education. By and large, they upheld higher standards for the moral conduct of their parishioners, especially for those participating in the sacraments, than did priests in non-Jansenist parishes.[8]

Yet the phenomenon known as *convulsionism* sprang, not from the wealthiest Left Bank parishes, but from six of the poorest Jansenist centers on the Right Bank: St.-Germain-l'Auxerrois (24 *convulsionnaires*), St.-Médard (24), St.-Etienne-du-Mont (17), St.-Gervais (15), St.-Jean-en-Grève (13), and St.-Nicolas-des-Champs (12). Likewise, 50 of the 116 (43%) reports of healing miracles came from eight lower class Right Bank parishes: St.-Eustache, Ste.-Marguerite, St.-Paul, St.-Germaine-l'Auxerrois, St.-Gervais, St.-Jacques-de-la-Boucherie, St.-Roch, and St.-Jean-en-Grève. Taken together, this phenomenon represented what Catherine Maire (1998) has called the "democratization" of Jansenism.[9]

The man indirectly responsible for the rise of convulsionism ministered quietly to the poor in the parish of St.-Médard in the poverty-stricken district of St.-Marceau, which the peripatetic observer Louis Mercier described as

> the quarter where the poorest people live, where the restless and most undisciplined of the capital dwell. There is more money in a single household in Saint-Honoré faubourg than in the whole agglomeration of Saint-Marceau. There hide the misfits, misanthropes, alchemists, maniacs, and several studious ones who seek solitude. These are a people who have no contacts with polite society on the banks of the Seine.[10]

In this poverty-stricken parish centered around the St.-Médard chapel lived a young deacon destined to become a Jansenist folk hero beloved for his piety, humility, penitence, liberality to the poor—and for the miracles that occurred at his tomb.

François de Pâris was born on 30 June 1690 to Nicolas de Pâris, a counselor in the Second Chamber of Inquests at the Paris Parlement, and Charlotte Roland, beloved for her kindness, affability, piety, and ascetic lifestyle. As the eldest son of a distinguished robe family whose magisterial roots stretched back nearly two centuries, François grew up amidst wealth, comfort, and the best that French education had to offer. From age seven to ten, he was tutored in Nanterre by Augustinian canons; they loved this "sweet scholar" who slept on a bed of straw and bemoaned his peccadilloes as if they were great sins. Destined to follow his father into Parlement, François at ten entered Mazarin's College of Four Nations to study philosophy, theology, and law.

But finding greater pleasure in reading the Bible, praying, and weeping over his sins, he ran away to join the Benedictine Congregation of St.-Maur at sixteen. His angry father rescued him and forced him to continue his legal studies. At 22, following an attack of smallpox that left his face horrible scarred, he lost interest in worldly things and longed for solitude. Against his parents' wishes, François transferred to the Jansenist Seminary of the Virtues at St.-Magloire to study theology and to pray. In August 1713 his life changed dramatically when he decided to give his annual family pension of 10,000 *livres* to the poor in the parish of St.-Jacques-du-Haut-Pas where he taught children's classes.

In June 1715 he became a tonsured monk and began studying Greek, Latin, and Hebrew to better understand sacred history and theology. After being promoted to sub-deacon and then canon at Reims in 1718, he left to attend the College of Bayeux, where he followed an austere lifestyle and sheltered persecuted Jansenists. There he taught the youth of St.-Côme from the Gospels and St. Paul's epistles and distributed most of his income as alms to the poor. In 1720 he was nominated as a deacon with promises of making him *curé* of St.-Côme, but he refused the honor, citing his unworthiness. When his parents died in 1723, François sold the family property, gave the money to the poor, and retired on a quarterly pension from his brother Jérome-Nicolas (a councilor at Parlement) to the *faubourg* St.-Marceau to live as a hermit among the poor he loved.[11]

Refusing the position of *curé*, he moved into a humble dwelling on the *rue* des Bourguignons close to Val-de-Grâce chapel (where the hearts of the Bourbon kings rested in porphyry urns) and near St.-Médard chapel in the heart of Jansenist territory. An *appelant* himself, Pâris saw the Bull *Unigenitus* as "the work of the devil" and protested against it in 1720. Like the solitaires, he lived with three or four men who assisted persecuted Jansenists. Here, in one of the capital's poorest districts, noisy, smelly, and over-crowded with grubby tanners and brewers, shopkeepers and traders, manufacturers and peddlers, the deacon ministered both to the spiritual and physical needs of his flock, who called him "Monsieur François." He helped them clean the streets and alleys, carried buckets of water to their homes, and knitted wool stockings to keep them warm in winter.[12]

Perhaps to atone for his privileged birth and many sins, Pâris increased the severity of his already ascetic lifestyle. Feeling unworthy, he refused to partake of communion from 1723 to 1725. He seldom left his tiny room except to attend services on Sundays and feast days; visitors infrequently darkened his doorstep. The *abbé* Nicolas Pommart, his spiritual advisor, forced him to sing in the choir at St.-Médard and to train younger clergy for holy orders. His bare feet became cut and bruised from walking on the paving stones in the course of fulfilling these duties. He slept on an old armoire, covered himself with a sheet bristling with iron wires that tore his flesh, arose at four every morning and retired at ten every evening. He wore a hair shirt, a spiked metal belt, and a chain around his right arm. He beat himself with an iron-tipped lash until the blood ran down his back. He lit no fire for warmth even during the coldest winter days. His diet of one meal a day consisted of bread, rice, and cabbage or vegetable soup prepared without seasonings, with bread and water for fast days and meat only at Christmas, Easter, and Pentecost.[13]

His body, tortured, undernourished, and overworked, rapidly deteriorated under the strain. Exhausting pilgrimages in 1726 and 1727 sapped his meager strength. By April 1727 he had developed a tumor on his knee and suffered from a high fever and severe gastrointestinal pains. Obeying a physician's order to get some rest, Pâris retired to his bed, nourished only by marmite boiled in water and his medicine, which he took every half hour. His brother Jérome visited him twice as he lay dying. François had the holy viaticum performed over him on Friday, May 1, at the same hour as Christ had died on the cross. He died in agony that evening just short of his thirty-seventh birthday.[14]

Ascetic even after death, Deacon Pâris requested a charity funeral without candles, bells, or wall hangings in the little chapel of St.-Médard. The burial of "the blessed Pâris" (as people were already calling him) in the cemetery (he refused to be buried in the chapel) on Sunday, May 3, cost the parish a mere 25 *livres*.[15] Scores of people from all over the capital—nobles, bourgeois, and laborers—attended his funeral service. "If angels could get sick and die," one remarked, "they would become ill & die just like he did."[16] As his body lay in state, shopkeepers, artisans, and laborers filed past, touching his corpse with rosaries, icons, bits of cloth, and devotional books. Bolder ones seeking relics snipped pieces of his hair and fingernails, threads from his clothing, wooden splinters from his casket, dirt, grass, and stones from his grave site, and fragments of his desk, bed, and armoire. Much to the chagrin of Church officials, these souvenirs became holy icons to *curés* and commoners alike.[17]

Revered as a martyr and saint, Pâris' grave soon became the site of pilgrimages. Bending to popular pressure, the pro-Jansenist Cardinal Noailles (who had himself attended Pâris' funeral) secretly began procedures for his canonization in 1728, but died without completing them in

1729. His successor, Archbishop Charles Gaspard de Vintimille du Luc, who opposed Jansenism, quickly halted the beatification process.[18]

To show his respect for his brother's memory and better mark his resting place, Jérome-Nicolas de Pâris erected a large rectangular slab of black marble raised on four stone supports over the grave in March 1728. Its Latin inscription, composed by the Jansenist Doctor of Theology Jandin, praised François as "one who employed his life in the service of God" and who had been "full of the Holy Spirit." His "rare piety" and "divine science" had made him a "model clergyman" full of faith, hope, and joy—"an innocent victim of penitence."[19]

But in the minds of Jansenists, Jesuits, and skeptics alike, Deacon Pâris' tomb soon became far more than the grave of a pious ascetic who had died in the odor of sanctity. Even the skeptical Voltaire recognized its significance as "the tomb of Jansenism in the minds of all honest people."[20] In his final "Profession of Faith," a spiritual testament dictated just days before he died, Pâris had outlined his theological views for posterity. In its pages, he denounced *Unigenitus* and the Jesuits as the authors of all the evils in the Church and encouraged the faithful to propagate the writings of Jansenist authors, especially those of the solitaires at Port-Royal des Champs.[21] This testament reflects the views expressed in his earlier *Compendium of Dogmatic and Moral Theology*, composed in 1714 when he was 24. The *Compendium* emphasizes his Gallicanism, his belief in the predestination (to heaven or hell) of all humanity, and the efficacious grace God grants to infants who die without baptism, to infidels beyond the pale of the Gospel, and to unrepentant sinners.[22]

Of much greater interest to his growing band of followers, however, were the deacon's many prayers to the Trinity. Invoking love, unity, peace, perfection, spiritual transformation, as well as poverty, humility, patience, hope, mercy and love for the truth, these beatitudes found their way into print and became a treasured legacy of his life and teachings.[23] Such pious prose soon inspired his admirers to write their own prayers in his memory. Only weeks after his death, Jansenists composed verses invoking his blessing, intercession, and healing ministry in their behalf.[24] One such prayer, addressing the deacon as "my holy protector, faithful child of the church . . . martyr of penitence," rejoices that although Pâris "has left us," he "has not abandoned us," but intercedes to help those who call on him.[25] Another lengthy petition filling thirteen pages gives homage to God, the angels, and the saints of all ages, including "the Holy Deacon [François] de Pâris."[26]

This popular adoration soon created a pious industry praising his merits. At least two hymns were composed in his honor ("Hymn to the Glory of the Blessed Pâris" and "Prayer to God by the Intercession of the Blessed François Pâris"). Two portraits were commissioned showing him as a saint with a dove over his head and the motto: "I will cover his enemies with shame and confusion and his crown will always flourish and never wither." Loyal followers discussed his life in hotels and salons and defended his teachings against the attacks of his Molinist opponents who considered him a "stubborn heretic" and even "an idiot" who filled his writings with "falsehoods and errors."[27]

By 1731 three biographies (or hagiographies), sold exclusively by 35 colporteurs in the streets of the capital, had been published by J.-L. Barbeau de La Bruyère, Barthélemy Doyen, and P. Doyer. Barbeau de La Bruyère's biography praised the deacon as "a great gift given to the church in these last days." Pâris had been "a great Saint in our century" and "the John the Baptist of our time."[28] Drawing on original documents and memoirs, Doyen's more detailed biography sought to prove that Pâris' sanctified life demonstrated not only God's approval of him, but also the righteousness of the *appelant* cause in its battle with Jesuits, Deists, atheists, and libertines.[29]

But the most frequent reason for invoking the humble deacon's name after 1727 was the expectation of miraculous healing. From its beginnings, this belief in miracles had played a significant self-justifying role both in Roman Catholic teachings in general and in Jansenist thought in particular. Before the Protestant Reformation began in 1517, miracles were so common and widely accepted that few Church officials kept written records of them. The Council of Trent (1545–1563), however, ruled that henceforth, bishops must hold formal investigations and compile declarations proving the divine origin of miracles. By the mid- to late-seventeenth century, amid a growing climate of skepticism and rationalism, Deists, philosophers, and scientists began raising doubts about the divine origin of such alleged cures as the "Miracle of the Thorn" (1656) at Port-Royal de Paris (see chapter 3).[30]

The Jansenists, however, never doubted God's ability and willingness to work miracles in the modern world. The same God who had healed the sick and resurrected the dead during the Apostolic "Golden Age of marvels and miracles" would, they believed, perform miracles again in the eighteenth century to comfort the afflicted (the *appelants*) and afflict the comfortable (their Jesuit enemies). As we have seen, nearly every time the Church or state officials threatened the Jansenists, healing miracles occurred to demonstrate the righteousness of their cause.[31] Miracles, which were "events contrary to nature," proved the Creator's "sovereign domain" over natural law.[32]

According to Antoine Arnauld, they proved much more than that. In his book *On the Authority of Miracles* (written after the "Miracle of the Thorn"), he states that miracles "provide solid proof of the veracity of doctrine to those who have not yet examined the doctrine." Citing patristic writings, ecclesiastical histories, and personal experience, he declares that genuine healing comes only from God.[33] Throughout his writings, Arnauld asserts that God never performs "true miracles" for "imposters," non-Catholics, or "the enemies of Port-Royal." Therefore, his cures demonstrate not only his divine authority and prove the veracity of his word, but also validate the innocence and orthodoxy of those healed.[34] Nonetheless, he cautions in *Frequent Communion* (1643), "God has not desired . . . that this great abundance of miracles that appeared at the birth of the Church should last forever."[35]

But Arnauld's eighteenth-century Jansenist descendants hoped he was wrong. One anonymous *appelant*, in the "Relation of Several Miracles Effected by the Intercession of the Blessed François Charines, *curé* of the Parish of La Tourette," listed four "Principles of Miracles." (1) God communicates his will through miracles, which (2) demonstrate his approval of the Christian Church and (3) of Catholic doctrines as well as (4) his disapproval of heretical sects (such as the Protestant ones) for whom he works no miracles. Jansenism, with its emphasis on grace, truth, millenarianism, and first-century purity is proved genuine by the healing miracles that show God's approval for the *appelant* cause.[36] After the healing of Marguerite Périer at Port-Royal in 1656 (see chapter 3), for example, the same thorn allegedly healed 80 more individuals in Paris.[37]

Unfortunately, the Jansenists' inward focus and desire for "signs and wonders" to validate their cause left them susceptible to miracles of any kind.[38] But the more cautious recognized that supernatural phenomena could be either divine or demonic. Some 40 years before the healing of Périer's eye, an outbreak of convulsions had occurred at Amou near present-day Acqs. This "sickness of Layra" struck 80 women and 40 men in 1613 with muscular contractions similar to epilepsy, leaving them rolling on the ground, beating the earth with their hands and feet, cutting themselves, and barking, whistling, mewing and braying. At the time, Church officials, blaming demonology, sought to exorcise the devil from these poor souls.[39] Although this outbreak bore no direct relation to Jansenism, the similarities between the "sickness of Layra" and the convulsions soon to occur in St.-Médard Cemetery no doubt prejudiced the minds of some officials who refused to accept the Jansenists' claim that these miracles came from God. After all, the term *thaumaturge* meant "a person who makes miracles"—and that "person" could be inspired by God, the devil, or their own selfish inclinations.[40]

The *appelants*, of course, gave God the credit for every miracle, healing, or convulsionary experience connected with the death of one of their own. And as officially sponsored persecution increased after 1679, so did the frequency of these healing phenomena. When Bishop Félix Vialard of Châlons (who had given his approval to Quesnel's writings) died in 1680, his tomb became the center of at least 40 healing miracles, duly witnessed by physicians and surgeons.[41] Several miracle cures allegedly occurred after the exhumation of corpses from the cemetery at Port-Royal des Champs in 1710–11 and their transfer to the cemeteries of St.-Jacques-du-Haut-Pas, St.-Etienne-du-Mont, and St.-Médard in Paris. At all of these sites, Jansenists reported healing miracles on the tombs of St.-Cyran, Mme. de Longueville, Racine, Boileau, Pascal, Nicole, and Le Maître de Sacy.[42] Even in distant Amsterdam, rumors had it that some had been healed of serious illnesses at the tomb of Pasquier Quesnel in 1719.[43]

As the controversy over the Bull *Unigenitus* grew hotter from 1713 to 1731 (see chapter 5), so did the frequency of healings and convulsions in and around Paris. To the embattled *appelants*, these phenomena provided tangible proof that God was blessing their cause. Their testimonies to that effect, filling thousands of manuscript and printed pages, were scattered like the leaves of autumn throughout Paris and the provinces.[44]

In Paris, these alleged miracles actually began two years before Deacon Pâris' death. In the parish of Ste.-Marguerite, Anne Charlier, 45, claimed that she had been healed instantly on 31 May 1725 of a bloody flux she had suffered for 20 years as she followed the Fête-Dieu procession. For many, this proved not only that the Holy Spirit was active in that parish, but also that the Jansenist cause Charlier espoused was right.[45] Later in July, healing miracles occurred in the Church of Ste.-Geneviève, and in November and December, several individuals claimed healing at the tomb of Monsieur Sauvage, an *appelant* priest of Boulogne. In January 1727, Archbishop Barchman and 170 witnesses testified to the immediate healing of a 45-year-old woman afflicted for twelve years with numerous illnesses. In March, *Père* Celoron of Lyons publicized the supernatural healing of a blind three-year-old who now could see.[46]

As the wave of cures increased, reports of miracles across central France began pouring into the capital. During the 1720s, the sick and infirm testified of being healed at the tombs of the *abbé* Desangins, the *abbé* Levier, the Bishop of Senez, the *duchesse* de Rochechouart, the marquise de Vieuxpont, and the prophetess Gabrielle Moulère. At the tomb of Deacon Gérard Rousse in Reims, several Jansenists claimed to have received instant cures in 1727. Thus, between 1725 and 1727 in Paris and the Ile-de-France, a surge of supernatural phenomena defended by the Jansenists as providential had already whetted the public's appetite for more miracles. Given the Deacon Pâris' ascetic life and pious death, it was only natural that his followers should anticipate similar miracles as they gathered around his grave.[47]

Yet before Deacon Pâris' death made St.-Médard a holy site for pilgrims, the parish had earned a rather unsavory reputation as a center of scandals. A 1726 letter from Inspector Guillotte to police chief Hérault indicated that "for a long time," the police had been arresting individuals near the chapel for indecency, immodesty, and "insolence in the sanctuary" (men had been chewing and smoking tobacco and behaving lewdly with girls and women). In June, agents armed with *lettres de cachet* had arrested four "bad spirits" inside the chapel itself.[48] To evaluate the alleged miracles at Pâris' tomb and the convulsions that followed, it is essential to keep in mind the Jansenists' belief in miracles as self-authenticating, previous patterns of supernatural phenomena in France, and the unsavory reputation of the St.-Marceau district and of the St.-Médard Cemetery in particular.

To the delight of François Pâris' friends and of Jansenists in general, the first miracle occurred during the deacon's funeral on May 3. As she knelt beside the grave, Louise Madéleine Beignet (or Beigney), 62, whose right arm had been paralyzed for 25 years, touched his coffin and experienced instant healing. Word of this event spread like wildfire around the city, and soon Pâris' grave became the foremost pilgrimage site in the capital. The sick came and lay on the black marble slab, while their attendants crowded around to pray, sing, recite passages from devotional books, and watch for miracles.[49] As the "Miracle of the Thorn" had shielded Port-Royal from destruction in 1656, the alleged healing of Louise Beignet infused Jansenism with new life.[50]

Although 39 alleged miracles occurred at St.-Médard from May 1727 through 1731,[51] only fourteen of the individuals involved were certified as incurable.[52] Nine of these deserve closer examination due to their notoriety and the claims made for their authenticity. The complete healing of Louise Beignet's paralyzed right arm on 3 May 1727 was recorded by notaries at the Châtelet court in Paris a few days later. Similarly, the wool carder Philippe Sergent, whose rheumatism and paralysis in his right arm rendered it completely useless, had sought assistance from physicians, surgeons, and hospitals for years without finding a cure. Near death, his skin turning blue, he came to St.-Médard in July 1731 and felt strength "rush" into the muscles of his arm. Physicians at the hospital at Bicêtre verified his complete recovery.

The Demoiselle Thibault (65), whose paralyzed body for years had swelled up with dropsy so bad that her ulcerated fingers appeared soldered together, had also sought the help of surgeons in vain. But before a crowd of witnesses at the cemetery, she was healed so completely that she jumped about and climbed stairs like a child, much to the amazement of the six surgeons who examined her and found no paralysis in her joints. A similar experience happened to the Demoiselle Hardouin, whose first stroke in 1725 had left her legs and left side partially paralyzed, but who by 1731 was totally paralyzed, unable to walk or talk. Near death and desperate, she had a surgeon take her to the cemetery on a stretcher. When laid on Pâris' tomb on 2 August 1731, her body twisted with convulsions, but soon "tranquility, repose, and peace replaced the violent tremors." Then before a crowd of onlookers, she walked back to her carriage.

But one did not have to be French or a Jansenist to be healed. Alphonse de Palacios, a Spaniard blinded by an accident, had sought the aid of Europe's leading oculists, but to no avail. On 1 July 1731, however, while kneeling at Pâris' tomb, his sight was restored and he spent the entire night writing about his cure. Marie-Anne Le Franc (67), a Protestant whose left side was paralyzed and who for 28 years had suffered from violent convulsions, high fevers, chest pains, and partial blindness, had been released from the Hôtel-Dieu as incurable. Twice before she had visited the Deacon's grave, but not until her third visit on 13 June 1731—and while she prayed for her mistress' recovery—did her own paralysis leave her before a crowd of witnesses. Praising God, she walked from the cemetery and began reading without glasses. Because Archbishop Vintimille and her brother, the *abbé* Le Franc, denounced her as a fraud and her healing as a hoax, Anne had a written copy of her experience signed by witnesses, physicians, and a notary, and filed an *appel comme d'abus* at the Parlement of Paris. Soon, her alleged miraculous recovery became a national *cause célèbre.*

On the other hand, not everyone who came received instantaneous healing. Marguerite-Françoise Duchêne, a physician's nightmare with ruptured blood vessels, inflamed tumors, apoplectic fits, and daily bloody vomit, experienced progressive healing during her visits to the cemetery between 16 and 21 July 1731.

Yet some experienced healing without going to the cemetery at all. In 1727, six individuals reported being cured after touching relics that had belonged to the Deacon, after saying novenas to him at home, or after relatives had prayed for them at his tomb. The Demoiselle Coirin, who since 1716 had suffered from breast cancer and paralysis in her side, asked friends to take some of her clothing to the Deacon's tomb and there to pray for her recovery. They did so, returning on 12 August 1731 with fresh soil from his gravesite. As a result, Coirin's cancer disappeared, the paralysis left her, and her limbs gained strength over the next two weeks. Pierre Gautier de Pézonas, who at age five had lost the sight in his left eye, was told by physicians that his condition was incurable. At seventeen he decided, however, to pray to the Deacon Pâris for the return of his eyesight, and during his third prayer in April 1733, his sight was completely restored. After examining the youth, the Bishop of Montpellier wrote to Louis XV describing the amazing cure.[53]

Among others whose cures were witnessed or notarized by officials between 1727 and 1731, many claimed healing from ulcerous sores, tumors, persistent fevers, paralysis, prolonged hemorrhaging, blindness, deafness, arthritis, and rheumatism. Still others came with nervous disorders, psychomotor disturbances, debilitating diseases, infections, disfigurements, fractures, hideous sores, and lingering cancers. Nearly all claimed complete recovery from these ailments within a few days or weeks (most of the cures after 1731 do not appear to have been immediate, unlike those before 1731).[54]

Catherine Maire's (1985, 1998) statistical studies of these alleged cures shows that exactly 50% (73) of the 146 individuals who claimed to be healed suffered from motor skill afflictions (paralysis, rheumatism, gout, epilepsy, convulsions). About 23% (33) had ulcers, abscesses, tumors, and cancers. Another 14% (20) had dropsy or bodily swellings. Approximately 9% (thirteen) had experienced respiratory illnesses, and 4% (seven) had problems with their eyesight. Her analysis of 106 cases in which cures happened shows that in only fifteen cases (14%) did individuals experience immediate healing. In the remaining 91 cases, twelve (11%) recovered within one day, 32 (30%) within nine days, 21 (20%) within eighteen days, thirteen (12%) within 27 days, and thirteen (12%) within 36 days.[55] Nine famous physicians, trained in the medical arts of that day, examined each of these cases.[56]

In the summer of 1731, the trickle of pilgrims to St.-Médard became a torrent. Nobles and *parlementaires*, bourgeois merchants and artisans, rich and poor, young and old, men and women—all crowded into this tiny cemetery to see for themselves if the rumors of healing were true. The flower of the aristocracy—the *princesse* de Rohan, the *princesse* de Conti, the *duchesse* de Montbazon, the *duchesse* d'Antin, the *comtesse* de Grignon, the marquise de La Branche, to mention a few—mixed with the unwashed multitude of laborers and servants who crammed the premises from 5 a.m. to 9 p.m. So did at least a dozen distinguished magistrates, councilors, and lawyers from Parlement, including Charles-Robert Boutin, the high court's president. On 18 August 1731 alone, the police reported 22 pilgrims at the cemetery, including three marquis, one princess, numerous priests and abbots, various gentlemen and demoiselles, and a Jewish banker.[57]

In their recent social histories of Jansenism, Catherine Maire (1985, 1998) and Françoise Hildesheimer (1992) have highlighted the broad social spectrum attracted to Deacon Pâris' tomb. Maire demonstrates that of the 116 who claimed miraculous healing, eight (7%) came from the clergy, 42 (36%) from the bourgeoisie (lawyers, merchants, master craftsmen), and 55 (48%) from the lower classes (tradesmen, apprentices, servants, shopkeepers, day laborers, etc.), with eleven (9%) from unknown backgrounds. In gender, 81 (70%) were women, 23 (20%) men, and twelve (10%) children under seventeen years of age. Among the women, the celibate (39) and widowed (fourteen) outnumbered those who were married (25) by more than two to one. In age, 51 (49%) of the adults were between eighteen and 39 years of age; 27 (26%) between 40 and 59; 21 (20%) over 60; and five (5%) of unknown age.[58]

Hildesheimer's table on the social origins of 606 individuals who experienced convulsions shows that only 100 (16.5%) of them came from clerical backgrounds, including priests, nuns, abbots, and curates. At least 200 (33%) had bourgeois origins (merchants, masters, magistrates, etc.). Another 174 (29%), who came from the lower classes, included tradesmen, artisans, laborers, servants, and peasants. The occupations of 132 (21.5%) are unknown.[59]

By and large then, the alleged miracles at St.-Médard and the convulsions that followed in their wake appealed to a politically unsophisticated, inexperienced, inarticulate populace, providing them with an alternative religious experience outside the Church's control. In the cemetery, the *menu peuple* could vent their inchoate feelings of discontent and alienation from the religious establishment and create "a new sacral community" of *frères et soeurs* united in egalitarian Christian fellowship.[60]

This informal fellowship, however, did not promote a worshipful atmosphere among the tombstones. Simultaneously, as some prayed, others sang, and still others writhed convulsively. A few arrived seeking healing of incurable afflictions; others came to meditate and pray; but the majority came from idle curiosity, seeking diversion and amusement. When Marie-Thérèse de Bourbon, *princesse* de Conti, sought healing from partial blindness, she brought 400 courtiers and friends to pray with her. With so many people milling about, talking, praying, laughing, crying, and occasionally shouting, the atmosphere inside the cemetery resembled the seventeenth-century Parisian "Court of Miracles" in reverse. Whereas that inner city district had transformed perfectly healthy men and women into blind and lame beggars for profit's sake, St.-Médard became famous for making the blind see, the deaf hear, the mute speak, the paralyzed walk, and the diseased healthy again. Soon wagons, carts, and carriages filled the streets around the graveyard; for six *sous*, one could rent a chair and be carried there to see the spectacles. One gentleman from Sens asked the girl who took his money, "Are we going to the opera?" Curiosity seekers packed the adjacent cafés, singing the popular new song "Here a Miracle, There a Miracle!" Adding to the carnival atmosphere, priests and abbots distributed bits of wool from Pâris' mattress and wood chips from his bed, while entrepreneurs hawked manuals of piety, relics, healing drugs, belts, crosses, bracelets, garters, iron bands, and portraits of the Deacon to pilgrims and souvenir hunters alike.[61]

By 1731, these alleged cures and the noisy hullabaloo surrounding them attracted the attention of government and Church officials. Minister Fleury saw the miracles of St.-Médard as nothing more than Jansenist imitations of the visionaries' convulsions in the Cévennes in the 1680s and again during the Camisard War (1702–1705). He perceived in both phenomena an emphasis on bodily shaking, alleged healing, apocalyptic prophesying, and violent reactions whenever the state forbade public assemblies.[62]

For their part, Church officials remained divided concerning the genuineness of these cures. Cardinal Noailles, who had attended Pâris' funeral and later visited his grave, ordered an official investigation into the alleged miracles in June 1728. From the reports he received, Noailles concluded that the cures had been "true and miraculous." When he attempted to publish his findings, however, Keeper of the Royal Seals Chauvelin intervened at the request of Minister Fleury, who thought this might complicate his efforts to reconcile the *appelants* and the *constitutionnaires*. "In times like these," Fleury advised, "it is important to do nothing that might give rise to new controversies and new pamphlets." At Noailles' death in 1729, no official inquiry was underway.[63] After reviewing the same documents, however, convinced that these phenomena came from the devil rather than from God, Archbishop Vintimille issued a mandate on 15 July 1731 condemning them as fraudulent miracles and ordering them to cease immediately. Instead, 70 more cures occurred at the cemetery that year.[64]

The police remained baffled and divided by what they witnessed at St.-Médard. With his spies in tow, Inspector Duval, secretary for police chief Hérault, made regular trips to the cemetery, and recorded the names and behavior of those who visited. These reports described the prayers, songs, speeches, relics, and cures they saw there. Yet in 1731, during the height of the phenomena, three-fourths of Hérault's officers and clerks thought the cures genuine.[65]

Defenders of the alleged miracles naturally viewed them as proof of God's blessing and his approval for the *appelant* cause. Because they saw these amazing cures as self-authenticating events, it proved increasingly easy to recruit new adherents to the Jansenist cause.[66] As early as July 1728, for example, the *Nouvelles Ecclésiastiques* had devoted two full pages to the miracles at Deacon Pâris' tomb, giving the names, ailments, prayers, and detailed accounts of the cures of those who came seeking healing.[67] Throughout the 1730s, the newspaper consistently presented these cures as miracles inspired by God through the intervention of Deacon Pâris. One writer boldly declared in 1733: "The more frequently miracles occur, the more those who want to crush them are faced with contradictions."[68]

If all this noise and confusion were not sufficient to thwart officials' attempts to preserve *le bon ordre*, deeper religious, political, and sociological issues threatened many of the fundamental values of the *ancien régime*. Despite Archbishop Vintimille's 1731 Mandate, a number of *appelant* priests and abbots supported this growing cult. Many clerics not only urged their parishioners to go to the cemetery, but themselves led prayers, said masses, and preached sermons there. A few laypersons, defying their bishops' orders not to honor the Deacon, wrote letters and signed petitions to have him beatified. Tracts and biographies written by religious and secular authors not only swelled the crowds at the cemetery, but also challenged the Church's orthodox position on miracles, *Unigenitus*, and Jansenism. As the emotional level of the debate escalated during the summer of 1731, many grew bored at seeing healing miracles produced "with mathematical regularity." Suddenly, a wave of convulsions broke out at the tomb.[69]

The first documented case involved Aimée (or Edmée) Pivert, 42, a servant from the Place Cambrai in Paris who suffered from a nervous disorder (possibly epilepsy). On 12 July 1731, when her friends laid her on the slab covering Pâris' tomb, she experienced involuntary spasms and contortions in her arms and legs almost (so observers said) as if demon possessed. The severity of her convulsions increased over the next three weeks until she left, allegedly cured, on August 3. A month later, two Parisian girls, a deaf-mute from Versailles and the *abbé* Bescherand of Montpellier, experienced violent convulsions at the Deacon's tomb. Twice a day the *abbé* went to the grave. During these visits his body was wracked by convulsions that lifted him into the air, his face was contorted by grimaces, and foaming at the mouth, he yelled and screamed for hours on end. Police reports described the sight as "terrifying," "scandalous," "diabolical," and "indecent and obscene."[70]

From September through November 1731, as the incidents of convulsions increased, onlookers rented chairs at six *sous* each to gawk in comfort at the moaning, yelling, whistling, caterwauling, convulsing participants. In addition to convulsions, many that autumn broke into versions of the *danse macabre*, twirling around and around until they fell exhausted to the ground.[71] This "theatre of divine miracles" soon filled the surrounding cabarets in the St.-Marceau district as hundreds of pilgrims and amusement seekers crowded into the parish to participate or simply stare at the bizarre phenomena unfolding before their eyes. Since physical convulsions often contorted women's bodies into indecent positions, some clever soul designed the *robe de convulsionnaire* to replace the tightly laced bodices and hoop skirts that prevented females from kicking and jerking.[72]

Why did the convulsions break out in the summer and fall of 1731? Was Deacon Pâris the "spiritual father" of this phenomenon (as Catherine Maire has stated)? To some extent, the answer is the same as why the alleged healing miracles occurred from 1727 to 1731. A strong Catholic and Jansenist belief in miracles; the conviction that these cures were divinely inspired; the argument that any healing, no matter how unusual, demonstrated the truth of Jansenism—all contributed to the descent into the bizarre. Interestingly, the convulsions broke out concomitantly with the issuing of Archbishop Vintimille's 15 July 1731 Mandate declaring the earlier healing of Anne Le Franc to be fraudulent, as if to counteract the Archbishop's influence by producing more miracles.[73]

A more immediate cause of this outbreak can be found in the writings of the *abbé* Etemare, whose prophetic views promoted the ideology of Figurism which saw in the convulsions the tangible mark of God's action on the bodies of the afflicted. Jean-Baptiste Le Sesne de Ménilles d'Etemare, born on 4 January 1682, entered the Oratorian College at Saumur at nine and the College des Grossins in Paris at eleven. He studied under the solitaire Le Nain de Tillemont for awhile before transferring to the College of St.-Magloire at fifteen, where he studied theology. Tonsured at eighteen, he became in 1709 the last priest to celebrate Mass at Port-Royal des Champs before its demise.[74]

Collaborating with other authors, Etemare wrote the *Hexaples, or Six Columns on the Constitution Unigenitus*, an attack on the 1713 Bull. By 1724, he had joined the schismatic party of *appelant* bishops and soon became a leading opponent of the Formulary and a prominent defender of Port-Royal's legacy. The convulsions controversy at St.-Médard freed him of his father's influence and enabled him to be his own man. He led a coterie of 60 men—the *Figuristes*—at his alma mater, the Seminary of St.-Magloire. Although few in number, from 1717 to 1732 these "Figurists" exerted a huge influence on religious and political affairs, especially in eight Paris parishes.[75]

When reports of healing miracles at St.-Médard began circulating in 1728, Etemare at first took a cautious stance. While he did not reject them as fraudulent, neither did he accept all of them as caused by God. For him, "celestial signs" outranked physical signs as proof of divine providence. Perhaps, he suggested, these miracle cures reflected both "the fruit of divine justice and divine mercy."[76]

Yet in his apocalyptic writings, Etemare provided a theological impetus for the convulsions. Salvation, he taught, can be found only within the *appelant* cause, where a remnant, last-day people preach God's true doctrines and prepare the Church for the return of Elijah (whom some identified as the *abbé* Vaillant, then ensconced at the Bastille). Soon, the Jews will be converted to Christianity and the "War on the Beast" (which began in 1730) will end in 1733. This impending anniversary of Christ's death in 33 AD raised many apocalyptic hopes and speculations. Since Deacon Pâris had been "a Jansenist to his fingertips" and since his body had been wracked by convulsions before he died (a phenomenon now repeated at his tomb), the Figurists adopted him as their spiritual father.[77]

Within weeks, this "theatre of spectacular bodily manifestations" had transformed the cemetery and parish of St.-Mêdard into a stage—and an urban battleground—where the quarrel between orthodoxy and heresy could be fought to its bloody finale. In a very real sense, the *convulsionnaire* phenomenon constituted the last great European affair to combine both politics and religion in a mass movement involving both the common people and the elite. Its denouement would mark the end of a world in which religion dominated politics.[78]

From the perspective of the participants themselves, how did it feel to have one's body wracked by convulsions? Marguerite de Roux-Sigy, better known as Sister Antoinette of the Assumption, described her experience this way: "There was not a single organ or nerve or joint in my body that did not feel its peculiar torment. My nerves began to snap." Next, she felt vibrations in her head, teeth, neck, shoulders, stomach, and abdomen. "From there, the convulsions descended to the nerves."[79]

When interviewed at the Bastille, Pierre Lalair told police that although the convulsions seized him "despite himself" and normally lasted 60 to 75 minutes, he could stop them when he wanted to by saying the *miserere* or some other prayer out loud to God.[80] On 27 August 1731, however, when Louise Hardouin experienced convulsions at St.-Médard, her trembling became so violent that even three men could not hold her down. With her "violent agitation" came unrestrained "emotions" and "anguish" that scared onlookers almost to death.[81]

Despite its frightening and bizarre nature, the convulsionist phenomenon spread like wildfire throughout Paris in 1731 and 1732. In addition to the parish of St.-Médard, the police reported outbreaks in the Place Maubert, near the Petit-Châtelet, and at the home of Carré de Montgeron, a major defender of the convulsions.[82] Monsieur Duguet, a police spy who had stated that "there are many more *convulsionnaires* in Paris than people realize," estimated their numbers at 270 (199 women and 71 men) in December 1731.[83] Soon, however, this number grew to between 400 and 800 twitching souls as 4000 people stared in disbelief from the sidelines.[84] Writing a decade later, the skeptical Madame Duguet-Mol cited a popular (but false) rumor that by 1732, Paris had 13,000 *convulsionnaires* running around![85]

Based upon their leaders and peculiar beliefs, the convulsionaries can be categorized into six broad groups. The "Figurists" sought to imitate the moments of Christ's passion, including the cock crowing at his trial, his death on the cross, his last words and cries, and his actual death. The "Visionaries" claimed to have dreams and visions in which they heard Deacon Pâris speak to them about angels and promise God's protection during a coming era of persecution. The "Thaumaturges" focused on healing miracles, especially the restoration of sight to the blind, utilizing dirt from Pâris' grave mixed with water from his well in imitation of Christ's miracles.

Female leaders called "Priestesses" specialized in celebrating the Mass, baptizing and ordaining new believers, hearing confessions, granting penitence, washing their disciples' feet, and speaking in unknown tongues (glossolalia). Those referred to as "Prophetesses" delivered ecstatic speeches concerning the evils in the Church and in individuals' lives and set dates for the future conversion of the Jews and the return of the Prophet Elijah. Finally, those who favored "spiritual marriages" left their spouses to become the partners of other married individuals with whom they professed to have greater spiritual affinity.[86] Regardless of their affiliation, however, the convulsionists called one another "Brother" and "Sister," seeing in each believer a sibling in Christ. In addition, they took new names like "Brother of the Cross," "Brother Blue," "Brother Isaiah," "Brother Innocent," "Little Brother White," "Sister Felicity," and "Sister Zion."[87]

Who were these people who exhibited such bizarre behavior? From what social classes did they come? What was their gender makeup? Léon Séché (1891), in a study of Jansenists from 1710 to 1870, described the movement as predominately a lower-class phenomenon led by women.[88] Nearly a century later, Robert Kreiser (1975) agreed, asserting that the *convulsionnaires* came primarily from the *menu peuple*. However, he added, the movement also included a sprinkling of priests, bishops, regular and secular clergy, robe and sword nobles, merchants and financiers, men of letters and royal functionaries, lawyers and notaries, medical men and theologians.[89] In his study of eighteenth-century religion, Dominique Julia (1991) found that as 70% of those healed at St.-Médard were women, so 65% of the Figurists within the convulsionist movement were also women.[90] Monique Cottret (1998) likewise discovered that working class members—and especially women—predominated in the movement, referring to this phenomenon as the "proletarisation" of Jansenism. Writers in the *Nouvelles Ecclésiastiques*, she pointed out, had argued that the convulsionaries' low social class origins proved the "enthusiasm, elegance, and greatness" of the movement.[91]

Daniel Vidal's (1987) statistical analysis of 564 convulsionists confirmed earlier qualitative studies. He found that of the 384 individuals whose class and gender were known, 231 (60%) were women and only 153 (40%) were men. At the two extremes of the social scale, the nobility represented only 8.5% of the men (thirteen) and 7% of the women (sixteen), while only 7.25% of the men (eleven) and 12% of the women (28) were peasants, domestics, or servants. The upper bourgeoisie (including rich merchants) claimed a larger slice of the men (65 or 42.5%) than of the women (73 or 31.5%). The opposite was true for the lower bourgeoisie and lower classes, which represented only 18.75% of the men (29) but 43% of the women (99). The percentage of male clerics (35 or 23%) outnumbered female religious (fifteen or 6.5%) almost four to one.[92]

Vidal discovered, however, that the gender and social class composition of those who *assisted* in convulsionary activities differed significantly from that of those who hosted such seances (as they called their meetings). Of the 395 helpers whose gender is known, only 87 (22%) were women while nearly four times that many (308 or 78%) were men. Assistants from the nobility represented only 18.25% of the men (56) but 39% of the women (37). The percentage of peasant and domestic helpers at the seances dropped even lower, to 2.75% of men (eight) and 10.25% of women (nine). Upper bourgeois assistants (including rich merchants) represented 26.5% of men (82) but only 18.5% of women (sixteen). Among the lower bourgeoisie and lower classes, however, men (31) comprised only 10%, less than half the percentage (23%) of women (20). Perhaps one astonishing fact that emerged from Vidal's study is that the female convulsionists who tortured and contorted their half-naked bodies relied five times more often on the help of celibate male ecclesiastics (131 or 42.5%) than on the assistance of female religious (eight or 9.25%).[93]

Yet the presence of so many clerics failed to bring healing to most of the afflicted souls at St.-Médard in 1731. In her study of eighteenth-century Jansenism, Catherine Maire (1998) found that of the 170 cases of convulsions at the cemetery, only 27 persons obtained healing while 30 received some relief from their pain; therefore, only about one-third of those who sought help received it.[94] Yet even those who claimed to be healed continued experiencing convulsions afterward: their disease might have been cured, but the trembling continued; it seemed that the convulsions had taken on a life of their own.[95]

As the convulsions escalated, *appelants* who saw God's hand in them took up their pens to defend them before a skeptical public. According to the *abbé* Marc-Antoine Reynaud, the small band of *convulsionnaires* produced some 37,200 separate works, including prayers, supplications, visions, parables, dialogues, figurative ceremonies, letters, songs, canticles, and poems. These writings, some printed, others handwritten, comprise hundreds of thousands of pages at the Archives Nationales, Bibliothèque Nationale, Bibliothèque de l'Arsenal, and in the Fonds Sainte-Beuve at the Bibliothèque de l'Histoire du Protestantisme Français.[96]

Their prose—bursting with figurative images, symbols, and metaphors—focused on three main themes: eschatology (especially the Jews' imminent conversion), figurative word games, and the convulsionists' relation to the monarchy. Like Jansenists in all ages, they loved discussing God, emulating the first-century Church, denying the world's pleasures, defending the truth, reveling in their sufferings, and meeting the attacks of their detractors.[97]

Yet the melodramatic tone, bizarre charm, and comic surrealism of their prose differs markedly from the pious pragmatism of earlier Jansenist writers such as Saint-Cyran, Arnauld, Quesnel, and Nicole. Convulsionist works reflect deep-seated fears and neuroses and a sense of alienation from the world around them. In their letters, poems, and songs, they see themselves as "God's orphans" and the "last-day remnant" in the Church. They alone uphold "the Truth" against the "sophisms" propagated by the Jesuits, Molinists, and *constitutionnaires* who defend *Unigenitus*. Not surprisingly, given the overwhelming number of women in the movement, their image of God is decidedly feminine—"the nourishing One" who suckles her infants. Like adolescents, their rhetoric of the body reveals an intense interest in oral and anal phenomena. At some seances, believers drank beef urine mixed with excrement as if it were coffee and milk; others arched their bodies like a bow, while some women's abdomens swelled up as if they were pregnant. The "Plan of Work" (a convulsionist manual) required believers to manifest convulsions to prove the genuineness of their experience.[98]

Their prayers, however, express calmer aspirations. "The Discourse of a Convulsionist Girl," addressing God as "Spirit, Consoler of our souls," speaks of a desire to "know the Truth." "Shine your light on me that I may love your Truth" is an oft-repeated phrase in *convulsionnaire* literature. Their prose reflects deep-felt emotions. "My cries are begging you for mercy," "embrace my heart with the divine fire of your love," "be not inflexible to my sobs," and "possess my mind and heart" are just a few examples. Beauty, light, heart, humility, innocence, and truth are frequent images employed. On the other hand, ignorance, stupidity, and low birth become virtues among those who will be "fools of love for Jesus Christ."[99]

If their prayers appeared to come from the New Testament, however, their prophetic utterances came straight from the Old Testament. Although the convulsionists never claimed to be prophets speaking God's words, so frequently did they invoke the name of Elijah that it was inevitable that someone—in this case, the *abbé* Vaillant—would claim to be the embodiment of that Israelite prophet. For them, the coming of Elijah (and later, the expulsion of the Jesuits) presaged the conversion of the Jews to Christianity and the Second Coming of Christ to punish the wicked and establish his kingdom on earth. "We wait for him and prepare our hearts to receive him," one prayer stated. "He will reveal holy mysteries to us. Send the prophet to us, Lord."[100]

One key element in Elijah's mission would be the restoration of the Jews to Palestine. Unlike European Catholics, who charged the Jews with deicide (killing Christ), the *convulsionnaires* believed that God would extend mercy to the Jews, who would repent of their past mistreatment of Christians, respond to "the call of Elijah," and convert to Christianity. Then, joining God's last-day remnant, they would repair the mistakes made by fallen humanity over the millennia and help save the current generation (the "wolves" and "dogs") from the future destruction of the world.[101]

The only way to unlock that future, of course, was through Figurism, a philosophy of history based on an elaborate system of types and anti-types (hence the term "figures" and "figurism"). Developed around 1710 by a few dozen "Defenders of the Truth" at the Seminary of St.-Magloire in Paris, this Figurist system of interpreting scripture sought contemporary applications for biblical terms and events. Predicated on a cyclical view of history, it suggested that Old Testament prophecies and events "prefigured" events that would occur either in the Apostolic Church or in the eighteenth-century Church (or both). For the Figurists, history was neither random nor trivial but predetermined and full of eternal significance. They sought the divine correlation between past and present.[102]

Pioneered by Jacques-Joseph Duguet and his disciples the *abbés* d'Etemare and Grégoire, this method of correlating the past and present to find "historical mysteries" attracted many adherents within the convulsionist camp. Like children seeking clues to the location of some buried treasure, Figurists searched their Bibles, trying to grasp the "double meaning" of nearly every Old and New Testament image. Employing this "theology of history," they drew spiritual lessons from the parallels they saw between the Israelites, the Maccabees, and the Jansenists—all of whom represented God's persecuted remnant. They saw the Jesuits as "the mystery of iniquity" condemned by Paul in the New Testament. During a coming time of mass apostasy, a faithful remnant (the Figurists) who preserved the Truth would be delivered.[103]

Theologically, Figurism and Jansenism overlapped in many respects, at least in the beginning. Both, emphasizing the importance of having faith in God, opposed the prevailing pessimism of the predestinarians. Both, wanting to restore the "tie" between heaven and earth, searched for tangible proofs of divine intervention in history. Both, to some extent at least, saw miracles of healing—including those at St.-Médard—as evidence of God's intervention in human affairs.[104]

Yet significant differences divided the two groups. The *convulsionnaires*, who saw history as a seamless robe, identified more with the first-century persecuted Christians in the Roman catacombs. Like those early Christians, the convulsionists lived in "cooperatives," shared their goods together, performed tasks for the common good (like gardening, cooking, cleaning, etc.), and practiced abstinence, austerity, and fasting. Etemare's *Essay Showing Parallels between the Times of Jesus Christ and Ours* demonstrated how the Catholic Church's persecution of eighteenth-century *appelants* paralled the Jewish synogogue's persecution of first-century Christians. The Jansenists, however, seeing a "rupture" between the first and eighteenth centuries, taught a theory based on "two falls": the Church had been corrupted by Constantine in the fourth century and again by the Jesuits in the sixteenth century. The convulsionists found inspiration in examples of sacrifice and persecution among Apostolic Christians, whereas the Jansenists valued the Middle Ages as a time of faith, purity, and unity in the Church.[105]

But by following the Figurist method of biblical interpretation, the convulsionists took the path least traveled and eventually parted ways with mainstream Jansenism. The *abbé* d'Etemare grounded his Figurist methodology in three principles of allegorical interpretation. First, a figure may be singular or represent the same thing (i.e., trees signify people so one tree represents one person, or sheep signify God's church so one sheep represents a single believer). Second, a figure may be literal and represent the same thing as in real life (flowers in the Temple, palms, carved cherubim). Third, one figure or object may have a relationship with another (the church may signify a village with its inhabitants as well as a group of faithful believers; its architects may be its builders as well as its spiritual pastors).[106]

As one might expect, this could lead to endless word games, riddles, and spiritual mysteries awaiting solutions by those savvy enough to crack the code. The *abbé* d'Etemare, one Figurist who certainly had a gift for unpacking "deeper meanings," wrote a *History of Religion Represented in Holy Scripture under Various Symbols* (not published until 1862) to help the faithful decipher biblical imagery. Here, for example, are a few of his Figurist "code words" and their underlying meanings:

Rome	Babylon of the Apocalypse & current Roman Catholicism
Maccabees	Solitaires of Port-Royal des Champs
Esther	the Jews who will be saved
Desert	this present world
Absalom & Leviathan	Jesuits who by probabilities make profits everywhere
Christ's crucifixion	the Bull *Unigenitus* which crucifies the Jansenists[107]

Knowing how to use and interpret these symbols placed one in a rather exclusive spiritual "club" composed of individuals who saw no realistic difference between the past (first century) and the present (eighteenth century). Instead, they reinterpreted the past to fit their needs in the present and also to create a comforting sense of unity between the "here and now" on earth and the "yet to come" in heaven above. Those who supported the St.-Médard miracle cures, who experienced convulsions, and who learned how to decipher the symbolic code contributed to a trend that Catherine Maire has called the "democratization of Figurism." Throughout 1731 and 1732, an increasing number of individuals crowded the St.-Médard cemetery to watch, participate, and learn.[108]

What lessons did they learn in the "seminary of St.-Médard"? First, they learned that miracle cures, attested by reputable physicians, demonstrated God's support for the truth in Jansenism and his disapproval of the evils in the Bull *Unigenitus*. Second, they discovered that, unlike the "diabolical order" of French hierarchical society, God is no respecter of persons; in his "democratic order," he heals women and men, peasants and nobles, poor and rich. Third, in the sick bodies of those who came to the cemetery, they saw tangible proof that a monstrous evil (which the Enlightenment denied) grows like a cancer in the world, that physical rottenness symbolizes the natural sinfulness of the soul, and that death is the diagnosis for all humanity. Fourth, they observed how healed bodies cast off that evil (via convulsions, spit, vomit, blood, urine, pus, or excrement). Fifth, they understood how human bodies could become "foyers for truth," demonstrating the transitory nature of evil which, through the convulsions, could be expunged from the body. Finally, they became convinced that convulsions ("the crucifixion of the body") demonstrated that true healing had taken place and that they could play a role in this collective "oblation of evil" through group solidarity with those who suffered.[109]

This curious blend of religious works, psychodrama and inspired theatre, eschatological prophecies and spiritual allegories, subjectivity and democracy was unique in its intensity, short duration, widespread publicity, social class mix, and the number of testimonies that it inspired. It might have done little harm to anyone had it not been for the progressively violent nature of its physical manifestations.[110] Despite an *arrêt* from the King's Great Council in June 1731 forbidding clerics to assemble at St.-Médard, many priests and abbots continued joining their parishioners there, lending an aura of ecclesiastical approval to the proceedings.[111]

In 1732, as the convulsions became increasingly contagious, men and women, old and young, *appelants* and *opposants* were seized with paroxysms, groans, and screams. They leaped into the air, danced around, swooned, and panted for breath. To prevent participants from hurting themselves, onlookers placed mattresses and cushions on the ground near the tomb. But as the shaking and writhing spread, others were struck down in the chapel, on nearby streets, even inside neighboring houses. Within a matter of weeks the entire parish of St.-Marceau appeared to be afflicted with a cacophony of singing, crying, barking, whistling, prophesying, and convulsing, particularly among girls and women.[112] When Monsieur Humbert, visiting from St.-Jacques parish, cynically inquired why the saintly Deacon did not bring convulsions to men as often as to women, onlookers beat him so badly that the police summoned the Swiss Guard to sneak him out the back gate.[113]

Responding to this growing atmosphere of social and spiritual chaos, officials sought ways to control the situation at St.-Médard. As early as August 1731, the authorities had established in the sacristy of the chapel an "office of verification" to protect the faithful from pious frauds. Staffed by a dozen medical experts, priests, and lay members, the bureau examined everyone who came to the cemetery for healing to determine the nature of their ailments and the effects of their cures. This group also took depositions from eyewitnesses, interviewed relatives and friends, and registered the cures that appeared to be genuine.[114]

This office, in part at least, represented Archbishop Vintimille's response to two requests made in August and October by 23 clerics who wished to have the "noise" (as they called it) concerning the convulsions investigated to determine whether they were genuine or fraudulent.[115] Employing the standard Catholic approach, Vintimille divided true from false miracles on the basis of whether the disease was incurable by known medical techniques and whether a recovery, which could not be attributed to natural causes, followed quickly and completely. On the basis of these tests, the Archbishop declared Anne Le Franc's healing fraudulent since her illness had been cyclical, hydrotherapy treatments had helped her walk before she went to St.-Médard, and some testimonies concerning her healing had been extorted with bribes. But Ann, refusing to accept Vintimille's judgment, asked Parlement to conduct its own investigation in September to restore her reputation.[116]

But appealing to civil authorities created a double-edged sword that could bring either justice or mercy. Since government and Church officials wanted to maintain order in society, the convulsionists should have known that their violent behavior would invite retaliation. During the late summer and fall of 1731, the police, who for months had been taking notes on every thing that happened in the cemetery, decided to intervene and restore order. Writing to Chancellor

D'Aguesseau in August, police chief Hérault described the alleged healing of Anne Thibaut from paralysis as fraudulent due to her severe one-hour beating and suggested that she should be arrested.[117] When fifteen "very violent" convulsions occurred on September 24, causing much turmoil in the parish, police attitudes began to harden noticeably.[118]

Yet not wanting to offend powerful Jansenist supporters, the police held back during the late fall and winter of 1731–32. They also reported that the convulsions bore some positive fruit. For example, Louis Sabinet, a Parisian rake whose drunken, violent behavior kept him in perpetual trouble with the police, had gone to Pâris' grave that autumn to ridicule the participants. Stunned by what he saw, Sabinet converted to Christianity, studied Catholicism with a priest, and devoted his remaining years to charitable works. Similarly, Monsieur Pinault, a skeptical lawyer and scientist who had gone seeking amusement, was seized with convulsions and became a convert, taking the nickname "Brother Peter." Similar stories of scoffers being converted filled police dossiers, causing even hardened law enforcement officers to wonder if there might not be some divine element in these bizarre events.[119]

The *convulsionnaires* answered that question for many when early in 1732 they published attacks against the pope, *Unigenitus*, and certain *constitutionnaire* bishops.[120] In addition, their increasingly aberrant behavior had become not only the talk of the town, but also the leading subject of gossip in the mirrored hallways of Versailles. As the police sent Minister Fleury more reports of the "pretended ill" gaining fraudulent cures, informing him that "everyone goes to St.-Médard all the time," the first minister decided he had heard quite enough about this weird sect.[121] Rumors spread of adults playing with dolls, wheeling toy carts around, barking like dogs or mewing like cats, stomping on Bibles, and babbling in unknown tongues at the cemetery. The police observed women writhing in pain on men's laps while other men walked on their hands. They watched in horror as *convulsionnaires* swallowed pebbles, glass, and hot coals. They were amused by those who whirled around on the balls of their feet while reading Quesnel's *Moral Reflections* for hours at a time. Minister Fleury, however, was *not* amused; he decided the time had come to put an end to this disorderly behavior.[122]

Jansenists themselves split into two camps over the convulsions: those who believed the St.-Médard phenomena to be divinely inspired ("the camp of Truth"), and a growing number who believed they were diabolical ("the camp of error"). Between 1732 and 1734, both sides published over 100 tracts and pamphlets defending or attacking the convulsions, precipitating a theological and metaphysical crisis within Jansenism.[123] Without a doubt, early Jansenists like the *abbé* de Saint-Cyran and Antoine Arnauld would have been disgusted with the convulsions for damaging the cause.[124] Although the *Nouvelles Ecclésiastiques* consistently defended them, the moderate Jansenist Jacques-Joseph Duguet, a consultant editor for the newspaper, condemned them, and by so doing, fell out of favor with his colleagues.[125]

One anonymous pamphlet, "Hypocrisy Unmasked, or Heresy Confounded in False Miracles" (1731), after examining counterfeit miracles of healing through the ages, condemned the St.-Médard convulsions as false. So did many other anonymous tracts.[126] The minor playwright P. Bougeant even included in his drama *The Holy Flushout* a line in Act 5, Scene 8 referring to St.-Médard: "Adieu, the miracle fair! All the merchants have been bankrupted!"[127]

While the *convulsionnaires* maintained that God inspired their cures and convulsions, the Archbishop of Paris saw them as "satanic healing" introduced by "rebellious heretics" to "trouble the Church." The police had also become convinced that these "miracles" were "fakes and simulated frauds." Moreover, a growing number of physicians believed that the convulsions were neither divine nor satanic, but "voluntary movements" on the part of the *convulsionnaires*.[128]

As formerly peaceful, orderly gatherings became increasingly disorderly, tumultuous ones, public opinion demanded that the police crack down. When one young neophyte desiring to join the sect was told to kneel down and don an iron necklace, bracelets, and belt with sharp metal points while assistants beat her over the head, she cried, "But one must be crazy to demand that [behavior]!"[129]

Anti-social behavior coupled with politically subversive ideas also prompted the police to intervene. While the convulsionists never openly attacked the king or the Church, they implicitly represented a growing mood of popular criticism and anti-establishmentarian independence that could not be tolerated in an absolute state. Many of their religious, political, and social ideas were not only incompatible with but also subversive of the most cherished values of the *ancien régime*: order, hierarchy, corporate privilege. By contrast, the "brothers and sisters" who met at Pâris' tomb represented a spiritual liberation, a fraternal, egalitarian society, a kind of "lay republic" every bit as threatening to the absolute monarchy as the seventeenth-century fear of a Huguenot republic had been. Their democratic, congregational polity constituted a serious indictment of the established, hierarchical order in both Church and state. By asserting that the convulsions were divinely inspired, the *convulsionnaires* threw down the gauntlet at the feet of the Bourbon monarchy and its dependent episcopacy, challenging both the king's exclusive power to heal ("the king's touch") and the Church's right to control religious activity.[130]

In so doing, they sparked a vigorous political discourse that offended a widening circle of important institutions and officials, including Louis XV and his ministers of state, courtiers at Versailles, the police, the pope, the Inquisition, and the Archbishop of Paris. By their immoderate words and immodest actions, they had so deeply disturbed the public tranquility, challenged the religious hierarchy, and offended the moral order that Minister Fleury felt compelled to send in the police.[131]

In reality, the police had maintained a visible presence in the cemetery since 1729. Police chief Hérault had posted at least one guard there at all times to observe the events taking place around the Deacon's tomb and to report in detail who came and what they did. While the officers had occasionally arrested peddlers for hawking proscribed items (relics, Jansenist tracts, biographies of Pâris), their presence rarely disrupted the services. But increasingly throughout 1731, police reports described "indecencies" and "scandals." As the guardians of law and order, the police felt that all this indiscriminate touching between males and females and the rising decible levels evinced by convulsions disturbed the public peace and offended the moral order.[132]

Although a few police officers had served as "double agents" both to spy on and to warn the convulsionists of police intentions, civic and religious officials in general had decided by the end of 1731 that there were far more "bad" than "good" convulsions coming from St.-Médard. Spies reported that "under the pretext of having convulsions," women "prostituted themselves" by allowing others to beat and torture their half-naked bodies, after which they preached and prophesied. Their propaganda—which described "seances," "sabbaths," "magical potions," and "flying on the winds"—increasingly blended Jansenist with satanic imagery.[133] In January 1732, Archbishop Vintimille informed Procurer-General Joly de Fleury that if this "fanaticism" were allowed to continue, "religion would be absolutely lost in Paris."[134]

One week later, bypassing Parlement's jurisdiction, Louis XV evoked all cases of alleged miracles at St.-Médard to his Council of State. In addition, he sent Hérault a copy of the 27 January 1732 Ordinance ordering the police to close the cemetery. The order cited "involuntary commotion and agitation" in which there was "nothing convulsive nor supernatural." Such events had "stretched the credulity" of the common people, given rise to "licentious discourse," and caused other "scandals" in the parish. Therefore, the cemetery's gates "will be and shall forever remain closed." All burials within and all assemblies nearby were forbidden. At 4 a.m. on January 29, the residents of the *quartier* St.-Marceau awoke to the sound of galloping horses as a detachment of 20 night watchmen and a horse guard led by the police chief himself surrounded the graveyard. Hérault replaced the cemetery's old gates with stronger ones, posted ten guards, and took the keys with him.[135] Shortly thereafter, someone nailed a handmade sign on the fence: "By the King's orders it is forbidden for God to make miracles in this place." And, as the *abbé* Terrasson quipped, "God obeyed."[136]

Despite these precautions, however, people continued gathering outside its locked gates, especially on May 1 (the anniversary of Pâris' death) and October 4 (the feast of his namesake, St. Francis of Assissi). So on December 3, Louis XV issued another *lettre de cachet* ordering the police to disperse the crowds and forbidding the *abbé* de St.-Médard to bury anyone inside the cemetery without royal permission. In addition, the police closed the chapel, filled in the well, and prevented followers from taking soil samples as relics from Pâris' grave.[137] A year later, the Ordinance of 17 February 1733 also forbade public spectacles of convulsionism.[138] This law had an unintended effect: by scattering the *convulsionnaires*, it encouraged them to meet in private homes and engage in even more violent behavior.[139]

If the government thought that closing the cemetery of St.-Médard would stop the *convulsionnaires* from meeting, it was sorely mistaken. Like self-propagating weeds, the sect multiplied across Paris and beyond. Within a few days, the police found one group of 30 at the convent of Ste.-Agathe, another meeting at the Filles de la Visitation, and a third joining with the Ursulines of St.-Jacques *faubourg*. Soon they had infiltrated the suburbs—Neuilly, Charenton, Vitry, Ecouen, Arpajon, Corbeil, Pontoise—with their anti-establishment attitudes and increasingly aberrant behavior.[140]

Within a few months, cells of *convulsionnaires* had taken root in the provinces at Champagne, Lyon, Accueil, Chapelle-Milon, Eure, Troyes, and Auxerre. Vigorous proselytizing added new members in such far-flung areas as Languedoc, Var, Provence, Metz, Aix, and Toulon. Disciples clustered around leaders like Brother Amable, Canon Boyer, Sister Manon, and Baron Legrand who provided them with visions, healed their illnesses, and preached the conversion of the Jews and the imminent return of Elijah. Far removed from the gaze of the police, members gathered in private homes for two-hour meetings and sang, prayed, convulsed, shouted, and witnessed healing miracles.[141] While most officials frowned on these clandestine enclaves, Charles Joachim Colbert de Croissy, Bishop of Montpelier, believed in their miracle cures and permitted them to continue unmolested despite Minister Fleury's labeling them as "trickery," "demonic operations," and "fanaticism" due to "overheated imaginations."[142]

In this laissez-faire climate when many officials turned a blind eye toward convulsionary activities if they did not disturb the public peace, the number observing or participating in the seances multiplied. From around 270 (211 women and 59 men) in 1732, the number of convulsionists more than doubled to between 600 and 700 in Paris alone by 1733. Beyond the capital, estimates ranged from the marquis d'Argenson's low of 2000, Barbier's guess of around 5000, to 8–10,000 (including 5–6000 participants and 3–4000 assistants), and even as high as 13,000 by late 1733.[143]

In her study of 432 *convulsionnaires* who actively participated in the *secours* (physical tortures), Catherine Maire (1998) found that 341 (79%) of them were males and 91 (21%) were females. In social class background, the percentage of noble women (20 or 22%) vastly exceeded that of men (twelve or 3.5%). On the other hand, male ecclesiastics (150 or 44%) outnumbered women religious (eight or 9%) by almost twenty to one. While very few participants were peasants or domestics (six men or 1.7% and eight women or 8.5%), artisans and day laborers represented roughly a tenth of each group (27 or 8% of men and nine or 10% of women). The two largest occupational groups among the participants were the masters and merchants (46 men or 13% and 23 women or 25%) and those who came from families with legal training (90 or 26.5% of men and 32 or 35.5% of women). Indeed, 70% of the men who participated in the *secours* were well-educated, wealthy professionals—including 52 lawyers and magistrates from the Parlement of Paris.[144]

But the picture changed somewhat when Maire examined the gender and social class backgrounds of all those who attended the *secours*. Now women (366 or 64%) far outnumbered men (204 or 36%). This time the percentage of men (fifteen or 7%) from the nobility basically equaled that of women (eighteen or 5%), although the male clergy (26 or 13%) outnumbered female religious (eight or 2%) by a three to one ratio. Again, few observers were domestics or peasants (nine men or 4.5% and 25 women or 6.5%). Twice as many female artisans and laborers (67 or 18%) attended the meetings as males from those groups (29 or 14%). Women (52 or 14%) from mercantile backgrounds are represented four times more often than male attendees (twelve or 6%) from the same group. But the largest group for men (56 or 27.6%) is that representing legal training (lawyers, *avocats*, magistrates). By contrast, Maire found no women attendees who came from legal backgrounds.[145]

About two-thirds (67%) of the women who led, participated in, or observed the seances were laity from the lower classes; 61% of them had been to St.-Médard to see the cures and convulsions between 1727 and 1732. Half of these women were under 40 years of age. Indeed, given the violent, sexual nature of the *secours*, it is surprising that young people were invited. Children as young as ten to sixteen years of age frequently attended these meetings. One laundry girl was only thirteen; a boy known as "Brother Balthazar" was only fourteen.[146]

With the passing of time, the gender composition at these seances shifted in favor of women, who played significant roles as hostesses, priestesses, preachers, healers, and organizers of the violent *secours*.[147] Many of the former nurse-nuns at the Hôtel-Dieu became celebrated leaders during the violent stage of the movement known as the *grand secours*. They included Sister Brigitte, Sister Félicité, Sister Cécile de la Croix, Sister de la Misericorde, Sister de l'Incarnation, and Mme. Ste.-Bazile.[148] In addition, Marguerite Périer, whose celebrated cure attributed to the "Miracle of the Thorn" in 1656 had already made her famous (see chapter 3), passed away at the height of the convulsionist movement. As she lay dying in 1733, she gazed upon a portrait of her Uncle Blaise Pascal on one wall—and a portrait of Deacon Pâris on the other wall.[149]

Like Périer, the convulsionists idolized Deacon Pâris and in their prayers, they asked for his intercession. But as the 1730s progressed and the movement splintered into dozens, then scores, and finally hundreds of tiny convulsing groups, they badly needed powerful patrons and charismatic leaders to protect, unify, and inspire them.[150] Members of these various sects (collectively known as "Friends of the Truth") gathered in dozens of private homes, hotels, and chateaux at night to elude police. They enjoyed the patronage of nobles like the *duchesse* de Rochechouart, the marquis d'Arbois, the *comte* de Tilly, the *comte* de La Bédoyère, the *comtesse* de Lampsac, the chevalier de Falord, and the retired royal secretary Louis Fontaine, who ate his meals kneeling. Prominent clerics who hosted seances included the priest Gaspard Terrasson, the *abbé* Jacques-Pierre Fleur, *abbé* Guillaume Boizon de La Courance, and even the *abbé* de Voltaire, the older brother of the philosophe François Marie Arouet de Voltaire.[151]

In keeping with their egalitarian nature, *convulsionnaires*, irrespective of social class, education, or wealth, called one another *Frère* (Brother) and *Soeur* (Sister), followed by a first name. Women often adopted the names of Old Testament Hebrew heroines like Ruth, Jael, Esther, Rachel and Rebekah, or took "Port-Royal names" like "Sister Angélique," "Sister Agnès," and "Sister Marie." Others chose more colorful monikers like "Sister Liguete," "Sister Orphelin," "Sister Plaeide," and "Sister de la Crois." Most men selected names of Old Testament Israelite heroes like Jephthah, Joseph, Manasseh, Ephraim, and Abraham, although (oddly enough) some chose names associated with evil and paganism like Cain and Nebuchadnezzar. Others, adopting Christian names, became "Brother Pierre," "Brother Michel," "Brother Thomas," and "Brother

Ottin." In a very real sense, the democratic ideals espoused by Edmond Richer in 1611 and recapitulated a century later by Pierre Quesnel triumphed in convulsionism, in which only "the body of the faithful" possessed dogmatic authority.[152]

For the most part, women served as hostesses for these gatherings and directed the seances, while men preached most of the sermons. With frequent references to Old and New Testament texts, they discoursed on a wide variety of topics, including "The Appearing of the Prophet Elijah," "Elijah's Soon Return to Reestablish All Things," "The Agreement of Fear and Love," and "The Search for Christian Truth."[153]

In the patriarchal society of the *ancien régime*, men took the lead. It should come as no surprise, therefore, that although women hosted and directed the seances, men organized and controlled the various sects around which these scattered convulsionary groups coalesced. Reflecting the names of their founders, these sects adopted names like *Augustinians, Margouillistes, Vaillantistes*, and *Ottinistes*.[154]

The *Augustinians*, for example, took their name from their founder, Jean-Robert Cosse de Montpellier, known as "Brother Augustine." A Jansenist student at the College of Ste.-Barbe and sacristan at the Petit Cordeliers, Montpellier soon became an active *convulsionnaire*. Extremely ascetic and mystical, he experienced convulsions and had eschatological fantasies following a 40-day fast. Allegedly able to heal the sick and paralyze skeptics, he considered himself (illogically) "The Fourth Person of the Holy Trinity." His followers called him "The Precursor of Elijah"; with becoming humility, he called himself "The Servant of the Servants of God." More orthodox convulsionists, however, charging him with blasphemy and sacrilege, called "Brother Augustine" a "ravishing wolf dressed in sheep's clothing" and shunned his group of fanatics as "half-mad visionaries" who perverted Deacon Pâris' legacy in their "synagogue of Satan."[155]

The *Vaillantistes* owed their beginning to the *abbé* Pierre Vaillant, who claimed to be the modern incarnation of Elijah (or *Elie*, from which their other title *Elisiens* is derived). Vaillant, an *appelant* priest from Troyes, had already been arrested, tried in 1726, and imprisoned at the Bastille (1728–31) for publicly opposing *Unigenitus*. At his release in 1731, he gathered some disciples around him at Pignons in Provence and predicted that the end of the world would come in September 1733 to mark the seventeenth centenary of Christ's death. When time proved him wrong, he refocused his energies on converting the Jews to Christianity, even preaching evangelistic sermons on the synagogue steps in Metz. But in 1734, for participating in convulsions and publishing the *Nouvelles Ecclésiastiques* in Paris (where he had 800 followers), the police arrested him and sent him to the Bastille (1734–56) and Vincennes (1756–61) where he died at age 73 after more than 30 years in detention.[156]

This self-proclaimed prophet, who signed his letters "V+J" ("Vive + Jesus" or "Long live Jesus"), continued setting new dates for the Second Coming of Christ, the last in 1747. From his prison chambers, Vaillant issued a torrent of letters and memoirs to encourage his followers (who gathered at the Bastille in 1736 to pray for his release) and to enlighten police chief Hérault concerning Bible prophecies. Some of his works deal with history ("The Secret Memoir on the Conduct of Cardinal de Noailles"), others with theology (with frequent allusions to the mission of Elijah), and still others with prophecy (focusing on apocalyptic themes of the destruction of Jerusalem and the end of the world). He also wrote sermons, homilies, and prayers in Latin and French for his followers ("My Dear Children") to read, as well as personal, diary-like "Reflections" and short spiritual "Lessons" for their devotionals. Only in his memoirs and letters did Vaillant come down to earth, expressing personal feelings (suffering, solitude, hopefulness) and needs (a handkerchief, a caged bird). Although his followers anticipated his resurrection shortly after his death in 1761, Vaillant disappointed them.[157]

Most convulsionary groups, however, did not enjoy the charismatic leadership of such luminaries as "Brother Augustine" and the "Prophet Elijah." Instead, they met secretly in tiny groups led by humble, often anonymous women. The format of their seances changed perceptibly after 1732. Instead of emphasizing prayer, singing, and healing miracles, believers now participated in "spiritual marriages" (which occasionally bore earthly children), encouraged violent convulsions (called "vuls"), and indulged in the *secours* (erotic and violent forms of torture), all of which reveals how neurotic the movement was becoming.[158]

Frequently, young women in their teens, twenties, or thirties served as hostesses, priestesses, preachers, and *thaumaturges* (healers). They staged plays (or tableaux) depicting scenes from Christ's life, the suffering of the martyrs, the conversion of the Jews, and various contemporary topics, and wrote character mimes representing drunkenness, adultery, bigamy, and other "sins of the Gentiles."[159] Both women and men led in "responsive readings" (in which a leader and the audience take turns reading a text) and delivered short "discourses" (usually one to five pages long). These homilies were based on prophecies, parables, prayers, biblical stories, or current events. In style they were simple, often repetitive, and full of symbols and allusions to biblical texts.[160]

Although some groups met in the morning (around 10:30 a.m.) and others in the afternoon (with 2:30 p.m., 4:00 p.m., and 5:30 p.m. being the most popular times), most gatherings took place in the evenings around 6–10 p.m. in order to accommodate the working schedules of the participants. Seances typically lasted about two or three hours. But at the home of five sisters near the Place Maubert, the "Elect of God" (who enjoyed prophesying, studying divine mysteries, and engaging in violent convulsions) began their meetings at 3 p.m. and continued them all night long. At a few homes, seances lasted two or three days, during which participants enjoyed a vaudeville show of preaching, praying, prophesying, illuminism, and physical torture.[161]

Their increasingly bizarre teachings soon led to violent anti-social behavior. *Père* Lambert, a Dominican priest who attended several of these seances, described the *secours* he observed in 1733. He witnessed fire that did not burn them, machines stretching them without pain, violent blows that left no bruises, and sword thrusts that did not pierce their skin. In this carnival-like atmosphere, he saw participants who rolled inside barrels lined with knives emerge unhurt, others who ate bent pins for Lent suffer no harm, while still others read books with their eyes tightly bandaged or spoke Arabic and other languages they had never learned.[162]

But all of this was mere child's play compared with what followed. With the introduction of the *petit secours* ("little aids" or "small assistance"), the movement degenerated from miracle working to masochism, from spiritual entertainment to social eroticism. Growing weary of miracle cures on demand and routine convulsions, participants began torturing one another. What began as a counter-irritant for the pain of violent convulsions soon became an end in itself, endowed with spiritual symbolism. During *secours* (dubbed "la petite" or "la Samaritaine"), often held on Catholic holy days such as Pentecost, Easter, and Christmas, participants beat each other with batons, tied tourniquets around each other's arms and legs, cut each other with knives, and pressed swords or spits into each other's chests, stomachs, and sides. Some lay on the floor while assistants trampled them, pressed heavy weights on them, or pinched them with tongs. Others crouched while participants beat them with heavy clubs.[163]

A few convulsionists gained renown for specializing in particular "aids." Marie Sonnet, known as "the Salamander" or "the Sister of Fire," lay down on a burning brazier filled with hot coals while helpers lowered a 50-pound weight ("the biscuit") on her chest. As he lay prostrate in the dirt, Brother Hilaire was whipped repeatedly in the chest and abdomen with an eight-ounce lead weight attached to a wire. One man was beaten with an oak cudgel for nearly an hour while another received 30,000 blows in one night. A girl permitted herself to be dragged face down on the floor for hours. To the *securistes*, this holy violence symbolized the pain of persecution which they, as the elect, endured in defense of "the Truth." In the end, they hoped divine grace would honor their "victorious resistance" by delivering them and punishing their foes.[164]

These bizarre actions clearly had sexual overtones as well. When male assistants pulled females' breasts, pierced their bodies with pins and swords, or pressed heavy weights upon their half-naked forms, spiritual torture became a substitute for actual sexual experience. Men inflicting pain on women derived a sadistic sense of pleasure from touching (albeit brutally) their bodies.[165] At one assembly in May 1736, the Benedictine *Dom* Samson reported seeing "girls of bad life" (i.e., prostitutes) performing "the most abominable actions" with "indecent postures." In a letter to police chief Hérault, he warned that "such abominations ["fornication and adulteries"] in the king's capital city" could bring down God's punishment on the entire kingdom.[166]

Yet like the Ancient Romans at the Coliseum, the spectators at the *petit secours* demanded more violence and blood. Instead of gladiators, however, they introduced the *grand secours* ("great aids" or "great assistance")—a realistic imitation of Christ's crucifixion. Because they believed that they could "triumph with Jesus Christ" only by suffering as he had, many *secouristes* sought to accomplish the *Opus Dei* (work of God) in their lives by risking death by crucifixion. Ironically, the appearance in Paris of a number of "bloody Christs"—crucifixes in which Christ's body appeared to shed (or be daubed with) real blood—may have reinforced this practice. In an attempt to "die a living death," participants had themselves strapped or nailed to wooden crosses, enduring hunger and thirst for hours or days at a time. Then an elaborately staged "resurrection" brought them back to life. Symbolically, by losing the self in death, they experienced rebirth; thus for some *secouristes*, death became an enjoyable experience.[167]

The *convulsionnaires*' brutal treatment of one another reveals their negative attitude toward the physical. For them, the body symbolized corruption. "All is sickness and death within me," the *secouriste* Gertrude Rachel exclaimed, "from the top of my head to the sole of my feet. All is corruption."[168] The theology behind the tortures taught that "suffering and persecution are our daily destiny, and we are free-will offerings. Our bodies are proof of that. But that is the price we pay for a general redemption, a glorious renovation." So "the more rigorous our loss, the more rich our salvation."[169]

To demonstrate the "poverty of the body" and its worthlessness, participants made their bodies into machines, accepting one torture after another until their nervous system shut down in protest, having reached the limits of its endurance. By self-torture, the *secouristes* made the symbols of pain, blood, and crucifixion real in their lives. Indeed, the word had become flesh, for "we no longer *represent*, we *are* the agony of Christ on the cross," nailed, whipped, bleeding, and (sometimes) dying. Thus metaphor became reality, the sacred came to earth in bodily ecstasy. At its core, the *secours* is "a foyer of death and the effusion of violence." Yet in order to crush the evil that inhabits the body, this "foyer" must be made public, for only by participatory social violence can the "social machine" be cleansed of sin.[170]

Consequently, both men and women participated in these crucifixions. As the victim lay prostrate on the cross, the "grand assistants" nailed their hands and feet to the wood beams and pierced their side in imitation of Christ's five "blessed wounds," thereby demonstrating "that Jesus Christ dwelt in the flesh of every *convulsionnaire*." These were not mock crucifixions. Edme Cellier ("Brother Innocent") had himself crucified eighteen times in five months using at least four nails and sometimes more.[171] Yet the beating, piercing, cutting, burning, and crucifying—which may at first have provided relief for those experiencing convulsions—soon became an end in themselves, a violent form of osteopathy.[172]

These *grand secours*, which stretch the credulity of readers today, also divided the Jansenist movement. As the cures at St.-Médard from 1727 to 1731 had polarized *appelants* into supporters and opponents, so the introduction of the *grand secours* split them into *Secouristes* and *Anti-*

Secouristes. The latter, calling such tortures immoral, scandalous, and contrary to the Ten Commandments (specifically "Honor thy father and thy mother" and "Thou shall not kill"), enlisted the aid of the king, Parlement, Sorbonne theologians, bishops, and laity to stop the *secours*. By the mid-1730s, all levels of French society expressed shock at the indecency, violence, and scandal exhibited by the *secouristes*. In the popular mind, their tortures had crossed the line between the self-denial of spiritual mystics and sexual brutality. Increasingly, people viewed this strange blend of millenarianism, eroticism, torture, and hysteria as a medical problem rather than a religious phenomenon. More often now, detractors referred to them as *convulsionnistes* to show the parallel with those who suffered from the medical problem of convulsions.[173]

Publications on the subject of convulsions had been almost nonexistent in France until the 1720s. Although in the 1650s, six works had discussed the "Miracle of the Thorn" (1656), from 1660 to 1720, no publications on healing miracles and convulsions had been printed. During the late-1720s, however, in the wake of the alleged cures at St.-Médard Cemetery, twelve works appeared. But during the 1730s, as the *petite* and *grand secours* increased, an astonishing 364 sources came from French presses. The number of sources on convulsions rapidly declined during the 1740s (43), 1750s (20), and 1760s (twelve) until they virtually disappeared in the 1770s (two) and 1780s (six). Thus, the tsunami of publications in the 1730s dealing with the convulsions represents 78 percent of the total output from 1650 to 1790. If one adds to that the works printed during the 1740s and 1750s, their total (424) accounts for 91 percent of all published writings on convulsionary phenomena in France for 140 years.[174]

As might be expected, the *convulsionnaires* and *secouristes* wrote many works defending their doctrines and themselves; most of these remain unpublished and are rarely read today. Some of their favorite themes included Christ's passion and sufferings, the evils within the Church, the life of the Deacon Pâris, oppression of the truth, and how one becomes nothing before God. Other works, drawing heavily on the Old Testament prophetic books of Daniel, Ezekiel, Hosea, Isaiah, and Amos, focused on eschatological and apocalyptic themes: the coming judgment, Babylon (or the Jesuits) destroyed, the conversion of the Jews, and the end of the world.

Whereas Jansenist authors in the seventeenth and early eighteenth century wrote works of a devotional, spiritual, almost mystical nature, the *convulsionnaires* preferred warnings, prophecies, and maledictions laced with Figurist symbolism. If seventeenth-century Jansenists served a New Testament God of grace, the eighteenth-century convulsionists worshiped an Old Testament God of vengeance. Their works, which reflect a fear of God's curses and the final destruction of sinners, frequently mention the cross, thorns, blood, suffering, and judgment.

In their use of the Bible, they also allude to more negative than positive images. Discourses and sermons frequently mention threatening animals (dogs, wolves, vipers), damaging natural elements (fire, storms, famine), and harbingers of destruction (war, poison, death). Their condemnation of the Jesuits as "wolves," "Ministers of Satan," and "Priests of Belial" exceeds the rhetoric used by most Jansenists. The *convulsionnaires* likewise preferred David's psalms of affliction, persecution, and penitence (favorites included Psalm 94 and 101) to his psalms of deliverance and rejoicing (like Psalms 19 and 91), because in this wicked world, they expected to suffer.[175]

As they despised and mistreated their bodies as sources of corruption, so the *convulsionnaires* viewed the world as "Babylon," the source of all evil. Like Jansenists everywhere, they criticized French society as corrupt and hypocritical for its theatre, dancing, gambling, and other amusements. They also condemned it for its lies, false compliments, hypocrisy, and pride. But the convulsionists' anti-intellectualism went even deeper, for in addition to attacking French society as morally corrupt, they also rejected the authority of earthly monarchs who were part of this temporal "Babylon." In an exhortation aimed at Louis XV, one convulsionist warned: "O Princes! O earthly kings! You arm yourselves and yet do you not see that the Savior will soon overthrow your scepters and crowns? . . . [My good angel] has shown me that he will have some kings killed . . . The death of these kings will precede the coming of the Holy Prophet [Elijah]."[176] Given their tragic vision of history, the convulsionists believed that earthquakes, meteorites, famines, droughts, and floods constituted God's apocalyptic warnings to kings and people that the end of the world was near.[177]

The *convulsionnaires*' gloom-and-doom message, alleged cures, and violent behavior sharply divided public opinion across class, occupational, and gender lines. Joachim Colbert, Bishop of Montpellier, issued a pastoral instruction in February 1733 expressing his firm belief in the genuineness of the healing miracles. When truth can no longer be freely spoken, he said, then God works miracles to affirm the truth "by marvels before our eyes." Clement XII, however, condemned Colbert's pastoral instruction as "scandalous, seditious, outrageous, absurd, blasphemous, schismatic, erroneous, and notoriously heretical."[178]

But many clerics, lawyers, and doctors strongly disagreed with the pope's condemnation. The *abbé* Languet, in a lengthy letter addressed to the Archbishop of Sens (a critic) in 1734, defended both the Deacon Pâris and the healing miracles as divinely inspired.[179] The following year, 23 lawyers who called themselves "defenders of the truth" signed a petition favoring both the miraculous cures and the convulsions.[180] Dr. Thieullier, regent of the faculty of medicine at the University of Paris and Louis XV's personal physician, after examining the Dlle. Masoron (healed of apoplexy during convulsions), called the healing a miracle of God. In a strongly worded response to Archbishop Vintimille (who had questioned the doctor's competency in 1735), Thieullier asserted, "I can distinguish the true from the false." He had personally examined Masoron before her healing and had declared her condition incurable, but when she prayed at the Deacon's tomb, her restoration came immediately. After examining her himself and interviewing her father and two witnesses, Thieullier assured the Archbishop that "I have not been duped."[181]

The convulsionists also enjoyed the protection of influential men in Parlement. In 1737, Louis-Adrien Le Paige, the silver-tongued orator and leader of the Jansenist party there, vigorously defended Figurism, the miracle cures, and even the *grand secours* as evidence that God was working on human bodies.[182] Likewise, Jérôme-Nicolas de Pâris, the brother of Deacon François de Pâris, abandoned his legal career as a counselor in the First Chamber of Inquest in Parlement and in 1732 joined the convulsionary movement, retreating to Clermont to live a life of extreme penitence and incredible austerity. As it had with his brother, this ascetic lifestyle brought him to an early grave on 16 August 1737. During his funeral at St.-Gervais, the crowds lining the streets, gazing out windows, and packing the church offered him public veneration. When police chief Hérault blocked his interment in the cemetery, Pâris' supporters buried him inside the church at St.-Gervais. Devotees took boards and dirt from the site, and soon miraculous cures were being attributed to these relics.[183]

But as the *convulsionnaires*' behavior grew more violent by the mid-1730s, even some of their friends began to repudiate them. Shocked by the brutality and indecency of the *grand secours*, which contrasted sharply with the austere practices and rigorous piety of Jansenism, many bishops, lawyers, *parlementaires*, and *appelants* in general began distancing themselves from the growing scandal in their midst.[184] Outspoken *Anti-Secouristes* among the clergy included Bishop Soanen, Bishop Colbert, and Bishop Caylus. In addition, 19 Paris *curés* and 30 doctors of theology at the Sorbonne condemned the convulsions as contrary to God's majesty, the spirit of holy worship, the honor of the Church, pure morals, and public decency.[185]

In a strongly worded pastoral instruction, Jean-Joseph Languet de Gergy, Archbishop of Sens, condemned the convulsions as diabolically inspired and their participants as "fanatics, visionaries, self-enlightened ones, fools, and demoniacs" (devil-possessed persons). To be genuine, he said, healing miracles must be attested by ecclesiastical authority (not popular acclaim), witnessed by persons of notable rank (educated and enlightened), investigated minutely (not "proven" by "certificates of healing," which were too easily obtained). Divine miracles, he asserts, are never bestowed upon "fanatics" and "fools" and seldom upon women because "illnesses" and "infirmities" are normal for their sex. Finally, he concludes, all so-called miracles except the resurrection of the dead are of "doubtful origin" because Satan can duplicate them.[186]

In his *Fair Judgment Concerning the Convulsions* (1733), the *abbé* Fourgon (a self-proclaimed Jansenist) separates the healing miracles at St.-Médard from the later convulsions. While he accepts the former as divinely inspired, he rejects the latter as satanic. Both scripture and Church tradition, he asserts, prove the convulsions false. In the Gospels and Pauline Epistles, convulsions always occur during demonic possession. Regarding miracle cures in cemeteries, Fourgon quotes St. Chrysostom's dictum that "the bones of the saints attract the power of the Demons." Demons enjoy inflicting pain on human bodies, he says, but God never works that way.

Instead, God created the body to be treated with decency and dignity, not to be subjected to the grimaces, contortions, indecencies, and "unnatural derangements" that characterize the convulsions. He gave humans life, integrity, and good health, but the convulsionists threaten the health and happiness of participants. God is the author of purity, continence, and chastity; by contrast, the convulsions promote indecency and immorality. God made mankind intelligent to distinguish them from the beasts; the *secours* deprive participants of their "liberty & reason." The "fruit" of the convulsions (falsehood, unjust judgments, blasphemies, and indecencies) proves their satanic origin.

Moreover, despite their prayers, songs, and miracle cures, the seances are still demonic because while Satan often mixes the good with the bad to achieve his goals, God employs only that which is good to fulfill his purposes. In fact, Fourgon avers, since Satan brings illness and evil into the world, the alleged healing miracles could simply be the cessation of his afflictions. In any case, just as the convulsionists' discourses reveal their ignorance and lies, so their *secours* destroy physical health rather than restore it. In the final analysis, Fourgon believes that the miracles wrought by Christ were infinitely superior in grandeur, fame, evidence, dignity and order, not only to those seen at Pâris' tomb, but also to those attributed to Moses, Elijah, and the Apostles. By contrast, the convulsions are totally satanic and devoid of Christian merit.[187]

Although brief, Fourgon's balanced, carefully reasoned tract mirrored the growing opposition to the *secouristes* that had developed by 1735. In his pastoral letter that year, Pierre de Guerin de Tencin, Archbishop of Embrun, called the "pretended miracles" and convulsions "fanaticism" and "the work of demons."[188]

Similarly, in his 100-page Ordinance on 8 November 1735, Archbishop Vintimille discounted Cardinal Noailles' earlier support for the miracles by asserting that his predecessor had failed to follow the proper channels for verification; therefore, his conclusions were null and void. Then Vintimille outlined the "rules" for judging genuine miracles. A healing could be defined as a divine miracle only if the illness failed to respond to natural remedies; if the cure was instantaneous, perfect, and complete; and if several "people of honor and probity" testified to its genuineness with no contradictory depositions.

According to these guidelines, nearly all the St.-Médard miracles and all of the current convulsionary ones were not only "pretended miracles" and "false healing," but also "scandalous & extravagant scenes which Religion & reason reject." Calling their seances "indecent," "obscene," "shameful spectacles," and "crimes" inspired by demons, the Archbishop told the faithful that convulsions never accompanied true miracles of healing. None of Christ's miracles had exhibited anything puerile, obscene, or cruel, he declared; instead, his miracles had all been dignified and noble.[189]

But could the convulsions be neither satanic nor divinely inspired, but humanly induced?

This proposal, first made by 30 Paris physicians in January 1735, attributed the convulsions to chance, to natural causes, or to the "overheated imaginations" of those participating in the seances. The only "evil" these medical doctors saw in the phenomenon was their tendency to produce indecencies, extravagances, and false predictions.[190]

This theory received some verification the following year when police chief Hérault interviewed Guillaume Antoine Maupoint, a 29-year-old convulsionist. Hérault asked him, "Can you induce these convulsions voluntarily?" Maupoint responded: "It is true that on several occasions, in order to satisfy the curiosity of those who want to see them in their alleged convulsions, [I have] induced them." Under normal circumstances, however, the shaking began following prayers and the reading of works attacking *Unigenitus* (whereas the convulsions ceased immediately when writings defending the Bull were read). On the day the police arrested him and took him to the Bastille, Maupoint's convulsions (which he saw as divinely inspired) began afresh.[191]

Despite the flood tide of opposition to the alleged miracles and seances, the *Nouvelles Ecclésiastiques* steadfastly defended them. This was true in part because many laymen and women who attended the seances also ran the clandestine presses that published the newspaper. Responding to the Archbishop of Sens' assertion that the convulsions constituted God's punishment for the Jansenists' refusal to submit to *Unigenitus*, one author declared that the recent healing miracles at the tomb of Monsieur Rouffe (which occurred without convulsions) "solidly refuted" the Archbishop's "supposition."[192] In celebration of Pâris' death on May 1, the newspaper attributed "the many prodigious miracles" that had occurred in Paris over the past decade to God's direct intervention.[193]

While many in the capital doubted God's intervention in the *secours*, they soon had concrete evidence that the police, responding to the shift in public opinion, intended to intervene and crack down on the movement. Since the closing of St.-Médard Cemetery in January 1732, the police had kept a watchful eye on convulsionist activities. Inspector Duval frequently sent police chief Hérault lists of names and addresses where their seances occurred.[194]

A year later, Louis XV decided the time had come to destroy the hydra of convulsionism before it grew new heads. On 17 February 1733 the Council of State issued an ordinance condemning those who "by a spirit of imposture" pretended to have convulsions, made a spectacle of themselves in private homes "to abuse the credulity of the people," and "gave birth to fanaticism already too widespread." For the good of religion and public tranquility, such disturbances would be stopped immediately. The penalty for having convulsions in a public place was 500 *livres*; men caught at the *secours* were sent to Bicêtre and women to La Pitié—both for five years at hard labor—as "seducers and disturbers of the public repose."[195]

Interestingly, whereas a century earlier Church and government officials had treated Jansenists as religious schismatics within Roman Catholicism (subject to canon laws), they now treated the *convulsionnaires* as social outcasts to be prosecuted to the fullest extent of the criminal laws. In April 1733, an *arrêt* established a tribunal of twelve commissioners at the Arsenal, chaired by Hérault, whose duty was to find, arrest, and imprison convulsionists.[196]

Using his vast network of spies, Hérault determined to crush these bizarre sects. He encouraged citizens to inform the police if their neighbors entertained convulsionists. He required priests and abbots to divulge confessional secrets that might provide tips for the police. Occasionally, officers even "planted" clerics inside prisons to spy on inmates, some of whom continued to convulse even in detention. A few former *convulsionnaires* (like Jean Le Bel) turned against their friends and told the police where they met. When Minister Fleury urged the police to bring the sect to heel and help pacify Paris, they tried to do so, but with mixed results.[197] In a letter to Hérault on 23 April 1733, Fleury bemoaned the fact that "there is something supernatural in the invincible stubbornness of all these sorts of people."[198] In August 1734, Fleury praised the police for making "a good capture," adding, "one could wish that there was no more to do" to crush the movement than to imprison the *convulsionistes*. In 1735, after the Minister restored Parlement's full authority to deal with the *convulsionnaires*, he rejoiced to see the Grand Chamber vigorously investigating and arresting the "Augustinistes." Yet despite the *parlementaires'* 50 *arrêts* against them, Fleury acknowledged that "fanaticism is growing instead of diminishing," expressing the fear that "it may yet gain the advantage."[199]

This prediction proved true, largely because neither Fleury nor Hérault understood the convulsionist mentality concerning persecution. Police harassment and imprisonment only convinced them that God had chosen them as his special elect to defend the truth against the "Gentiles" (government ministers, the police, clerics). As the remnant, nothing predisposed them to believe more in the supernatural than persecution, especially when miraculous cures and convulsions accompanied their misfortunes and authenticated their message and mission. Therefore, the harder the state bore down on them, the stronger their faith became and the larger their numbers grew. Whereas the *abbé* de St.-Jean had estimated their membership to be about 400 in 1733, their defender Carré de Montgeron claimed between 3000 and 4000 by 1745 (with only 500–600 actually participating in the *secours*). By 1750, despite two decades of police repression (see chapter 8), the marquis d'Argenson believed that 2000 *convulsionnaires* still lived in or near Paris.[200]

Therefore, although *lettres de cachet, arrêts,* and ordinances curtailed the convulsionary movement after 1735, they did not extinguish it. Like crabgrass, underground sects multiplied in secrecy. Some moved from violent behavior to political discourse, attacking Louis XV as "that impious prince" and "Pharaoh of hardened heart." Those who favored numerology accused the king of being the Anti-Christ of Revelation 12 because the Roman numerical value of his Latin name LUDOVICUS was 666. Others pointed out that the numerical value of his full title (LUDOVICUS DECIMUS QUINTUS FRANCIAE ET NAVARRE REX) signified 1733, a year when "the beast" began persecuting "the innocent ones." In May 1736, the police foiled an alleged convulsionary plot to overthrow Parlement and the king and establish a body resembling the Estates-General. The 25 or 30 plotters planned to shoot Louis XV while he was hunting or blow up his carriage during a royal procession. One sect, somewhat less dangerous, invented the "mysterious calendar" full of millennial hopes and apocalyptic predictions regarding the imminent return of Enoch, Elijah, or Christ.[201]

Another more pacifist group appealed to Louis XV for clemency:

> Prince, we wish to strengthen your crown by supporting your rights, and [yet] you take for disturbers of the public order those who are the most zealous for the interests and the peace, the honor and the glory, of their King and their native land! You knock down, you torment, and you crush those who have the greatest affection for you; you reject your most faithful subjects; you hold them of no account.[202]

But as law enforcement officials spread their nets farther afield after 1735, they caught some rather big fish at the *secours* who definitely were not "of no account." To the great surprise of the police and the embarrassment of his family, one raid on a seance caught the all-too-curious son of Sieur Adam Antoine Royer, sub-delegate for the *intendant* of Paris. Sent to Vincennes, the youth faced deportation from France, but his father's political connections saved him. The family's eight-page *placet* pleading for his detention rather than exile includes nine letters from such powerful figures as Secretaries of State D'Argenson and Phélyppeaux, Minister of War Pontchartrain, *Intendant* Biguoy of Paris, and Chancellor D'Aguesseau—all of whom had family ties to the Royers.[203]

The increased police surveillance in the capital drove many "Augustinian *convulsionnaires*" (as the police called them after 1736) to seek safer pastures in the countryside. A few groups migrated to the abandoned grounds of Port-Royal des Champs. There they preached and prophesied, communed and convulsed in all-night sessions ending at dawn. In January 1736, the police arrested 26 individuals and their family members there, incarcerating the women at Petit-Châtelet and the men at For-l'Evêque before putting them on trial at the Conciergerie.[204]

Such public trials and longer prison terms (see chapter 8) demonstrated not only the government's determination to crush the movement, but also its strategy of undermining these sects' popularity with pro-Jansenist sympathizers. Even the case of the widow Catherine Lefebvre (whose 27 May 1736 *placet* begged for the release of her convulsionist daughter Anne to care for her paralytic mother) failed to move Hérault. Because Anne continued having convulsions at Salpêtrière and the Bastille, the police chief denied her release in 1742.[205] Louis XV's Ordinance of 17 February 1737, blaming the "pretended convulsions" on the Jansenists' "unhealthy imagination" and "spirit of imposture," clearly signaled the government's intentions to crush the movement.[206]

Before the police could congratulate themselves on bringing the convulsionaries to heel, however, the movement received a shot in the arm from the imprisonment of one of its most prominent defenders. Louis-Basile Carré de Montgeron, a wealthy *parlementaire* in the Second Chamber of Inquest at Paris, had been a Deist and a libertine until a visit to St.-Médard on 7 September 1731 made him a believer in healing miracles. After experiencing a four-hour trance himself, Montgeron became an indefatigable missionary for the movement, defending the convulsionaries in Parlement, serving as a *secouriste* at their seances, giving pensions to poor members, visiting those imprisoned, and defending their beliefs. His influence, in fact, protected many of them from being arrested, because Hérault "hesitated to inconvenience" him by detaining his friends.[207]

But on 29 July 1737, Montgeron overstepped the bounds of propriety. Clutching a copy of his 900-page book *The Truth of the Miracles Performed by the Intercession of Monsieur de Pâris & Other Appelants* (recently published in Utrecht), he took a carriage to Versailles. Dressed in his magisterial robes, he presented the startled king with a gold-embossed, green leather-bound copy of his defense of convulsionism, briefly explaining that it contained "several truths which are being kept hidden from you" by government ministers. Without even giving his name, Montgeron strode from the palace, pausing only long enough to distribute four more copies to the *duc* d'Orléans, Procurer-General Joly de Fleury, First President of Parlement Le Peletier, and Advocate-General Gilbert de Voisins. At 2 a.m. the following day, the police arrested him for his impertinence and sent him to the Bastille. From his window, he watched the police burn 5000 copies of his book—but Montgeron had already arranged for a new printing in Holland.[208]

Despite protests from his colleagues in Parlement and a vigorous defense from the editorial staff of the *Nouvelles Ecclésiastiques* (who praised him as "a new Justinian"), Montgeron spent the next seventeen years in prison. He was first sent to the Bastille (July-October 1737), briefly to the Benedictine monastery of St.-André-de-Villeneuve, then to the Fortress of Viviers, and finally to the Fortress of Valence (1738–1754). During his detention, he published a second edition of his book in Holland (1741) and corrected a third edition in his cell at Valence (1747). If Minister Fleury had prevailed, however, he would have been sent to St.-Lazare, an institution for youthful offenders and the insane in Paris. Instead, he died in 1754 at Valence.[209]

In his book, Montgeron defends the St.-Médard miracles as "God's voice" speaking to humanity in defense of his divinity, his true church, and its message. Such miracles build faith, convert Deists, separate the orthodox from the heretical, and prove God's presence in these last days. Montgeron also highlights the role God has called the *convulsionnaires* to play in France as "instruments" of his mercy and justice, to "instruct & persuade Kings," and to clarify the difference between "true" and "false" miracles.[210]

His defense of their violent *secours*, however, cost him the support of mainstream Jansenists.

In 1742 the editors of the *Nouvelles* repudiated his views as "arbitrary, untenable, contrary to Scripture and [Catholic] rituals." But Montgeron's writings would outlive their author and bring new converts to the cause during the 1740s and '50s.[211]

In conclusion, the *appelant* conviction that miracles demonstrated divine approval of Jansenist truth spawned bizarre offspring that split the movement. Antoine Arnauld's support for the "Miracle of the Thorn" (1656) and the cult surrounding Deacon Pâris after his death (1727), produced alleged healing miracles at his grave in St.-Médard. But as this noisy phenomenon degenerated into convulsions, it further split the Jansenist movement and brought police repression. As the *convulsionnaires'* private seances became more violent and their writings more subversive of Church and state authority, officials sent increasing numbers of them to the Bastille and other prisons, further radicalizing the movement, as chapter 8 demonstrates.

Chapter 8

Crucifying Jansenism: *Grands Secours* and the Death of Convulsionism, 1741–1799

"[*Convulsionnaires* are] rowdy characters who go from attic to attic performing miracles, roasting little girls without doing them harm, hitting them with stakes and whips for the love of God, and yelling against the Pope."—*Voltaire*[1]

With most of its leaders dead, exiled, or imprisoned by 1741, the convulsionist movement had passed its hysterical peak and by the mid-1740s, entered a period of relative calm.[2] In a letter to her anonymous friend M***, Madame Duguet-Mol stated in 1743 that "the fad of the convulsions begins to pass." In Paris at least, many of them either hide their "indecencies" or deny their participation in the *secours*. Duguet-Mol expresses her satisfaction that such "indecent, horrible spectacles" and "excesses and insulting excitements" have notably declined. Although she believes some participants have actually been "possessed by demons," she also recognizes that others, whom she calls "rascals," "false prophets," and "pretenders," have perpetrated fraudulent cures and false miracles on a gullible populace.[3]

As convulsionism entered its final, most bizarre phase, it could no longer mobilize public opinion in its favor. Even the *Nouvelles Ecclésiastiques*—previously a staunch defender of the *secours*—disavowed Carré de Montgeron's second volume, *The Continuation of the Demonstrations of the Miracles Operating by the Intercession of M. de Pâris and Other Appelants*. By 1742, it was printing letters both for and against the violent *secours* from bishops, theologians, and *appelants* across France. But when the *convulsionnaires* began behaving as if they were really first century Christians persecuted in the catacombs of Ancient Rome, they soon embraced sadomasochism. Abolishing time and history, they sought to identify more closely with the suffering Christ by inscribing on their bodies the marks of his physical suffering. Consequently, the movement developed a savage liturgy that included beating, piercing, cutting, and crucifying participants.[4]

As the alleged healing miracles at St.-Médard and the rise of violent convulsions had twice before divided the Jansenist movement into supporters and opponents, so in the 1740s, the adoption of the *secours meurtrier* (killing aids) split the convulsionist camp into three opposing sects. The *secouristes* embraced the more violent *secours*, finding ever more creative ways to beat, bruise, and bloody the human body. The *mélangistes* or moderates, who opposed such brutality, remained the mainstream supporters of the *Nouvelles Ecclésiastiques*. The "Religious Enlightened Ones," including the Sorbonne theologian Louis de Bonnaire, the physician Philippe Hecquet, the seminary director Philippe Boidot, and the academician Etienne Mignot, disagreed with both of the above groups and wanted to find common ground with the philosophes. Acrimonious infighting broke out among these sects, with the *mélangistes* calling the "Enlightened Ones" "Libertines," "Socinians," and "Deists" while both the *mélangistes* and the "Enlightened Ones" considered the *secouristes* "fanatics," "enthusiasts," and "illuminati" and their "murderous *secours*" demonic.[5]

These three squabbling groups, who met mostly at night in the 1740s, were but a shadow of the movement's strength in the 1730s. Police dossiers show tiny bands of two or three or ten believers assembling together, with the 25 or 30 women and children meeting near the Church of St.-Marine in 1744 being perhaps the largest group. One cell led by "John the Baptist" awaited the return of the "new Elijah"; another group nurtured an infant whom they called "Jesus of Cyre"; several *mélangiste* sects focused their efforts on printing issues of the *Nouvelles Ecclésiastiques*. The members of one tiny group met only in cemeteries at the tombs of the *abbés* Tissart, Jube, and Roussel for worship and miracle cures. With most of their men imprisoned, exiled, or dead, these scattered pockets of believers consisted mostly of women, priests, abbots, and children.[6]

The preponderance of women in the movement left an imprint on the seances, which grew more creative and emotional during the 1740s. One Figurist group, for example, reckoned time by the Hebrew calendar. They met to sing, pray, and preach in Hebrew, believing that this would be the language that the "New Elijah" would speak when he set up his kingdom. Their leaders experienced "ecstasies," had visions at 4 a.m., and delivered "lectures" that left listeners weeping. Glossolalia (speaking in unknown tongues) was the featured attraction at the seances held in the home of Armand de Voltaire, the philosophe's older brother. At other seances, members engaged in "dialogues" with "Nebuchadnezzar," offered prayers to the "Holy Prophet" (Elijah), and concluded their meetings with hugs, kisses, and the "Go in Peace" farewell.[7] In a letter to the Bishop of Auxerre, however, M. Le Blanc felt that "such dangerous novelties" promoted "disobedience, insubordination, and schisms" in the Church and divided convents and monasteries. They must be stopped, he added.[8]

Church and government officials agreed. To that end, after 1742, the government transferred all responsibility for arresting convulsionists to the police. Instead of sending them to comfortable chambers in the Bastille or Vincennes by a royal *lettre de cachet*, law officers used *ordres de police* (police warrants) to incarcerate them in the dungeons of the St. Martin prison. This increased police role represented a concomitant decrease in Parlement's involvement (either by issuing *arrêts* or by protesting convulsionaries' treatment) in the social control of Jansenism. In 1744 police chief Hérault congratulated himself that these measures had forced the movement to "go up in smoke."[9]

But a few convulsionary embers continued to burn in Paris and beyond despite the best efforts of police to extinguish them. In 1747 several members met at the Hôtel de Chavigny, the home of *Sieur* Baudin, wealthy bourgeois notary at the Châtelet, until police chief Berryer sent the septuagenarian to the Bastille for two years and then banished him from Paris.[10] Another group met with the teenage Moulère sisters until they were arrested and sent to prison—Gabrielle to La Salpêtrière and Jeanne to Ste.-Pélagie—for nine years.[11] A handful of others helped Lioutaud Ebeniste hawk water from Pâris' well, claiming that it cured all kinds of illnesses, until the police arrested him and posted a guard at the well in 1751.[12]

One cell, directed by Pierre La Barre, an advocate at the Parlement of Rouen, met in Paris' Marais district for regular crucifixions supervised by "Sisters" Félicité, Marie, Madéleine, and Rachel. Its attendees included the *princesse* de Kinski, the prince de Monaco, the *comte* de Strarember*g*, the marquis de Bousales, the chevalier de Sarsfield, the chevalier de Forbin, and numerous military officers and physicians.[13] Jean-Lambert Dulong ("Brother Gideon"), a well-known mathematician, organized seances at his home where convulsions and religious tortures occurred from 1740 to 1783.[14] At yet another seance, "Brother Pierre" held "conversations" with the "sisters" about Elijah's coming, how the prophecies of Ezekiel and Isaiah fit contemporary circumstances, and what God's restored kingdom would be like. Afterwards, participants enjoyed watching "extraordinary miracles" and "prodigies of humiliation" (the violent *secours*).[15]

At many seances, the violence of these "killing aids" increased dramatically. For example, in one meeting, "Sister Thérèse" had herself lowered headfirst into a fire 300 times. "Sister Rachel," bound with four iron bands, allowed participants to trample on her body 84 times and on her face 60 times, after which they beat her on the head 350 times, on the stomach 85 times, and on her breasts 30 times. "Sister Catin," bound on her back in a doorway (as two men pushed the door against her body), received 171 blows on her back and chest before being trussed up in midair and dropped to the floor. One wonders who counted each of the 184,000 blows Catherine Lefèvre allegedly received at one séance.[16]

Although these sadomasochistic exercises appear (to the twenty-first century reader) utterly devoid of spiritual meaning, the *convulsionnaires* defended them in their clandestine publications. In a "Letter on the murderous aids" written about 1741, the author asserts that "the first violent *secours* were far inferior to those performed today. The gradation [of pain] is now sensible, and one sees that the participants in the convulsions move always forward by events more striking and more amazing." Today, he adds, the *secouristes* make certain that the body can endure various increments of pain before they administer more of it. When the willing victim "is capable of supporting things above ordinary forces," then participants "move to the next level of the *secours*." Moreover, he said, "they let nature heal the old wounds before inflicting new ones."[17]

Sensing, perhaps, that such assurances would not convince skeptics, the author justifies the violent *secours* on spiritual grounds in his "Response," a question-and-answer catechism aimed at critics. The convulsionists have "the moral certainty" that God wishes them to stage these spectacles because the Bible is full of miracles, the Holy Spirit performs miracle cures through the convulsions, unbelievers are converted thereby, the truth is spread abroad, and they bring many blessings in their wake. Furthermore, he adds, the *secours* are voluntary, break no laws, show love for God, and demonstrate trust in one's friends. Spiritually, they promote humility, purity, and grace. Moreover, the beatings "relieve them, heal them, and invigorate them." "They promote vigor, good health, and the more abundant life," he declares. Finally, he asserts, in the past eight years (1733–1741), not one person has died receiving the tortures—certainly proof of God's blessing.[18]

To first-time observers shocked by what they saw, however, receiving God's blessing may not have been uppermost in their minds. Perhaps to prepare newcomers for what lay ahead, therefore, a typical "conference" (as the *secouristes* called them) began with prayers, responsive readings, and vigorous preaching in which the leader (ironically named "Sister Dove") evoked vivid images of Babylon, wolves, mercenaries, hell, false prophets, blind enemies, sinners, tyranny, and punishment. Then came the convulsions, during which "Sister Dove" shouted encouragement using positive imagery focusing on Jerusalem, sheep, infants of God, God's glory and mercy, prophets (Elijah or Isaiah), and the "stones speaking out." Gradually, her shouting rose in volume as she encouraged bystanders to get involved and "beat your spouse . . . give her blows as it is said, Unnatural children, I urge you to oppress your mother." As the participants began beating the victim, he or she cried out, "My God, the hour of my suffering has not yet come; I have not yet suffered the loss of my blood." During the "grand finale," as the victim lost blood during repeated torture or crucifixion, assistants gave them water.[19]

As the brutality of the *secours meurtrier* increased, the intellectual and spiritual content of the discourses decreased correspondingly. Obviously, attendees had become more interested in seeing naked bodies tortured than in listening to sermons. At times, leaders lapsed into repetitive, meaningless phrases and even infantile gibberish. "Hear us, O great God, Hear the sinner, Hear us, O great God, Hear him, O great God" is an example of the former, while "Ba be bi bo bu" (repeated three times) and "Ba ga va la sa og ma lo tem be be bi bo bu" illustrates the latter. In such seances, worship had degenerated into mindless entertainment and amusement.[20]

Although the Figurist groups (led by the two "J.-B.'s"—D'Etemare and Poncet des Essarts) rejected such meaningless gibberish, their services, too, had become repetitive. As in the 1730s, members looked for the coming of Elijah and the conversion of the Jews. While they waited, their leaders shared discourses full of hackneyed phrases and spiritual word games concerning Nebuchadnezzar, Babylon, the white horse, the coming flood, the desert, Egyptian slavery, Elijah's cave, and Rachel in tears. As political storm clouds gathered over Paris, the *convulsionnaires'* apocalyptic rhetoric and bloody visions assumed darker hues, predicting the downfall of the Roman Catholic Church and the overthrow of Europe's monarchs. Before Elijah's coming to restore world peace, "abominations" (pestilence, famine, war, earthquakes, floods, and fire) would afflict the earth. But during those terrible times, the Jews would be converted and the *convulsionaires* miraculously delivered.[21]

In the present, however, such convictions did not deliver them from punishment. Despite the *secouristes'* scattered, clandestine existence and growing tendency to commit their writings to code,[22] their hostile attitude toward the state soon brought reprisals. One prayer offered at a seance in 1743 made reference to Louis XIV and added: "How I tremble for your next in line [Louis XV] so holy and so sacred!" The prayer then predicted that "the Lord will undermine what you have built . . . and crush your house . . . that superb palace which for such a long time has been the seat of injustice and iniquity." The "errant and fugitive criminal" (Louis XV), the supplicant stated, would suffer God's wrath and "seek his crown and scepter on the ruins" of his palaces.[23] In 1744, "Sister Dove" predicted not only that Louis XV would fall, but also that kings in Italy and Spain and many archbishops across Europe would be "ravaged and devastated." Three years later, "Brother Isoré" warned that Paris itself would burn to the ground.[24]

Such talk constituted treason, and government officials took it very seriously. At police headquarters, Inspector Duval took charge of all cases involving the "Augustinian *convulsionaires*." The police, with mounting frustration (and poor spelling), labeled these miscreants *convultioners* and their trembling "alleged (*prétendues*) convulsions." In most cases, they hustled them off to the prisons of St. Martin or La Salpêtrière.[25]

By the 1750s, police repression and the Grim Reaper had taken a heavy toll on *convulsionnaire* leadership and defenders. Bishop Colbert de Montpellier died in 1738; Bishop Soanen of Senez in 1740; and Bishop Caylus d'Auxerre in 1754—the same year in which the convulsionaries' chief defender, Carré de Montgeron also died in prison.[26] Nonetheless, a few scattered sects met secretly in Paris. One group gathered at the grave of the priest *Père* Dory. Another group of six convulsionists (mostly *curés*), however, finally submitted to *Unigenitus* in April 1752 and dispersed.[27] The silver-tongued *parlementaire* Adrien Le Paige—after 1756 a bailiff at the Temple of Malta for the prince de Conti—continued serving unofficially as a secretary-archivist for the convulsionist sects in the capital during the 1750s and '60s. He amassed a collection of some 15,000 documents dealing with important political, religious, and parlementary controversies during the last 50 years of the Old Regime.[28] Manuscripts 196 and 197 at the Bibliothèque de l'Histoire du Protestantisme Français (Paris) indicate that perhaps 30 convulsionists gathered in Reims during the 1750s and '60s as well. Yet another tiny band met with the priest *Père* Joly in Troyes in the late-1750s. But by 1755, the total number of convulsionaries had dwindled below 800 across France.[29]

Overall, one gets the impression that rigor mortis was rapidly overtaking the movement, despite the allegiance of those who swore to uphold the "Confession of Faith" of January 1752. In taking this oath, believers, who claimed to be both "Christian" and "Catholic," defended Quesnel's *Moral Reflections* and professed their belief in the genuineness of the St.-Médard miracles and in the "truly supernatural convulsions and *grand secours* which all appear to be equally divine prodigies." The Confession also portrayed the convulsions as the "forerunner" of God's renewing the Church, converting the Jews, sending forth Elijah, and bringing an end to human history.[30]

If the convulsionary seances at Reims typified those being held by scattered groups across France during the 1750s, the emphasis in their meetings had shifted somewhat. Instead of the bloody "killing aids," this group (of five or six members and 30 attendees) focused on discourses (much longer now), baptisms (when surnames were bestowed), interpreting dreams (called "voyages") and visions (called "mountain-top experiences"), and singing psalms and other songs (*cantiques*)—mainly in Latin. Some unique features included the holding of communion services (when participants were served eggs, bread, wine, and vinegar) and "aspersions" (quasi-magical exorcisms to purify demon-possessed members).

Their homilies focused on the need to imitate the "Port-Royal virtues": charity, truth, humility, silence, retreat, hopefulness, and penitence. In their devotional exercises, leaders emphasized the need for confession, communion, penitence, fasting, baptism, and veneration of Christ, the Virgin, and the cross (which had a magical ability to ward off evil). Sermons routinely drew inspiration from the Bible (especially the Old Testament books of Daniel, Ezekiel, Hosea, Amos, and Isaiah), Quesnel's *Moral Reflections*, Agnès Arnauld's "Secret Chapelet," and Bishop Bossuet's writings. Their imagery was more positive and reassuring ("The Elect," "Infants of God," "the lamb," "diamond crowns," and "my palace in heaven") than in the 1730s and '40s. Yet much of it continued to be negative and threatening as well (Nebuchadnezzar, Sodom & Gomorrah, "hardened hearts," blood, death, purgatory, sacrifices, and enslavement). Speakers always concluded their discourses with the words "He who has ears to hear, let him hear."

While they continued practicing convulsions (known as "vuls" or "conditions") and *secours* (now called "prodigies"), the records seldom mention crucifixions. Unusually zealous, this sect in Reims met two or three times a week, most often in the morning (at 6 a.m., 11 a.m., or ll:30 a.m.) or mid-afternoon (3 p.m.) rather than late at night. Many of their seances lasted three to five hours and occasionally, all night long. Another interesting development was that while many of their female leaders adopted feminine names as before ("Sister Nanette," "Sister Judith," "Sister Ruth," "Sister Marcele"), some now assumed male nicknames ("Sister Alexis," "Sister Joseph," "Sister Abra[ham]"). Their primary leaders—"Sister Orpheline," "Sister Nanette," and "Brother Ottin"—served as prophets and visionaries for the members, called "Children of God" (also "instruments" or "tools"). Ottin specialized in predicting the destruction of the Society of Jesus (whose members he called "ardent wolves," "ministers of Satan," and "priests of Belial"). Based on what his "good angel" had told him, Ottin declared that sometime after 1758, "God's fire" would descend from heaven and destroy the Jesuits' buildings, after which princes and kings would expel them.[31]

Therefore, when Robert Damiens (allegedly inspired by the Jesuits) tried to assassinate Louis XV in 1757, the convulsionaries resurrected their *secours meurtrier*. Believing their king in mortal danger, at least 20 of them (mostly women) had themselves crucified, dedicating their pain to the monarch. Two of these, Françoise Obillard (who died in 1760) and Denise Regnier (who died in 1759), lived in Paris. According to the record, the assistants (or "laborers") first beat (or "worked") Françoise with garden spades, iron chains, hammers, and brooms. They then jabbed her body with swords, pelted her with stones, and buried her alive. Finally, they crucified her, using nails, awls, and needles. Françoise survived this sadistic torture. Denise was cut with a knife numerous times in her back, side, waist, arms, fingers, neck, feet, chest, and face, her tongue turned black, and gangrene set in, contributing to her early demise.[32]

To prevent the convulsionists from repeating these activities publicly at St.-Médard, the police closed the chapel on May 1 (the anniversary of Deacon Pâris' death) and October 4 (the feast day of his namesake, St. Francis of Assisi) from 1732 to 1757. But on 4 October 1757, the churchwardens themselves held a small service and no riots resulted. When they requested the privilege of holding a Mass in Pâris' honor in 1758, police chief Bertin, procurer-general Joly de Fleury, and the first president of Parlement consulted together concerning "measures to take to avoid a scandal." Apparently, they granted the wardens' request. Two years later on 4 October 1760, eight Masses were celebrated at St.-Médard "with great tranquility" (according to police chief Sartine) between 5 a.m. and noon. This time, the Deacon had been honored without miracle cures, convulsions, or crucifixions.[33]

Yet beneath this surface respectability lurked violent, anti-political strains within the convulsionary movement that made officials anxious. One cause for concern was the martyrdom complex many convulsionists evinced. Seeing themselves as "miserable sinners" on the one hand yet "instruments of God's justice" on the other, they focused their attention almost exclusively on end-time events and how they, as laborers preparing the earth for Elijah's coming, should face the apocalypse. While they hoped to become "Children of the Promised Land" above, if necessary, they were ready to become martyrs on earth if by so doing they could usher in God's kingdom. Because they saw themselves as first century Christians, *convulsionnaires* embraced punishment and affliction joyfully. "If it is necessary," they said, "we will expend all our blood for the salvation of our brothers and sisters." White-robed baptismal candidates were routinely asked: "Are you willing to die for the truth?" The correct response was: "To the degree that God gives me the grace to do it, such are [my] sentiments."[34]

Even more threatening than their penchant for martyrdom, the convulsionists' political views made them deeply suspect. The police accused the "Augustinians" of preaching against the laws of the state and holding secret commerce with the Jews. They saw the "Margouillists" as a cabal threatening government security and almost as much to be feared as the "Vaillantists," but less than the "Ottinists" whom the police saw as drunkards. The Church charged all of these sects with profaning the sacraments, abolishing penance, abandoning the Mass, using French-language Bibles, dispensing with priests, and denouncing the primacy of the pope.[35] In general, because the *convulsionnaires* believed in divine right monarchy as the proper model of God on earth, they never attacked the king directly; only in the name of "the All Powerful King" of heaven (God) did they point out Louis XV's shortcomings. Moreover, they saw themselves as "mediators" between God and the king to warn him of coming events.[36]

Yet sometimes government officials found their "warnings" offensive. In 1750, for example, "Sister Dorothée," alluding to Louis XV, declared: "Impure monarch, your days are numbered. You will perish with your scepter, you and your mistress will be struck by a tragic death."[37] In one terrible dream, "Sister Alexis" saw the Palace of Versailles in flames and the king surrounded by four lions. Interpreting her dream, she predicted that Parlement would cause the king much trouble, imposters would attack him, but Louis XV, after "converting and doing penitence," would "run to the convulsionists" for help.[38] Another discourse exclaimed: "Do you see the King, broken, not by God's voice but by politics, by the Parlement? . . . Accordingly, the conversion of this hardened sinner is next; he will no longer be able to resist Parlement, and God himself will speak to him without his knowledge of it."[39] Another sternly declared: "I come to you by the Spirit who inspires me to speak against your throne, your Diadem, O King. I command you to descend from your throne; I command you by the Spirit within me to make your penitence, without which you will see God's arms of vengeance exterminate you."[40]

The *convulsionnaires*' cataclysmic visions also embraced the future of the Church and the Society of Jesus. In their writings, they saw the Catholic Church as corrupt and in need of reform, brought to a state of ruin by its "unworthy ministers" (often called "beasts," "wolves," and "dogs") whose hands were "soiled with the blood of iniquity." "Sister Nanette's" vision of four cats predicted the imprisonment of Archbishop Beaumont. Others, based on their dreams, foretold the downfall of the Jesuits (usually described as "serpents," "priests of Belial," and "ministers of Satan"). The convulsionaries even attacked Jansenist doctors of theology for their elitism and "rational disputations" that replaced the "light of faith" with human reason.[41] In response, 30 Sorbonne doctors rejected the convulsions as contrary to God's commandments.[42]

Convulsionist sects, like the dodo bird, had become nearly extinct by the 1760s. One group, a "distinguished company" of old men, young girls, and parents with children led by "Sister Rachel"—all dressed informally in their chamber robes and bonnets—met in a home on the *rue* des Trois Virtus in Paris. An outside observer, admitted to one particular seance in February 1760, saw convulsions (with sobs and "trembling respiration"), "states of ecstasy" approaching "derangement," and the *grand secours* (with violent blows nearly suffocating the victim). Finally, the observer witnessed the crucifixion of a female participant during which assistants drove large nails into her hands (between the third and fourth metatarsals) and pierced her tongue. Showing no signs of pain, the young woman testified that "it felt good [to be] on the cross." As the girl's tongue swelled and her wounds gushed blood, "Sister Felicity," an older woman, calmly talked about the Church while off to one side, "Sister Sion" had a convulsion so violent that someone had to step on her chest to restrain her. Some participants stood while being beaten on the back, others lay prone while being pressed with heavy weights on their chest, and still others received the five stigmata of Christ (wounds in their hands, feet, and side). Just as the seance reached what the observer called "external disorder," however, the police arrived and packed everyone off to the Bastille and the Grand-Châtelet.[43] Two years later, Parlement issued an *arrêt* forbidding the *grand secours* as "potentially dangerous" to human life; those caught participating in it would be imprisoned.[44]

With the exception of Vincennes and the Bastille (royal "prisons of state"), Louis XV and his ministers left the choice of where the convulsionaries would be incarcerated up to the police. Basic considerations of decency and good order, not heresy or family honor, sparked a police crackdown in Paris after 1735.[45] The statistics of incarceration make it clear that officials intended to sweep the capital clean of convulsionists. Between 1732 and 1774, they sent 176 of them to the Bastille, 74 to the Grand-Châtelet, and 300 to the chateau of Vincennes. Women made up about 90 percent of those arrested.[46] Lower class offenders were incarcerated at the Petit-Châtelet, the Conciergerie, For-l'Evêque, St.-Lazare (for youth), La Salpêtrière (for women), and Bicêtre (for men). The government sent others to the provinces to be exhibited as curiosities before crowds who paid to see them at citadels and castles.[47]

After 1732, when arrests intensified, the outlook for the convulsionaries darkened perceptibly. In January 1736 alone, the police arrested 80 convulsionist "pilgrims" beating and cutting each other around a table at Port-Royal des Champs. The usual penalty was five hours in the *carcan* (stocks) or several weeks in prison.[48] Occasionally, they spent time in several prisons. For continuing her convulsions in detention, the police in 1734 moved Pélagie Rousseau from the Petit-Châtelet to the Bastille to Vincennes—all within one week. Her convulsions inspired the visitor Carré de Montgeron, horrified her guards, and disgusted police chief Hérault.[49] Similarly, the officers moved La Gallois from the Petit-Châtelet to Vincennes because "she was still capable of creating disorder among the prisoners" with her continued convulsions. Several weeks on a bread-and-water diet, however, starved her convulsons and secured her release.[50]

Male convulsionists went to Bicêtre, a prison within the vast Hôpital-Général complex for beggars, vagabonds, and lower-class criminals. Typically, these men worked thirteen-hour days knitting, weaving, and sewing to help defray their expenses; they ate mainly bread and soup and slept on straw ticks. In an effort to rehabilitate inmates, prison officials forced them to attend Mass, hear daily prayers, and read their catechism and pious books.[51] For resisting his arrest and fighting with police, Monsieur Moquion was sent to Bicêtre in January 1732.[52] Jacques Blanchet, a master shoemaker who had done time at the Bastille in 1692 for conspiring against Louis XIV, found himself at Bicêtre in 1736 for leading convulsionary assemblies and distributing copies of the *Nouvelles Ecclésiastiques*. The police sent 20 other convulsionists there in May for trying to overthrow the king and Parlement and reestablish the Estates-General.[53] Convulsionism mixed with treason usually brought longer prison terms.

But the regimen at the women's prison of La Salpêtrière proved so harsh that many *convulsionistes* died.[54] Part of the Hôpital-Général complex, Salpêtrière admitted lower-class prostitutes, beggars, and female criminals who spent fifteen hours a day knitting and weaving. They attended mandatory Mass on Sunday, heard daily prayers and catechism lectures, and listened to pious books being read while they worked. Poorer inmates ate only bread and soup, slept on straw ticks, and if disobedient, were whipped, branded, chained, tortured, and put in the stocks or in dark, cold, damp isolation cells. Because of harsh treatment, overcrowding, and unhygienic conditions, scores of women died every year.[55]

The first female convulsionary entered La Salpêtrière in 1731 when Minister of State Maurepas ordered the orphan Margueritte Dousson (eighteen) detained for counterfeiting spurious miracle cures at St.-Médard and for faking convulsions. At different times, Dousson had come to St.-Médard pretending to have a lame leg, a twisted arm, a lump in her throat, and a discharge of blood, then claimed instant healing at the Deacon's grave. After her friend Bonabel Lorisse revealed this hoax to Minister Fleury and police chief Hérault, however, they sent Dousson to La Salpêtrière.[56]

For holding convulsionist seances in their home, teenaged sisters Jeanne and Gabrielle Moulère spent almost twelve years (1737–1748) in the Bastille, Salpêtrière, and the hospital-prison of La Force. Gabrielle died at Salpêtrière in 1748 at age 26; her sister Jeanne was transferred to Ste.-Pélagie, where she died shortly thereafter.[57] Convulsionist leader Jeanne Marie Coutelier was more fortunate. Incarcerated at Salpêtrière in 1742, she endured a "long and hard detention" of nearly 20 years, but was released in 1761 when police chief Sartine felt she had "expiated her faults."[58] Several female *convulsionnaires* staged an "epidemic of convulsions" inside Salpêtrière in 1764, but when the police threatened to whip them and put them on "starvation diets" (bread and water), the convulsions ceased.[59]

Male convulsionaries sent to For-l'Evêque endured a harsh regimen similar to that imposed on women at La Salpêtrière. Situated on the *rue* St.-Germain-l'Auxerrois near the Seine with dungeon cells ten or twelve feet underground, this prison was often plagued by flooding, "putrid miasmas," poor light and ventilation, and general decay. In the Middle Ages, "the Fort" had been a Church prison for heretics, debtors, and actors, but Louis XIV made it a prison of state for *lettre de cachet* detainees. By the 1740s, however, it had become a police prison, and police chiefs Feydeau de Marville and Nicolas Berryer sent several convulsionists there.[60]

The first Jansenists detained there had been arrested for hawking portraits of the Deacon Pâris in 1731. Those incarcerated included Jean Le Roux, a soldier in the Regiment of Saillant, Jacques Guillebert (only fourteen), and his friends Duval, Le Maistre, and Verdive. Oddly enough, the police sent the thirteen-year-old girl Margueritte Hamelin, who had been arrested with these young men, to For-l'Evêque as well, but released all of them after only four days.[61] But the prior Brayer spent two months at "the Fort" for attending convulsionist seances in 1739.[62]

Normally, the police sent children and youth to the prison of St.-Lazare. A leper hospital during the Middle Ages, by the 1630s, the reforming monk Vincent de Paul had transformed it into a seminary, hospital, insane asylum, and correctional institution for juvenile delinquents in the *faubourg* St.-Denis. During the eighteenth century, however, it held primarily young libertines, elderly pensioners, and the mentally ill. Here, youthful convulsionists followed a militaristic regimen: they rose early, said their prayers, made their beds, exercised, worked, and retired early. Depending on the seriousness of their infractions, inmates were deprived of meat or whipped. St.-Lazare's motto was not to punish, but to reform.[63]

Given the limited number of children attending the seances, however, and the sketchy nature of St.-Lazare's records, one could surmise that officials sent very few *convulsionnaires* to this prison. But in 1737, when a police sweep caught the *comte* d'Avernes and his five-year-old son at a seance, they sent the boy to St.-Lazare for several weeks to reform his life.[64]

Although the record is incomplete, officials probably sent his father the count to Vincennes, formerly a royal residence. The Bourbon kings transformed this chateau into a prison of state reserved for rebellious nobles, leaders of religious sects, poison plotters, and wealthy bourgeois. Located in southeastern Paris near the Bois de Vincennes, this sister chateau to the Bastille had thick, impregnable walls, four tall towers, and many humid chambers. But its upper-class clientele enjoyed better food, clothing, furniture, and social privileges than inmates in other Paris prisons.[65]

For participating in a convulsionary seance, police arrested the young student Paul François Langlade and sent him to Vincennes in April 1734. But after three months, with his mind "absolutely deranged," Minister Maurepas transferred him to Charenton, a hospital-prison that specialized in treating mental illness. Treatments there "completely restored his health." After promising to have no further relations with his convulsionary friends, Langlade was released. But for "falling into the same excesses" at the Church of Ste.-Marine, he was rearrested in November and sent to Bicêtre. His dossier contains no *lettre de cachet* of release, only the notation that he "is tranquil and not dangerous."[66]

A police sweep in August 1735 sent ten *convulsionnaires* to Vincennes, most of them women who had participated in a seance. Caught in their net, however, was the only son of *Sieur* Adam Royer, the sub-delegate for the *intendant* of Paris and hunting master for the *duchesse* de Vendôme. In their nine-page placet, which included letters from Secretaries of State D'Argenson and Phélypeaux, Minister of War Pontchartrain, Chancellor D'Aguesseau, and *intendant* of Paris Beiguoy, the distraught parents asked that their (unnamed) son remain at Vincennes rather than be exiled from Paris. This request was granted.[67]

Typically, when the police arrested someone, they conducted a thorough search of their premises to find incriminating evidence that could be used in court. Seldom, however, did they succeed so well as in the case of the *abbé* Jacques Pierre Guillani Fleur de Rouvroy. When he entered Vincennes in November 1735, so did 778 pieces of his correspondence, poems, sermons, essays, eulogies, devotional writings, and polemical works which today fill three rolls of microfilm at the Bibliothèque de l'Arsenal.[68]

Without a doubt, two anonymous convulsionists—one man and one young girl—hold the record for the longest period of detention. When Louis XVI's Minister of the Household Lamoignon de Malesherbes released them in November 1775, these two had already spent 41 years (1734–1775) at the Conciergerie prison in Paris. It is likely that, in addition to their convulsionary activities, they were guilty of more serious crimes. However, such lengthy incarcerations were not typical during the reign of Louis XV.[69]

Convulsionnaires at the Bastille, 1731–1774: A Quantitative and Qualitative Analysis

Because of incomplete records on convulsionist detentions for all of the above prisons except the Bastille, the following statistical analysis is valid only for that chateau. What follows, however, may shed light on larger trends that could be valid for other prisons during this era.

During the reign of Louis XV, 176 convulsionaries entered the Bastille, slightly more than half the number (326) of Jansenists for the same period. [Graph 12] Yet whereas 85% of the Bastille's Jansenists had been men and only 15% women, 55% (97) of the convulsionists were women and 45% (79) men. [Graphs 5 and 11] As previously seen, this gender reversal reflected the more prominent roles women played in the convulsionary movement as sufferers at St.-Médard, hostesses at seances, and participants in the *secours*.

The peak years for their incarceration—the 1730s and 1740s—comprised the decades of the greatest Jansenist and convulsionist activity in Paris. [Graph 4] Between 1729 and 1738, 82 *convulsionnaires* entered the Bastille (about eight per year), and from 1739 to 1748, 102 more entered (about ten per year). But from 1749 to 1774, only eighteen convulsionists entered the chateau (less than one per year) as government repression waned and splits within the various sects caused the movement to die out. Although no convulsionaries entered the Bastille during Louis XVI's reign, the unduly long detention of one leader, Nicolas-Antoine Leguay (from 1757 to 1786), extended into his reign.

Of those whose occupations and status are known [Table 4], only eighteen (10.3%) of the convulsionists sent to the Bastille were from the First Estate (thirteen abbots, four monks, and one priest). Only six (3.6%) of those arrested came from the Second Estate, for very few nobles stayed with the movement during its violent *secouriste* stage. Consequently, most of the convulsionaries at the Bastille (75 or 42.3%) came from the Third Estate. At least sixteen (9.2%) represented the respectable middle class: merchants, gentlemen, lawyers, writers, and so forth. Although the status of 77 (43.8%) is unknown, police records make it likely that most of these came from the capital's blue-collar tradesmen. Most (98.3%) of these had been arrested and charged with fraudulent miracles of healing, holding convulsionist assemblies, or simply supporting the movement in some way. Of the three charged with other offenses, two entered for assisting another prisoner with convulsions and one for Jansenist writings.

Despite the harsh treatment of some *convulsionnaires* at the prison, on the whole, Louis XV did not detain them nearly as long as he did Jansenists. For example, whereas the mean term for Jansenists between 1715 and 1774 had been 324 days (almost eleven months), the mean stay for the convulsionaries amounted to only 252 days (8.5 months) [Tables 5 and 8]. The difference between the Jansenist median stay (133 days or 4.5 months) and the convulsionists' median stay (63.5 days or two months) is even more striking, given the often violent behavior of the latter. But the government leaned in the opposite direction when it came to releasing these inmates. Whereas Louis XV had freed 83.4% of the Jansenist detainees and transferred only 3.1% of them to other prisons, he granted complete freedom to only 74.4% (131) of his convulsionaries and transferred almost six times more of them—17.6% (31)—to other penal institutions. A further thirteen (7.4%) were exiled and one went to the galleys [Tables 11 and 12].[70]

While computer-generated statistics contribute precise quantitative information about *convulsionnaire* inmates over long periods of time, personal anecdotes provide human interest details and insights into the qualitative differences in their treatment during the long reign of Louis XV (1715–1774). Pro-Jansenist writers like Augustin Gazier (1924) have asserted that the vast majority of convulsionists sent to the Bastille endured "very harsh" treatment, being denied the right to exercise, write, and receive the sacraments.[71] Such generalizations, however, do not fit the reality for the treatment of most eighteenth-century convulsionaries according to the cases discussed below.

Thérèse Langlois (1731)

For peddling copies of the *Nouvelles Ecclésiastiques*, Thérèse Langlois and her niece Ursule Lombard, both from printing families, entered the Bastille in September 1731. After the police arrested and imprisoned her husband, their printing business went bankrupt and Thérèse suffered a physical and mental breakdown. Out of consideration for her condition, officials released her in December after only three months' detention.[72]

Marguerite Giroux (1732)

Arrested for going to St.-Médard several times seeking relief from her asthma, Marguerite Giroux (41) entered the Bastille in January 1732. But because her severe asthma attacks continued at the chateau, she was released after only two weeks there.[73]

Denise Régnier (1733–1756)

For her participation in the violent *secours*, Denise Régnier spent 23 years at the Bastille, Vincennes, the Conciergerie, and St.-Martin prisons. In her autobiography, *A Relation of Singular and Interesting Facts* (published posthumously in 1761), Régnier (or more likely, a ghostwriter) makes some rather preposterous statements about her treatment there. She claims to have been put in a dungeon chamber (they were almost never used in the eighteenth century), locked behind five doors (chambers only had double doors), and interrogated by 100 men in black robes (only the police chief or the governor conducted interviews at the Bastille). Police chief Hérault allegedly whipped her twice a day (no one was tortured or beaten there in the eighteenth century) and allegedly threatened her with chains, poison, and burning at the stake if she had convulsions. She claims the governor fed her on bread and water (never true at the Bastille) and denied her the right to attend Mass and receive visitors (probably true, given her aberrant behavior). Her frequent conferences with the Bastille's governor, police, magistrates, and Jesuits probably did not occur. Her litany of complaints regarding her eyes, stomach, head, and back ailments were likely due to her participation in the violent *secours*. Her allegations of being "miraculously healed" from cancer and of being chained to the dungeon walls four times have about as much truth to them as her claim that these one inch thick chains "miraculously" broke every night. In short, Régnier's alleged autobiography, while entertaining, reflects her hysterical state of mind rather than historical truth.[74]

Antoinette and Galois Prudhomme (1734)

For participating in convulsions three times a week in the *faubourg* St. Martin, the sisters Antonette and Galois Prudhomme went to the Bastille in February 1734. Their vicar, who considered convulsions "a common sickness" which could be healed over time, believed their detention would bring them and his parish "tranquility" from "these scandalous spectacles." Due to their father's mental incapacity and physical paralysis, however, the sisters asked to be released to nurse him. Antoinette's signed declaration that "in the future, I promise that I will have no more convulsions" secured her freedom after only eight days, while Galois (who did not sign a promise) was transferred to Vincennes.[75]

Milord Edward Donald Drummond (1739, 1748, 1750–55)

Certainly one of the most bizarre characters to enter the Bastille was Milord Edward Donald Drummond (50) of Perth, a Roman Catholic colonel in a regiment of Reformed Scottish Cavalry. He had been arrested several times for attending convulsionary seances in the homes of Mlle. de Vieupont, the *comte* d'Avernes, and Monsieur D'Angervilliers, the treasurer of France. Following his arrest in October 1739, he was sent first to the Bastille and then to the Chateau of St.-Germain-en-Laye for two weeks. The police, who tracked Drummond after his release, reported that he continued attending *secours* between 1750 and 1755 when, ill and hemorrhaging, he died with an English priest at his side.[76]

Alexandre Fleury (1741–1742)

Sometimes individuals with no connections to convulsionism attended seances merely out of curiosity, but during police chief Marville's crackdown in the 1740s, they suffered the same fate as participants. When Alexandre Fleury went to a seance, his curiosity got him nine weeks' detention at the Bastille (December 1741 to March 1742). His brother and two sisters wrote multiple letters to police chief Marville and Minister D'Argenson to eventually secure his release.[77]

Charles Hébert Family (1746–47)

Under rare circumstances, an entire convulsionary family could be caught in a police sweep. This happened to the iron merchant Charles Hébert, his wife Marie Charlotte, and their twelve-year-old daughter Marie-Madéleine-Charlotte when in September 1746, police arrested them along with three women and two men at a seance directed by the Héberts. All three Héberts ended up at the Bastille—the parents for six months and their little daughter (whom the police said "participates in the convulsions") for one month. Only after Charles (and his brother) wrote several letters to Inspector Duval and Minister Maurepas pleading that "this long captivity is so harmful to my family, my finances, and the training of my minor children" were he and his wife finally released.[78]

Pélagie Rousseau (1747–48)

Police had previously sent "Sister Pélagie" Rousseau, a leading convulsionist married to a clockmaker, to the Bastille and Vincennes with her eight-year-old daughter for misbehavior at St.-Médard Cemetery. Even though she was pregnant in November 1747, they sent her back to the chateau for continued convulsionary activity. But as the time approached for her to give birth, they transferred her to the Hôtel-Dieu hospital. After she gave birth in April 1748, officials sent the mother and son back to the Bastille but released the daughter to live with her father. Weeks later, they transferred Pélagie and her infant son to La Salpêtrière and then to the Hôtel-Dieu. Finally, on July 21, Minister Phélypeaux granted them their freedom after eight months.[79]

Claude De S____ and Sieur Baudin (1747–49)

If the police nets caught the very young at the *secours*, they also nabbed the very old. Officers arrested Claude de S____, 64, and *Sieur* Baudin, 72 (both of whom were convulsionist leaders) in 1747 and sent them to the Bastille. Because of Claude's age and feeble health, however, Inspector Duval transferred him to a monastery after only a few days. But Baudin, a notary at the Châtelet, remained at the chateau enjoying abundant food in his lavishly furnished room, writing letters to his many friends, and exercising in the prison garden. In June 1749, after Baudin had been detained 21 months, police chief Berryer granted his release on condition that he live outside Paris and stop holding seances.[80]

Abbé Vaillant (1728, 1734–61)

The prominent Figurist and *convulsionnaire* leader *abbé* Vaillant had already been sent to the Bastille in 1728 for his "extravagances" (to use police chief Hérault's word). Claiming to be the "true Elijah," he was sent back to the chateau in 1734. "I think that it will always be necessary to keep him imprisoned because of his weak mind," Hérault advised. Nonetheless, during his long tenure at the chateau, Vaillant enjoyed frequent visits from his wife, son, sister, brother, nephew, lawyer, and assorted friends. Among other gifts, they brought him clothing (shirts, vests, trousers, bonnets, shawls, and shoes) and lots of food (white wine, macaroons, cookies, spices, oil, butter, anise, cakes) and tobacco. He wrote letters (in Latin and French) to his family and friends and to Minister Fleury requesting his freedom. In short, he lived as comfortable a life at the

Bastille as any noble ever enjoyed there. On 19 February 1761, after suffering a stroke, Vaillant received the last rites and died that afternoon. He was buried at midnight under the name "*comte* d'Ipsum, foreigner" (a common practice at the Bastille).[81]

Susanne Raubeau Duchenne (1748)

Sometimes the quickest way out of the Bastille was to sign a confession of guilt and promise to abandon one's convulsions. Typical of many such pledges is the confession signed by Susanne Duchenne on 15 March 1748:

> I, Susanne Raubeau, wife of Duchenne, declare in the sincerity of my heart and without any force being applied that my convulsions have been purely voluntary on my part, believing them good to do, and that I would not have had them if I had known they are simply an illusion that I created on my own, which is why I promise Monsieur Lieutenant-General of Police [Nicolas Berryer] to do them no more and to renounce the work of convulsions and never again to attend their assemblies nor associate with particular *convulsionnaires* . . . as [convulsions are] dangerous things only too human and an invention of myself.[82]

Yet release from the Bastille did not guarantee one freedom, for as the statistics cited above show, one-fourth of the convulsionists released from the chateau were either transferred to other prisons or exiled. In 1732, Marie Beaubourg was sentenced to five years banishment from Paris for distributing copies of the *Nouvelles Ecclésiastiques*.[83] Those who printed the newspaper, however, were sent farther away for longer periods of time. The printer *Sieur* Earotanacq, for example, spent only twelve days at the Bastille in 1733, but Minister Maurepas banished him to Toulouse for an indefinite period of time.[84] Convulsionary leaders, on the other hand, could be exiled from France forever. In 1734, when the *intendant* of Moulin banished Jeanne Desbarbert, she fled to Holland and changed her name to Delamarre.[85] The convulsionary leader Pierre de La Barre, a lawyer in the Parlement of Rouen, could consider himself lucky when Minister Phélypeaux signed an order exiling him for only nine years (1761–70) for holding seances in his home.[86] When he came to the throne in 1774, however, Louis XVI freed all the remaining *convulsionnaires* at the Bastille and banished only priests and *curés* who refused to give the sacraments to their Jansenist parishioners.[87]

Yet freedom from persecution, far from inspiring growth and spiritual vitality, had the opposite effect on the convulsionary movement. The few remaining sects grew more rigid, less spiritual, and more violent. As Catherine Maire (1998) explained, by the late 1770s, the convulsionists had lost the sense of a theology focused on a "hidden God." They had also suppressed all forms of individual or institutional mediation by their doctrine of grace. Although the certainty of their faith was stronger than that of the Protestants, convulsionaries offered members no chance of redemption by works (as Calvinists did) or any hope of recovering a sense of union with God.[88]

Instead, their *secours*, bloodier and more violent than ever before, offered an endless variety show of sadomasochistic tortures. During one three-week series of seances from 20 September to 10 October 1772, one woman cut herself 479 times with a stiletto, hit herself 1,143 times with a shovel, pierced her skin 244 times with a pair of scissors, beat her back and groin innumerable times with sticks and a hammer, and carved the sign of the cross into her flesh with a razor. One observer remarked: "Her blouse was full of blood."[89] And during this shocking scene, no one offered a discourse interpreting the deeper spiritual meaning of this self-inflicted brutality or led the group in songs or prayers. One suspects that for many convulsionary sects in the 1770s, the *secours* had degenerated into violence for its own sake. Lust for the bloody, erotic spectacle had replaced love for spiritual communion and healing miracles.

As the *convulsionnaire* craze waned in Paris, it spread to the provinces. Two decades before the

French Revolution, tiny, scattered sects—called the *Petites Eglises* (the "Little Church") after 1776—met intermittently at Lyons, Forez, and a few other locations. Altogether, their numbers probably never exceeded 100. Their leaders included *Père* Michel Pinel ("pontiff of the order"), the Bonjour brothers, "Sister Babet" (also called "Sister Angélique"), "Sister Anne" ("the Servant of the Highest"), and the mysterious "Mme. S." Their seances featured bizarre visions, more violent convulsions, and bloodier tortures. In addition, some groups added sorcery and exorcism to their programs; a decade later, others would introduce mesmerism and "animal magnetism" into their seances.[90]

Written records of seances during the 1770s are as scarce as hen's teeth, but at the Bibliothèque de l'Histoire du Protestantisme Français (Paris), the Fonds Ste.-Beuve contains a transcript (manuscript 130) of one tiny sect that met between 1770 and 1775. Led by "Sister Angélique Rachel" with the help of "Sister Madéleine Esther," "Sister Judith Moz," and "Sister Jocabed," this democratic group also included a number of male "assistants": "Brother Jacob-Job," "Brother Azarias Joseph," "Brother Bonan," "Brother Jonas," "Brother Augustine," and "Brother Joseph Samuel."[91]

The discourses and letters written by these convulsionaries contain vivid images, themes, and symbols. Positive themes include the fact that Jesus entrusts his "Infants of God" with "hidden truths," that God's kingdom will soon be reestablished, and that one can obtain victory through Christ's crucifixion. On the other hand, frequent references to being exiled from home and enduring earthly sacrifices and sufferings, injustice and violence, the terror of the judgment, and persecution evoke negative themes and imagery. Symbols are both positive (Judah, Israel, Elijah, Joseph, the Temple, sheep, God's spouse, bread, the "living seed") and negative (the "smoke of iniquity," prostitution, a "letter of death"). While on the one hand, members eagerly anticipate the coming of Elijah and the conversion of the Jews, on the other hand, they tremble at the "divine vengeance [soon to fall] upon our criminal nation" as God "humiliates" France, "perhaps in a war."[92]

This doom-and-gloom outlook obviously clashed with the optimistic spirit of the Enlightenment and made the *convulsionnaires* personae non grata with the philosophes. Although Monique Cottret (1998) was not entirely correct when she asserted that all the philosophes "without exception" saw the convulsionists as fanatics and denounced them as such,[93] most of them did see these sects as the incarnation of irrationality, superstition, enthusiasm, obscurantism, and imposture.[94]

A few philosophes, however, made positive comments about them. David Hume (who allegedly did not believe in miracles), in his *Inquiry Concerning Human Understanding*, stated that the St.-Médard cures were better attested than the healing miracles performed by Christ.[95] The baron de Montesquieu praised the convulsionist Carré de Montgeron as "a great visionary and a great Jansenist," although he felt he had been "too audacious" to present his book to Louis XV in person without an invitation.[96] The *abbé* Tingault, who wrote articles for the *Encyclopédie*, was a convulsionary. D'Alembert, La Condamine, and Grimm occasionally attended seances; at one, D'Alembert observed the bloody *secours* of Françoise Obillard (described above). La Mettrie not only frequented convulsionary assemblies, but assisted at one seance in St.-Malo. In his book *Man the Machine*, La Mettrie's theory of man as a "plastic machine" and his emphasis on the decisive importance of muscles, oscillation, and irritability may have been influenced by his experience at these *secours*.[97]

The philosophe François Arouet de Voltaire, however, saw the *convulsionnaires* as his personal enemies, the epitome of irrationality, superstition, and fraud. In his *Philosophical Dictionary* he attacked their convulsions as "a gangrenous and incurable sickness."[98] In *The Century of Louis XIV*, he described them as "enthusiasts" struck by "frenzy" and by "epidemic illnesses" such as "dementia" and "extravagances." To him, Carré de Montgeron had been "an absurd man, a mouthpiece for and a victim of absurdities." He realized, however, that what "has become ridiculous can no longer be dangerous."[99] In his *Seventh Discourse in Verse on Man: On True Virtue*, he called the convulsionaries "lazy fanatics" whose "convulsive enthusiasm," "contorted hands," and "false healing" produce "deaf ones who stupidly listen but understand nothing.[100] In his "Treatise on Tolerance," Voltaire called the convulsions "a lousewort illness to which only the most vile populace are attached."[101]

Yet Voltaire hid a family secret: His own brother Armand Arouet, receiver of court fees, fines and taxes at the Paris Chamber of Accounts, was a staunch defender of convulsionism. Armand enjoyed attending their assemblies and participating in the "fantastic and bizarre" rituals, some of which occurred at his home. Yet Armand was never arrested or imprisoned for his involvement with these sects, although his name was slandered in the popular press. François never spoke or wrote about his older brother, no doubt embarrassed that this seminary-educated man with a killjoy attitude and a humorless approach to life belonged to the same family.[102] Their father, however, once quipped: "I have two fools for sons, one in prose and the other in verse."[103]

Other philosophes shared Voltaire's negative views of the convulsionists. After attending one or two of their *secours*, D'Alembert called them "disgusting farces" that deserved to be "unmasked" so that they would lose whatever "little merit that remains" in them. Because of their bizarre and brutal practices, he predicted that "soon the name Jansenist will be forgotten."[104] Despite his Jansenist education at the Collège d'Harcourt, Denis Diderot, repulsed by the convulsions occurring in his neighborhood, called the movement "a sect of fools" and rejected their miracles as "cheats" and "deceits."[105] As would be expected, therefore, articles in the *Encyclopédie* attacked the convulsionists as a hysterical, "fanatical sect" and condemned their alleged healing miracles and *secours* as "the worst excesses" of human devising, neither satanic nor divine. One author even suggested that women staged these "spectacles" for financial gain.[106]

While no archival sources show women being paid for enduring the *secours*, neither financial gain nor love of the truth could keep the sinking movement afloat. By the 1780s, the Grim Reaper had removed its charismatic leaders and police repression had scattered most of its members. Except for a handful led by Catherine-Françoise Moreau ("Sister Brigitte"), a religious at the Hôtel-Dieu, and her helper "Sister Babet," they had become nearly extinct in the capital. In 1780, on his way to attend an Easter liturgy with the Carmelite friars, the peripatetic author Restif de la Bretonne met Edme Rapenot, a convulsionist bookseller, and persuaded him to accompany him to the service.[107] Most, however, had scattered to the four winds. Provincial sects meeting at Toulouse, Lyons, Marseilles, Pignons, Le Forez, Le Vivarais, and in the Ursuline convent at Charlieu in the Loire Valley attracted a handful of diehard adherents. Their *secours*, however, had ceased to be virtuous and had become vicious. Seances, which routinely lasted five or six hours, featured naked, bloody participants reciting the psalms as assistants rained hundreds of blows upon their trembling flesh (one woman endured 440 blows at one seance). It took months for *secouristes* to recover from such brutal treatment.[108]

By 1787, the convulsionists meeting at Lyons—certainly one of the longest-lasting sects on record—had disintegrated. One of their leaders, the curate Claude Bonjour, was imprisoned at Tanloy, while the other, his brother François (a vicar), was exiled for predicting the fall of the Catholic Church, Christ's Second Coming, and other "quasi-insurrectionary ideas."[109]

Seeing the end of the world drawing near, other *convulsionnaires* issued their own dire warnings. In 1783, one announced the imminent arrival of pestilence and fevers that would kill thousands in Paris. "Sister Cathay," predicting many "great evils" in 1784, warned that several French cities would be swallowed up "without a trace" in the earthquake to follow in 1785. A year later, Anne Elisabeth Fronteau (who, as "Sister Hulda" had been convulsing for 44 years since the age of fourteen), prophesied that the Gallican Church would soon be destroyed. Her contemporary, "Brother Athanase," declared: "I am the prophet Micah; I announce only calamities." In 1787 "Sister Aile" predicted that one of those "calamities" would be a revolution in Paris. "It is necessary that the Revolution come," she exclaimed. "I see only an ambush . . . the blood swirling around me; I hear the noise of guns, the king's palace is taken, his crown is snatched from him. I find myself plunged into the pits of the abyss in the midst of such a great revolution."[110] When the agricultural innovator Arthur Young dined with a handful of convulsionaries in 1788, they told him that within a short time, not one stone of the Palace of Versailles would remain atop another, for Christ would topple them all.[111]

In the face of such impending doom, some *convulsionnaires* sought hope while others searched for entertainment. After starving themselves and donning iron belts with spikes piercing their flesh, one group of Parisian convulsionists dressed as pilgrims walked barefoot to Port-Royal des Champs (an eight-hour journey) to sing, pray, and torture themselves in 1788.[112] Another group, caught up in the popular fad of "animal magnetism" advocated by the Viennese doctor Franz Anton Mesmer, incorporated "mesmerism" (a form of hypnotism) into their seances. Adrien Le Paige, Antoine Court de Gebelin, and Charles Devillers defended the convulsions in 1784 as a form of "animal magnetism" or "somnabulism" (sleepwalking) and tried to explain the miraculous cures in terms of the psychological laws of human nature.[113]

But neither "animal magnetism" nor psychology could keep France from descending into the abyss of revolution. Amidst growing social and political unrest, the convulsionaries reacted the only way they knew how—with violence. In Tours, a nine-year-old girl whose tongue had already been pierced 12,000 times with needles was crucified in 1788, but she survived. Marguerite Bernard was not so fortunate. Crucified earlier in 1787, she submitted to crucifixion again on 6 January 1789, and died as a result—the last documented convulsionist to die in the *secours*.[114]

Other convulsionaries, however, would die in the French Revolution. Despite their dire predictions, the convulsionists appeared confused by the Revolution. While Suzette Labrousse and Catherine Théot saw it as the fulfillment of God's promises of regeneration, "Sister Victoire" interpreted it as "God's anger" against "Sodom" (France), whose "corruption was even worse at the foundation than it had appeared on the surface."[115] Some, like the *abbé* Grégoire, expected the Revolution to bring the conversion of the Jews, the return of Elijah, and the Second Coming of Christ. Because the execution of Louis XVI, the Civil Constitution of the Clergy, the crowning of Napoleon Bonaparte as emperor, and the Concordat did not fit within Grégoire's prophetic schema, he, like many convulsionists, voted against all those events.[116]

As the French Revolution raged around them, a few diehard convulsionists assembled now and then for seances. In Paris, Marie-Gilles Bouzenet, who from childhood had participated in convulsions, *secours*, and crucifixions as the daughter of "Mother Macchabée" and close friend of "Sister Hulda," hosted one group that met until 1790. Several Benedictine and Dominican monks, a councilor in Parlement, and the secretary of the papal nuncio to France assisted at her *secours*.[117] At another assembly, "Sister Suzanne," who spoke Hebrew, received visions from the prophet Elijah, and announced the imminent return of the Jews to Palestine, baptized Jewish children in anticipation of the conversion of all Jews to Christianity.[118]

From the sketchy evidence extant, it appears that the *convulsionnaires* continued preaching their Figurist message to the very end. In 1793, Bernard de la Plaigne Lambert, a Dominican priest and one of the last partisans of the convulsions and *secours*, taught that the Jews' conversion and the Second Advent of Christ were two coinciding events that would usher in the end of the world.[119] At the end of the 1790s, "Sister Isaac" presented the same message in Lyon.[120]

Although Jansenists in general and the *Nouvelles Ecclésiastiques* in particular chose to ignore the French Revolution, it nonetheless left its mark on the convulsionary movement. In addition to taking the lives of many convulsionists, the Revolution radicalized their doctrines. By 1799, many of them taught that baptism was superfluous, that one could confess one's sins directly to God without priestly mediation, that the regular clergy and the cult of the Virgin Mary should be abolished, and that a common lecture and moral reflection should replace the Mass. When members of their various sects died, the convulsionists buried them anywhere, without tombstones or crosses. By advocating these beliefs and following such unorthodox practices, they alienated potential recruits and further widened the gulf between a resurgent Roman Catholicism and a dying Jansenism and convulsionism at the dawn of the nineteenth century.[121]

As this chapter has shown, by mid-century, convulsionism had entered its most violent stage as extremists embraced forms of sadomasochism, beating, piercing, and cutting one another in the *secours* and finally crucifying some of their members during the *secours meurtrier.* Such violence further split the movement into *secouristes* (who supported crucifixions), *mélangistes* (moderates who opposed them), and "Enlightened Ones" (who opposed both groups and sought common ground with the philosophes). By the 1760s, dwindling groups meeting in private homes at night to avoid police detection characterized the movement. Its handful of writers made doomsday predictions about the overthrow of the French monarchy, the downfall of the Catholic Church as "Babylon," and the imminent return of "Elijah." Surrounded by a growing number of enemies (including Louis XV, Parlement, the police, and the Archbishop of Paris), these radical *convulsionnaires*, increasingly obsessed with martyrdom in the 1770s, lost even the support of writers in the *Nouvelles Ecclésiastiques*. Following several decades of intense police repression, the movement all but expired in the 1780s, with the last recorded crucifixion occurring in 1788.

CHAPTER 9

Jansenism and Convulsionism, 1650–2000: An Historiographic Essay

"I am totally stupefied and extremely astonished at what I have seen. Some say that it's all a game acted out . . . only time will verify everything; if the work is of God, it will endure; if not, then it will collapse of itself."—*Dr. Jean-François Chomel*[1]

While the previous two chapters have focused on the convulsionary movement mainly in terms of its enemies and friends, a third group—those who sincerely tried to understand, diagnose, or explain the miracles and convulsions taking place—deserves closer attention. After examining its alleged miracle cures and convulsions, some of these individuals became proponents of the movement while others became opponents. To better understand this bizarre movement, therefore, one should examine the writings of those who have studied its causes, manifestations, and effects.

Over 70 years before Deacon Pâris' death, Antoine Arnauld laid the foundation for the Jansenists' acceptance of miracles. In 1657 he asserted: "God has only performed miracles in favor of those who are defenders of His truth." Consequently, miraculous cures provided "certain proof" not only of the orthodoxy of those healed, but also of the injustice and falsehood of those who persecuted them.[2]

Blaise Pascal agreed, stating in his *Thoughts* (1662): "Miracles enable us to judge of doctrine, and doctrine enables us to judge of miracles." Yet he acknowledged that both true and false miracles existed. False ones, however, were performed "in the devil's name" and did not impart "inward grace" as true miracles did. But scientific tests could not be used to tell the difference. "It is not possible to have a reasonable belief against miracles," he declared, for even false ones "prove the existence of true ones." Like Arnauld, Pascal believed that healing miracles could occur only within the context of orthodox (Roman Catholic) belief; God would not perform them for groups teaching false doctrines (Protestants and Jesuits). Thus, he concluded, miracles "are more important than you think. They have served for the foundation [of the Church], and will serve for the continuation of the Church until the end."[3]

In his war of words against the Jesuits and rationalist-materialists like Hobbes, Malebranche, Spinoza, and Simon, Jansenist writer Pierre Nicole argued in his *Essays* (1680s) that miracles demonstrated God's activity in the world to "convince the obdurate." While public miracles, he admitted, were rare, "secret and invisible" ones occurred frequently. Nicole defended the miracle of the "Holy Thorn," stating that it showed the "mark of its authenticity" in Marguerite Périer's holy life.[4]

These seventeenth-century theological and philosophical arguments set the stage for widespread acceptance of the events that occurred after 1727 in St.-Médard Cemetery. As far as the Jansenists were concerned, the miraculous cures at Pâris' grave demonstrated the sanctity of the Deacon's life, and proved the truthfulness of Jansenism.[5]

Two books and a letter written in 1731 illustrate how Jansenists used these themes in their self-defense. The anonymously written *Miracles* asserted: "It is one of the promises of Jesus Christ to his Church that miracles would result from the faith of those who believe in him." Far from being limited to the Early Church, such miracles would reoccur to the end of time. As examples of genuine miracles, the author cited the 25 cures wrought beside Pâris' tomb from 1727 to 1730. Not content with internal, self-authenticating criteria to prove their divine origin, this writer further argued that the testimonies of a host of witnesses and physicians demonstrated the supernatural nature of the cures and "prove that the cause of the *Appelants* is God's cause."[6]

In his *Life of Monsieur Pâris, Deacon*, the Jansenist Pierre Boyer called the St.-Médard miracles "God's design," declaring them just as genuine as any others connected with Catholic saints through the ages. Not only did their existence prove the Deacon's sanctity, but for six years they also "came as a much-needed help from Heaven" to confound their enemies (the Jesuits) and strengthen the faith of believers.[7]

But in a 12 December 1731 letter to Armand Wallon, the physician Jean-François Chomel, administrator of a hospital at Vichy, reflected a more cautious tone. Having witnessed the healing of at least two persons, he confessed to his friend that

> I am totally stupefied and extremely astonished at what I have seen. Some say that it's all a game acted out . . . Several sick persons are attacked with convulsions after their prayers and, despite their paroxysms, are not tired, which is extraordinary. For me, I do not know what to say; only time will verify everything; if the work is of God, it will endure; if not, then it will collapse of itself . . . I think the best thing to do is to live as a good Roman Catholic and not philosophize on these matters because there is much so extraordinary that I do not understand.[8]

This remarkably balanced observation came from one who did not consider himself either a Jansenist or a skeptic. The following year, after making several visits to observe the events at St.-Médard, Inspector Duguet was equally cautious: "God has operated in the course of these convulsions . . . to intervene and heal all manner of sickness," he wrote. Yet while many had found relief from their symptoms, some had not; therefore, he concluded, not all the miracles were genuine. What truly puzzled him, however, was how so many could be convulsed for days at a time, yet come through the experience "refreshed and tranquil."[9]

The answer, according to *Frère* Augustin, was because this was God's work of grace and not a sickness or devil possession. In a speech before Parlement in January 1736, Augustin declared that God himself had chosen the convulsionists to receive visions and to suffer for his truth.[10]

Doubtless the leading proponent for the divine origin of the miracle cures and convulsions was Louis Baptiste Carré de Montgeron, councilor at the Paris Parlement. He had come to St.-Médard in 1731 seeking amusement, but after being struck with paralysis at Pâris' tomb for four hours, he left the cemetery a believer. From 1737 to 1747, he allegedly spent over 100,000 *livres* in researching, writing, and publishing three ornate volumes (*The Truth about Miracles*) to prove the genuineness of the cures there.[11]

The Truth about Miracles was Montgeron's magisterial reply to the Archibishop of Sens' attack on the St.-Médard phenomena as false miracles. Marshalling first-hand testimonies from physicians, surgeons, notaries, and nobles, Montgeron employed the techniques of the historian, the scientist, and the apologist in his defense of the *convulsionnaires*. For the believer, he established parallels between the "Holy Thorn" miracle and the cures at St.-Médard. To convince the skeptic, he quoted from the letters and interviews of witnesses, giving specific details concerning the sufferers' symptoms before and after being healed. For the sake of the devout, he mentioned the various relics attending these cures and told where they might be seen. For the scientifically minded, he showed how these miracles followed natural law. For his legal colleagues, he used juridical logic to persuade them. By treating miracles as facts, Montgeron implied that they could be discerned both by faith and reason.[12]

Montgeron, who dedicated his book to Louis XV, strengthened his case with the king by focusing on eight of the most remarkable cures. To appeal to the king's spiritual nature, he emphasized God's role in the cures and how these miracles had combated Deism and doubt and "rendered glory to God." To satisfy the monarch's judicial bent, he focused on the thorough investigations of 60 *curés* from Paris to Reims. He also showed how genuine miracles fostered morality and developed good citizenship.[13]

But Montgeron also used the miracles to defend Jansenism and attack the Bull *Unigenitus.* He not only informed the king that miracles were superior to Church doctrine, but also that they proved the orthodoxy of *appelant* teachings. Therefore, since God could not bestow his miracle-working power on any church holding erroneous doctrines, the fact that he had honored the Jansenists must show that he did not approve of the Bull because it was not consistent with Catholicism.[14] These heretical assertions landed Montgeron in four different prisons over the next seventeen years.

Basically, those who defended the miracle cures and convulsions between 1650 and 1750 did so primarily on religious grounds, citing examples of miraculous healing from the Bible, Church history, and recent events. But some writers in the seventeenth century offered other explanations for convulsionary behavior, and skeptics based their opposition on those arguments. While some saw the convulsions as the result of demon possession or religious melancholy (the fear of hell), others blamed them on epilepsy, hypochondria, nervous affections, or "dance mania."[15]

For Church officials to employ such arguments, however, posed problems in that a denial of the divine origins of *some* miracles could lead many to question the genuineness of *all* miracles. This could even cast doubt on the miracles of Christ himself. Thus, for Archbishop Vintimille to repudiate the cures attributed to Pâris while defending the miracles attributed to other saints forced him to walk a tightrope between faith and reason.[16] On the other hand, skeptics saw his assertion that only the Church could define true and false miracles and that the former occurred only within the context of true doctrine as a circular, self-serving argument.[17]

Nonetheless, that is exactly what Vintimille stated in his Ordinance of 1735. By declaring that genuine miracles must be instantaneous and complete and that they must be accompanied by spiritual acts (prayers, Mass) and witnessed by persons whose orthodoxy and probity were beyond question, the Archbishop explicitly denied that any healing could be providential if it happened to a Jansenist. His narrow definition thus permitted him to condemn the St.-Médard phenomena as false cures on the grounds that they did not meet his eight criteria.[18]

While some eighteenth-century opponents of those cures portrayed them as the work of demons, impostures, or female fanaticism, the majority defined them as symptomatic of an illness. Given the widespread interest in medicine and Mesmerism during the Enlightenment, such diagnoses ran the gamut from the serious to the absurd. Some suggested that the convulsions were psychosomatic in origin, possibly caused by epileptic seizures, organic neuropathy, or hyperventilation. Others saw them as group-induced behavior, the result of "sympathetic contagion" (imitation and suggestion). Still others diagnosed them as a nervous disorder, either from sensory deprivation or from over-stimulation of the nervous system. But as the debate shifted from theological to medical grounds, many anti-Jansenists continued to employ circular reasoning, judging the miracles on a priori principles which themselves were in dispute. Wanting to believe the cures fraudulent or demonic, opponents paraded the convulsionists' "bizarre, absurd antics" as proof of the "degeneration and decadence" of Jansenism itself. Because of participants' violence and indecency, these cures could not come from God and therefore must be due to natural causes, willful fraud, or mental derangement.[19]

One anonymous author of a pamphlet entitled "The Infallible Rule for Discerning True from False Miracles" argued in the 1730s that such aberrant behavior proved, in fact, that these Jansenist cures were inspired by the devil. Since God would never perform a miracle for a heretical group (Protestants, Jansenists, and Jews), these "illusory cures" must be satanic. God permitted them only to test the faith of his saints.[20] This was the argument advanced by the Archbishop of Sens, Jean-Joseph Languet de Gergy, in his long-standing debate with the Bishop of Montpellier, Colbert de Croissy (who defended the miracles). For the Archbishop, anyone who disagreed with the pope, *Unigenitus*, and Catholic doctrines had to be of the devil. In the same vein, Bishop Caylus of Auxerre wrote two letters calling convulsionism "an illusion & an enthusiasm." Behind its so-called miracles stood "the serpent Satan," feeding "false & pernicious ideas" into the movement and inspiring its demonic *secours*.[21]

Leaving theological debates to the clergy, secular writers in the 1730s began focusing on medical explanations for the convulsions. One of the earliest to do so was Philippe Hecquet, Dean of the Medical Faculty at Paris and a physician at Port-Royal. While he venerated Deacon Pâris and had personally verified some of the cures at St.-Médard, he believed that most genuine miracles had occurred before his death in 1727. Hecquet also noted that sometimes the convulsions occurred apart from healing miracles. In his *Naturalism of the Convulsions in the Maladies of the Convulsionnaire Epidemic* (1733), the doctor drew upon observation, Cartesian logic, and scientific experimentation to suggest several natural explanations for them. The convulsions could be due to "vapors," "nervous disorders," "nocturnal hypochondria," melancholy, or "animal magnetism." He personally saw magnetism as the cause, arguing that in its natural state, the body fluids maintained equilibrium in the "hydraulic machine," but in a state of disequilibrium, convulsions could occur. Because the female nervous system was more sensitive than that of the male, it was more susceptible to "uterine vapors" which caused convulsions, especially once "erotic passions" were aroused. This resulted in "scandals" and "obscenities." Noting the elements of crowd psychology, fanaticism, and eroticism in the St.-Médard miracles, Hecquet suggested isolating males from females, refusing them financial support, and giving them cold douches, opium, bleedings, and whippings to cure them.[22]

To explain the convulsions, physicians and curates often borrowed from each other's disciplines. In his "Theological Letters XIX" (1737), for example, Dom La Taste believed that the convulsions demonstrated "the diabolic spirit" and that their "prodigious frenzies and incredible excesses" showed symptoms of mental derangement.[23] Doctor of Theology Louis de Bonnaire at the Sorbonne stated in his *Polemical Treatise on the End of the World* (1738) that the convulsionists' mental derangement was probably caused by their focus on Figurist exegesis, numerology, Christ's sufferings, and end-time prophecies. Consequently, an unbalanced spiritual focus led to an unhealthy mental, emotional, and physical life.[24]

In his book *Vain Efforts of the Mélangistes or Discernants in the Work of the Convulsions* (1738), the *abbé* d'Asfeld amplified this theme. As an *Augustiniste*, he believed that while a few of the cures and convulsions had been "good," many others had been fraudulent and therefore "shameful." If the former came from God, the latter, then, must have come from Satan. The problem, however, was to determine which was which. Asfeld suggested that any convulsions connected with indecency, fanaticism, or heresy could not be genuine. He further stated that these fraudulent miracles must be caused either by demons or by "specious invention" of human minds. It was even possible, he argued, that the minds of many *convulsionnaires* had become unbalanced, throwing them into "tranquil deliriums" (paralysis), "furors" (violent shaking), or "true madness." Their deranged minds caused the "violent agitation" of their bodies, leading to indecent postures and shameful actions. Such violence could itself be proof of devil possession.[25]

Less analytical than the *abbé*, Bishop Pierre-François Lafiteau, in his *History of the Constitution*

Unigenitus (1738), simply called all convulsions "tricks" played on the "gullible public" by "false prophets, Fanatics, heretics, and Imposters." Neither from God nor the devil, these violent convulsions had been man-made to "seduce simpletons" and gain fame for the Jansenist movement. Instead, Lafiteau said, they had "made the Angels blush" and brought scandals into the Church.[26]

Replying to Carré de Montgeron's 1737 defense of the movement, Antoine Vinchon Des Voeux penned his two-volume *General Critique . . . on the Miracles of MR. the abbé de Pâris or New Letters on the Miracles* (1740). Seeing too much "deceit & trickery" in the movement, he argued that healing did not always establish the truth of one's doctrines nor the divine origins of one's miracles. Healing attributed to a dead man proved nothing, especially to Protestants who did not believe in the intercession of the saints. Besides, miracles could just as well be satanic as divine in origin; the former certainly could not be classified as "true," while the latter might have been due to the operation of natural principles or medical science. Des Voeux attributed some of the convulsions to nervous disorders, melancholic humors, and unhealthy imaginations.[27]

In the 1750s, the *encyclopédistes* took a cautious stance regarding supernatural phenomena. The article on "Miracles" defined one as "an extraordinary event that surprises us by its novelty" (the popular meaning) and "an effect that does not follow any of the known laws of nature" (the philosophical meaning). Miracles could come either from God or from demons.[28] Less restrained in tone, the article on "*Convulsionnaires*" described them as "a sect of fanatics . . . who still exist" and whose alleged miracles were either "the work of the devil" or "an imposture."[29]

On the eve of the French Revolution, Louis-Sébastien Mercier, the secular-minded man-about-town, reflected on the convulsionary experience in the light of the current Mesmerism craze. Although his multi-volume *Scenes of Paris* (1782–1788) expressed admiration for Pâris as a "Jansenist saint," it had little good to say about those who came to "grimace & convulse on his tomb." The "alleged miracles," he argued, were caused by the "extreme force of imagination" and the "delirium" of "maniacs going to extremes." Once "folly bit genius," the feeble brains of some snapped. "They have danced on the tomb of deacon Pâris; they have eaten the dirt from his grave. What greater miracles [are there] than this frenzy?" he inquired. While he found this "enthusiasm" inexplicable, Mercier blamed "electrical commotion" and "fermentation" in their minds as the reason why the "flame of reason" appeared to be "extinguished" in most convulsionaries' brains.[30]

Nineteenth-century commentators, repeating the explanations of their eighteenth-century predecessors with slightly different terminology, could not agree as to the cause of the convulsions. Bishop Grégoire of Blois argued in his five-volume *History of Religious Sects* (1828) that all of the St.-Médard miracles had been "the work of Satan." Attacking their "bizarre opinions," "indecent acrobatics," and "immodest acts," he called the whole movement a "sacrilege and madness" counterfeited by Satan, who worked through "organic perturbations" to cause "delirium and imbecility."[31]

Non-theologians made the word "delirium" the centerpiece of their diagnoses of the convulsionaries' behavior. Dr. L. F. Calmeil, for example, asserted in his book *On Madness* (1845) that convulsionism was a form of delirium called *théomanie extato-convulsive monomania*. This mania particularly afflicted Jansenists who got little sleep, seldom bathed or changed their clothes, exposed themselves to the cold and heat, and spent hours kneeling in prayer. Such behavior, he said, caused spasms of the pharynx and esophagus, ecstasy, sleepwalking, catalepsy, and in extreme cases, madness.[32] Dr. J. M. Carcot of the Hôpital de Salpêtrière added another explanation in his book *On the Permanent Hysterical Contractions* (1872) when he suggested that "nervous contractions" and "hysterical attacks" often caused convulsions, too. Other nineteenth-century physicians modified Charcot's terminology, referring to this phenomenon as "crucifixion hysteria," "hysterical epilepsy," and "hysterical contractions."[33]

But a growing cadre of professional historians and scholars at the end of the century took a more cautious view of the movement. In his three-volume history, *The Last Jansenists from the Ruin of Port-Royal to Our Day, 1710–1870* (1891), Léon Séché frankly admitted that the convulsionary phenomenon puzzled him. One either believed that God healed the eight individuals whose cures had been notarized at St.-Médard or one denied that a supernatural power existed. "Between the two solutions," he said, "I admit that my reason hesitates . . . It is one of those subjects one can never get to the bottom of without losing either one's faith or one's reason."[34] Séché concluded, however, that the miracles had been "complete nonsense" and "charlatanism" most likely caused by the "nervous and fevered condition" of those who had been listening too long to the "magnetic" sermons of their leaders (Du Guet, D'Asfeld, and D'Etemare).[35]

Early twentieth-century writers found the diagnosis of hysteria to be the most convincing explanation for the convulsions. In an article on "The *Convulsionnaires*" (1908), André Maricourt and Georges Firmin-Didot attributed this "veritable religious folly" to hysterical women.[36] Likewise in his article "The Faith That Healed at Saint-Médard" (1909), the physician Julien Noir asserted that in at least 45 cases, these miracles were "scientifically explicable" as hysteria or "mystical madness."[37]

In his magnum opus on *Jansenism* (1909), Jules Paquier, a professor at the Catholic Institute of Paris, denied that the convulsions stemmed from providential or natural causes. Yet he seemed unsure whether to attribute them to hypnosis and hysteria or to demon possession. In the end, he straddled the fence between theology and psychology, concluding that God had used the "Holy Thorn" miracle of 1656 to try to bring the Jansenists back to Catholic orthodoxy. When they persisted in their errors, he allowed Satan to possess their bodies (via hysterical convulsions) so that they might see the importance of obeying God and his Church.[38]

But this contrived explanation satisfied no one. Instead, with some emendations, the hysteria theory prevailed during the Interwar Era (1919–1939). In an article on the "Convulsionnaires" in the *Dictionary of Catholic Theology* (1923), L. Loevenbruck ascribed the "false and illusory" cures at Pâris' grave to purely natural causes such as hysteria and other nervous afflictions commonly found among "fanatical sects."[39] The following year, August Marie, a physician at the asylum of Ste.-Anne, compared the convulsions of St.-Médard to the juggling and conjuring seen among the Fakirs, but he also saw elements of sadism in the *secouristes*. This abberant behavior was due either to pseudo-paralysis and spasmodic contractions or other nervous disorders.[40]

Writing about *The Jansenist Quarrel* in 1924, the *abbé* Léon Bournet posited three possible explanations for the convulsions: some were supernatural (but from God or Satan? he wondered); others stemmed from imitation or deceit; while still others could be attributed to hysteria. Because their doctrines as well as their cruel behavior had been condemned by the Church, Bournet preferred to believe that "the action of a demon inside a human life" explained their "diabolic actions."[41] In an article on the *convulsionnaires* for the *Apologetic Dictionary for the Catholic Faith* (1925), G.-J. Waffelaert agreed with Bournet in attributing the convulsive attacks not only to hysteria and nervous disorders, but also to demon possession. By their "rebellion against legitimate authority," the Jansenists had exposed themselves to Satan's control in their lives. At. St.-Médard he had led them into immorality, cruelty, and sacrilege.[42] In his major study of religious *Enthusiasm* (1950), R. A. Knox, concurring with Waffelaert and Bournet, blamed the convulsions and *secours* on "diabolism" which "can persist, even where men and women . . . are using religious formulas and invoking the name of God."[43]

As psychiatry and psychology became more sophisticated after WWII, so did the explanations relating to the convulsions and *secours*. In his 1953 article "Did the Convulsionaries of

Saint-Médard Surpass the Limits of Human Power?," Dr. Jean Vinehon asserted that the convulsions were medically explicable. Some of them had been due to mental illnesses (schizophrenia, melancholic anxiety, maniacal excitation, frenzy, or nervous crises), others to sadism (the *secours*), while still others demonstrated participants' preference for eroticism and magic.[44]

In their two-volume survey of *The Political and Doctrinal Struggles to the 17th and 18th Centuries* (1955), Edmond Preclin and Eugene Jarry explained that while some of the convulsions had been caused by spontaneous and involuntary spasms, others had been due to premeditated actions, imitation, or the desire for fame.[45] Abandoning this psychological explanation in *The Strange History of the Convulsionnaires of St.-Médard* (1953), Albert Mousset traced the intellectual heritage of the sect from Renaissance mysticism through eighteenth-century Freemasonry, Mesmerism, and the Illuminism of Adam Weishaupt. He considered the convulsionists "unique" but "absurd."[46]

The most recent interpretations of the convulsions have focused more attention on their psychosomatic nature than on spiritual, physical, and psychological dimensions. In her 1970 biography of Pope Benedict XIV, Renée Haynes, noting the "definite pattern" of violent convulsions followed by quick healing, labeled them "psychosomatic illnesses."[47] While admitting that Jansenists had many high ideals, John McManners (1975) described convulsionism as "a strange spiritual underworld of masochism and miracles," a "degradation of the original Jansenist ideal."[48]

In his *Miracles, Convulsions, and Ecclesiastical Politics in Early Eighteenth Century Paris* (1978), Robert Kreiser attempted to understand the mentality of the sect. After hours of "enthusiastic phenomena," he said they had experienced "a profound emotional catharsis." They felt divine acceptance and consolation, release from tension, spiritual liberation, and personal exaltation. Many felt deep inner peace and intense joy. Not only did the experience bring personal satisfaction; it also built religious solidarity.[49] Then Kreiser faced the baffling question of genuineness:

> Probably the most difficult problem with which one is faced on a subject of this sort is to try to make a determination of what was 'contrived' and what was 'real'; who went to the cemetery out of pure spiritual motives and who was prompted by appellants and others; who had real 'cures' and, later, real 'convulsions' and who merely pretended to have them; and, in all these cases—why?[50]

Then, tucked away in a footnote, Kreiser gave his personal response to this question:

> I have assumed that, whatever their actual cause, 'real' cures and 'real' convulsions occurred at Pâris' tomb and that most of the people who frequented the cemetery or the church of Saint-Médard did so out of sincere conviction and faith in the thaumaturgic powers of François de Pâris.[51]

No non-Jansenist for 250 years had been willing to admit that some of the St.-Médard cures might in fact have been genuine miracles.

In the 1980s and 1990s, the two leading authorities on the convulsionary movement—Daniel Vidal and Catherine Maire—have both treated it with deep respect and understanding. Vidal, in *Miracles and Jansenist Convulsions in the 18th Century* (1987), provided a comprehensive, balanced history of the movement. His book contained several charts and tables giving the number, gender, and social class of those who participated in the movement. Without taking sides, he devoted several pages to discussing those who saw the convulsions as satanic, fraudulent, hysterical, insanity, a biological imbalance, eroticism, menstrual disorders, fevers, and hallucinations.[52]

In *The Convulsionnaires of Saint-Médard* (1985) and *From the Cause of God to the Cause of the Nation* (1998), Maire attacked the "imposture thesis" (that the miracles and convulsions were fraudulent) because the facts contained in police reports showed otherwise. The convulsions were the latest development in the history of the "collective language of the body" from the medieval dances of St. John, St. Vitus, and St. Guy; the *danse macabre* of the fourteenth century; witchcraft in the sixteenth century; and the miracle cures in Paris. All to some degree focused on the body, the emptying of self, and the desire to have God (or Satan) in one's soul. Psychology was therefore the "key" to understanding their hysterical behavior. The convulsionists simply went farther than their predecessors by mixing private devotion with political action (opposition to *Unigenitus*). And when the state repressed them, these sects opposed the monarchy itself and advocated freedom of conscience for all.[53]

As this chapter has shown, over the past 350 years, interpretations of Jansenist-Convulsionist phenomena have followed basically four trends. In the seventeenth and eighteenth centuries, Jansenist writers like Arnauld (1657), Pascal (1662), Nicole (1680s), Boyer (1731), and Carré de Montgeron (1737) developed a spiritual defense of the miracles, seeing them as evidence of God's approval for Jansenist truth and consequently proof of the genuineness of the movement. Conversely, their enemies saw Jansenism and convulsionism as inspired by the devil.

During the Enlightenment, writers such as Hecquet (1733), Lafitau (1738), and Des Veaux (1740) sought physical explanations for the convulsions. Laying aside God and the devil as immediate causes, they emphasized the role played by Mesmerism, epilepsy, and nervous disorders in these bizarre phenomena.

During the nineteenth and early twentieth centuries, as more physicians and psychologists examined the history of convulsionism, they in turn interpreted it on the basis of mental or psychological disorders. Calmeil (1845), Carcot (1872), Séché (1891), Noir (1909), Paquier (1909), and Bournet (1924) emphasized delirium, hysteria, and hypnosis as possible explanations.

Finally, in the second half of the twentieth century, historians highlighted psycho-somatic causes. Vinehon (1953), Preclin and Jarry (1955), Haynes (1970), Kreiser (1978), Vidal (1987), and Maire (1998) focused on schizophrenia, sadism, eroticism, spasms, insanity, and hallucinations as possible explanations for the convulsions. As the twenty-first century unfolds, no doubt new explanations will arise for this endlessly fascinating historical phenomenon.

Conclusion
The Impact of Jansenism in France

"It is certainly true that of all our freedoms, it is the one of religious conscience that has been the most painful and taken the longest to achieve. No other freedom has a higher price."—*Jacques Galland*[1]

The story is told about a *curé* who asked a dying laborer if he was a Jansenist.
"No, father," the man replied.
"Then are you a Molinist?" the priest asked.
"No more, father," the laborer said.
"What are you then?" asked the surprised *curé*.
"I am a cabinet maker," the naïve man responded.[2]

Whether true or apocryphal, this anecdote illustrates how the teachings of Cornelius Jansen that troubled the theological landscape of the *ancien régime* for a century and a half barely registered in the consciousness of most citizens after the Revolution. But Jansenism had left its mark on French religion, society, and culture.

Léon Bournet (1924) believed that Jansenism had had both negative and positive impacts on French culture. Physically, its extreme austerities had separated individuals from congregational worship, the sacraments, and the Mass. Theologically, its doctrines of grace and liberty defied good sense, while its over-emphasis on the corruption of human nature had made it easier for many to accept the Enlightenment's ideal of the innocence of mankind. Its attacks on the Church had diminished the prestige and authority of popes, bishops, and priests and introduced the "spirit of revolt" into Catholicism. The expulsion of the Jesuits brought the "triumph of philosophy" and destroyed the last Catholic bulwark against deism. While Jansenists and Jesuits quarreled, doubt gained ground in France. Finally, the convulsions at Pâris' tomb had discredited all miracles in the eyes of many Catholics.[3]

On the positive side, however, Bournet believed that the Jansenist controversy had sharpened intellectual life in the Old Regime. Jansenism had kept alive the utopian ideal of a "divine society on Earth" at Port-Royal. It had also provided a counter-weight to the laxity, latitudinarianism, and casuistry of the age by encouraging Catholics to seek a deeper piety and devotion to God in their private worship. The Jansenists had furthered the cause of separating Church from state to keep the latter from harassing the former.[4]

Wallace K. Ferguson (1927) likewise believed that Jansenism had brought both positive and negative results. It had succeeded in establishing a higher standard of personal morality. But Jansenist polemics had discredited many Catholic teachings that kept some members in the Church without offering them acceptable alternatives. Moreover, its bitter theological controversies, legal quibbles, and fine distinctions (between "fact" and "right") encouraged skepticism and bred contempt for dogmatic creeds. Finally, its "warfare" against the Society of Jesus opened the door to the deism and skepticism that both groups despised.[5]

Justin Godart (1934) considered the *Affaire Jansénius* and the *Affaire Dreyfus* the "two great collective leaps of honesty . . . demonstrating . . . the continued existence of the sensibility and uprightness of the French conscience." Although three centuries apart, both "affairs" demonstrated that in the end, truth could prevail despite the opposition of pope, king, Parlement, university, and clergy. In Godart's words, both Cornelius Jansen and Alfred Dreyfus struggled for "moral causes" against "passionate evil" and prevailed.[6]

Although the Jansenists' notions of efficacious grace, moral rigorism, and Holy Communion have been repudiated, R. A. Knox explained (1950) that their devotion to the Sacred Heart of Jesus has spread throughout the world and become imbedded in Catholic liturgy. But their joyless morality overlaid the eighteenth-century Church and their love of controversy infected its discourse adversely. As a result, thousands of Catholics stopped going to Communion regularly. In the end, the Jansenist controversy weakened the Church, rendering it incapable of mounting an offensive against the philosophes and the French Revolution.[7]

Ellen Weaver (1978) posited that "Jansenism has come to have a pejorative connotation in Catholicism: it symbolizes all that is harshly moralistic and legalistic in Catholic practice and attitudes, particularly in regard to the sacraments of confession and communion." Although some have applied this negative judgment to Port-Royal, Weaver's positive portrayal of the nuns' fidelity to Cistercian ideals showed that this was "not fully warranted."[8]

Conversely, Dominique Dinet (1983) viewed Jansenism as the chief "agent of dechristianizaiton" in France. Its endless theological controversies had "enfeebled the faith" and caused "the near total disappearance of the [Catholic] faith" in Nantes, Yonne, Bourgogne, Auxerrois, and other regions. She emphasized declining clerical recruitment, ordination patterns of priests and monks, growing opposition to the Sacred Heart cult, increased arrests of Jansenists, falling church attendance, and rising illegitimate births. In the end, Dinet blamed Jansenism for rising indifference and drunkenness and declining attendance at catechism classes, vespers, and the Eucharist. By weakening members' confidence in the clergy, Jansenism had brought dechristianization in France.[9]

Yet on the positive side, Alexander Sedgwick (1990) declared that in defending their beliefs, the *appelants* had developed arguments based on freedom of conscience and reason that anticipated themes—reason, natural science, individual judgment, religious liberty—advanced by the Enlightenment.[10] Centuries later, even the Church recognized this legacy of liberty of conscience. On 8 September 1991, the 400th anniversary of *Mère* Angélique Arnauld's birth, Cardinal Jean-Marie Lustiger celebrated a Mass in the chapel of Port-Royal de Paris. During the service, he praised Port-Royal for its "extraordinary spiritual efflorescence," its "quest for God," and its promotion of "liberty of conscience." *Mère* Angélique, he said, had exemplified the ideals of poverty, obedience, purification, and humility" which are "truly the fruits of God." In his concluding remarks, Cardinal Lustiger stated that "our century, tormented and traversed with contradictions, has need of this bubbling source of purity and truth to empower it to accomplish its task . . . Let us affirm respect for liberty of conscience," he added, and not force others into martyrdom.[11]

In two books (1991, 1992), Françoise Hildesheimer depicted the Jansenist legacy as divided between positive and negative effects. In its own time, Jansenism caused a decline in attendance at Communion and in the number of French priests willing to serve. Yet it also defended the individual's right to search for truth and in 1789 became a symbol of resistance to Church and state tyranny. On one hand, the movement advanced the search for truth, grace, Gallicanism, Richerism, human liberty, Church reform, and freedom of conscience. On the other, it opposed the Jesuits, ultramontanism, royal absolutism, the Renaissance, and the Enlightenment. Its long-term legacy, she asserted, included Augustinian determinism, Stoic morality, the integrity of the individual's conscience, and the defense of religious liberty. Moreover, after 1962 Vatican II revived Jansenism's "style of spirituality" and "psychological temperament."[12]

Leszek Kolakowski (1995) blamed *both* Jesuits and Jansenists for "the enfeeblement of Christian values" in France: the former by their "leniency" and the latter by their "intransigence." Whereas the Jesuits made the Christian life easy, the Jansenists made it "so exacting as to be practically inaccessible to the overwhelming majority of mortals." He saw both groups as "the two dangerous diseases" within Catholicism. What the Gallican Church needed, he said, was "the middle way" of Bishop Bossuet.[13]

Finally, Dale Van Kley (1996) has asserted that the failure of the Jansenist movement in the seventeenth century brought mostly negative consequences. These included the persistence of a privileged Catholic Church (more dependent than ever on the king) and the reinforcement of the monarchy's sacral identity (with its more invasive absolutism and intrusive censorship). In the end, the Jansenist controversy led to the repudiation of Christianity during the Revolution.[14]

While one can argue the pros and cons of each of the above interpretations, when taken together, they illustrate the complex, controversial nature inherent in Jansenism, which, like a kaleidoscope, presented the viewer with different pictures of itself as its theological, social, and political milieus changed. In the seventeenth century, for example, its founders as well as the nuns and solitaires at Port-Royal des Champs portrayed an image of saintly suffering. Rejecting worldly comforts, they embraced ascetic lifestyles, praised self-denial in others, found comfort in hard labor and severe penance, and focused on death and dying. They believed that their regimen of fasting, praying, silence, solitude, self-discipline and minute self-examination would bring them closer to God and his truth.

Unfortunately, their boldness in defending Augustinian truth, with its emphasis on efficacious grace and moral rigorism, brought them into conflict with Church and state institutions. By their persistent refusal to sign the Formulary mandated by several papal bulls, they crossed swords with popes, kings, archbishops of Paris, General Assemblies of the Clergy, and Parlement, thus insuring that the history of Jansenism would be a history of almost constant conflict.

The complex makeup of Jansenism—theologically, socially, and politically—in part explains its controversial nature. In addition to Augustinianism, the fabric of Jansenism included threads of Gallicanism, Richerism, and conciliarism. These ideals led *appelants* to deny papal infallibility, favor Church councils, advocate electing bishops, and eventually, to urge the separation of Church and state functions. Naturally, their willingness to suffer and even die for these ideals drew them into constant battles with kings (Louis XIV and Louis XV), popes (Innocent X, Alexander VII, Clement XI), and Archbishops of Paris (Péréfixe, Harlay de Champvallon, Noailles, de Beaumont).

Yet in addition to these external conflicts, Jansenism's internal diversity created further tensions. Within its ranks one could find robe nobility, bourgeoisie, artisans and craftsmen. Over a century and a half, the movement embraced liberals like Robert Arnauld d'Andilly and the Bishop of Comminges, moderates like Antoine Arnauld and Pierre Nicole, conservatives like Saint-Cyran and Angélique Arnauld, and extremists like Jacqueline Pascal. The rise of convulsionism further split the movement into Figurists, Visionaries, Thaumaturges, Margouillistes, Vaillantistes, and Ottinistes, while the practice of crucifixion pitted *secouristes* (who favored such sado-masochistic practices) against *anti-secouristes* (who opposed them).

Because a suffering saint was never a silent saint, Jansenists in each of these groups defended their brand of truth through the printed word. Today thousands of their letters, speeches, sermons, books, petitions, remonstrances, and lawsuits demonstrate how they used the written word to preach their version of truth, resist the Jesuits, and practice civil disobedience to government and Church authority. Using "the feminine paradox," the sisters at Port-Royal crafted a strategy of passive resistance to forestall signing the Formulary and to defy Louis XIV's attempts to close the convent. During the eighteenth century, their example inspired Jansenists in Parlement, the General Assembly of the Clergy, and the Sorbonne to block approval of papal bulls, resist royal orders, and defy the commands of archbishops and bishops.

And this human drama, with all its pathos, humor, anguish, ecstasy, controversy, joy, and brutality, shows how these suffering saints were real people, not cardboard saints. They experienced love, happiness, and awe as well as sorrow, pain, and loss, just as we do today. I hope that this book will help readers better understand the ideals the Jansenists advocated, the holy experiment they established at Port-Royal, the church–state controversies in which they engaged, their bizarre descent into violence, and their gradual support of toleration. Although the social, political, religious, and economic reforms brought by the French Revolution made Jansenism largely irrelevant to the modern world, no understanding of the *ancien régime* would be complete without grasping its impact on seventeenth and eighteenth-century France.

Notes

Introduction: Jansensim in France

1 Antoine Arnauld, "Requête des ecclésiastiques de Port-Royal [au Roi]," 19 May 1668, in *Oeuvres de Messire Antoine Arnauld, docteur de la maison et société de Sorbonne* (Paris and Lausanne: Sigismond d'Arnay, 1775–1783; reprint, Bruxelles: Culture et Civilisation, 1964–1967), 24:471.

2 Antoine Arnauld to Port-Royal nuns, 10 January 1668, in *Lettres de Monsieur Antoine Arnauld, Docteur de Sorbonne* (Paris: n.p., 1655; reprint, Nancy: Joseph Nicolai, 1727), 2:288–89.

3 Weaver, *Port-Royal*, 41; see especially Marilynn Dunn, *The Emergence of Monasticism: From the Desert Fathers to the Early Middle Ages* (Melden, MA: Blackwell Publishers, 2000), 3, 6, 8, 14, 25, 42, 60–64, 111–27.

4 Angélique Arnauld's letters to the *princesse* de Guéménée and to her brothers Henri and Antoine Arnauld, quoted in Fabian Gastelier, *Angélique Arnauld* (Paris: Librairie Arthème Fayard, 1998), 266, 269, 407, 408.

5 Pasquier Quesnel, *Instructions chrétiennes et élévations à Dieu sur la passion avec les octaves de Pasque, de la Pentocoste, du S. Sacrement de Noel* (Paris: André Pralard, 1702), Preface.

6 Elizabeth Raplay, *A Social History of the Cloister: Daily Life in the Teaching Monasteries of the Old Regime* (Montreal and Kingston: McGill–Queen's University Press, 2001), 198–205.

7 Angélique Arnauld to unknown friend, 1643, quoted in Alexander Sedgwick, *The Travails of Conscience: The Arnauld Family and the Ancien Régime* (Cambridge, MA: Harvard University Press, 1998), 136.

8 Jacqueline Pascal to Angélique de Saint-Jean, 22 June 1661, in Jacqueline Pascal, *A Rule for Children and Other Writings* (1665), ed. and trans. John J. Conley (Chicago and London: University of Chicago Press, 2003), 146–52.

9 Roxane Kural, "Contribution à l'Histoire des mentalités de l'Occident pré-industriel: Etude de deux manuscrits de Convulsionnaires Jansénistes du milieu du XVIIIème siècle" (Paris: TMs photocopy at the Bibliothèque de l'histoire du protestantisme français, 1970–71), ff. 164–65.

10 Edmond Préclin, "Edmond Richer," *Revue d'histoire moderne* 5 (1930):321–33.

11 Antoine Arnauld, *Considerations sur les affaires de l'Eglise* (1681), cited by Bernard Chédozeau, "Port-Royal, les Gallicans et les Politiques à la veille de la *Déclaration des Quatres Articles* (1679–1681)," *Revue des sciences philosophiques et théologiques* 77 (1993):535–41.

12 Muchembled, ed., *Dictionnaire*, 22; Cabourdin and Viard, *Lexique historique*, 24; Marion, *Dictionnaire*, 103–108; and Bernard Barbiche, ed., *Les institutions de la monarchie français à l'époque moderne* (Paris: Presses Universitaires de France, 1999), 96–98.

13 Jacques Gres-Gayer, *Le Gallicanisme de Sorbonne: Chroniques de la Faculté de Théologie de Paris, 1657–1688* (Paris: Honoré Champion, 2002), 54–55, 179–80, 320–21, 435–39.

14 Saint-Cyran, quoted in Aimé Richardt, *Le Jansénisme de Jansénius à la mort de Louis XIV* (Paris: François-Xavier de Guibert, 2002), 72.

15 Antoine Arnauld, *Quartre Factums pour les neveux de Jansénius* (1694), in *Oeuvres*, 30:532; Pierre Nicole and Antoine Singlin, cited by Frédéric Delforge, *Les petites écoles de Port-Royal, 1637–1660* (Paris: Les Editions du Cerf, 1985), 132.
16 Antoine Arnauld, *Considerations sur les affaires de l'Eglise* (1681), cited by Chédozeau, "Port-Royal," 535–41.
17 Séance of 20 December 1743, Bibliothèque de l'histoire du protestantisme français, Fonds Ste.-Beuve, ms. 117, ff. 439–44.
18 Catherine Laurence Maire, *De la cause de Dieu à la cause de la Nation: Le jansénisme au XVIIIe siècle* (Paris: Editions Gallimard, 1998), 531–34; Durand Echeverria, *The Maupeou Revolution: A Study in the History of Libertarianism, France, 1770–1774* (Baton Rouge and London: Louisiana State University Press, 1985), 45–46; and Monique Cottret, *Jansénismes et Lumières: Pour un autre XVIIIe siècle* (Paris: Editions Albin Michel, 1998), 148–50, 153, 172–73, 177.
19 This scene at Court is reconstructed from memoirs in François Bluche, *Le Journal secret de Louis XIV* (Paris: Editions du Rocher, 1998), 40.
20 Unnamed Port-Royal girl to Archbishop Péréfixe, quoted in Félix Cadet, *L'éducation à Port-Royal* (Paris: Librairie Hachette, 1887), 66.
21 Antoine Arnauld, *Oeuvres*, 24:158.
22 Antoine Arnauld, Index to *Oeuvres*, 43:227.
23 Angélique Arnauld to unknown, 1653, quoted in Jérome Besoigne, *Histoire de l'abbaye de Port-Royal* (Cologne: Aux dépens de la Compagnie, 1752–53), 1:357.
24 Daniella Kostroun, "A Formula for Disobedience: Jansenism, Gender and the Feminist Paradox," *Journal of Modern History* 75 (September 2003): 485–89, 493–94.
25 Bull *Ad sacram*, quoted in Aimé Richardt, *Le Jansénisme de Jansénius à la mort de Louis XIV* (Paris: François-Xavier de Guibert, 2002), 82.
26 Emile Jacques, *Les années d'exil d'Antoine Arnauld, 1679–1694* (Louvain: Publications universitaires de Louvain, 1976), 491.
27 Antoine Arnauld to Prince Ernest of Hesse-Rhinfels, 19 April 1683, in *Oeuvres*, 2:238.
28 *Les Nouvelles Ecclésiastiques*, 28 May 1788, Bibliothèque de l'histoire du protestantisme français, ms. 522, pp. 85–86.
29 Rabaut de Saint-Etienne, speech before the Constituent Assembly, 1790, quoted in Cottret, *Lumières,* 200.
30 *Nouvelles Ecclésiastiques*, 1790, quoted in ibid., 199.

1 Who Were the Jansenists?

1 Antoine Arnauld, "Requête des ecclésiastiques de Port-Royal [au Roi]," 19 May 1668, in *Oeuvres*, 24:471.
2 J. D. Crichton, *Saints or Sinners? Jansenism and Jansenisers in Seventeenth Century France* (Dublin: Veritas Publications, Criterion Press, 1996), 278.
3 Cottret, *Lumières*, 308–309; Catherine Maire, "Port-Royal: The Jansenist Schism," in *Realms of Memory: Rethinking the French Past*, vol. 1: *Conflicts and Divisions* (NY: Columbia University Press, 1966), 302.
4 For a discussion of these historiographic views, see Richard Golden, *The Godly Rebellion: Parisian Curés and the Religious Fronde, 1652–1662* (Chapel Hill, NC: University of North Carolina Press, 1981), 124–25.
5 H. G. Judge, "Church & State under Louis XIV," *History* (U.K.) 45 (1960):217.
6 Ibid., 141; Pierre Chaunu, "Jansénisme et frontière de Catholicité (XVIIe et XVIIIe siècles)," *Revue Historique* 227 (1962):118; Pierre Chaunu, Madeleine Foisil, and Françoise de Noirfontaine, *Le Basculement religieux de Paris au XVIIIe siècle* (Paris: Fayard, 1998), 141.
7 Philippe Loupès, *La vie religieuse en France au XVIIIe siècle* (Paris: SEDES, 1993), 14.
8 David A. Bell, *The Cult of the Nation in France: Inventing Nationalism, 1680–1800* (Cambridge, MA: Harvard University Press, 2001), 28.
9 Jean-Paul Charlot, quoted in Richardt, 5.
10 René Taveneaux (1992), quoted in Richardt, 7.

11 Marc Venard and Anne Bonzon, *La religion dans la France moderne, XVIe–XVIIIe siècle* (Paris: Hachette, 1998), 3–4.

12 Richardt, *Jansénisme*, 12. If one accepts a recent estimate of US $40 per *livre*, the Church's revenues amounted to a staggering $4,000,000,000 in 1662 and $6,000,000,000 in 1674.

13 Maire, *Cause de Dieu*, 14.

14 Jacques LeGoff and René Rémond, *Histoire de la France religieuse*, vol. 2, *Du Christianisme flamboyant à l'aube des Lumières (XIVe–XVIIIe siècle)*, ed. François Lebrun (Paris: Editions du Seuil, 1988), 2:361.

15 Richardt, 14–15.

16 Golden, *Godly Rebellion*, 124, 126–27; Albert de Meyer, *Les Premières Controverses jansénistes en France, 1640–1649* (Louvain: Imprimerie Veuve Joseph Van Linthout, 1917), 475; and Jacques Plainemaison, "Pourquoi 'les Provinciales' ou une guerre purdue d'avance," *Revue historique* 287 (1992): 120–28.

17 Robert Remsberg, *Wisdom and Science at Port-Royal and the Oratory: A Study of Contrasting Augustinianisms* (Yellow Springs, OH: Antioch Press, 1940), 76.

18 Philippe Sellier, "Port-Royal: Un emblème de la Réforme Catholique," in *Chroniques de Port-Royal* (Paris: Bibliothèque Mazarine, 1987), 37:15–18.

19 David Hudson, "The *Nouvelles ecclésiastiques:* Jansenism and Conciliarism, 1717–1735," *Catholic Historical Review* 70 (1984): 399. On Jansenism in the religious orders, see also Augustin Gazier, *Histoire générale du mouvement janséniste depuis ses origines jusqu'à nos jours* (Paris: Librairie Ancienne Honoré Champion, 1924), I: 320–21, 331–33.

20 René Taveneaux, "Jansénisme et vie sociale en France au XVIIe siècle," *Revue d'Histoire de l'Eglise de France* 54 (1968): 27; Lucien Ceyssens, "Le jansénisme: Considérations historiques préliminaires à sa notion," *Analecta gregoriana* 71 (1952):5–6.

21 Guy Droppier to André Rivet, 16 January 1642, quoted in Jean-Robert Armogathe, "Le 'Phantôme du Jansénisme' ou la rhétorique de la déviance," in *Vie ecclesiale, communauté et communautés* (Paris: Didier-Erudition, 1989), 96.

22 Charles François Abra de Reconis, *Continuation des Examens de la doctrine du feu abbé de S. Cyran et de sa cabale* (1645), quoted in ibid., 97.

23 François Vavasseur, *Cornelis Jansenius Iprensis Suspectus* (1650), quoted in ibid., 96.

24 Mersenne, *Lettre à un ami touchant le jansénisme* (1651), quoted in ibid.

25 Golden, *Godly Rebellion*, 126.

26 Ceyssens, "Jansénisme," 7–8.

27 François Pinthereau, quoted in Armogathe, "Phantôme," 97.

28 Richelet, *Dictionnaire* (1695) and *L'Arte de penser* (n.d.), quoted in Armogathe, ibid., 98.

29 Jacques-Philippe Lallemant, *Jansénius condamné par l'église, par luy-mesme et ses défenseurs, et par S{aint} Augustin* (Bruxelles: François Van den Abbeelen, 1705), preface.

30 Jacques Fouillou, *Chimère du Jansénisme ou Dissertation sur le sens dans lequel les cinq Propositions ont été condamnées* (N.p., 1708), preface.

31 Silvester Jenks, *A Short Review of the Book of Jansenius* (1710), quoted in H. G. Judge, "Louis XIV and the Church," in *Louis XIV and the Craft of Kingship*, ed. John C. Rule (N.p.: Ohio State University Press, 1969), 244.

32 Pasquier Quesnel, quoted in Jean Laporte, "Le Jansénisme," in *Etudes d'histoire de la philosophie française au XVII siècle* (Paris: Librairie philosophique J. Vrin, 1951), 88.

33 Pasquier Quesnel, quoted in J. Dedieu, "Le déssarroi janséniste pendant la période du Quesnellisme," in *Introduction aux études d'histoire écclésiastique locale,* ed. V. Carrière (Paris: Libraire Letouzey et Ané, 1936), 513 (n. 3).

34 Pierre Nicole, *Lettres sur l'hérésie imaginaire* (1665), cited by Maire, *Cause de Dieu*, 11.

35 Robert Arnauld d'Andilly to Anne of Austria (no date), quoted in Golden, *Godly Rebellion*, 187 (n. 1).

36 Antoine Arnauld, "Lettre à une personne de condition," 1655, in *Oeuvres*, 19:331.

37 Antoine Arnauld, "Première et seconde lettres à un duc et pair," 1655, in *Oeuvres*, 19:369.

38 Antoine Arnauld to Claude Auvry, Bishop of Coutances, 15 March 1656, quoted in Paule Jansen, *Arnauld d'Andilly, défenseur de Port-Royal (1654–1659): Sa correspondance inédite avec la Cour conservée dans les Archives du Ministère des Affaires Etrangères* (Paris: Libraire Philosophique J. Vrin, 1973), 92–93.

39 Antoine Arnauld, *Apologie pour les Religieuses de Port-Royal* (1664), in *Oeuvres*, 23:274, 475.

40 Antoine Arnauld to unknown, 20 October 1682, quoted in "Lettres de Grand Arnauld (1682–1694)," Bibliothèque Nationale, Manuscrits Français 19723, f. 8 [hereafter cited as BN, Ms. Fr.].
41 See, for example, Antoine Arnauld's letters of 19 December 1680, 20 December 1682, 22 January 1683, 31 January 1687 in BN, Ms. Fr. 19727, ff. 18–19, 85, 139, 148–49, 181; letters of 9 January, 31 January, 20 February, 27 March 1687 in BN, Ms. Fr. 19724, ff. 2, 4, 12, 29; letter to M. Du Vaucel, 8 July 1689, in *Oeuvres*, 32:223; letters to Paolo Walloni in Rome, 15 June and 4 August 1689 and 22 September 1690, in BN, Ms. Fr. 19725, ff. 62, 80, 92; letters to unknown, 6 and 21 March, 1 August 1692, in BN, Ms. Fr. 19726, ff. 13, 16, 64; and "Phantom" entry in Index to *Oeuvres*, 43:129–30.
42 Antoine Arnauld to Prince Ernest of Hesse-Rhinfels, 10 May 1683, in *Oeuvres*, 2:255.
43 Antoine Arnauld to M. Du Vaucel, 31 July 1685, in *Oeuvres*, 2:543–44.
44 Antoine Arnauld, *Le Phantôme du jansénisme* (1686), quoted in Edmond Préclin and Eugène Jarry, *Les luttes politiques et doctrinales aux XVIIe et XVIIIe siècle*, in *Histoire de l'Eglise depuis les origines jusqu'à nos jours*, eds. Augustin Fliche and Victor Martin (Paris: Bloud & Gay, 1955–56), 19:212. See chapter 2 for a detailed discussion of the Five Propositions.
45 Antoine Arnauld, "Heresie," in the Index to *Oeuvres*, 43:120.
46 Jacques Fouillou, *Histoire abrégée du Jansénisme, et Remarques sur l'Ordonnance de M. L'Archevêque de Paris* (Cologne: Jean Druckerus, 1698), unpaginated.
47 Fouillou, *Chimère du Jansénisme*, 276, 278, 284.
48 Jean Carreyre, "La Doctrine janséniste," in *Introduction aux études d'histoire ecclésiastique locale*, ed. Victor Carrière (Paris: Libraire Letouzey et Ané, 1934), 3:515. In essence, Carreyre reiterates the earlier argument made by Augustin Gazier in *Histoire générale du mouvement janséniste* (1924).
49 Catherine-Laurence Maire, *Les convulsionnaires de Saint-Médard: Miracles, Convulsions et prophéties à Paris au XVIIIe siècle* (Paris: Gallimard, Julliard, 1985), 23–24.
50 Antoine Arnauld, *Seconde Lettre à un Duc et Pair de France*, 1655, in *Oeuvres*, 19:392–94.
51 Antoine Arnauld, Index to his *Oeuvres*, 43:251; see also Bruno Neveu, *Erudition et religion aux XVIIe et XVIIIe siècles* (Paris: Editions Albin Michel, 1994), 16.
52 Alexander Sedgwick, "Jansen and the Jansenists: Grace and the Free Will Controversy in 17th Century France," *History Today* 40 (July 1990):39; Cottret, *Lumières*, 271–72 ; and B. Robert Kreiser, *Miracles, Convulsions, and Ecclesiastical Politics in Early Eighteenth Century Paris* (Princeton: Princeton University Press, 1978), 3–4.
53 Antoine Arnauld, "Verité" in the Index to *Oeuvre* 43:276.
54 Antoine Arnauld, "Considerations sur l'enterprise Faite par Maître Nicolas Cornet," 1649, in *Oeuvre* 19:3.
55 David Garrioch, *The Making of Revolutionary Paris* (Los Angeles: University of California Press, 2002), 151.
56 Pierre Chaunu, Madeleine Foisil, and Françoise Noirfontaine, *Le basculement religieux de Paris au XVIIIe siècle* (Paris: Fayard, 1998), 85–86.
57 *Mémoires secrets numero xxxiv*, 2 March 1787, p. 230, quoted in Geoffrey Adams, *The Huguenots & French Opinion* (Atlantic Highlands, NJ: Humanities Press International, 1991), 275.
58 Giovanni Marchetti, *Che importa ai preti?* (1798), quoted in Robert Shackleton, "Jansenism and the Enlightenment," *Studies on Voltaire and the Eighteenth Century* 57 (1967): 1388–89.
59 Jean Carreyre, *Le Jansénisme durant la Régence* (Louvain: Bureau de la Revue, 1929–1933), 3:391.
60 Bell, *Cult of the Nation*, 194.
61 Jean de Brisacier, *Les Jansénistes reconnus Calvinistes* (Paris: Sébastien Cramoisy et Gabriel Cramoisy, 1652), 3–5, 8, 26, 45, 68, 72, 76, 81–84.
62 Nicolo di Bagno, 7 August 1656 dispatch to Rome, cited by Pierre Blet, "Le nonce Nicolo di Bagno et le Jansénisme, 1651–1656," in *La vie, la mort, la foi, le temps*, ed. Jean-Pierre Barde and Madeleine Foisil (Paris: Presses Universitaires de France, 1993), 436.
63 W. H. Lewis, *The Splendid Century: Life in the France of Louis XIV* (N.p.: William Morrow, 1954), 88.
64 Pierre Jurieu, *L'Esprit de MR. Arnauld: Tiré de sa conduite & des Ecrits tant de lui que de ses Disciples; particulièrement de l'Apologie pour les Catholiques* (Deventer: Jean Colombius, 1684), 2:4, 7, 9, 11.

65 Dale K. Van Kley, *The Religious Origins of the French Revolution: From Calvin to the Civil Constitution, 1560–1791* (New Haven, CT: Yale University Press, 1996), 100–102.

66 John McManners, *French Ecclesiastical Society under the Ancien Régime: A Study of Angers in the Eighteenth Century* (Manchester: Manchester University Press, 1960), 174.

67 L. Patouillet and D. Colonia, *Dictionnaire des Livres jansénistes ou qui favorisent le Jansénisme* (Anvers: Jean-Baptiste Verdussen, 1754), 52–53.

68 Carreyre, *Régence,* 2:391; Robin Briggs, "The Catholic Puritans: Jansenists and Rigorists in France," in *Communities of Belief: Cultural and Social Tension in Early Modern France* (Oxford: Clarendon Press, 1989), 362; Alexander Sedgwick, *The Travails of Conscience: The Arnauld Family and the Ancien Régime* (Cambridge, MA: Harvard University Press, 1998), 257; Auguste Sabatier, "Port-Royal et le protestantisme," *Révue Chrétienne* 2 (1897):82; John D. Woodbridge, *Revolt in Prerevolutionary France: The Prince de Conti's Conspiracy against Louis XV, 1755–1757* (Baltimore: Johns Hopkins University Press, 1995), 35; Henry Phillips, *Church and Culture in Seventeenth-Century France* (Cambridge: Cambridge University Press, 1997), 193; and R. A. Knox, *Enthusiasm: A Chapter in the History of Religion with Special Reference to the XVIIth and XVIIIth Centuries* (Oxford: n.p., 1950; reprint, Westminster, MD: Christian Classics, 1983), 176.

69 Carreyre, *Régence,* 2:390–91; Briggs, *Communities,* 362; Sabatier, "Port-Royal," 87; Chaunu et al., *Basculement,* 117; Henri-Jean Martin, *The French Book: Religion, Absolutism, and Readership, 1585–1715,* trans. Paul and Nadine Saenger (Geneva: n.p., 1969; reprint, Baltimore and London: The Johns Hopkins University Press, 1996), 18; and Norman Ravitch, e-mail to H-FRANCE listserv, 17 June 1996.

70 Robert R. Palmer, *Catholics and Unbelievers in Eighteenth-Century France* (Princeton, NJ: n.p., 1939; reprint, New York: Cooper Square Publishers, 1961), 29.

71 Ibid., 25, 101.

72 Athanase Coquerel, *Les forçats pour la foi: Etude historique, 1684–1775* (Paris: Michel Lévy Frères, 1866), 15.

73 Knox, *Enthusiasm,* 186; Fabian Gastelier, *Angélique Arnauld* (Paris: Librairie Arthème Fayard, 1998), 41–42; Daniella J. Kostroun, "Undermining Obedience in Absolutist France: The Case of the Port-Royal Nuns, 1690–1709" (Ph.D. diss., Duke University, 2000), 48; and Sedgwick, *Travails,* 12–16.

74 Sedgwick, *Travails,* 17, 228; Kostroun, "Port-Royal Nuns," 49–51.

75 Sedgwick, *Travails,* 4, 116; Henri Perruchot, *Port-Royal* (Paris: Livre de Paris, 1947), 94.

76 Meyer, *Controverses,* 14–16.

77 Réne Taveneaux, *Jansénisme et politique* (Paris: Armand Colin, 1965), 17–19; Maire, *Cause de Dieu,* 351–53.

78 Nicole Lemaitre, *Histoire des curés* (2002), quoted in Joseph Bergin, *Crown, Church and Episcopate under Louis XIV* (New Haven and London: Yale University Press, 2004), 218.

79 Antoine Arnauld to [Paolo Walloni?] at Rome, 2 April 1688, BN, Ms. Fr. 19724, f. 97.

80 Cottret, *Lumières,* 234.

81 Jonathan Wright, *God's Soldiers: Adventure,Politics, Intrigue and Power—A History of the Jesuits* (New York: Doubleday, 2004), 169.

82 Jotham Parsons, e-mail to H-FRANCE netserv, 14 June 1996; Jurieu, *Esprit,* 2:168–76.

83 Léonard de Marandé, *Inconvénients d'estat procedans du Jansénisme, adressez à Mr. Arnauld* (Paris: Sébastien et Gabriel Cramoisy, 1653), 305–22.

84 Jeffrey W. Merrick, *The Desacralization of the French Monarchy in the Eighteenth Century* (Baton Rouge, LA: Louisiana State University, 1990), 136–37; Palmer, *Unbelievers,* 26–27.

85 Antoine Arnauld to M. Du Vaucel, 20 October 1685, in *Lettres de Monsieur Antoine Arnauld,* 4:233.

86 Neveu, *Erudition,* 412–13.

87 Patouillet and Colonia, *Dictionnaire,* volumes 1–4.

88 Untitled list of sixteen major Jansenists writers, Fonds Sainte-Beuve, ms. 116, Bibliothèque de l'Histoire du Protestantisme Français (Paris) [Hereafter cited as BHPF].

89 Jennifer Speake and Thomas G. Bergin, eds., *Encyclopedia of the Renaissance and the Reformation* (Aylesbury, United Kingdom: Market House Books Ltd., 2004), 41; Charles Poulet, *Histoire de l'église de France* (Paris: Beauchesne, 1946–1949), 2:132–33; William Doyle, *Jansenism: Catholic Resistance to*

Authority from the Reformation to the French Revolution (New York: St. Martin's Press, 2000), 9; and Maire, *Cause de Dieu*, 17–18.

90 Maire, *Cause de Dieu*, 18–19; Speake and Bergin, eds., *Encyclopédie*, 41; Doyle, *Jansenism*, 9; Poulet, *Eglise* 2:133–34; M. Haillant, "Jansenius et ses défenseurs dans *l'Instruction* pastorale de Fénelon, archevêque de Cambrai, portant condamnation du *Cas de conscience*, le 10 février de l'an 1701," in *L'Image de C. Jansénius jusqu'à la fin du XVIIIe siècle*, ed. Edmond J. M. Van Eijl (Leuven: University Press, 1987), 119.

91 Le Goff and Rémond, *France religieuse* 2:361.

92 Luis Molina, *De Concordia liberi arbitrii cum gratiae donis*, 1588, cited by Richardt, *Jansénisme*, 47; Speake and Bergin, eds., *Encyclopédie*, 320; Doyle, *Jansenism*, 10.

93 Richardt, *Jansénisme*, 48; Doyle, *Jansenism*, 10–11.

94 Edmond Préclin, "Edmond Richer," *Revue d'histoire moderne* 5 (1930): 242–44, 250–52.

95 Ibid., pp. 321–33; Doyle, *Jansenism*, 14; and Dale K. Van Kley, *The Damiens Affair and the Unraveling of the Ancien Régime, 1750–1770* (Princeton: Princeton University Press, 1984), 176.

96 Préclin, "Richer," 258–69; Robert Muchembled, Ann Conchon, Bruno Maes, Isabelle Paresys, eds., *Dictionnaire de l'Ancien Régime* (Paris: Armand Colin, 2004), 257.

97 Venard and Banzon, *Religion*, 186. Ultramontanists could usually be found among the Jesuits, the theology faculty at Paris, the mendicant orders, most lay congregations (such as the Company of the Most Holy Sacrament), and the majority of the clergy in Spain, Portugal, and Italy. Gallicans, on the other hand, included the Jansenists, French *politiques* and *parlementaires*, and conciliarists everywhere. See Bernard Chédozeau, "Port-Royal: les Gallicans et les Politiques à la veille de la *Déclaration des Quatres Articles* (1679–1681)," *Revue des sciences philosophiques et théologiques* 77 (1993): 534.

98 Maire, *Cause de Dieu*, 369–70; McManners, *Angers*, 10; Muchembled et al., eds., *Dictionnaire*, 137–38; Judge, "Church and State," 219–22, 231; and Bernard Chédozeau, "Port-Royal et le jansénisme: la revendication d'une autre forme du tridentinisme?," *XVIIe siècle* 171 (1991): 119–20. For example, regarding doctrinal orthodoxy, king, pope, and Jesuits would be pitted against the Jansenists. On the *régale* (the right enjoyed by the Crown to appropriate revenues of a vacant see and to nominate bishops and *curés* to benefices), however, king, Jesuits and Gallicans opposed the pope and Jansenists. Yet the Jansenists backed the king, pope, and Gallicans against the Quietists. In the politically charged atmosphere of eighteenth-century *Jansénisme*, however, kings and popes often took sides against the Jansenists and Gallicans in the Paris Parlement.

99 Taveneaux, *Politique*, 37–38; Carreyre, "Quesnellisme," in *Introduction*, 3:574–75; and Joseph Dedieu, "Le désarroi janséniste pendant la période du quesnellisme," in *Introduction aux études d'histoire écclesiastiques locales*, ed. Victor Carrière (Paris: Librairie Letouzey et Ané, 1936), 3:592–93.

100 Richardt, *Jansénisme*, 17–31; Lucien Ceyssens, "Que penser finalement de l'histoire du jansénisme et de l'anti-jansénisme?," *Revue d'histoire ecclésiastique* 88, no. 1 (1993):112–13; Jean Orcibal, *Jansénius d'Ypres, 1585–1638* (Paris: Etudes Augustiniennes, 1989), 57–69; Henri Fouqueray, *Histoire de la Compagnie de Jésus en France des origines à la suppression, 1528–1762* (Paris: Bureaux des Etudes, 1910–1925), 391; and Léopold Willaert, *Les Origines du jansénisme dans les Pays-Bas catholiques*, vol. 1, *Le milieu: Le Jansénisme avant la lettre* (Gembloux: Editions J. Duculot, 1948), 338–41.

101 Richardt, *Jansénisme*, 32–37; Ceyssens, "Jansénisme et anti-jansénisme," 113–14; Yves de La Brière, "Le Jansénisme de Jansénius. Etude critique des Cinq Propositions," *Recherches de science religieuse* 6 (1916):298; and Antoine Arnauld, *Oeuvres*, 14:780.

102 Richardt, *Jansénisme*, 71.

103 Willaert, *Jansénisme*, 336–38.

104 Orcibal, *Jansénius*, 193, 200–204. See, for example, Jansen's *Alexipharmacum, Notarum Spongia,* and *Grand Perpétuité.*

105 Orcibal, *Jansénius*, 223, 228, 232, 235, 241–43; Henri Grégoire, *Oeuvres de l'abbé Grégoire,* vol. 12, *Les Ruines de Port-Royal en 1801* (Paris: Imprimerie-librairie chrétienne, 1801), 146.

106 Jean Orcibal, *Saint-Cyran et le jansénisme* (Paris: Editions du Seuil, 1961), 28.

107 Gérard Ferreyrolles, "Jansénius politique: le *Mars Gallicus*," *Actes du colloque de Clermont-Ferrand*, 20–23 September 1990, pp. 95–100.

108 Meyer, *Controverses*, 86; Achille Maulvault, *Répertoire alphabétique des personnes et des choses de Port-Royale* (Paris: Honoré Champion, 1902), 63.
109 Richardt, *Jansénisme*, 39–41.
110 Antoine Arnauld, *Apologie pour Monsieur Jansénius* (1644), in *Oeuvres*, 16:56.
111 Orcibal, *Jansénius*, 207–208.
112 Ibid., 282–83.
113 Jansen, quoted in Jean-Pierre Laporte, *La doctrine de Port-Royal: La Morale d'après Arnauld* (Paris: Libraire Philosophique J. Vrin, 1951–1952), 2:1.
114 Jansen to Saint-Cyran, 15 October 1620, quoted in Richardt, *Jansénisme*, 39.
115 Jansen, *Augustinus*, cited by Richardt, ibid., 64, 66.
116 Neveu, *Erudition*, 454, 462–63.
117 Antoine Arnauld, *Seconde Apologie pour M. Jansénius* (1645), in *Oeuvres*, 17:187–88.
118 Pierre Bayle, *Dictionnaire*, quoted in Neveu, *Erudition*, 451–52.
119 Neveu, *Erudition*, 459–61, 480; idem, "Augustinisme janséniste et magistère romain," *XVIIe siècle* 135 (1982):199.
120 Gestelier, *Angélique*, 245.
121 Kostroun, "Port-Royal Nuns," 170.
122 Cornelius Jansénius, *Augustinus; Réforme de l'homme interieur*, trans. Robert Arnauld d'Andilly (n.p.: Joannis Berthelin, 1643); Richardt, *Jansénisme*, 41–44; and Meyer, *Controverses*, 89–110.
123 Richardt, *Jansénisme*, 42–44.
124 Neveu, *Erudition*, 464–65; idem, "Augustinisme," 204–205.
125 Richardt, *Jansénisme*, 90–91.
126 Neveu, "Augustinisme," 200.
127 A. Janssen, "Un Polémiste anti-janséniste. Le Père Fr. Annat, S.J.: son role dans la condamnation des cinq propositions de l'Augustinus," in *Melanges d'histoire offerts à Charles Moeller* (Louvain and Paris: Van Linthout, 1914), 349–58. See chapter 2 for a detailed discussion of these Five Propositions.
128 Bishop Bossuet to the *maréchal* de Bellefond, undated, quoted in Richardt, *Jansénius*, 79.
129 Antoine Arnauld, *Seconde lettre à un duc et pair de France* (1655), cited by Doyle, *Jansenism*, 27; Jean Mesnard, *Pascal, His Life and Works* (New York: Philosophical Library, 1952), 126–27.
130 Neveu, *Erudition*, 489.
131 *Père* Annat, *Augustinus a Baianis vindicatus*, quoted in ibid., 452.
132 Jean Paul Sartre, quoted in J. Walgrave, "L'*Augustinus* de Jansénius," *Jansénius et le Jansénisme dans les Pays-Bas*, eds. J. Van Bavel and M. Schrama (Leuven: University Press, 1982), 38.
133 Dedieu, "Désarroi," 515; Jean Orcibal, "Jansenius et Rome," *Actes du colloque sur le jansénisme organisé par l'Academia belgica, Rome* (Louvain: Editions Nauwelaerts, 1973), 32.
134 Louis Cognet, *La Mère Angélique et Saint François de Sales, 1618–1626* (Paris: Editions Sulliver, 1951), 223–24, 235, 240–41.
135 Louis Prunel, *Sébastien Zamet, évêque, duc de Langres, pair de France (1588–1655): Sa vie et ses oeuvres* (Paris: Thèse, Librairie Alphonse Picard, 1912), 200–205; Edmond Préclin, *Sébastien Zamet, sa vie et ses oeuvres: Les origines du Jansénisme* (Paris: Librairie Alphonse Picard et Fils, 1912), 200–201.
136 Prunel, *Zamet*, 206, 209; Préclin, *Zamet*, 208–10, 220–26, 237–39; and Barbara Diefendorf, *From Penitence to Charity: Pious Women and the Catholic Reformation in Paris* (New York: Oxford University Press, 2004), 167–68.
137 Anthony Levi, *Cardinal Richelieu and the Making of France* (New York: Carroll and Graf, 2000), 158–59; Préclin, *Zamet*, 228–32; and Diefendorf, *Penitence to Charity*, 167–68.
138 Préclin, *Zamet*, 233–34; Diefendorf, *Penitence to Charity*, 170.
139 Levi, *Richelieu*, 158–59; Diefendorf, *Penitence to Charity*, 168, 170; and L.-Frédéric Jaccard, *Saint-Cyran, précurseur de Pascal* (Lausanne: Editions La Concorde, 1945), 108.
140 Richardt, *Jansénisme*, 19–25; Jean Orcibal, *Les Origines de Jansénisme*, vol. 3, *Jean Duvergier de Hauranne, abbé de Saint-Cyran et son temps, 1581–1638* (Paris: Librairie Philosophique J. Vrin, 1948), 201–23; and Cognet, *Angélique*, 170.
141 Kostroun, "Port-Royal Nuns," 125–26; Meyer, *Controverses*, 334–35, 340; and Crichton, *Jansenisers*, 41, 52–55.

142 Antoine Arnauld to M. Du Vaucel, 15 February 1692, *Oeuvres*, 3:427; Jean Lesaulnier, "Petite galerie des personnalités familières de Port-Royal," *Chroniques de Port-Royal* 40 (1991):177–40.
143 Préclin, *Zamet*, 251–60.
144 Kostroun, "Port-Royal Nuns," 161; see also Richardt, *Jansénisme*, 17.
145 Crichton, *Jansenisers*, 57; Jaccard, *Saint-Cyran*, 67; Orcibal, ed., *Correspondance*, 1:ix; and Jean Laporte, *Saint-Cyran* (Paris: Presses Universitaires de France, 1922), 44–49.
146 Saint-Cyran, quoted in Richardt, *Jansénisme*, 72.
147 H. Bremond, *Histoire littéraire du sentiment religieux en France*, vol. 4, *L'école de Port-Royal* (Paris: Bloud, 1923), 39–43, 63–68; Gastelier, *Angélique*, 173, 176, 184, 187; and Albert Rivaud, "Claude Lancelot, éducateur janséniste," *Revue des Deux-Mondes* 13, no. 13 (July 1951):306–308.
148 Meyer, *Controverses*, 27.
149 Jean Du Vergier de Hauranne, *Oeuvres chrétiennes et spirituelles de Messire Jean Du Vergier de Hauranne, abbé de Ssaint-Cyran* (N.p.: 1645; reprint, Lyon: Thomas Amaulry, 1679), 4: Table of Contents; Antoine Arnauld, *Théologie familière* (1643), cited by Meyer, *Controverses*, 330–31.
150 Meyer, *Controverses*, 332; Antoine Arnauld, *Moral pratique des Jesuites* (1689), in *Oeuvres*, 33:66; idem, *Oeuvres chrétiennes*, I: "Approval" list.
151 Annie Barnes, ed., *Lettres inédite de Jean Duvergier de Hauranne, abbé de Saint-Cyran* (Paris: Librairie Philosophique J. Vrin, 1962), *passim*; Robert Arnauld d'Andilly, "Preface," in Antoine Arnauld, *Oeuvres chrétiennes*, 1 and volumes 1–3: *passim.*
152 Bremond, *Ecole*, 129–34, 139–47, 151–56.
153 Maire, *Cause de Dieu*, 23; Sedgwick, *Travails*, 127–28.
154 Saint-Cyran, quoted in Richardt, *Jansénisme*, 16.
155 Maire, *Cause de Dieu*, 23; Jaccard, *Saint-Cyran*, 137, 140–42; and Claude Lancelot, *Mémoires touchant la vie de Monsieur de Saint-Cyran par M. Lancelot pour servir l'éclaircissement à l'histoire de Port-Royal* (Cologne: Aux dépens de la Compagnie, 1738), 2:425–26.
156 Saint-Cyran to Angélique Arnauld, 1647, quoted in Jaccard, *Saint-Cyran*, 103.
157 Jaccard, ibid., 105–107.
158 Saint-Cyran, quoted in ibid., 115.
159 Antoine Singlin, quoted in Antoine Arnauld, *Oeuvres*, 21:CXIX.
160 Laporte, *Saint-Cyran*, 15–17.
161 Bernard Dorival, *Pascal et les Provinciales. Catalogue de l'exposition du Musée national des Granges de Port-Royal* (Paris: Editions des Musées nationaux, 1963), 62; Lucien Goldmann, ed., *Correspondance de Martin de Barcos, abbé de Saint-Cyran avec les abbesses de Port-Royal et les principaux personnages du groupe janséniste* (Paris: Presses Universitaires de France, 1956), 603–604; and Sedgwick, *Travails*, 133.
162 Goldmann, ed., *Corresponance*, 1, 10–12, 19, 25–26, 51.
163 Ibid., 31–35, 44.
164 Richardt, *Jansénisme*, 23–24; Jaccard, *Saint-Cyran*, 60–61; Sedgwick, *Travails*, 32; and "Necrologe de Port-Royal des Champs," BHPF, ms. 120, p. 493.
165 "Preface Historique et Critique" to Antoine Arnauld, *Oeuvres*, 21:XVI (note b); Sedgwick, *Travails*, 124–26, 137; and Lesaulnier, "Galerie," 137.
166 Antoine Arnauld, quoted in Sedgwick, *Travails*, 130.
167 Jaccard, *Saint-Cyran*, 66; Antoine Arnauld, *Oeuvres*, 10:I; and Angélique Arnauld, *Relation écrite par la Mère Angélique Arnauld sur Port-Royal*, ed. Jean Lesaulnier (Paris: Bibliothèque Mazarine, 1992), 55–56. Saint-Cyran's first words to Angélique were that he had "seen many abbesses who reformed their convents, but few among them [had] reformed themselves" as she had.
168 Antoine Arnauld to Saint-Cyran, 24 December 1638 and 14 January 1639, in *Oeuvres*, I:2–11.
169 Antoine Arnauld to Saint-Cyran, 15 September and September 1641, in *Oeuvres*, I:17–23.
170 See, for example, subtitles under "Vergier, Jean du" in the index for Antoine Arnauld, in *Oeuvres*, 43:275–76.
171 Antoine Arnauld, *Apologie pour Messire Jean du Vergier de Hauranne, abbé de Saint-Cyran* (1644), in *Oeuvres*, 29:173–390.
172 Catherine Arnauld to Antoine Arnauld, 1639, quoted in Jean Lesaulnier, *Images de Port-Royal* (Paris: Nolin, 2002), 339.

173 Antoine Arnauld to Paolo Walloni, 19 September 1691, BN, ms. fr. 19725, f.190.
174 Antoine Arnauld to unknown, 9 May 1692, BN, ms. fr. 19726, f. 31.
175 De Lamoignon, "Certificat," 9 April 1696, quoted in Antoine Arnauld, *Oeuvres*, 5:LXVI.
176 Antoine Arnauld to unknown, 10 September 1682 and 22 January 1683, BN, ms. fr. 19727, ff. 159, 181.
177 Knox, *Enthusiasm*, 196–98; Crichton, *Jansenisers*, 175, 179.
178 Crichton, ibid., 183–84.
179 Antoine Arnauld, *Oeuvres*, 21:LXX, LXXX–LXXXII; idem, "Seconde Lettre à un duc et pair" (1655), in *Oeuvres*, 19:456, 466; and idem, *Sur les disputes internes entre les Théologiens de Port-Royal, au sujet du Livre de Jansénius & du l'acceptation des Bulles d'Innocent X & d'Alexandre VII* (1656), in *Oeuvres*, 22:667–832.
180 Sedgwick, *Travails*, 153.
181 Antoine Arnauld, *Oeuvres*, 10:VII (The oath in Latin ends with "usque ad effusionem sanguinis").
182 Antoine Arnauld, *Apologie de Monsieur Jansénius, evesque d'Ipres & de la Doctrine de S. Augustin, expliquée dans son Livre, intitulé AUGUSTINUS* (Paris: n.p.,1644) and *Seconde apologie de Monsieur Jansénius, evesque d'Ipres & de la Doctrine de S. Augustin, expliquée dans son Livre, intitulé AUGUSTINUS* (Paris: n.p., 1645), *passim*; idem, *Seconde Apologie*, 93; see also Sedgwick, *Travails*, 130–31.
183 Antoine Arnauld, "Seconde observations sur la fausse Bulle" (1643), quoted in *Oeuvres*, 16:5.
184 Archbishop of Philippi, quoted in Antoine Arnauld, "Preface" to the *Apologie pour Monsieur Jansénius* (1644), in *Oeuvres*, 16:58.
185 Doctors of Theology at Paris, quoted in ibid.
186 Antoine Arnauld, "Dessein des Jesuites contre S. Augustin" (1654), in *Oeuvres*, 19:201.
187 Antoine Arnauld, "Secondes observations sur la fausse Bulle" (1643), in *Oeuvres*, 16:5.
188 Antoine Arnauld, "Considerations sur la lettre de M. de Vabres" (1649), in *Oeuvres*, 19:54–55.
189 Antoine Arnauld, *Seconde Lettre de M. Arnauld Docteur de Sorbonne à un duc et pair de France* (1655), in *Oeuvres*, 19:335, 455–56, 465; Antoine Arnauld, cited by Sedgwick, *Travails*, 165–66.
190 Antoine Arnauld, Index to *Oeuvres*, 43:92.
191 Antoine Arnauld, *Apologie pour les Religieuses de Port-Royal* (1664), in *Oeuvres*, 23:214; idem, Index to *Oeuvres*, 43:92–93.
192 Antoine Arnauld, *Ecrits sur les Bulles d'Alexandre VII* (1664), in *Oeuvres*, 22:138–39, 209–12; Antoine Arnauld, cited by Phillips, *Church and Culture*, 203.
193 Antoine Arnauld, *Ecrits sur les bulles d'Alexandre VII et les Formulaires du clergé de France* (1657), in *Oeuvres*, 21:65, 22:443; idem, *Dix Mémoires sur la Cause des évêques qui ont distingué le fait du droit* (1668), in *Oeuvres*, 24:193–94; idem, "Defense de la lettre circulaire des quatre evêques" (1668), in *Oeuvres*, 24:428–29; and idem, Index to *Oeuvres*, 43:88.
194 Richardt, *Jansénisme*, 89.
195 Antoine Arnauld to Queen Anne, 2 March 1656, cited by Jansen, *Andilly*, 87–91.
196 Antoine Arnauld, *Ecrits sur les Bulles d'Alexandre VII* (1663), in *Oeuvres*, 21:199.
197 Antoine Arnauld to *Père* Salesse, 7 April 1657, quoted in *Oeuvres*, I:164–65.
198 Antoine Arnauld to Assembly of Bishops at Grands Augustins, 1660, quoted in Pierre Blet, "Louis XIV et les Papes aux prises avec le Jansénisme," *Archivum Historiae Pontificiae* 31 (1993):169.
199 Antoine Arnauld to *abbé* de La Lone, 28 August 1663, in *Oeuvres*, I:329–30; see also idem, *Lettres*, 2:56–75, 218–20.
200 Antoine Arnauld, *Apologie pour les religieuses de Port-Royal du Saint-sacrement* (1665), in *Oeuvres*, 23:165, 496–500.
201 Richardt, *Jansénisme*, 67–68; N. D. Kurland, "Antoine Arnauld's First Controversy: *De la Fréquente Communion*," in *The Dawn of Modern Civilization*, ed. Kenneth A. Strand (Ann Arbor, MI: University of Michigan Press, 1962), 239–40; and Louis Cognet, *Claude Lancelot, Solitaire de Port-Royal* (Paris: Editions Sulliver, 1950), 61. The full title of Arnauld's controversial book was *De la fréquente communion, où les sentimens des pères, des papes, et des Conciles, touchant l'usage des Sacramens de Pénitence & d'Eucharistie, sont fidélement exposéz* (Paris: n.p., 1643; reprint, Lyon: C. Plaignard, 1739).
202 Perle Bugnion-Secretan, *La Mère Angélique Arnauld (1591–1661), d'après ses écrits: Abbesse et réformatrice de Port-Royal* (Paris: Les éditions du Cerf, 1991), 182.

203 Antoine Arnauld, "Declaration de M. Antoine Arnauld touchant son Livre de *la Fréquente Communion*," 14 March 1644, in *Oeuvres*, 28:36–37.
204 Lesaulnier, *Images*, 351–59.
205 Fabio Chigi, letters of 1 February and 15 April 1644, cited by Antoine Arnauld, in *Oeuvres*, 28:620.
206 Antoine Arnauld, *Communion*, 830, 832, 836, 848; Orcibal, "Port-Royal," 269.
207 Honoré de Balzac, quoted in Lesaulnier, *Images*, 55.
208 Kurland, "Controversy," 244.
209 Meyer, *Controverses*, 222.
210 René Rapin, quoted in Kurland, "Controversy," 244.
211 Meyer, *Controverses*, 222, 225.
212 Antoine Arnauld, *Communion*, passim; Richardt, *Jansénisme*, 69; Kurland, "Controversy," 240–41; and André Tuilier, *Histoire de l'Université de Paris et de la Sorbonne* (Paris: Nouvelle Librairie de France, 1995), 2:13–14.
213 Venard and Bonzon, *Religion*, 185.
214 Arnauld, *Communion*, 168–79, 259, 274, 780–85.
215 Ibid., 381–86.
216 Ibid., 793–97, 801.
217 Ibid., 803, 810, 817–19.
218 Abra de Raconis, *Examen*, Preface; Parts I & II:63–114, 132–54, 343–77; Part III:18–25.
219 Léonard de Marandé, *Inconvénients d'estat procedans du Jansénisme, adressez à Mr Arnauld* (Paris: Sébastien and Gabriel Chamoisy, 1653), Preface, 1–69, 116–81, 192–220, 305–28.
220 Meyer, *Controverses*, 269–72.
221 Antoine Arnauld to *Mère* Constance, c. 1676, in *Oeuvres*, 24:588; idem to M. Du Vaucel, 20 October 1682, in *Oeuvres*, 2:165; idem to Prince Ernest, Landgrave of Hesse-Rhinfels, 29 January 1683, in *Oeuvres*, 2:197.
222 Cardinal Tanora, July 1690, as reported by M. Hennebel, Doctor of Theology at Louvain, quoted in Antoine Arnauld, *Oeuvres*, 28:667.
223 Antoine Arnauld, "Relation Touchant le livre de *la Fréquent Communion*" (1695), in *Oeuvres*, 28:710–11.
224 Antoine Arnauld, "Relation de M. Bourgeois docteur de Sorbonne . . . pour la Défense du Livre de la *Fréquente Communion*" (1695), in *Oeuvres*, 28:713.
225 Doyle, *Jansenism*, 23–24.
226 Antoine Arnauld, *Seconde lettre à Duc et Pair* (1655), in *Oeuvres*, 19:372.
227 Pierre Nicole, *Imaginaire* (1664), quoted in Antoine Arnauld, *Oeuvres*, 26:XCII.
228 Antoine Arnauld to Cardinal Cibo, September 1677, in *Oeuvres*, 2:11.
229 Antoine Arnauld to M. Du Vaucel, 29 November 1685, *Oeuvres*, 2:574; same to same, 11 November 1689, *Oeuvres*, 3:254; idem, *Difficultés proposées à M. Steyaert* (1691), in *Oeuvres*, 8:558.
230 Guy Basset, "Eclats de vie d'Henri Arnauld: Rencontres, accords et affrontements," *Chroniques de Port-Royal* 32 (1983):80–92.
231 Henri Arnauld, "Reflexions sur le livre de Jansénius et le Jugement qu'on en doit porter après qu'on en a fait une Lecture exacte," BN, ms. fr. 17758, ff. 94–124.
232 Jansen, ed., *Andilly*, 12–24; Antoine Arnauld, *Oeuvres*, 43:14.
233 Cornelius Jansen to Robert Arnauld d'Andilly, 16 August 1625, quoted in Jean Orcibal, ed., *Correspondance de Jansénius* (Louvain: Bureaux de la Revue, 1947), 1:287.
234 "Lettre à Messeigneurs les Archevêques et evêques de France," 1645, quoted in Saint-Cyran, *Oeuvres*, 1: (unpaginated).
235 Robert Arnauld d'Andilly to Cardinal Bentivoglio, December 1643; 3 March, 15 April, 15 May, 16 June, 24 June, 26 June, 11 July, 10 December, 18 December 1644; 13 March 1645; in Antoine Arnauld, *Oeuvres*, 28:621–27, 634–45.
236 Jansen, ed., *Andilly*, 9.
237 Robert Arnauld d'Andilly to duchesse de Chevreuse, 1 January 1654, quoted in ibid., 33–36.
238 Robert Arnauld d'Andilly to Cardinal Mazarin, 10 January 1654, quoted in ibid., 36–39.
239 Robert Arnauld d'Andilly to Cardinal Mazarin, 26 October 1655, quoted in ibid., 72–73.

240 Robert Arnauld d'Andilly to Queen Maria Theresa, 2 March 1656, quoted in ibid., 87–91.
241 Cardinal Mazarin to Robert Arnauld d'Andilly, 24 March 1656, quoted in ibid., 102–103.
242 Robert Arnauld d'Andilly to Cardinal Mazarin, 30 March, 2 and 9 May 1656, quoted in ibid., 103, 108–10; Mazarin to Arnauld d'Andilly, 5 May 1656, quoted in ibid., 109.
243 Robert Arnauld d'Andilly to Cardinal Mazarin, 12 February 1656, quoted in ibid., 77–81.
244 Robert Arnauld d'Andilly to Bishop of Coutances, 18 February 1656, quoted in ibid., 83–84.
245 Robert Arnauld d'Andilly to Bishop of Coutances, 24 March, 26 and 29 April 1654; 25 August, 11 September 1655; 15 and 21 March 1656; quoted in ibid., 42–44, 52–54, 67–71, 92–93, 101.
246 Jansen, ed., *Andilly*, 24.
247 René Cerveau, *L'Esprit de M. Nicole, ou Instructions sur les Vérités de la Religion tirées des Ouvrages de ce Grand Théologien tant sur les Dogmes de la Foi et les Mystères, que sur la Morale* (Paris: G. Desprez, 1765), v; Bernard Chédozeau, "Les années de jeunesse de Pierre Nicole et son entrée à Port-Royal, 1625–1654," *XVIIe siècle* 101 (1973):51–53, 61–62; and Lesaulnier, "Galerie," 169.
248 Antoine Arnauld, *Oeuvres*, 19:LXIX-LXXIV; André Hallays, *Le pélerinage de Port-Royal* (Paris: Libraire Academique Perrin, 1914), 220–24; and Lesaulnier, "Galerie," 170. The original titles of these two works are *Dissertatio quadripartita* and *Apologie pour les religieuses de Port-Royal.*
249 Lesaulnier, "Galerie," 170; Chédozeau, "Nicole," 62–67.
250 Antoine Arnauld, *Oeuvres*, 24:157.
251 Antoine Arnauld to Prince Ernest, 17 December 1685, BN, ms. fr. 19727, f. 34.
252 Pierre Nicole, Diary (c. 1649), BHPF, ms. 109, ff. 1–77.
253 Pierre Nicole, *Eclaircissement de quelques difficultés des Religieuses de Port-Royal sur la signature du Formulaire* (October 1668), in Antoine Arnauld, *Oeuvres*, 23:XXVI–XXVII.
254 Pierre Nicole, *Traité de l'éducation d'un prince*, 2d ed. (Paris: Chez la veuve Chas. Savreux, 1671), 1–15, 19–27, 38–51, 69.
255 Privilège du Roi and Approbation des Docteurs de Théologie, 3 July 1670, in ibid.
256 Pierre Nicole, *Traité de la Prière Divisé en sept Livres* (Paris: Louis Josse et Charles Robustel, 1714), 1:Preface.
257 Ibid., 1:1–282.
258 Ibid., 2:1–347.
259 Richardt, *Jansénisme*, 121; Maire, *Cause de Dieu*, 52–53; Joseph Anna Guillaume Tans and Henri Schmitz DuMoulin, *Pasquier Quesnel devant la Congregation de l'Index* (La Haye: Martinus Nijhoff, 1974), VII–XI, XVIII; and Jacques-François Thomas, *Querelle de l'Unigenitus* (Paris: Presses Universitaires de France, 1950), 37–38.
260 Patouillet and Colonia, *Dictionnaire*, 4:67; Richardt, *Jansénisme*, 129–30; Loupès, *Vie religieuses*, 34; and Bluche, *Journal secret*, 263.
261 Popular French quatrain (1703), quoted in Richardt, *Jansénisme*, 129.
262 Antoine Arnauld to Madame de Fontpertuis, 23 October 1693, in *Oeuvres*, 3:684. Arnauld had previously given Quesnel 380 *livres*.
263 Antoine Arnauld, *Oeuvres*, 24:593–94.
264 Pasquier Quesnel to *Père* de La Chaise, 1704, quoted in Antoine Arnauld, *Oeuvres*, 24:594.
265 "Lettre du Père Quesnel Au Roy," 1704, BN, ms. fr. 15595, ff. 33–38.
266 Patouillet and Colonia, *Dictionnaire*, 3:143–44; Richardt, *Jansénisme*, 130; Chaunu, *Basculement*, 118; and J. A. G. Tans and H. Schmit du Moulin, eds., *La Correspondance de Pasquier Quesnel, inventaire et index analytique* (Bruxelles: Editions Nauwelaerts, 1989), 1:XI–XIII.
267 Pasquier Quesnel, "Last Testament," December 1719, quoted in Albert Le Roy, *Un Janséniste en exil: Correspondance de Pasquier Quesnel, prêtre de l'Oratoire sur les affaires politiques et religieuses de son temps* (Paris: Librairie Academique Perrin, 1900), 2:438–40.
268 Bishop of Châlons, *Mandement* of 9 November 1671, in a foreword to Pasquier Quesnel, *Instructions chrétiennes et élévations à Dieu sur la passion avec les octaves de Pasque, de la Pentecoste, du S. Sacrement de Noel* (Paris: André Pralard, 1702).
269 Quesnel, ibid., Preface.
270 "Lettres Patentes du Roi," 27 March 1677, and "Approbation" of Sorbonne, 15 February 1687, cited by Quesnel, *Instructions Chrétiennes*; John McManners, *Church and Society in Eighteenth Century France*,

Vol. 2, *the Religion of the People and the Politics of Religion* (Oxford: Clarendon Press, 1998), 354.

271 Antoine Arnauld to Madame de Fontpertuis, 5 June 1691, in *Oeuvres*, 3:355.

272 Marcel Brongniart, *La Paroisse Saint-Médard au faubourg Saint-Marceau* (Paris: A. et J. Picard, 1951), 67; McManners, *Church and Society*, 2:354.

273 Pasquier Quesnel, *Le Nouveau Testament en François avec des Réflexions morales sur chaque verset, pour en rendre la lecture plus utile, & la Meditation plus aisée* (Paris: André Pralard, 1698), *passim*; Maire, *Cause de Dieu*, 65; Dedieu, "Désarroi," 546–47; and Carreyre, "Quesnellisme," 543–48.

274 Maire, *Cause de Dieu*, 51–52, 61; Dedieu, "Désarroi," 573–55; and Pierre Blet, *Le Clergé de France: Louis XIV et le Saint-Siège de 1695 à 1715* (Vatican: Archivio Vaticano, 1989), 382–85.

275 Maire, *Cause de Dieu*, 66–67.

276 J. A. G. Tans, ed., *Pasquier Quesnel et les Pays-Bas: Correspondance publiée avec introduction et annotations* (Paris: Librairie Vrin, 1960), 62, 64, 79, 84–87, 95–97. In these letters, Quesnel employs at least nine code names in Latin, French, and Dutch for Antoine Arnauld alone.

277 Carreyre, "Quesnellisme," 550–55, 567–71; Dedieu, "Désarroi," 567.

278 Antoine Arnauld, *Oeuvres*, 43:200.

279 Lesaulnier, "Galerie," 170–73; Marvin R. O'Connell, *Blaise Pascal: Reasons of the Heart*. Library of Religious Biography, eds. Mark A. Noll, Nathan O. Hatch, Allen C. Guelzo (Grand Rapids, MI: William B. Eerdmans, 1997), 108–9; and Howard Clive Barnard, *The Little Schools of Port-Royal* (Cambridge: Cambridge University Press, 1913), 37–38.

280 Blaise Pascal, quoted in Jean Laporte, *La Doctrine de Port-Royal: Essai sur la formation et le développement de la doctrine: Saint-Cyran* (Paris: Presses Universitaires de France, 1923), 1:XL.

281 O'Connell, *Pascal*, 109–10; Richardt, *Jansénisme*, 90; and Jean Mesnard, *Pascal et les Roannez* (Paris: Desclée de Brouwer, 1965), 1:404.

282 Jacqueline Pascal to Blaise Pascal, January 1655, quoted in Jean Mesnard, "Les séjours de Pascal à Port-Royal des Champs," *Chroniques de Port-Royal* 1(1951):18.

283 O'Connell, *Pascal*, 118–20; Mesnard, "Pascal," 18–21, 25.

284 Blaise Pascal, *Lettres Provinciales* (number 16) and *Pensées sur les miracles*, quoted in Jerome Besoigne, *Histoire de l'abbaye de Port-Royal* (Cologne: Aux dépense de la Compagnie, 1752–1753), 1:385–87.

285 Blaise Pascal, *Lettres provinciales*, quoted in F. Ellen Weaver, *Mademoiselle de Joncoux: polémique janséniste à la veille de la bulle Unigenitus* (Paris: Les Editions du Cerf, 2002), 158.

286 Richardt, *Jansénisme*, 104.

287 Knox, *Enthusiasm*, 201–3.

288 Mesnard, *Pascal*, 176–77.

289 Luisa Borella, *Plaidoyer pour Arnauld: Lecture des trois premières 'Provinciales' de Pascal* (Parme: Edizioni Universitaire, 1988), 39–40.

290 Mesnard, *Pascal*, 75–76.

291 Plainemaison, "Provinciales," 61–62, 68.

292 Ibid., 70–87; Antoine Arnauld, *Oeuvres*, 30:XII. No layperson was required to sign the Formulary.

293 Richardt, *Jansénisme*, 89–95; Blaise Pascal, *Lettres provinciales* (1656), cited by Mesnard, *Pascal*, 76–85. In Catholic tradition, probabilism dictated that when theologians differed on a subject, they should adopt the most certain view when the opposing opinion was equally probable. In 1577, however, the Dominican Barthélémy de Médina argued that one could with a clear conscience prefer the least probable opinion. By 1598 the Jesuits had adopted this view, convinced that it was sufficient in reason to have the support of only one writer to render an opinion probable.

294 Blaise Pascal, *Lettres provinciales* (1656–57), cited by Mesnard, *Pascal*, 86–91; Préclin and Jarry, "Luttes politiques," 198–99; and Richardt, *Jansénisme*, 95–97.

295 Richardt, *Jansénisme*, 95; Borella, *Arnauld*, 35.

296 Wallace K. Ferguson, "The Place of Jansenism in French History," *Journal of Religion* 7(1927):29

297 Antoine Arnauld, *Oeuvres*, 43:201; Mesnard, *Pascal*, 91, 101–102; Plainemaison, "Provinciales," 86; and M.E. Lowndes, *The Nuns of Port-Royal as Seen in Their Own Narratives* (Oxford: Oxford University Press, 1909), 355–57.

298 Antoine Arnauld, *Quatre Factums pour les neveux de Jansénius* (1694), in *Oeuvres*, 30:532. See also the introduction to volume 30, pages XII–XIII.

299 Pierre Nicole and Antoine Singlin, cited by Frédéric Delforge, *Les petites écoles de Port-Royal, 1637–1660* (Paris: Les Editions du Cerf, 1985), 132.
300 Richardt, *Jansénisme*, 104.
301 "Necrologe de Port-Royal," volume 2 (July to December), BHPF, Fonds St.-Beuve, Ms. 120, 342.
302 Jean Orcibal, "L'enfance de Racine," *Revue d'histoire littéraire de la France* 51 (1951):3.
303 Orcibal, "Racine," 4–13; Lesaulnier, "Galerie," 174.
304 Orcibal, "Racine," 13.
305 Antoine Arnauld to Prince Ernest, Landgrave of Hesse-Rhinfels, 13 March 1689, in *Oeuvres*, 3:175; idem to M. Du Vaucel, 18 March 1694, in *Oeuvres*, 3:758–60.
306 Racine to Boileau, 8 April 1692, BN, ms. fr. 12886, f. 92; J. H. Shennon, *Louis XIV* (London: Routledge, 1986), 31.
307 Bluche, *Journal*, 237; Racine's final will, 10 October 1698, BN, ms. fr. 12886, f. 269.
308 "Necrologe de Port-Royal des Champs," volume 2 (July–December), BHPF, Fonds St.-Beuve, ms. 120, 336.
309 List of Racine's books and manuscripts, BN, ms. fr. 12886.
310 Jean-Baptiste Racine, *Abrégé de l'histoire de Port-Royal* (N.p.: 1695; reprint, n.p.: Editions d'aujourdhui, 1981), 190 pages.
311 Racine's letters are collected in BN, ms. fr. 12886.
312 Maire, *Cause de Dieu*, 27–28.
313 Knox, *Enthusiasm*, 189–202.

2 What Was Jansenism?

1 *Mère* Agnès de St. Paul Arnauld to her brother Robert Arnauld d'Andilly, 26 November 1635, BN, ms. fr. 23481, f. 6.
2 Ibid.
3 Lucien Goldmann, *Le Dieu caché {The Hidden God}*, trans. Philip Thody (Paris: Gallimard, 1955; reprint, NY: The Humanities Press, 1964). Others who discuss these four groups include Richard Golden, *Godly Rebellion*, 126, and Gérard Namer, *L'Abbé Leroy et ses amis: Essai sur le Jansénisme extrémiste intramondain* (Paris: SEVPEN, 1964), 8–9.
4 Albert N. Hamscher, "The Parlement of Paris and the Social Interpretation of Early French Jansenism," *The Catholic Historical Review* 63 (July 1977):393–405.
5 Ibid., 405, 410.
6 William Ritchey Newton, *Sociologie de la communauté de Port-Royal, Histoire, économie* (Paris: Klincksieck, Collection "Port-Royal," 1999), 120; Jean Mesnard, "Fideles de Port-Royal en France et en Hollande du XVII au XIXe siècle," *Chroniques de Port-Royal* 35 (1986):18–24.
7 Besoigne, *Port-Royal*, 1:422–23; Lesaulnier, "Galerie," 148.
8 Louise-Marie de Gonzague, Queen of Poland, quoted in Lesaulner, "Galerie," 149.
9 *Mère* Angélique Arnauld, 1647, quoted in Crichton, *Jansenisers*, 133.
10 Pierre Goubert, *Mazarin* (Paris: Fayard, 1990), 397; Jacques Wilhelm, *La Vie Quotidienne: Des Parisiens au temps du Roi-Soleil, 1660–1715* (Paris: Hachette, 1977), 232–33.
11 Cécile Gazier, *Les Belles amies de Port-Royal* (Paris: Perrin et Cie, 1930), *passim*; Lesaulnier, "Galerie," 149–53, 165–69, 175–76; Léon Bournet, *La querelle janséniste* (Paris: Pierre Téqui, 1924), 150–70; and J. H. M. Salmon, *Cardinal de Retz: The Anatomy of a Conspirator* (New York: The Macmillan Company, 1969), 35.
12 Lesaulnier, "Galerie," 163; Hallays, *Pélerinage*, 108; and René Taveneaux, *Jansénisme et Réforme catholique* (Nancy: Presses Universitaires de Nancy, 1992), 41–43.
13 Bournet, *Querelle*, 178–79.
14 Bruno Neveu, "Un Parlementaire parisien érudit et janséniste: Jean Le Nain (1609–1698)," *Paris et Ile-de-France. Mémoires* 16–17 (1965–1966):191–213.
15 Bruno Neveu, "Un ami de Port-Royal: Guillaume Du Gué de Bagnols (1616–1657)," *Chroniques de Port-Royal* 15–16 (1966):45–49, 55–72.

16 Durand Echeverria, *The Maupeau Revolution: A Study in the History of Libertarianism, France, 1770–1774* (Baton Rouge and London: Louisiana State University Press, 1985), 8–9.
17 Henri Lefebvre, *Pascal* (Paris: Les éditions Nagel, 1949), 1:52.
18 Golden, *Godly Rebellion*, 137, 143, 150.
19 Anthony Levi, *Louis XIV* (New York: Carroll & Graf Publishers, 2004), 290.
20 Maire, *Cause de Dieu*, 473; Briggs, *Communities*, 345; and Chaunu, "Jansénisme," 124, 133–34.
21 Antoine Arnauld, *Apologie pour Monsieur l'Abbé de St.-Cyran* (1644), in *Oeuvres*, 29:187.
22 Antoine Arnauld, "Remonstrance aux Pères Jésuites" (1651), in *Oeuvres*, 29:495.
23 Antoine Arnauld, *Seconde lettre à un duc et pair* (1655), in *Oeuvres*, 19:394, 445–47.
24 Antoine Arnauld, *Difficultés proposées à M. Steyaert* (1691), in *Oeuvres*, 8:560.
25 Kreiser, *Miracles*, 4.
26 F. Ellen Weaver, "Jansenist Bishops and Liturgical-Social Reform," in *Church, State and Society under the Bourbon Kings*, ed. Richard M. Golden (Lawrence, KS: Coronado Press, 1982), 25–33, 47–62; William Ritchey Newton, "Port-Royal and Jansenism: Social Experience, Group Formation and Religious Attitudes in Seventeenth-Century France" (Ph.D. diss., University of Michigan, 1974), 9, 33, 39.
27 Crichton, *Jansenisers*, 28; Alexander Sedgwick, *Jansenism in Seventeenth-Century France: Voices from the Wilderness* (Charlottesville: University Press of Virginia, 1977), 194, 196, 201.
28 Guy Cabourdin and Georges Viard, eds., *Lexique historique de la France d'Ancien Régime* 2d ed. (Paris: Armand Colin, 1990), 177; Ceyssens, "Jansénisme," 28; Doyle, *Jansenism*, 87; Lefebvre, *Pascal*, 72–73, 78; and Knox, *Enthusiasm*, 176.
29 Knox, *Enthusiasm*, 212; Sedgwick, *Travails*, 1, 136, 254; idem, "Jansenism," 130; and James Van Horn Melton, *The Rise of the Public in Enlightenment Europe* (Cambridge and New York: Cambridge University Press, 2001), 164–65.
30 Knox, *Enthusiasm*, 212.
31 Sedgwick, "Jansenism," 129–33; Cerveau, *Esprit de M. Nicole*, 181–85.
32 Pierre Corneille, quoted in Jacqueline Michel, *"L'aventure janséniste" dans l'oeuvre de Henry de Montherlant* (Paris: A. G. Nizet, 1976), 19, 21–24.
33 "Supplement au Nécrologie de Port-Royal," BN, ms. fr. 23482, ff. 140, 145.
34 "Dispositions de Mlle. La Duchesse de Liancourt pour passes sa vie chrétienment," BN, ms. fr. 23482, ff. 168–70.
35 Edmond Préclin, "Les Conséquences sociales du jansénisme," in *Introduction aux études d'histoire ecclésiastique locale*, ed. Victor Carrière (Paris: Letouzey et Ané), 3:591–92, 595, 610–14; Cottret, *Lumières*, 245; and Kreiser, *Miracles*, 7.
36 Crichton, *Jansenisers*, 28–29; Lefebvre, *Pascal*, 52–55; and Merrick, *Desacralization*, 117.
37 Golden, *Godly Rebellion*, 127; Cerveau, *Esprit de M. Nicole*, 306–70; "Pièces relatives à l'histoire de Port-Royal," BHPF, Ms. 108, pp. 383–94. Within the same Ms. 108 collection, see also "Sentimens de Piété pour une personne malade" (83 pages), "Maximes Chrétiennes" (12 pages), and "Questions sur les affaires du tems" (70 pages).
38 Ceyssens, "Jansénisme et anti-Jansénisme," 109; Crichton, *Jansenisers*, 37; David C. Hudson, "The Regent, Fleury, Jansenism and the Sorbonne," *French History* 8 (1994):136.
39 Kostroun, "Port-Royal Nuns," 19; Levi, *Louis XIV*, 227; Marcel Raymond, "Du jansénisme à la morale de l'intérêt," *Mercure de France* 330 (June 1957):240–43.
40 Muchembled et al., *Dictionnaire*, 157; Augustin Gazier, "Les Christs prétendus Jansénistes," *Revue de l'art chrétien* 60 (1910):77–94. Gazier, who disproves this myth by showing that while the convent of Port-Royal in Paris had a crucifix with Christ's arms stretched horizontally, the Jesuit missionary St. Francis Xavier possessed one with the Savior's arms stretched vertically, therefore concludes: "There never was a Jansenist crucifix."
41 Du Verger de Hauranne, abbé de Saint-Cyran, *Considerations chrétiennes sur la Mort*, 3d ed. (Paris: Veuve de Guillaume Desprez, 1710), *passim*.
42 Jean Vallier, quoted in Blet, "Nonce," 423.
43 Venard and Benzon, *Religion*, 179, 181; Daniel Vidal, *Miracles et convulsions jansénistes au XVIIIe siècle: Le mal et sa conaissance* (Paris: Presses Universitaires de France, 1987), 23.

44 Monique Cottret, "Les Représentations mythique de l'Eglise primitive dans les polémiques entre les jansénistes et les jésuites, 1713–1760" (Université de Paris, Thèse de 3e cycle, 1979),1:134–36.
45 Neveu, *Erudition*, 476–77; Cottret, *Lumières*, 270; Monique Cottret, "Aux origines du républicanisme janséniste: le mythe de l'église primitive et le primitivisme des lumières," *Revue d'histoire moderne et contemporaine* 31 (1984):99–100.
46 Neveu, *Erudition*, 14, 17.
47 Ibid., 17.
48 Antoine Arnauld, cited by Jean Orcibal, *Louis XIV contre Innocent XI: Les appels au futur concile de 1688 et l'opinion française* (Paris: Librairie Philosophique J. Vrin, 1949), 78; Antoine Arnauld, Introduction to *Oeuvres*, 1:I.
49 Antoine Arnauld, *Ecrits sur les Bulles d'Alexandre VII et les Formulaires du clergé de France* (1658), in *Oeuvres*, 21:103–104, 237, 402.
50 Antoine Arnauld, "Lettre pastorale de l'evêque d'Alet" (20 July 1668), in *Oeuvres*, 37:10, 15–17.
51 Antoine Arnauld, *Considerations* (1681), cited by Chédozeau, "Port-Royal," 544–46.
52 Antoine Arnauld to unknown, 22 January 1683, BN, ms. fr. 19727, f. 178.
53 Antoine Arnauld, Index to *Oeuvres*, 43:197–98. Although many seventeenth-century clergy and magistrates accepted papal infallibility, it had no dogmatic or canonical authority until 18 July 1870. Consequently, theologians and church leaders frequently debated among themselves which papal judgments, bulls, etc. should be considered infallible and which not. See Neveu, *Erudition*, 392.
54 Michel Dupuy, quoted in Richardt, *Jansénism*, 7.
55 Guillaume Le Roy, "Lettre sur la constance et le courage" (1665), quoted in Pierre Deyon, "Perspectives et limites d'une 'sociologie' du jansénisme," *Annales: Economies, Sociétés, Civilisations* 21 (1966):429.
56 *Duc* de Saint-Simon, *Mémoires*, quoted in J. A. G. Tans, "Les Idées politiques des jansénistes," *Neophilologus* 40 (January 1956):1.
57 Pasquier Quesnel, *Abrégé de la Morale de l'Evangile* (1672), *Reflexions Morales* (1692), and *La Souvereinété des rois défendue* (1696), cited by Tans, ibid., 1–5.
58 Antoine Arnauld, *Traité sur la soverainété des rois*, cited by Tans, ibid., 7–14.
59 Golden, *Godly Rebellion*, 127–30; Tans, "Idées politiques," 16–18; and Orcibal, *St.-Cyran et Jansénisme*, 156–57.
60 Benoît Fourgon, quoted in John McManners, "Jansenism and Politics in the Eighteenth Century," a review of Derek Baker, ed., *Church, Society and Politics* (Oxford: Basil Blackwell, 1975), in *Studies in Church History* 12 (1975):262.
61 Pasquier Quesnal, *La discipline de l'Eglise tirée du Nouveau Testament et de quelques anciens conciles* (1689), cited by Cottret, "Républicanisme janséniste," 103.
62 Pierre Barral, *Maximes sur le devoir des Rois* (n.d.), cited by Cottret, ibid., 106.
63 Cottret, ibid., 107–13.
64 Ibid., 114.
65 Golden, *Godly Rebellion*, 127–28.
66 Antoine Arnauld, "Lettre d'un docteur en théologie à un de ses amis" (2 April 1644), *Oeuvres*, 28:462.
67 Antoine Arnauld, Index to *Oeuvres*, 43:227.
68 Antoine Arnauld, *Ecrits sur les Bulles d'Alexandre VII* (1657), *Oeuvres*, 21:51–52, 440–41.
69 Antoine Arnauld to Mme. de Fontpertuis, 24 March 1692, *Oeuvres*, 3:456.
70 Melton, *Rise of the Public*, 50.
71 Antoine Arnauld to M. Perrier, 28 June 1674, in *Oeuvres*, 1:723.
72 Cardinal Giovanni Bona, quoted in Louis Cognet, *Le Jansénisme* (Paris: Presses Universitaires de France, 1961), 124.
73 Crichton, *Jansenisers*, 17.
74 Golden, *Godly Rebellion*, 127.
75 Elfrieda T. Dubois, "A Jesuit History of Jansenism," *The Modern Language Review* 64 (1969):773; Remsberg, *Wisdom*, 73; Sedgwick, *Travails*, 128.
76 Kurland, "Controversy," 243–44; Briggs, *Communities*, 340–44.
77 Kreiser, *Miracles*, 4; Maire, *Cause de Dieu*, 201–202; and Wright, *God's Soldiers*, 165, 169.

78 In Roman Catholicism, casuistry refers to the solving of special cases of right and wrong in conduct by applying general principles of ethics and deciding how far circumstances alter cases. Probabilism is the doctrine that in matters in which there are two opinions, both probable but neither decisive, it is lawful to follow the one preferred. The Jansenists criticized the Jesuits for using such subtle but morally evasive reasoning in questions of Christian duty.
79 Georges Pirot, "Extraict de quelques propositions tirées d'un livre intitulé *Apologie pour casuistes contre les calomnies des Jansénistes* (Paris: n.p., 1657), 1–10.
80 Angélique Arnauld to Marie des Anges, 1626, cited by Knox, *Enthusiasm*, 188.
81 Angélique Arnauld to Archbishop of Paris, 17 December 1651, cited by Antoine Arnauld, in *Oeuvres*, 29:557.
82 Antoine II Arnauld , quoted in Sedgwick, *Travails*, 21–22, 25.
83 Antoine Arnauld, "Considerations sur la lettre de M. de Vabres" (1650), in *Oeuvres*, 19:59.
84 Antoine Arnauld, "Remonstrance aux Pères Jésuites" (1651), in *Oeuvres*, 29:531.
85 Antoine Arnauld, *L'Innocence et la Verité défendues* (1652), in *Oeuvres*, 30:144–45; idem, *Ecrits sur les Bulles d'Alexandre VII* (1663), in *Oeuvres*, 22:310. It would appear that for Arnauld, the only good Jesuit was a suffering Jesuit!
86 A thesis sustained at the College of the Jesuits at Paris, 12 December 1661, in the Introduction to Antoine Arnauld, *Oeuvres,* 21:LIV–LV.
87 Antoine Arnauld, "Lettre à un ami" (1662), in *Oeuvres*, 1:301–2.
88 Antoine Arnauld, *Morale Pratique des Jésuites* (N.p., 1683), 2:1–45.
89 Antoine Arnauld to Prince Ernest, 9 April 1683, BN, ms. fr. 19727, f. 10.
90 Antoine Arnauld to unknown, 22 January 1683, BN, ms. fr. 19727, f. 183; Arnauld to Prince Ernest, 30 May 1683, in *Oeuvres*, 2:268; Arnauld to unknown persons, 2 November 1684, 14 September and 18 October 1685, 22 March 1686, BN, ms. fr. 19723, ff. 89, 110, 114, 119, 133, 198; Arnauld to Prince Ernest, 1 August 1685, in *Lettres* 4:206–209; Arnauld, *Jésuites* 2:1–45.
91 Antoine Arnauld to M. Du Vaucel, 13 December 1685, in *Lettres* 4:245; Arnauld to Paolo Walloni, 8 July 1688, BN, ms. fr. 19724, f. 118; Arnauld to Paolo Walloni, 10 November 1690, BN, ms. fr. 19725, f. 150; idem, *Morale pratique des Jésuites* (1689)*, in Oeuvres*, 33:73–75, 203–4.
92 Antoine Arnauld to Paolo Walloni, 22 September 1689, 10 March and 29 September 1690, BN, ms. fr. 19725, ff. 94, 125, 136; same to same, 11 April 1692, BN, ms. fr. 19726, f. 24.
93 Antoine Arnauld, *Jésuites* 3: Preface and Table of Chapters.
94 Antoine Arnauld to Madame de Fontpertuis, 24 March 1692, in *Oeuvres*, 3:456–57.
95 Neveu, *Erudition*, 415; Doyle, *Jansenism*, 21; Richardt, *Jansénisme*, 63; and Fouqueray, *Compagnie de Jésus*, 5:406.
96 François Annat, *La conduitte de l'Eglise et du Roy justifiée dans la condamnation des jansénistes* (Paris: Sébastien Cramoisy, 1664), "Preface," 121–350.
97 Patouillet and Colonia, *Dictionnaire*, 3:203.
98 Ibid., 1:133–40; 2:398–401; 3:340; 4:83–88.
99 Ibid., 1:118–19, 145–46; 2:144–47; 3:362–63.
100 Ibid., 2:32, 177–80, 223–28; 3:302; 4:2–3, 45–48.
101 Ibid., 1:120–24, 131.
102 Ibid., 3:53–54.
103 Kurland, "Controversy," 242–43.
104 Introduction to Antoine Arnauld, *Oeuvres*, 26:XXXV–XXXVI.
105 Patouillet and Colonia, *Dictionnaire*, 1:74–77; 2:236–37, 338, 414–17.
106 Ibid., 1:25–26; 2:51, 158, 191, 221, 271, 472–73; 3:242, 475.
107 Ibid., 4:52–59.
108 Ibid., 2:495–98.
109 Ibid., 3:52.
110 Ibid., 1:97–100; 2:149–51, 252–54; 4:45–52, 215–16.
111 Ibid., 1:18–19; 3:251–56.
112 Ibid., 2:291–93, 403, 524–25; Richardt, *Jansénisme*, 191.
113 Besoigne, *Port-Royal*, 3:561–62.

114 Racine, *Port-Royal*, 59, 80.
115 Felix Cadet, *L'éducation à Port'Royal* (Paris: Librairie Hachette, 1887), 78.
116 Antoine Arnauld, Letters for 1687–1688, BN, ms. fr. 19724, *passim.*
117 Meyer, *Controverses*, XII–XIII; Lucien Ceyssens, "Que penser finalement de l'histoire du Jansénisme et de l'antijansénisme?" *Revue d'Histoire ecclésiastique* 88 (1993):119–20.
118 Meyer, *Controverses*, 445–48, 480–82.
119 Levi, *Richelieu*, 36–37, 158–60.
120 Martin, *French Book*, 48.
121 Cardinal Richelieu, quoted in G. R. R. Treasure, *Cardinal Richelieu and the Development of Absolutism* (New York: St. Martin's Press, 1972), 221–24; Lowndes, *Nuns*, 256–58.
122 Introduction to Antoine Arnauld, *Oeuvres*, 19:XXXVI; 21:VII; idem, *Ecrits sur les bulles d'Alexandre VII* (1657), in *Oeuvres*, 21:443.
123 Golden, *Godly Rebellion*, 131–33, 570–80.
124 Cardinal de Retz, quoted in Cadet, *Education*, 74.
125 Paule Jansen, *Le Cardinal Mazarin et le mouvement janséniste français, 1653–1659* (Paris: Libraire philosophique J. Vrin, 1967), 28–29; Maire, *Cause de Dieu*, 30.
126 Richard M. Golden, "The Mentality of Opposition: The Jansenism of the Parisian *Curés* during the Religious Fronde," *The Catholic Historical Review* 64 (1978):565–69; Phillips, *Church and Culture*, 200–201.
127 Golden, *Godly Rebellion*, 129–31; Phillips, *Church and Culture*, 201–202; and Maire, *Cause de Dieu*, 29.
128 Jean Racine, *Abrégé de l'histoire de Port-Royal*, 91–92, quoted in Sedgwick, *Jansenism*, 58.
129 Sedgwick, ibid., 57–59.
130 *Mère* Angélique to unknown, 16 April 1654, quoted in Bugnion-Secretan, *Mère Angélique*, 194; Sedgwick, *Travails*, 141.
131 Sedgwick, *Travails*, 146.
132 Ibid., 148–49; Hurbert Carrier, "Port-Royal et la Fronde: Deux Mazarinades inconnues d'Arnauld d'Andilly," *Revue d' histoire littéraire de la France* 75 (1975):3–5.
133 Robert Arnauld d'Andilly, *Avis d'Etat à la Reine sur le gouvernement de sa Regence* (1649) and *La Verité toute nue* (1652), cited by Carrier, "Fronde," 6–21.
134 Colbert to Mazarin, 1657, quoted in Golden, "*Curés*," 568.
135 Jean François Paul de Gondi, Cardinal de Retz, *Memoirs of Cardinal de Retz,* with an introduction by David Ogg (London: J. M. Dent, 1917; reprint, Paris: Pléiade, 1956), vii–x; Antoine Arnauld, "Discours Historique et Apologétique," in *Oeuvres*, 20:817.
136 Mazarin to M. de Laigues, 15 April 1652, and Mazarin to *abbé* Fouquet, 30 April, 7 May, and 21 June 1652 in *Lettres du Cardinal Mazarin pendant son ministère* (Paris: Imprimerie Nationale, 1872–1906), 5:83, 100, 108, 131.
137 Sedgwick, *Travails*, 150–52.
138 Mazarin to Nicolas Foucquet, 6 September 1652, in *Lettres*, 5:211–12.
139 Mazarin to Le Tellier, 7 September 1652, in *Lettres*, 5:214–16.
140 Mazarin to Le Tellier, 5 October 1652, in *Lettres*, 5:345.
141 Cardinal Retz, *Memoirs*, 1:66–67, 314.
142 Ibid., 2:171.
143 Both sides of this sordid affair are described in Mazarin's letters for 1652–1655, found in his *Lettres*, volumes 5–7; in Le Paige and Du Rey, *Retz*, 3–56; and in various documents at the Bibliothèque Nationale, especially the *lettre de cachet* of 16 April 1655, BN, ms. fr. 17589, f. 236; the *lettre de cachet* of 14 September 1656, BN, ms. fr. 13894; and Retz's "Open Letter" to the French bishops, 14 December 1654, BN, Nouvelles Acquisitions Français 1525, ff. 56–84 (hereafter cited as NAF).
144 Louis-Adrien Le Paige and J. B. F. Du Rey de Meinières, *Histoire de la détention du Cardinal de Rets, Archevesque de Paris, et de ses suites* (Vincennes: n.p., 1755), 129–31, 136, 143–45, 153.
145 Anonymous "Mémoire" (c. 1650s), BN, ms. fr. 17589, ff. 349–50.
146 Augustin Gazier, *Les Dernières années du cardinal de Retz (1655–1679): Etude historique et littéraire* (Paris: Ernest Thorin, éditeur, 1875), 142–47.
147 Introduction to Antoine Arnauld, *Oeuvres*, 5:LVI.

148 Retz, *Memoirs*, 1:12, 29.
149 Louis Batiffol, *Biographie du Cardinal de Retz* (Paris: Librairie Hachette, 1929), 188–89; Cardinal de Retz, "Appeal to the General Assembly of the Clergy," 28 March 1657, BN, NAF 1525, ff. 91–99.
150 Robert Arnauld d'Andilly to Cardinal de Retz, 1658, quoted in Salmon, *Retz*, 312.
151 Salmon, ibid., 313, 316.
152 See letters from Mazarin to Le Tellier, 16 July, 5 and 9 August, 8 October 1659, and to the Bishop of Coutances, 17 October 1659, in Mazarin, *Lettres*, 9:180, 182, 222, 229, 342, 375.
153 Cardinal de Retz to Alexander VII, 1661, quoted in Salmon, *Retz*, 321–22.
154 Batiffol, *Retz*, 202–5. The Jansenists allegedly gave Retz the princely sum of 700,000 *livres* in 1653 alone.
155 Le Paige and Du Rey, *Rets*, 121–23.
156 This scene at Court is reconstructed from memoirs in Bluche, *Journal*, 40.
157 Le Paige and Du Rey, *Rets*, 124.
158 Salmon, *Retz*, 29, 67.
159 Cardinal de Retz to Guillaume Charrier, *abbé* de Chage, 9 February 1652, quoted in Salmon, *Retz*, 206.
160 Robert Arnauld d'Andilly to Mazarin, 9 March 1655, quoted in Jansen, *Andilly*, 59–60.
161 Robert Arnauld d'Andilly to Mazarin, 25 August 1655, quoted in ibid., 63–66.
162 Robert Arnauld d'Andilly to Mazarin, 12 February 1656, quoted in ibid., 77–80.
163 Antoine Arnauld to Bishop of Coutances, 21 March 1656, quoted in ibid., 99–101.
164 Mazarin to Robert Arnauld d'Andilly, 24 March 1656, quoted in ibid., 102–103.
165 Robert Arnauld d'Andilly to Queen Anne and to Mazarin, 2 May 1656, quoted in ibid., 107–8.
166 Mazarin to Robert Arnauld d'Andilly, 5 May 1656, quoted in ibid., 108–109.
167 Robert Arnauld d'Andilly to Mazarin, 9 May 1656, quoted in ibid., 109–10.
168 Mazarin to Bishop of Coutances, 21 November 1658, quoted in Mazarin, *Lettres*, 9:749.
169 Mazarin to Chancellor Le Tellier, 17 October 1659, quoted in ibid., 9:369–72.
170 Mazarin to *Mère* Angélique Arnauld, 22 March 1660, quoted in ibid., 9:934.
171 Louis XIV, quoted in Andrew Lossky, *Louis XIV and the French Monarchy* (New Brunswick, NJ: Rutgers University Press, 1994), 185.
172 Lucien Ceyssens, "Autour de la bulle Unigenitus: Louis XIV," *Bulletin de l'Institut historique belge de Rome* 55–56 (1985–1986):124–44.
173 Shennon, *Louis XIV*, 29; Pierre Goubert, *Louis XIV and Twenty Million Frenchmen* (NY: Vintage Books, 1966), 75; Anne York, "Religious Aspiration and Janséniste Confrontation," paper presented at the Western Society for French History conference, Orcas Island, Washington, 15 October 1992.
174 A *Bull* is a solemn document published by the pope and sealed with two small lead balls, called "bulls"; the proper term for it is "constitution" (as with the Constitution *Unigenitus* of 1713). A *Mandement* is a circular addressed by a bishop to the faithful of his diocese. A *Placet* is an act by which the king authorizes the execution in France of an act given by the pope. See Venard and Bonzon, *Religion*, 180, 183–84.
175 Jacques M. Grès-Gayer, *Le Jansénisme en Sorbonne, 1643–1656* (Paris: Klincksieck, 1996), 130–32.
176 Neveu, *Erudition*, 409.
177 Ceyssens, "Jansénisme et anti-jansénisme," 116–17; Meyer, *Controverses*, 128–31; and Yves de La Brière, "Les premiers contradicteurs de l'*Augustinus*," *Recherches de science religieuse* 1 (1910):497–98.
178 Neveu, *Erudition*, 460; Doyle, *Jansenism*, 24.
179 Meyer, *Controverses*, 132–36; Grès-Gayer, *Jansénisme*, 23–26.
180 Meyer, ibid., 436.
181 *Père* Brisacier, *Jansénisme confoundu* (1651), cited by Louis Gorin de Saint-Amour, *The Journal of Mons. de Saint Amour, Doctor of the Sorbonne, containing a full Account of all the Transactions both in France and at Rome concerning the Five Famous Propositions Controverted between the Jansenists and the Molinists from the beginning of the Affair till the Popes {sic} Decision, 1646–1653* (London: T. Ratcliff, 1664), 137.
182 Ibid., 256–57.
183 Grès-Gayer, *Jansénisme*, 175, 280.
184 Ibid., 21; Antoine Arnauld, "Nicolas Cornet," in *Oeuvres*, 43:65.

185 Préclin and Jarry, *Luttes politiques*, 194–95.
186 Richardt, *Jansénisme*, 75–77; Maulvault, *Répertoire*, 64; and Tuilier, *Sorbonne*, 2:23–25. See chapter 2 for a detailed discussion of the five propositions.
187 Tuilier, *Sorbonne*, 27.
188 Antoine Arnauld, "Considerations sur l'enterprise de M. Cornet" (1649) and "Considerations sur l'assemblée du 4 Novembre 1655" (1655), in *Oeuvres*, 19:11, 613.
189 Angélique Arnauld, quoted in Tuilier, *Sorbonne*, 2:27.
190 St. Amour, *Journal*, 10.
191 Meyer, *Controverses*, 421; Hamscher, *Fronde*, 112.
192 Sedgwick, *Travails*, 138; Antoine Arnauld, *Mémoires sur la cause des Quartre Evêques* (1668), in *Oeuvres*, 24:258–60.
193 Antoine Arnauld, "Relation touchant le livre de *la Fréquente Communion*" (1695), in *Oeuvres*, 28:689–90.
194 Antoine Arnauld, *Ecrits sur les Bulles d'Alexandre VII* (1663), in *Oeuvres*, 22:211.
195 Antoine Arnauld to Henri, Bishop of Angers (?), January 1664, in *Oeuvres*, 1:462.
196 Antoine Arnauld, *Ecrits sur les Bulles d'Alexandre VII* (1663), in *Oeuvres*, 22:212, 219; idem, *Oeuvres*, 19:XII.
197 Paul Sonnino, *Louis XIV's View of the Papacy, 1661–1667* (Berkeley: University of California Press, 1966), 22–24, 27–28.
198 Bull *Ad sacram*, quoted in Richardt, *Jansénism*, 82–83; Lucien Ceyssens, "Les Cinq propositions de Jansénius à Rome," *Revue d'histoire ecclésiastique* 66 (1971):459–65, 473–75, 826, 836, 847–48.
199 Ceyssens, ibid., 867.
200 St. Amour, *Journal*, 365–68.
201 Maire, *Cause de Dieu*, 30; Jansen, *Mazarin*, 40–41; and Crichton, *Jansenisers*, 35.
202 Blet, "Louis XIV," 117; St. Amour, *Journal*, 440.
203 Mazarin, quoted in Richardt, *Jansénism*, 84; Kostroun, "Port-Royal Nuns," 163.
204 Levi, *Louis XIV*, 231.
205 Antoine Arnauld, Introduction to *Oeuvres*, 21:CXVIII–CXIX.
206 Maire, *Cause de Dieu*, 31–32.
207 Richardt, *Jansénism*, 85; Hamscher, *Fronde*, 112; Chaunu, *Basculement*, 87–89; and Paule Jansen, "L'Assemblée générale du clergé de 1655 et l'affaire janséniste," *Chroniques de Port-Royal* 32 (1983):162–65, 176.
208 Grès-Gayer, *Jansénisme*, 109.
209 Jansen, *Mazarin*, 173; Hamscher, *Fronde*, 113.
210 Godefroi Hermant, *Mémoires de Godefroi Hermant sur l'histoire ecclésiastique du XVIIe siècle (1630–1663)*, ed. A. Gazier (Paris: Plon-Nourrit, 1905–1910), 2:568–70.
211 Tuilier, *Sorbonne*, 2:35–36; Richardt, *Jansénius*, 86–87; Kostroun, "Port-Royal Nuns," 29–30; and Hermant, *Mémoires*, 3:123. Arnauld prayed: "Since they [the Theology Faculty at the Sorbonne] have persecuted me only for the Truth, support me, Lord, so I can fight for the truth to the day I die."
212 Richardt, *Jansénism*, 85.
213 Phillips, *Church and Culture*, 278–81.
214 Doyle, *Jansenism*, 28; Gastelier, *Angélique*, 13; and Jansen, *Mazarin*, 133, 140.
215 Neveu, *Erudition*, 424–25; Doyle, *Jansenism*, 31.
216 Hermant, *Mémoires*, 3:323–25.
217 Ibid., 345; Jansen, *Mazarin*, 163.
218 Colbert to Mazarin, 1657, quoted in Hamscher, *Fronde*, 114.
219 Introduction to Antoine Arnauld, *Oeuvres*, 21:XVI; Jansen, *Mazarin*, 163–67, 177; and Hermant, *Mémoires*, 3:580–81, 585. While Arnauld dates the *lit de justice* as the 14th of December, Jansen and Hermant put it on the 19th of December 1657.
220 Isaac Le Maistre, letter of 1 June 1657, cited by Richardt, *Jansénisme*, 99–100.
221 Emanuel S. Chill, "The Company of the Holy Sacrament, 1630–1666: Social Aspects of the French Counter-Reformation" (PhD diss., Columbia University, 1960), 174–77, 183; Alain Tallon, "Prière et charité dans la Compagnie du Saint-Sacrement (1629–1667)," *Histoire économie et société* 10 (1991):122–23.

222 Jaccard, *Saint-Cyran*, 134; Delforge, *Ecoles*, 138–40; and Raoul Allier, *La cabale des dévôts, 1627–1666* (Paris: n.p., 1902; reprint, Geneva: Slatkine Reprints, 1970), 159–63, 167–71, 175, 179, 182, 187–89.
223 Kostroun, "Port-Royal Nuns," 186–87.
224 Jacques Nouet, quoted in ibid., 192.
225 Allier, *Cabale*, 189–92; Alfred Rébelliau, "Deux ennemis de la Compagnie du Saint-Sacrement, Molière et Port-Royal," *Revue des Deux-Mondes*, 2d ser., 53 (15 October 1909):914–23.
226 Jules Paquier, *Le Jansénisme* (Paris: Librairie Bloud, 1909), 471–72.
227 Ibid., 473; Françoise Hildesheimer, *Le Jansénisme en France au XVII et XVIIIe siècles* (Paris: Publisud, 1991), 63; Jean Lhermitte, *Le problème des miracles*, 7th ed. (Paris: Gallimard, 1956), 60; and Kreiser, *Miracles*, 71.
228 Lhermitte, ibid., 70; Crichton, *Jansenisers*, 243–44; Samuel P. Tregelles, *The Jansenists: Their Rise, Persecutions by the Jesuits, and Existing Remnant: A Chapter in Church History* (London: Samuel Bagster, 1851), 23 (see note).
229 Paquier, *Jansénisme*, 469.
230 Blaise Pascal, quoted in Jean-Robert Armogathe, "A propos des miracles de Saint-Médard: Les preuves de Carré de Montgeron et le positivisme des Lumières," *Revue de l'histoire des religions* 180 (1971):135. A century later, Jean-Jacques Rousseau retorted: "I do not need miracles in order to be a Christian."
231 Mary Aanne Schimmelpenninck, ed., *Select Memoirs of Port Royal*, 5th ed. (Philadelphia: Henry Longstretch, 1853),1:233.
232 Kreiser, *Miracles*, 71.
233 Ibid., 72.
234 Maire, *Cause de Dieu*, 35.
235 La Brière, "Jansénisme," 274.
236 Maire, *Cause de Dieu*, 36–37.

3 Sunrise Over Port-Royal, 1600–1661

1 *Mère* Angélique Arnauld, March 1608, quoted in Gastelier, *Angélique*, 73.
2 Lefebvre, *Pascal*, 64, 67.
3 Orcibal, "Port-Royal," 261–65.
Bugnion-Secretan, *Mère Angélique*, 65.
5 Chédozeau, "Tridentinism," 123–25.
6 Chaunu et al., *Basculement*, 65–68.
7 Bruno Neveu, "Preface," in Lesaulner, *Images*, 8–9.
8 Barnard, *Schools*, 6; Gastelier, *Angélique*, 55.
9 Ed. Finot, *Port-Royal et Magny* (Paris: Georges Chamerot, 1888), 1–2.
10 *Abbé* Grégoire, *Oeuvres de l'Abbé Grégoire*, vol. 12, *Les Ruines de Port-Royal des Champs en 1801* (Paris: Imprimerie Librairie Chrétienne, 1801), 77; Marguerite Tollemache, *French Jansenists* (London: Kegan Paul, Trench, Trübner, 1893), 253; and Thérèse Monthéard, *Le Guide de la vallée de Chevreuse et de Port-Royal* (Besançon: Editions de la Manufacture, 1992), 119, 125–30; and Angélique Arnauld, *Relation*, 24.
11 Phillips, *Church and Culture*, 46; Delforge, *Ecoles*, 23. The Saint-Honoré district included the convents and monasteries for the Dominicans, Reformed Cistercians, Capuchins, Capuchines, Dames of the Assumption, Daughters of St. Thomas, Daughters of the Conception, and the Chapel of the Feuillants.
12 Raoul Berenguier, *Port-Royal et la vallée de Chevreuse* (Paris: Nouvelles Editions Latines, [c. 1962]), 3; Racine, *Port-Royal*, 13–15; and Gastelier, *Angélique*, 53–54.
13 Gastelier, *Angélique*, 56–58; André Hallays, *Les solitaires de Port-Royal* (Paris: Plon, 1927), 5; and Charles Clémencet, *Histoire générale de Port-Roïal, depuis la réforme de l'abbaïe jusqu'à son entière destruction* (Amsterdam: Jean Vanduren, 1755–1757), 1:cxxxix–clv.
14 Diefendorf, *Penitence to Charity*, 7; François Bayrou, *Ils portaient l'écharpe blanche: L'aventure des premiers réformés, des guerres de religion à l'Edit de Nantes, de la Révocation à la Révolution* (Paris: Editions Grasset

& Fasquelle, 1998), 237; and Elizabeth Rapley, *The Dévotes: Women and Church in Seventeenth-Century France* (Montreal and Kingston: McGill–Queen's University Press, 1990), 5.

15 Bayrou, *L'Aventure*, 233.

16 Bugnion-Secretan, *Mère Angélique*, 108.

17 Diefendorf, *Penitence to Charity*, 8–9, 17.

18 Bugnion-Secretan, *Mère Angélique*, 10; Sedgwick, *Travails*, 35–37; and Gastelier, *Angélique*, 27–35.

19 Gastelier, ibid., 45–47.

20 Ibid., 47; Richardt, *Jansénisme*, 25–26; and Sedgwick, *Travails*, 38.

21 Kostroun, "Port-Royal Nuns," 42.

22 Angélique Arnauld, quoted in Gastelier, *Angélique*, 43, 68, 71.

23 Gastelier, ibid., 52; Kostroun, "Port-Royal Nuns," 44; and Ethel Romanes, *The Story of Port-Royal* (London: John Murray, 1907), 7.

24 Gastelier, ibid., 47–48; Sedgwick, *Travails*, 38–40; Newton, "Port-Royal," 154; and May 1601 Bull, BN, ms. fr. 15806, ff. 96–99.

25 Sedgwick, ibid., 40–41; Gastelier, ibid., 48–50, 65.

26 The abbesses were Marie Angélique de Ste. Madeleine Arnauld, Agnès de St. Paul Arnauld, and Angélique de St. Jean Arnauld d'Andilly. The prioresses were Françoise-Louise de Ste. Claire Arnauld, Anne-Eugénie de l'Incarnation Arnauld, Marie-Angélique de Ste. Thérèse Arnauld d'Andilly, and Marie-Charlotte de Ste. Claire Arnauld d'Andilly. The solitaires were Antoine Arnauld, Henri Arnauld, Robert Arnauld d'Andilly, and C. H. Arnauld de Luzancy. See lists in J. Bruggeman and A. J. Van de Ven, *Inventaire des pièces d'archives françaises se rapportant à l'abbaye de Port-Royal-des-Champs et son cercle et à la résistance contre la bulle Unigenitus et à l'appel* (La Haye: Martinus Nijhoff, 1972).

27 Sedgwick, ibid., 41–43.

28 Gastelier, *Angélique,* 72–73.

29 Angélique Arnauld, March 1608, quoted in ibid., 73.

30 Angélique Arnauld, *Relation* (1655), 11–13; Ruth Clark, *Strangers & Sojourners at Port-Royal* (Cambridge: University Press, 1932), 14; and J. L. A. A. Frencken, *Agnès Arnauld* (Nimègue-Utrecht: N. V. Dekker en Van de Vigt en J. W. Van Leeuwen, 1932), 20–24.

31 Arnauld, *Relation*, 14–20.

32 Richardt, *Jansénisme*, 26; Angélique Arnauld, quoted in Sedgwick, *Travails*, 43–44.

33 Gastelier, *Angélique,* 69, 80–81, 85; Sedgwick, *Travails*, 44; and Kostroun, "Port-Royal Nuns," 33–35.

34 *Père* Bernard, quoted in Gastelier, ibid., 73.

35 *Père* Pacifique and Catherine Dupont, quoted in ibid., 73–74.

36 Kostroun, "Port-Royal Nuns," 81–82; Gastelier, ibid., 87.

37 Sedgwick, *Travails*, 47.

38 Hallays, *Solitaires*, 6–7; Gastelier, *Angélique*, 74; Kostroun, "Port-Royal Nuns," 84–85; Rapley, *Cloister*, 131–46; Louis Cognet, *La Réforme de Port-Royal, 1591–1618* (Paris: Editions Sulliver, 1950), 192–93; and F. Ellen Weaver, *The Evolution of the Reform of Port-Royal from the Rule of Cîteaux to Jansenism* (Paris: Editions Beauchesne, 1978), 31–34, 44–46, 55, 154–56.

39 Kostroun, ibid., 50, 59–60.

40 Angélique Arnauld's nine letters, which cover the period from November 1640 to June 1653, are found in BN, ms. fr. 23481, ff. 12–23.

41 Angélique Arnauld, *Relation*, 25–27, 30–33, 37–38, 43, 47, 54, 61, 66–73.

42 Bugnion-Secretan, *Mère Angélique*, 23; Kostroun, "Port-Royal Nuns," 87.

43 Newton, "Port-Royal," 154, 176, 185, 192.

44 Kostroun, "Port-Royal Nuns," 55; Gastelier, *Angélique*, 120–21; and "Pièces originales sur Port-Royal: Bulles et brevets," BN, ms. fr. 15805, f. 28.

45 "Pièces originales sur Port-Royal," BN, ms. fr. 15806, ff. 151–52; Gastelier, *Angélique*, 122–23.

46 Gastelier, ibid., 137.

47 Ibid., 104–106; Kostroun, "Port-Royal Nuns," 82; and Besoigne, *Port-Royal*, 1:84–85.

48 Gastelier, ibid., 124–27; Richardt, *Jansénisme*, 27.

49 François de Sales to Madame de Chantel, 11 October 1621, quoted in Cognet, *Angélique,* 140.
50 Angélique Arnauld, 1622, quoted in Richardt, *Jansénisme*, 49.
51 Angélique Arnauld to Queen Anne of Austria, 1661, quoted in Cognet, *Angélique*, 103–6.
52 François de Sales, quoted in Kostroun, "Port-Royal Nuns," 108–10.
53 Lesaulnier, *Images*, 11–17; Richardt, *Jansenism*, 49.
54 Richardt, ibid, 49–51; Kostroun, "Port-Royal Nuns," 118–21; and Sedgwick, *Travails*, 51–53.
55 Kostroun, ibid., 122–23; Phillips, *Church and Culture*, 195.
56 André Fraigneau, *Port-Royal des Champs* (Paris: Editions Sun, 1949), 3.
57 Madame de Ligny to Angélique Arnauld, quoted in Victor-L. Tapié, *France in the Age of Louis XIII and Richelieu*, trans. and ed. D. McN. Lockie (New York: Praeger Publishers, 1975), 284.
58 Augustin Louis Gazier, *Jeanne de Chantal et Angélique Arnauld d'après leur correspondance, 1620–1641* (Paris: Librairie Ancienne Honoré Champion, 1915), 113.
59 Angélique Arnauld to Robert Arnauld d'Andilly, 7 January 1621, in Jacqueline Marie Angélique Arnauld, *Lettres de la Reverende Mère Marie Angélique Arnauld, abbesse et réformatrice de Port-Royal, 1620–1661* (Utrecht: Aux Depens de la Compagnie, 1742), 1:13 [hereafter cited as *Lettres*].
60 Crichton, *Jansenisers*, 65; Le Goff and Rémond, *French Religion*, 2:362–63.
61 Kostroun, "Port-Royal Nuns," 134–35.
62 Laporte, *Doctrine*, 1:XX–XXIV, XXXVI.
63 Angélique Arnauld to Robert Arnauld d'Andilly, in *Lettres*, 1:13, 21, 111.
64 Angélique Arnauld to M. Macquet, 24 May 1638, in ibid., 139.
65 Agnès Arnauld to Antoine Arnauld, 21 April 1639, in Jeanne-Catherine-Agnès Arnauld, *Lettres de la Mère Agnès Arnauld, abbesse de Port-Royal*, ed. M. P. Faugere (N.p., 1626 ; reprint, Paris: Ernest Thorin, 1866), 1:89.
66 Angélique Arnauld to M. Macquet, 31 January 1640, in *Lettres*, 1:183.
67 Angélique Arnauld to M. Macquet, 27 February 1643, in *Lettres*, 1:231.
68 Angélique Arnauld to M. Macquet, 6 March 1643, in *Lettres*, 1:232–33.
69 Angélique Arnauld to *princesse* de Guéménée, October 1643, in *Lettres*, 1:234.
70 Kostroun, "Port-Royal Nuns," 112–13, 116; Cognet, *Angélique*, 247; and François Calot and Louis-Marie Michon, *Port-Royal et le Jansénisme* (Paris: Albert Morancé, 1928), 29–30.
71 Louis XIII, letters patent, December 1623, BN, ms. fr. 15805, f. 50.
72 Kostroun, "Port-Royal Nuns," 114.
73 Letter of Jean-François de Gondi, Archbishop of Paris, 14 August 1625; letters patent establishing Marie de Medicis as "founder" of Port-Royal de Paris, December 1625, BN, ms. fr. 15805, f. 51; *arrêt* of Parlement, 16 February 1626, BN, ms. fr. 15805, f. 52; Gastelier, *Angélique*, 141–43; and Crichton, *Jansenisers*, 122.
74 Brief of Urban VIII, 15 June 1627, BN, ms. fr. 15806, ff. 1, 122–23; approval of the *abbé* of Citeaux, 16 December 1624, BN, ms. fr. 15806, ff. 116–17; and *lettre de cachet* of Louis XIII, 31 July 1627, BN, ms. fr. 15806, f. 2.
75 Letters patent from Louis XIII, January 1629, BN, ms. fr. 15806, f. 6; register of the Grand Conseil du Roy, 20 February 1629, BN, ms. fr. 15809, f. 2; Gastelier, *Angélique*, 153–54; Maulvault, *Répertoire*, 22–23; Weaver, *Port-Royal*, 44; and Kostroun, "Port-Royal Nuns," 79–80.
76 Sedgwick, *Travails*, 50; Crichton, *Jansenisers*, 122.
77 Gastelier, ibid., 148.
78 Besoigne, *Port-Royal*, 1:138–40.
79 Kostroun, "Port-Royal Nuns," 116–17; Frencken, *Agnès Arnauld*, 61–62.
80 Bugnion-Secretan, *Mère Angélique*, 38.
81 Sedgwick, *Travails*, 54.
82 Robert Arnauld d'Andilly's wife (name not given), quoted in ibid., 60.
83 Frencken, *Agnès Arnauld*, 62; Gazier, *Port-Royal*, 107.
84 Kostroun, "Port-Royal Nuns," 140–44; Sedgwick, *Travails*, 55–56, 59.
85 Ibid., 130 (n. 92); Richardt, *Jansénisme*, 50.
86 Antoine Arnauld, *Apologie pour Monsieur de St. Cyran* (1644), in *Oeuvres*, 29:190–91; idem, "Defense de la Censeur contre Le P. Brisacier" (1652), in *Oeuvres*, 29:575–77. A century later, Charles

Clémencet, in "Works Falsely Attributed to M. de St.-Cyran" (c. 1750), also denied this charge. See Charles Clémencet, "Histoire littéraire de Port-Royal," BHPF, Fonds Ste.-Beuve, ms. 101, f. 128.

87 Kostroun, "Port-Royal Nuns," 130–31; Richardt, *Jansénisme*, 50–51.

88 Gastelier, *Angélique*, 162–66.

89 Mlle. de Joncoux, quoted in Weaver, *Joncoux*, 159.

90 Lesaulnier, *Images*, 25–37.

91 Angélique Arnauld to unkown, September 1634, quoted in Bugnion-Secretan, *Mère Angélique*, 54.

92 "Act of Election," 1657, BN, ms. fr. 15806, ff. 54–57; Frencken, *Agnès Arnauld*, 100–3.

93 Elections at Port-Royal de Paris, 1633–1658, BN, ms. fr. 15806, ff. 14–18, 58–61; Newton, *Port-Royal*, 59.

94 Richardt, *Jansénisme*, 54–55; Louis Cognet, "La direction de conscience à Port-Royal," *Supplément de la vie spirituelle* 8 (1955):295–301.

95 Cognet, *Lancelot*, 47–48; Fouqueroy, *Compagnie de Jésus*, 400.

96 Crichton, *Jansenisers*, 39.

97 Gastelier, *Angélique*, 189, 193, 205, 214; Newton, *Port-Royal*, 16–18.

98 Martin, *French Book*, 47–48.

99 Bishop Henri Arnauld to President Barillon at the Rouen Parlement, 6 October 1641, BN, ms. fr. 15611, f. 282.

100 Delforge, *Ecoles*, 45.

101 Anne of Austria to *princesse* de Guéménée, 1643, cited by Salmon, *Retz*, 67.

102 Delforge, *Ecoles*, 46.

103 Gastelier, *Angélique*, 285–88; Newton, "Port-Royal," 178–79; and Ellen Weaver, "The Bible and Port-Royal," *Cîteaux* 41 (1990):91.

104 Angélique Arnauld to M. de Fleury, 5 January 1650, in *Lettres*, 1:447–48; Delforge, *Ecoles*, 72–73.

105 Antoine Adam, *Du mysticisme à la révolte: Les jansénistes du XVIIe siècle* (Paris: M. Fayard, 1968), 189–92.

106 See Sedgwick, *Jansenism*, 61–66, for a discussion of Robert Arnauld d'Andilly's pamphlets.

107 Ibid., 106.

108 Sedgwick, *Travails*, 161.

109 Gastelier, *Angélique*, 303.

110 Angélique Arnauld to Agnès Arnauld, 13 January 1649, in *Lettres*, 1:406; Frencken, *Agnès Arnauld*, 160–61.

111 Angélique Arnauld to Queen of Poland, 12 May 1649, in *Lettres*, 1:420–22; Ellen Weaver, *Madame de Fontpertuis: une dévote janséniste, amie et gérante d'Antoine Arnauld et de Port-Royal* (Paris: Klincksieck, 1998), 29.

112 Bugnion-Secretan, *Mère Angélique*, 157, 160, 169; Gastelier, *Angélique*, 334, 346.

113 Angélique Arnauld to M. de Fleury, 21 September 1651, in *Lettres*, 1:582–83.

114 Angélique Arnauld to Agnès Arnauld, March 1652, in *Lettres*, 2:62; idem to Le Maître, 14 June 1652, in *Lettres*, 2:131.

115 Angélique Arnauld to Queen of Poland, 16 May 1652, in *Lettres*, 2:111–14; idem to M. Le Maître, 23 May 1652, in *Lettres*, 2:119; and Dominique de Courcelles, *Le Sang de Port-Royal*, ed. de l'Herne (Paris: L'Herne, 1994), 87.

116 Angélique Arnauld to M. le Maître, May 1652, in *Lettres*, 2:123.

117 Angélique Arnauld to Queen of Poland, 28 June 1652, in *Lettres*, 2:139–40.

118 Ibid., 141–44.

119 Angélique Arnauld to M. le Maître, June 1652, in *Lettres*, 2:144–46; Delforge, *Ecoles*, 77–78.

120 Angélique Arnauld to Queen of Poland, 28 June 1652, in *Lettres*, 2:143–44; Delforge, ibid., 80–84.

121 Angélique Arnauld to Queen of Poland, 5 July 1652, in *Lettres*, 2:152–54; idem to M. de Barcos, 24 September 1652, in *Lettres*, 2:184–86.

122 Angélique Arnauld to Queen of Poland, 1 August 1653, in *Lettres*, 2:354.

123 Angélique Arnauld to *Soeur* Angélique Magdeleine Annonciade, 10 August 1653, in *Lettres*, 2:360.

124 Sedgwick, *Travails*, 62, 240.

125 Ibid., 63–75; Antoine Arnauld, *Oeuvres*, 43:141, 23:180; de Courcelles, *Sang*, 52; Knox, 195–96; Gastelier, *Angélique*, 71, 77, 149, 256; and Goldmann, *Hidden God*, 411.

126 Kostroun, "Port-Royal Nuns," 148.
127 Antoine Arnauld, *Oeuvres,* 23: II; Levi, *Louis XIV*, 228; O'Connell, *Pascal*, 68; and Hildesheimer, *Jansénisme*, 38.
128 Angélique de Saint-Jean Arnauld d'Andilly, *Relation de captivité d'Angélique de Saint-Jean Arnauld d'Andilly*, ed. Louis Cognet (Paris: Gallimard, 1954), 7–17; "Pièces pour l'histoire litteraire des solitaires de Port-Royal," BHPF, Fonds Sainte-Beuve, ms. 115, f. 65.
129 De Courcelles, *Sang*, 52–53; Sedgwick, *Travails*, 120.
130 Sedgwick, ibid., 92; BHPF, Fonds Sainte-Beuve, ms. 115, f. 231; Robert Arnauld d'Andilly, *Mémoires,* in *Collection des Mémoires relatifs à l'histoire de France*, ed. M. Petitot (Paris: Foucault, Libraire, 1824), 1:286–91; and Kostroun, "Port-Royal Nuns," 77–78.
131 Angélique Arnauld to Robert Arnauld d'Andilly, 15 August 1625, in *Lettres*, 1:24.
132 Arnauld d'Andilly, *Mémoires*, 2:78.
133 Ibid., 100, 291; Robert's six daughters became Sister Catherine de Sainte Agnès, Sister Angélique de Saint Jean, Sister Marie Charlotte de Sainte Claire, Sister Marie Angélique de Sainte Therèse, Anne Marie d'Andilly (a novice), and Elisabeth d'Andilly (a pensioner). One son—Simon, marquis de Pomponne—served Louis XIV as *sécretaire d'état* and an ambassador to several European countries.
134 Antoine Le Maître, quoted in Sedgwick, *Travails*, 82–86; Lesaulnier, "Galerie," 158–59; and BHPF, ms. 115, f. 217.
135 Sedgwick, ibid., 86–87.
136 Isaac-Louis Le Maître de Sacy, quoted in ibid., 88; Lesaulnier, "Galerie," 159–60; Schimmelpenninck, *Port-Royal*, 1:452; and Geneviève Delassault, *Le Maistre de Sacy et son temps* (Paris: Librairie Nizet, 1957), 7–9.
137 Ibid., 113–14, 118–19.
138 Schimmelpenninck, *Port-Royal*, 1:245–46; Kostroun, "Port-Royal Nuns," 154.
139 Angélique Arnauld, *Lettres*, 2:110–11; Cognet, *Lancelot*, 82; and Taveneaux, *Jansénisme et Réforme*, 36–40.
140 Delforge, *Ecoles*, 196–204; Cognet, *Lancelot*, 34–35; and Lesaulnier, "Galerie," 180–82. Charles Clémencet's lengthy manuscripts "Histoire littéraire de Port-Royal" and "Histoire littéraire des Religieuses de Port-Royal des Champs" (BHPF, ms. 101) give a detailed history of each of the solitaires (name, title, position, education, outstanding qualities, friendship network, years at Port-Royal, major events, significant writings, date and cause of death, encomiums, etc.).
141 Bruggeman and Van de Ven, *Inventaire*, #462–#917; Gastelier, *Angélique*, 153; Sedgwick, *Travails*, 144; and John J. Conley, *The Suspicion of Virtue: Women Philosophers in Neoclassical France* (Ithaca and London: Cornell University Press, 2002), 12–13, 20–24.
142 Monsieur Benoise, *Mémoire* (c. 1650s), BN, ms. fr. 17750, f. 13; Jean Racine's essay on Port-Royal, BN, ms. fr. 12887, ff. 107, 118.
143 Louis de Pontis, *Mémoires du Sieur de Pontis officier des Armées du Roi contenant plusieurs circonstances des guerres et du gouvernement sous les règnes des rois Henri IV, Louis XIII et Louis XIV*, ed. Andrée Villard (N.p., 1676; reprint, Paris: Honoré Champion, 2000), 9–15, 46, 636–37, 689–710.
144 Jean de La Fontaine, *Recueil de poésies Chrétiennes et diverses* (1671), quoted in Lesaulnier, "Galerie," 153–54.
145 Pierre Magnard, "Angélique de Saint-Jean ou l'Esprit de Resistance," in *Chroniques de Port-Royal* 34 (1985):13–15, 18–26.
146 Gastelier, *Angélique*, 354–57.
147 *Père* Annat, *Cavilli jansenianorum* (1654), cited by Delforge, *Ecoles*, 99.
148 Kostroun, "Port-Royal Nuns," 206.
149 Angélique Arnauld to *abbé* de Fleury, 24 July 1653, *Lettres*, 2:352–53.
150 Angélique Arnauld to Queen of Poland, 22 August 1653, *Lettres*, 2:363–64.
151 Angélique Arnauld to M. de Fleury, 22 August 1653, *Lettres*, 2:365–66; Angélique Arnauld to unknown, 22 August 1653, quoted in Richardt, *Jansénisme*, 84.
152 Angélique Arnauld to Queen of Poland, 4 February 1654, *Lettres*, 2:441.
153 Angélique Arnauld to unknown, 1653, quoted in Besoigne, *Port-Royal*, 1:357.
154 Angélique Arnauld to Queen of Poland, 4 February, 13 March, 17 June 1654, *Lettres*, 2:441, 453, 507; Gastelier, *Angélique*, 365.

155 Angélique Arnauld to Queen of Poland, 5 February 1655, *Lettres*, 2:563.
156 Angélique Arnauld to Queen of Poland, 5 March 1655, *Lettres*, 2:571.
157 Angélique Arnauld to M. le Maître, 5 March 1655, *Lettres*, 2:573.
158 Angélique Arnauld to Queen of Poland, 11 March 1655, *Lettres*, 2:575.
159 Angélique Arnauld to Queen of Poland, 28 May 1655, *Lettres*, 2:620–21.
160 Angélique Arnauld, August 1655, quoted in Gastelier, *Angélique*, 369.
161 Robert Arnauld d'Andilly to Jules Mazarin, 10 January 1654, quoted in Jansen, *Andilly*, 39.
162 Alexander VII, quoted in the introduction to Antoine Arnauld, *Oeuvres*, 19:XXXIX–XLI.
163 Jean Orcibal, *Port-Royal entre le miracle et l'obéissance: Flavie Passart et Angélique de Saint-Jean Arnauld d'Andilly* (Paris: Desclée de Brouwer, 1957), 8.
164 Gastelier, *Angélique*, 392.
165 Justin Godart, *Le Jansénisme à Lyon; Benôit Fourgon, 1687–1773* (Paris: Félix Alcan, 1934), 22.
166 Formulary of 1656, quoted in Gabriel Gerberon, *Histoire générale du Jansénisme, contenant ce qui s'est passé en France, en Espagne, en Italie, dans les pais-bas . . .* (Amsteredam: Chez J. Louis de Lorme, 1701), 4:32.
167 Alison Forrestal, *Fathers, Pastors and Kings: Visions of Episcopacy in Seventeenth-Century France* (Manchester and New York: Manchester University Press, 2004), 127; Claude Quétel, *De Par Le Roy: Essai sur les lettres de cachet* (Toulouse: Privat Editeur, 1981), 63.
168 Phillips, *Church and Culture*, 204; Conley, *Suspicion*, 26; and Kostroun, "Port-Royal Nuns," 30, 207–8.
169 Antoine Arnauld, *Ecrits sur les Bulles d'Alexandre VII* (1657), in *Oeuvres*, 21:207–209, 213–36, 485; 22:IV, 125.
170 Antoine Arnauld to *Père* Feret, 22 July 1658, in *Oeuvres*, 1:185, 518, 586.
171 Blaise Pascal, cited in the introduction to Antoine Arnauld, *Oeuvres*, 21:CXXVIII–CXXIX.
172 Gastelier, *Angélique*, 378–79, 383.
173 Angélique Arnauld to the Queen of Poland, 24 March 1656, in *Lettres*, 3:199.
174 Angélique Arnauld to M. le Maître, 27 March 1656, in *Lettres*, 3:201–202.
175 Angélique Arnauld to the Queen of Poland, 1 June 1656, in *Lettres*, 3:248; Cognet, *Lancelot*, 132, 147, 178.
176 Delforge, *Ecoles*, 119.
177 Angélique Arnauld to Saint-Cyran, 29 April 1652, in *Lettres*, 2:87.
178 Tetsuya Shiokawa, *Pascal et les miracles* (Paris: Librairie A.-G. Nizet, 1977), 79–83; Jacqueline Pascal, *A Rule for Children and Other Writings*, ed. and trans. John J. Conley (N.p., 1665; reprint, Chicago and London: University of Chicago Press, 2003), 141–42.
179 Pascal, ibid., 95, 142–43; Jean Pommier, "Port-Royal et la Sainte-Epine," *Mercure de France*, 1 March 1956, pp. 445–50; and Gastelier, *Angélique*, 380.
180 Gastelier, ibid., 382.
181 Blaise Pascal, quoted in Shiokawa, *Pascal*, 119–20, 128.
182 Antoine Arnauld, *Reponse à un écrit publié sur le sujet des miracles qu'il a plu à Dieu de faire à Port-Royal depuis quelque temps par une Sainte Epine de la Couronne de Notre Seigneur* (1656), in *Oeuvres*, 23:10–12.
183 Angélique Arnauld to unknown, 1656, quoted in Gastelier, *Angélique*, 380–81.
184 Angélique Arnauld to Mlle. Joffe, 22 June 1656; idem to the Queen of Poland, 30 June and 14 July 1656, in *Lettres*, 3:263–73; Besoigne, *Port-Royal*, 1:364–82.
185 Angélique Arnauld to the Queen of Poland, 14 July 1656, in *Lettres*, 3:272–73; idem to the Queen of Poland, August 1656, quoted in Sedgwick, *Travails*, 157.
186 Antoine Arnauld to Angélique Arnauld, c. August 1656, quoted in Sedgwick, *Travails*, 169. Miracles could fill a convent's coffers as well. A grateful Princess Palatine, healed of "a great illness" by the thorn, sent 1000 *livres* to Port-Royal.
187 Angélique Arnauld to Angélique de Sainte-Agnès de Marle de Falaire, December 1656; idem to the Queen of Poland, 1 and 28 December 1656; idem to Mme. Joffe, 12 January 1657; idem to *Mère* Dorothée de l'Incarnation le Conte, June 1657; idem to the Queen of Poland, 3 and 30 August 1657, in *Lettres*, 3:308, 318–19, 329–30, 339–40, 403, 406, 413–15.
188 Shiokawa, *Pascal*, 97–102.
189 Queen Anne to Robert Arnauld d'Andilly, June 1659, quoted in Sedgwick, *Travails*, 159.
190 Kostroun, "Formula," 492.

191 Sedgwick, *Travails*, 157–58.
192 Jean Brisacier, *Le Jansénisme confondu* (1651), cited by Sedgwick, ibid., 152.
193 Lucien Ceyssens, "La lettre circulaire du Port-Royal: un faux indestructible," *Bulletin de l'Institut historique belge de Rome* 43 (1973):509–44.
194 Agnès Arnauld to unknown, 6 November 1657, quoted in Frencken, *Agnès Arnauld*, 164.
195 Charles A. Sainte-Beuve, *Port-Royal* (Paris: Hachette, 1867), 4:374. Although I have found no primary source supporting this emigration plan, R. A. Knox credits it in *Enthusiasm*, 206.
196 Angélique Arnauld to Anne the Queen Mother, 25 May 1661, in *Lettres*, 3:536–45.
197 Angélique Arnauld, 6 August 1661, quoted in de Courcelles, *Sang*, 23.
198 Pierre Guilbert, *Mémoires historiques et chronologiques sur l'Abbaye de Port-Royal des Champs* (Utrecht: n.p., 1755–56), 1:524.
199 Newton, "Port-Royal," 173–74; Pierre Leclerc, *Histoire des persécutions des Religieuses de Port-Royal, écrites par elles-mêmes* (Villefranche: n.p., 1753), xi–xiii.
200 Weaver, *Joncoux*, 102; Conley, *Suspicion*, 25.
201 Conley, ibid., 26.
202 Pierre Thomas Du Fossé, in *Mémoires pour servir à l'histoire de Port-Royal* (Cologne and Utrecht: Aux depens de la Compagnie, 1739), 176–79, asserts that the Assembly of the Clergy on 1 February 1660 sent a deliberation to Louis XIV requesting that Port-Royal des Champs be closed. An *arrêt* of the Council of State on 13 April 1661 ordered all novices, pensioners, and postulants who refused to sign the Formulary to leave the convent. Du Fossé maintains that in August, the *Procureur du Roi* and the *lieutenant civil* actually came to Port-Royal des Champs to enforce this *ordre du roi.*
203 Kostroun, "Formula," 485–89, 493–94.
204 Ibid., 496.
205 Ibid., 497–98, 520.
206 Phillips, *Church and Culture*, 195; Sedgwick, *Travail*, 88–90; Cognet, "Jansénisme," 394–97; and Cécile Gazier, *Ces Messieurs de Port-Royal* (Paris: Perrin, 1932),V–VII.
207 Antoine Le Maître, quoted in Jean Félicissime Adry, "Histoire littéraire de Port-Royal," BN, ms. fr. 15271, ff. 4–7. A slightly different version appears in Françoise Hildesheimer, *Le Jansénisme: L'histoire et l'héritage* (Paris: Desclée de Brouwer, 1992), 42.
208 Pierre Pascal, "L'abbé de Saint-Cyran, les Chartreux et les Solitaires de Port-Royal," *Revue historique* 191 (April 1941):235.
209 Angélique Arnauld, quoted in Gastelier, *Angélique*, 9. This is a reference to Christ's parable of the five wise and five foolish virgins in Matthew 25.
210 Louis Cognet, "Le mépris du monde à Port-Royal et dans le jansénisme," *Revue d'ascétique et de mystique* 41 (1965):387.
211 Paule Jansen, "Les Travaux et les jours," *Chroniques de Port-Royal* 37 (1987):50.
212 Knox, *Enthusiasm*, 206, 211; Cognet, "Jansénisme," 393; and Maulvault, *Répertoire*, 19.
213 Laporte, *Doctrine*, 1:XIV.
214 Marcelle Tinayre, "Une journée à Port-Royal-des-Champs (1654)," *Revue de Paris* 2 (1902):833–34.
215 Jansen, "Travaux," 46–49; Finot, *Port-Royal*, 58–63; and Weaver, *Port-Royal*, 59–63, 76–79, 85–93 "After a good director," *Mère* Angélique said, "there is nothing more essential than a good physician." M. Pally (1650s–1664), Jean Hamon (1664–1669), M. Hecquet (1669–1670s), and M. Dodart (1670s–1680s) served as Port-Royal's doctors.
216 Newton, *Port-Royal*, 3–4.
217 Cognet, *Réforme*, 142–43; Crichton, *Jansenisers*, 112; and Jansen, "Travaux," 51–52.
218 Jansen, "Travaux," 50–51.
219 Ibid., 51; Romanes, *Port-Royal*, 139, 144, 148, 155; and Gastelier, *Angélique*, 110–11.
220 Clémencet, *Port-Roïal,* 2:495–99; Crichton, *Jansenisers*, 116; and Gastelier, *Angélique*, 112.
221 Janson, "Travaux," 52–53; Hildesheimer, *Jansénisme*, 87.
222 Crichton, *Jansenisers*, 40; Bremond, *Ecole*, 282–83, 288; and Bernard Chédozeau, "Idéal intellectuel et vie monastique à Port-Royal," *Chroniques de Port-Royal* 37 (1987):57–65.
223 Delforge, *Ecoles*, 284–85, 352; Cottret, *Lumières*, 253.
224 Cottret, ibid., 255–57; Dedieu, "Désarroi," 614–15; and Delforge, *Ecoles*, 73–75, 90, 102.

225 Edmond Préclin, "Les conséquences sociales du jansénisme," *Revue d'Histoire de l'Eglise de France* 21(1935):375–78.
226 Delforge, *Ecoles*, 157–59; Henry Charles Perrier, "Quelques Remarques sur les écoles de Port-Royal" (Paris: Thèse de la Faculté libre de théologie protestante de Paris, 1911), 12.
227 Adry, "Histoire littéraire de Port-Royal," BN, ms. fr. 15271, ff. 15–22.
228 Delforge, *Ecoles*, 17–24, 30–33, 41, 55–59; Harold Clive Barnard, *The Port-Royalists on Education: Extracts from the Educational Writings of the Port-Royalists* (Cambridge: Cambridge University Press, 1918), 54–55; and Antony McKenna, "Les petites écoles de Port-Royal," *Chroniques de Port-Royal* (1975):13, 15, 21.
229 Gastelier, *Angélique*, 222; Barnard, ibid., 22.
230 Grégoire. *Ruins de Port-Royal*, 89.
231 Adry, *Port-Royal*, ff. 2–4; Delforge, *Ecoles*, 9.
232 Delforge, ibid., 50, 195–96.
233 Sources differ regarding the exact number of professors. Barnard, *Education*, 36–51, mentions only fourteen, but McKenna, "Petites écoles," lists eighteen. In one setting (BN, ms. fr. 15271, ff. 54–57, 58–68), Adry gives 21, but in his "Histoire littéraire de Port-Royal," suggests 23 teachers. While Delforge, in *Ecoles*, page 173 states that there were 20 teachers "whose names are known," he earlier (7) set that number at 27 teachers.
234 Saint-Cyran, quoted in Jaccard, *St.-Cyran*, 289.
235 Ibid., 284–86; Cadet, *Education*, 81; and Bruno Neveu, *Un historien à l'école de Port-Royal: Sébastien LeNain de Tillemont, 1637–1698* (La Haye: Martinus Nijhoff, 1966), 34, 46.
236 Delforge, *Ecoles*, 51, 193, 269–72.
237 Ibid., 193–94.
238 Ibid., 191–92; Lesaulnier, *Images*, 378.
239 Cadet, *Education*, 202–19; Charles Clémencet, "Notice de la vie et des ouvrages de Claude Lancelot et principalement de ceux qu'il a composés pour les Petites Ecoles de Port-Royal" (c. 1750s), BHPF, Fonds Ste. Beuve, ms. 107, f. 9.
240 Lancelot, *Mémoires*, 1:XII–XXIX; Antoine Arnauld to M. Du Vaucel, 17 March 1689, in *Oeuvres*, 2:177; Delforge, *Ecoles*, 188–91; Clémencet, "Notice," ff. 2–13, 16–54; Cognet, *Lancelot*, 215; and Rivaud, "Lancelot," 306–12.
241 See the various lists in Delforge, ibid., 50, 96, 63, 102, 213–15; Adry, *Port-Royal*, ff. 41–42; and Barnard, *Schools*, 163–64.
242 Barnard, ibid., 166.
243 Delforge, *Ecoles*, 218–65. See also Adry, *Port-Royal*, ff. 24–90.
244 BN, ms. fr. 15271, f. 10.
245 Adry, *Port-Royal*, ff. 39–60 [actually ff. 69–90].
246 Du Fossé, *Port-Royal*, 31–32, 41, 50.
247 Besoigne, *Port-Royal*, 4:298–300.
248 Lesaulnier, *Images*, 423–24; Martin R. P. McGuire, "Louis-Sébastien Le Nain de Tillemont," *The Catholic Historical Review* 52 (July 1966):188–99; and "Tillemont (Sébastien Le Nain de)," *Dictionnaire de Théologie Catholique* (Paris: Librairie Letouzey et Ané, 1946), cols. 1029–33.
249 "Cahiers d'étudiant Jean Racine à Port-Royal," BN, ms. fr. 12887, ff. 1–234; Delforge, *Ecoles*, 65–66, 85, 133–36, 258–61.
250 Jean Racine, *Abrégé de l'histoire de Port-Royal*, 58.
251 Hallays, *Solitaires*, 118–20.
252 Barnard, *Schools*, 216; Delforge, *Ecoles*, 8, 321–25; and Rapley, *Dévotes*, 239 (n. 114).
253 Phillips, *Church and State*, 80.
254 Adry, *Port-Royal*, ff. 15–18.
255 Ibid., ff. 29–30; Remsberg, *Wisdom*, 86.
256 Knox, *Enthusiasm*, 221; Delforge, *Ecoles*, 320, 326; Perrier, "Ecoles," 50–54; and Edouard Paradis, *La Pédagogie janséniste comparée à la pédagogie catholique* (Lyon and Paris: Librairie Catholique Emmanuel Vitte, 1910), 68, 97.
257 Delforge, ibid., 160–61; Charles Daniel, "Les méthodes de Port-Royal et les jésuites," *Etudes religieuses, philosophiques, historiques et littéraires* 42 (1880):126; and Barnard, *Education*, 240–41.

258 Delforge, *Ecoles*, 292, 310–19; Daniel, "Méthodes," 133.
259 Delforge, ibid., 294, 303–9; Daniel, ibid., 122–23; and Tuillier, *Sorbonne*, 2:139–40.
260 Delforge, ibid., 165–68, 274–79.
261 Monsieur Cousin, quoted in Cadet, *Education*, 54.
262 Jean Racine, quoted in ibid., 55.
263 *Abbé* Fromageau, 1679, quoted in ibid. (n. 1).
264 Cottret, *Lumières*, 254–55.
265 Jean Racine, *Abrégé de l'Histoire de Port-Royale*, quoted in Barnard, *Education*, 191.
266 Pascal, *Children*, 1–8; Delforge, *Ecoles*, 200–1.
267 Pascal, ibid., 10–13; Delforge, ibid., 120.
268 Pascal, ibid., 6, 69–70.
269 Ibid., 7, 72–88, 95–96.
270 Ibid., 95; Barnard, *Education*, 202–3, 211.
271 Pascal, ibid., 116; Cadet, *Education*, 61.
272 Cadet, ibid., 62–64.
273 Agnès Arnauld, "Rules," quoted in Barnard, *Education*, 194–96.
274 Pascal, *Children*, 108.
275 Ibid., 7, 97–99.
276 Unnamed Port-Royal girl to Archbishop Péréfixe, quoted in Cadet, *Education*, 66.
277 Adry, "Port-Royal," BN, ms. fr. 15721, ff. 1–4.
278 Knox, *Enthusiasm*, 204.
279 Perrier, "Ecoles," 39.
280 Barnard, *Education*, 11–13; idem, *Schools*, 44–45; and Wright, *God's Soldiers*, 54–55.
281 Barnard, *Education*, 14, 65–70; Delforge, *Ecoles*, 353–54; and Paradis, *Pédagogie*, 81, 84, 90.
282 Cottret, *Lumières*, 263.
283 Ibid., 262–63.
284 Delforge, *Ecoles*, 70, 88–89.
285 Ibid., 106–10, 129, 146–52; McKenna, "Petites écoles," 22–24.
286 Barnard, *Schools*, 49–51; Loupès, *Vie religieuse*, 53.
287 Delforge, *Ecoles*, 354–55.
288 Jacques de Sainte-Beuve to Bishop Bossuet, quoted in Kostroun, "Port-Royal Nuns," 289.
289 Frencken, *Agnès Arnauld*, 140.
290 Clémencet, "Histoire littéraire de Port-Royal," BHPF, ms. 115.
291 Crichton, *Jansenisers*, 39.
292 *Bibliothèque Janséniste* (Bruxelles: Chez Simon T'Sertetevens, 1740), 1:9–39.
293 Dominique de Colonia, *Dictionnaire des livres jansénistes, ou qui favorisent le jansénisme* ([Antwerp]: Chez Jean-Baptiste Verdussen aux duex Cicognes, 1752), 5 vols.
294 Sedgwick, *Travails*, 173–74, 188; Charles Clémencet, *Histoire générale de Port-Roïal, depuis la réforme de l'abbaïe jusqu'à son entière destruction* (Amsterdam: Jean Vanduren, 1755–1757), and "Histoire littéraire de Port-Royal," BHPF, Fonds Ste.-Beuve, mss. 101A, 101B, 101C.
295 Angélique Arnauld to the Queen of Poland, 22 March and 4 July 1647, *Lettres*, 1:327–29, 335–36; idem to Antoine Arnauld, December 1651, *Lettres*, 1:603–4.
296 Neveu, *Erudition*, 99; Knox, *Enthusiasm*, 200; and Mita Choudhury, *Convents and Nuns in Eighteenth-Century French Politics and Culture* (Ithaca, NY: Cornell University Press, 2004), 36–37, 43.
297 The exact number of her letters probably exceeded 1,500. Her three-volume collection of *Lettres*, published at Utrecht in 1742, includes 1,040 letters from 1620 to 1661, but Dominique de Courcelles, in *Le Sang de Port-Royal* (1994), 128, states that from 1640 to 1660, Angélique sent over 1,500 letters to her niece Angélique de St. Jean alone. Not all of these have been collected and published.
298 Perle Bugnion-Secretan, "La Mère Angélique Arnauld à Travers ses écrits," *Chroniques de Port-Royal* 37 (1987):78–87.
299 Angélique Arnauld to unknown friend, 1643, quoted in Sedgwick, *Travails*, 136.
300 Angélique Arnauld to Archbishop François de Gondi, 19 September 1653, quoted in de Courcelles, *Sang*, 140.

301 Angélique Arnauld to M. de Fleury, 26 March 1654, *Lettres*, 2:462–63.
302 Angélique Arnauld to the *princesse* de Guéménée, quoted in Gastelier, *Angélique*, 266.
303 Angélique Arnauld to Antoine Arnauld, quoted in ibid., 269.
304 Angélique Arnauld to Antoine Arnauld, February 1644, *Lettres*, 1:246.
305 Angélique Arnauld to Antoine Arnauld, May 1644, *Lettres*, 1:260.
306 Angélique Arnauld to Antoine Arnauld, 28 November and 8 December 1655, *Lettres*, 3:100, 108.
307 Angélique Arnauld to unknown nun at Port-Royal des Champs, 4 February 1656, *Lettres*, 3:174; idem to Mme. de Bellisi, 18 March 1656, *Lettres*, 3:196–97; idem to *Mère* de l'Incarnation, May 1657, *Lettres*, 3:386; idem to M. de Sevigné, 30 December 1660, *Lettres*, 3:501; idem to *abbesse* de Xaintes, 19 January 1661, *Lettres*, 3:509–10; idem to *Mère* Marie de Sainte Magdelaine du Fargis, 25 and 28 April, 3 May 1661, *Lettres*, 3:526–30.
308 Angélique Arnauld to Isaac Le Maître, November 1653, *Lettres*, 2:392.
309 Angélique Arnauld, letters for 1660 and 1661, cited by Gastelier, *Angélique*, 401.
310 Angélique Arnauld to M. de Contes and M. Bail, 12 July 1661, quoted in Lowndes, *Nuns*, 377.
311 Guilllaume Dall, *La Mère Angélique, abbesse de Port-Royal, d'après sa correspondance* (Paris: Librairie Académique Didier, 1893), 303–305; Lowndes, *Nuns*, 370.
312 Angélique Arnauld to Anne of Austria, 26 May 1661, BN, NAF 1525, ff. 5–12; also in Leclerc, *Port-Royal*, 20–22.
313 Angélique Arnauld, quoted in Gastelier, *Angélique*, 407.
314 Angélique Arnauld to Henri Arnauld, 14 July 1661, cited by ibid., 408.
315 Angélique Arnauld to Agnès Arnauld, 1661, quoted in Sedgwick, *Travail*, 170.
316 Agnès Arnauld, quoted in ibid., 171.
317 Angélique Arnauld, 1656, quoted in Gastelier, *Angélique*, 386.
318 Angélique Arnauld, 1657, quoted in Le Goff and Rémond, *French Religion*, 2:367.
319 Dall, *Mère Angélique*, 295.
320 Isaac Arnauld, *Le Mépris du monde; résolution vertueuse de l'obéissance deu au roy; Meditations sur la veillesse* (N.p., 1618; reprint, Genève: Pour Jean Ant. & Samuel De Tournes, 1670), *passim.*
321 Robert Arnauld d'Andilly, *Journal de Robert Arnauld d'Andilly*, 1620–1626, Bibliothèque de l'Arsenal, mss. 5180, 5181, 5182 [hereafter cited as BA].
322 Robert Arnauld d'Andilly, 1645, quoted in Gastelier, *Angélique, 277–78.*
323 Phillips, *Church and Culture*, 278–81.
324 Cognet, *Jansénisme*, 76; Cécile Gazier, *Histoire du monastère de Port-Royal* (Paris: Perrin, 1929), 154–55.

4 Sunset Over Port-Royal, 1661–1711

1 Louis XIV (1661), *Mémoires for the Instruction of the Dauphin*, ed. and trans. Paul Sonnino (NY: Free Press, 1970), 54.
2 Agnès Arnauld, *Lettres*, 1:489 (n. 2); "Nom[s] de[s] Religieuses qui etaient à Port-Royal en 1661 au Commencement de la Persecution," BHPF, ms. 124.
3 Dedieu, "Déssarroi," 634.
4 Namer, *Abbé Leroy*, 12–13, 97–103.
5 Newton, "Port-Royal," 30–31. Ironically, thanks to his recent treatise on the education of a prince, the Jansenist Robert Arnauld d'Andilly received serious consideration as the dauphin's first confessor in 1644. But his ties with Saint-Cyran and his brother Antoine Arnauld's recent publication of *Frequent Communion* displeased the Jesuits and doomed his chances of being appointed to that position. See Georges Bordonove, *Les Rois qui ont fait la France: Les Bourbons.* Vol. 3: *Louis XIV* (Paris: Pygmalion, 1982), 35.
6 François Annat, *Chicanes des Jansénistes* (1654), cited by Georges Minois, *Le confesseur du roi: Les directeurs de conscience sous la monarchie française* (Paris: Fayard, 1988), 389–91; idem, *La conduitte de l'Eglise et du Roy justifiée dans la condamnation des jansénistes* (Paris: Sébastien Cramoisy, 1664), Preface, 268–319, 329–47.
7 Marc Escholier, *Port-Royal: The Drama of the Jansenists* (NY: Hawthorn Books, 1968), 276. For the

sake of decency, Escholier renders this colorful phrase as "my pitch-pot," which destroys the earthy fragrance of the expression altogether.

8 Minois, *Confesseur du roi*, 456–57.

9 Théodore Delmont, *Bossuet et le Jansénisme d'après les plus récentes publications* (Arras: Sueur-Charruey, 1899), 30; Dorival, *Musée,* 134; and Alfred Rébelliau, *Bossuet* (Paris: Hachette, 1900), 59.

10 Louis XIV, quoted in Paul Fargues, *Histoire du Christianisme*, vol. 5: *De l'Edit de Nantes à la Révolution* (Paris: Librairie Fischbacher, 1938), 198.

11 Louis XIV, *Mémoires*, 1661, quoted in Sonnino, ed., *Mémoires*, 25.

12 Kostroun, "Port-Royal Nuns," 17–19; Réné Taveneaux, *Le Catholicisme dans la France classique, 1610–1715* (Paris: Société d'Edition d'Enseignement Superieur, 1994), 322–23.

13 Louis XIV to *Père* de La Chaise, quoted in Briggs, *Communities*, 349.

14 Levi, *Louis XIV*, 230; Sedgwick, *Travails*, 214; and John B. Wolf, *Louis XIV* (NY: The Norton Library, 1968), 600. In fact, the *duc* de Saint-Simon stated in his *Mémoires* that Louis XIV saw the Jansenists as "little different from the Huguenots and nearly as heretical." See Loupès, *Vie religieuse,* 35.

15 René Taveneaux, *La Vie quotidienne des jansénistes aux XVIIe et XVIIIe siècles* (Paris: Hachette, 1973), 85.

16 *Duc* de Saint-Simon and *princesse* de La Palatine, quoted in Richardt, *Jansénisme*, 101.

17 Louis XIV, *Mémoires*, cited by Levi, *Louis XIV*, 223; Sonnino, ed., *Mémoires*, 161.

18 William Shipton Browning, *History of the Huguenots, from 1598 to 1838* (London: W. Pickering, 1839), 187–88.

19 Louis XIV to *comtesse* de Gramont, quoted in Prince Michael of Greece, *Louis XIV: The Other Side of the Sun*, trans. Alan Sheridan (NY: Harper & Row, 1983), 359.

20 Kostroun, "Port-Royal Nuns," 14–15, 24.

21 Sedgwick, *Travails*, 189; Richardt, *Jansénisme*, 102.

22 *Arrêt* of the General Assembly of the Clergy, published by the *Conseil d'état*, 13 April 1661, quoted in G. E. de Falguerolles, "La Tour de Constance dans la lutte pour le rétablissement des libertés de pensée et de réunion," *Bulletin de la société de l'histoire du protestantisme française* 114 (1968):175.

23 Leclerc, *Port-Royal*, 1–3; Gastelier, *Angélique*, 402; Christine Rogelet, *Port-Royal des Champs en notre temps* (Paris: Editions du Temps, 1969), 12; and *lettres de cachet* for 2 and 9 May 1661, BN, NAF 1525, ff. 1–3.

24 Leclerc, ibid.,15–17; Frencken, *Agnès Arnauld*, 165.

25 Antoine Arnauld to Godefroi Hermant, 21 April 1661, quoted in Hermant, *Mémoires*, 4:655.

26 Agnès Arnauld to Louis XIV, 6 May 1661, BN, ms. fr. 13894, ff. 28–30. Slightly different versions can be found in BN, ms. fr. 15595, ff. 65–66 and in *Mère* Agnès, *Lettres*, 1:493–96.

27 Levi, *Louis XIV*, 283.

28 *Mère* Agnès to Mme. de Foix, 26 April 1661, *Lettres*, 1:487–88; Kostroun, "Port-Royal Nuns," 230–31; and Frencken, *Agnès Arnauld*, 167–69.

29 Richardt, *Jansénisme*, 103; Sedgwick, *Travails*, 166.

30 Jacqueline Pascal to Angélique de Saint-Jean, 22 June 1661, in Pascal, *Children*, 146–52. A slightly different version of this stirring letter is found in Hildesheimer, *Jansénisme*, 68.

31 Knox, *Enthusiasm*, 177.

32 Henri Arnauld to Angélique Arnauld, 27 June 1661, BN, ms. fr. 19734, f. 36.

33 Henri Arnauld to Louis XIV, 17 September 1662, BN, ms. fr. 17750, ff. 193–97; Henri Arnauld to papal nuncio, 17 September 1662, BN, ms. fr. 17750, ff. 101–208.

34 Kostroun, "Port-Royal Nuns," 232, 241.

35 Namer, *Abbé Leroy*, 14–16; *Defense des Religieuses de Port-Royal et de leurs directeurs, sur tous les faits alleguez par M. Chamillard Docteur de Sorbonne dans ses deux libelles contre ces Religieuses* (N.p., 1667).

36 Jacqueline Pascal, quoted in Kostroun, "Port-Royal Nuns," 240.

37 Angélique de St.-Jean, quoted in ibid., 243–46.

38 Agnès Arnauld, quoted in Claude Cochin, *Henry Arnauld, evêque d'Angers, 1597–1692* (Paris: Auguste Picard, 1921), 351.

39 Marie Angélique Arnauld, "Sur les affaires de la Signature," BHPF, ms. 106, ff. 87–88.

40 Robert's letters for 1657 to 1661 show that he spent at least seven months (and possibly nine months)

at Port-Royal des Champs in 1656, up to eleven months in 1657, over two years from 1657 to 1659, and several weeks in 1661, doubtless to be with his sister Angélique Arnauld who died that summer. See BA, ms. 6035, ff. 71–95, 100–383, ms. 6036, ff. 22, 64, ms. 6037, ff. 214, 372–78.

41 Robert Arnauld d'Andilly to marquise de Sablé, 9 December 1659, 20 August 1660,12 July 1661, BN, ms. fr. 10587, ff. 35, 52, 74.

42 Robert Arnauld d'Andilly, "Que l'on doit preferer son Ami à sa Patrie," BN, ms. fr. 10587, ff. 123–26.

43 Robert Arnauld d'Andilly to Louis XIV, 26 March 1661, BN, ms. fr. 13894, ff. 70–73.

44 Robert Arnauld d'Andilly to marquise de Sablé, 7 August 1661, BN, ms. fr. 10587, f. 145.

45 Albert N. Hamscher, *The Parlement of Paris After the Fronde, 1653–1673* (Pittsburgh, PA: University of Pittsburgh Press, 1976), 111, 116; idem, "Parlement," 410.

46 Préclin and Jarry, *Luttes politiques*, 203.

47 Taveneaux, *Vie*, 91.

48 André Corvisier, *Louvois* (Paris: Fayard, 1983), 414; Jean Bérenger, "Charles Colbert, Marquis de Croissy," in *Le Conseil du roi, de Louis XII à la Révolution*, ed. Roland Mousnier (Paris: Presses Universitaires de France, 1970), 193.

49 Louis André, *Michel Le Tellier et Louvois*, 2d ed. (Paris: Armand Colin, 1943), 443–46.

50 Corvisier, *Louvois*, 412–15.

51 *Mère* Agnès Arnauld, *Lettres*, 2:61 (notes 1 and 2); Frencken, *Agnès Arnauld*, 171; and Bergin, *Crown*, 219. Because circumstances delayed Péréfixe's arrival until April 1664, however, seven grand vicars performed his duties for 20 months.

52 Kostroun, "Port-Royal Nuns," 252; Richardt, *Jansénisme*, 107.

53 *Lettre de cachet*, 28 August 1662, cited by Cochin, *Arnauld*, 377–78.

54 Agnès Arnauld to Henri Arnauld, 4 November 1662, in *Lettres*, 2:71.

55 Agnès Arnauld to Mme. de Foix, 5 March 1662, in *Lettres*, 2:42.

56 Agnés Arnauld to Mme. de Foix, 10 December 1662, in *Lettres*, 2:76.

57 "Journal des Six derniers Mois de l'Année 1663," BN, ms. fr. 17775, ff. 1–3.

58 Ibid., ff. 5–7, 19, 24, 38–39.

59 Ibid., f. 39.

60 Ibid., f. 89.

61 Ibid., f. 87.

62 Sister Dorothée to Archbiship Péréfixe, 17 December 1663, ibid., ff. 146–54.

63 Port-Royal prayer for 1663, ibid., f. 132.

64 See the collection of these written protests from 5 July 1664 to 28 June 1669 in BN, ms. fr. 17776.

65 Claude de Sainte-Marthe, *Déffense des religieuses de Port-Royal et de leurs directeurs sur tous les faits alleguez par M. Chamillard, Docteur de Sorbonne, dans ses deux libelles contre ces Religieuses* (N.p., 1667).

66 Augustin Gazier, "Claude Lancelot d'après sa correspondance inédite (1664–1665)," *Revue hebdomadaire*, 8 August 1908, p. 196.

67 Antoine Arnauld to unknown, 11 September 1664, quoted in ibid., 197.

68 Cognet, *Lancelot*, 136; Geneviève Delassault, *Choix des lettres inédites de Louis-Isaac Le Maistre de Sacy, 1650–1683* (Paris: Librairie Nizet, 1959), 104, 124; and idem, *Sacy*, 112.

69 Cognet, ibid., 128.

70 Lancelot, *Mémoires*, 502–7, 517–18.

71 Agnès Arnauld to Mme. de Foix, 16 April 1664, quoted in Richardt, *Jansénisme*, 108.

72 Agnès Arnauld, "Advis sur la conduite qu'il faudra tenir au cas qu'il arrive du changement dans le gouvernement de la Maison," 1664, BHPF, ms. 126, ff. 1–4.

73 *Lit de justice* of 29 April 1664, in Introduction to Antoine Arnauld, *Oeuvres*, 1:XC; "Lettres Patentes du Roy en forme d'edict," 29 April 1664, BN, NAF 1525, ff. 248–56.

74 Kostroun, "Formula," 499.

75 Richardt, *Jansénisme*, 109.

76 M. de Ste.-Marthe to Archbishop Péréfixe, June 1664, quoted in Anna Catharina Marie Duinker, *Claude de Sainte-Marthe, prêtre et confesseur de Port-Royal* (Haarlem, Netherlands: N/V H. D. TjeenkWillink, 1932), 66, 68.

77 Agnès Arnauld to Mme. de Foix, 13 July 1664, in *Lettres*, 2:166; Kostroun, "Port-Royal Nuns," 269.

78 Agnès Arnauld to Mme. de Foix, 20 July and 6 August 1664, in *Lettres*, 2:169, 171, 174–75.
79 Archbishop Péréfixe, 21 August 1664, quoted in Bluche, *Journal*, 41; Kostroun, "Port-Royal Nuns," 269; and BHPF, Fonds Ste.-Beuve, ms. 115, ff. 253–54.
80 BHPF, ms. 115; Hallays, *Pélerinage*, 59–60, 65–69; Phillips, *Church and Culture*, 204; Sedgwick, *Travails*, 181–82; and Richardt, *Jansénisme*, 111–12.
81 Although most historians state that twelve nuns were dispersed to other convents, Clémencet's "Pièces pour l'histoire littéraire des solitires de Port-Royal," in the BHPF, Fonds Sainte-Beuve, ms. 115, states that fifteen nuns were transferred elsewhere.
82 Hallays, *Pélerinage*, 69–71; Richardt, *Jansénisme*, 111.
83 Kostroun, "Port-Royal Nuns," 270, 285–88.
84 Antoine Arnauld, *Apologie pour les religieuses* (1664), 3–12, 37, 80.
85 Claude de Sainte-Marthe to unknown friend, August 1664, quoted in Duinker, *Ste.-Marthe*, 27–28.
86 Claude de Sainte-Marthe, "Requeste des Religieuses de Port-Royal du Saint Sacrement," 7 October 1664, in Sainte-Marthe, *Deffense*, 1–4.
87 Antoine Singlin, quoted in Pierre Magnard, "De l'obéissance en temps de persecution," *Chroniques de Port-Royal* 37 (1987), 89–100.
88 Robert Arnauld d'Andilly to the marquise de Sablé, 8 October 1664, BN, ms. fr. 10587, f. 4.
89 Robert Arnauld d'Andilly to the marquise de Sablé, 26 April 1664, f. 9; 29 January, 3 May, 17 August 1665, BN, ms. fr. 10587, ff. 11, 13, 15.
90 Catherine Agnès de St. Paul to Archbishop Péréfixe, 20 September 1664, BN, ms. fr. 17775, ff. 111–12.
91 "Requests" from the sisters of Port-Royal des Champs, 6, 23, and 30 December 1664, in Antoine Arnauld, *Apologie pour les Religieuses de Port-Royal*, 81–86, 88–94.
92 Archbishop Péréfixe to Port-Royal des Champs nuns, 24 December 1664, in ibid., 87–88.
93 Archbishop Péréfixe to Port-Royal des Champs nuns, 31 December 1664, in ibid., 95.
94 Archbishop Péréfixe to Marguerite de Sainte-Gertrude Dupré, 10 June 1664, quoted in Kostroun, "Formula," 485; Levi, *Louis XIV*, 283.
95 Kostroun, ibid., 501–9.
96 Ibid., 324–26, 506.
97 Frencken, *Agnès Arnauld*, 173–74; Arnauld, *Captivité*, 17–18.
98 "Relation faite par La Mère Angélique de St. Jean, Soeur de Mr de Pomponne," 11 November 1665, BHPF, Fonds Sainte-Beuve, ms. 104, ff. 1–5, 33, 59, 88, 99, 147, 260, 325; Arnauld, *Captivité*, 69, 70, 76, 84, 99, 104, 105, 107, 138, 156, 160, 181, 182, 213, 225.
99 Arnauld, *Captivité*, 27–67.
100 Frencken, *Agnès Arnauld*, 175–77.
101 Besoigne, *Port-Royal*, 2:9–10.
102 Sainte-Beuve, *Port-Royal*, 2:343.
103 Bishop of Aleth to Louis XIV, 1664, quoted in Richardt, *Jansénisme*, 112.
104 Nicolas Pavillon to Henri Arnauld, 5 September 1664, BN, ms. fr. 19734, f. 25.
105 Nicolas Pavillon to "My very dear Sisters," 3 June 1665, BN, ms. fr. 19734, ff. 4–5.
106 Nicolas Pavillon to unknown recipients, 9 November 1665 and 15 September 1666, BN, ms. fr. 19734, ff. 7, 11.
107 Nicolas Pavillon to "My very dear Sisters," 8 February 1666 and 23 July 1668, BN, ms. fr. 19734, ff. 6, 15.
108 Henri Arnauld to Archbishop Péréfixe, 12 April 1664, quoted in Antoine Arnauld, *Oeuvres*, 23:428–38.
109 Hardouin de Péréfixe to Henri Arnauld, 5 November 1664, in Antoine Arnauld, *Oeuvres*, 23:441–65.
110 Antoine Arnauld, *Apologie pour les Religieuses de Port-Royal* (1664), in *Oeuvres*, 23:278–79.
111 Antoine Arnauld, "Justification des Actes des religieuses de Port-Royal, au Sujet des violences exercisées par M. de Péréfixe dans ce Monastère," October 1664, in *Oeuvres*, 23:147–49.
112 Antoine Arnauld, *Apologie pour les Religieuses de Port-Royal*, in *Oeuvres*, 23:202–203, 272–74.
113 Antoine Arnauld, "Mémoire ou Remarques sur la Déclaration du Roi du 29 avril 1664" (May 1664), *Oeuvres*, 22:525–26.

114 Antoine Arnauld, *Apologie pour les Religieuses de Port-Royal* (1664), cited by Kostroun, "Port-Royal Nuns," 272.
115 Ibid., 273–76.
116 Antoine Arnauld, "Requête Présentée au Roi par les Ecclésiastiques qui ont été à Port-Royal," 19 May 1668, *Oeuvres*, 24:466, 473.
117 Antoine Arnauld to Bishop of Alet, 16 February 1664, *Lettres*, 2:168–76.
118 Antoine Arnauld to *Soeur* Françoise Louise de Sainte-Claire, 5 July 1664, *Lettres*, 2:195–97.
119 Cochin, *Arnauld*, 191.
120 Formulary of 1665, quoted in Doyle, *Jansenism*, 91.
121 Written procedures for signing the Formulary of 1665, BN, ms. fr. 19734, f. 8; Doyle, ibid., 33.
122 Bluche, *Journal*, 46; Chaunu et al., *Basculement*, 92; and Hamscher, *Fronde*, 116–17.
123 BN, ms. fr. 17750, ff. 56–59, 70–73; Richardt, *Jansénisme*, 113.
124 Richardt, ibid., 113.
125 Gerberon, *Jansénisme*, 5:38–39.
126 Gazier, "Lancelot," 198–202, 208, 225–27.
127 Claude Lancelot to Isaac Le Maître de Sacy, 1 January 1665, quoted in Maire, *Cause de Dieu*, 476.
128 Protest of the religious of Port-Royal des Champs, 29 May 1665, cited by Cognet, *Lancelot*, 161–62.
129 Catherine-Agnès de Saint-Paul to the sisters at Port-Royal de Paris, 27 June 1665, in *Lettres*, 2:201–2.
130 Besoigne, *Port-Royal*, 2:269–72, 339–43, 359–66; Gazier, *Histoire générale*, 1:169–74; and Georges Guitton, *Le Père de la Chaize, confesseur de Louis XIV* (Paris: Beauchesne et ses fils, 1959), 1:209–10.
131 Antoine Arnauld, *Apologie pour les religieuses de Port-Royal* (1665), in *Oeuvres*, 23:275.
132 Antoine Arnauld to M. de Sevigné, 1666, in *Lettres*, 2:282–83.
133 Mme. de Longueville to *Mère* Agnès, 24 January 1667, BN, ms. fr. 23481, f. 79.
134 Accusations of M. Chamillard, cited by Saint-Marthe, *Déffense des Religieuses*, 12–18, 22–35, 42–81, 87–124, 129–33.
135 Ibid., "Preface."
136 Antoine Arnauld, "Requête Présentée au Roi par les Ecclésiastiques qui ont été à Port-Royal," 19 May 1668, in *Oeuvres*, 24:466–78.
137 Antoine Arnauld to Port-Royal nuns, 10 January 1668, in *Lettres*, 2:288–89.
138 Kostroun, "Port-Royal Nuns," 306; Marie-José Michel, *Jansénisme et Paris, 1640–1730* (N.p.: Klincksieck, 2000), 182.
139 Agnès Arnauld, 1668, quoted in Kostroun, "Port-Royal Nuns," 302.
140 Dorival, *Musée*, 77.
141 Sedgwick, *Travails*, 190–91; Levi, *Louis XIV*, 284; and Jacques Parguez, *La bulle Unigenitus et le Jansénisme politique: Avant-coureur de la Révolution Française* (Paris: Librairie Maurice Glomeau, 1936), 23–24.
142 Marquise de Sablé to Cardinal de Raspigliosi, unknown date, quoted in Conley, *Suspicion*, 28.
143 *Duchesse* de Longueville to Clement IX, 25 July 1667, in Arnauld, *Oeuvres*, 24:140–41.
144 Angélique de St.-Jean Arnauld d'Andilly to Antoine Arnauld, 17 May 1668, quoted in Guilbert, *Mémoires*, 1:21–22.
145 Agnès Arnauld to Antoine Arnauld, July 1668, in *Lettres*, 2:261.
146 Antoine Arnauld to Archbishop of Sens, 3 July and September 1668, in *Oeuvres*, 1:612, 627. See also *Oeuvres*, 24:151–52.
147 Pierre Nicole to Antoine Arnauld, 5 July 1668, quoted in Guilbert, *Mémoires*, 1:37.
148 Ibid., 38.
149 Agnès Arnauld to Antoine Arnauld, 21 October 1668, in *Lettres*, 2:268–70.
150 Antoine Arnauld, *Oeuvres*, 24:163, 168–69; Bluche, *Journal*, 66.
151 Antoine Arnauld, *Oeuvres*, 24:157; Bluche, ibid., 65.
152 Arnauld, ibid., 158; Bluche, ibid., 65–66; and Guilbert, *Mémoires*, 1:281–84.
153 Arnauld, *Oeuvres*, 25:331–57; Louis XIV to Cardinal Raspigliosi, September 1669, quoted in Blet, "Louis XIV," 147.
154 Louis XIV to Bishops of Sens and Châlons, 1669, quoted in Arnauld, *Oeuvres*, 24:154.
155 Ibid., 155.

156 Préclin and Jarry, *Luttes politiques*, 205.

157 Clement IX to Archbishop of Sens and Bishops of Châlons and Laon, 19 January 1669, quoted in Arnauld, *Oeuvres*, 24:578.

158 Clement IX, 1672, quoted in the introduction to Antoine Arnauld, *Oeuvres*, 5:LIV–LV.

159 *Duchesse* de Liancourt to Agnès Arnauld, 16 October 1668, BN, ms. fr. 23481, ff. 79–81; Agnès Arnauld to the *duchesse* de Liancourt, November 1668, in *Lettres*, 2:278–79.

160 Agnès Arnauld to Louis de Bourbon, prince de Condé, 19 March 1669, in *Lettres*, 2:292.

161 Dominique de Ligny to Agnès Arnauld, 5 February 1669, BN, ms. fr. 19734, f. 69; Agnès Arnauld to Dominique de Ligny, Bishop of Meaux, March 1669, in *Lettres*, 2:297.

162 Agnès Arnauld to Louis-Henri de Pavillon de Gondrin, Archbishop of Sens, 22 March 1699, in *Lettres*, 2:293–94.

163 *Arrêt* of the *Conseil du Roi*, 23 October 1668, BN, NAF 1525, ff. 264–65; Antoine Arnauld, "Preface Historique et Critique" (c. 1669), *Oeuvres*, 24:167, 585; Port-Royal des Champs nuns to Archbishop Péréfixe, 14 February 1669, BN, ms. fr. 17778, ff. 11–14; *Placet* (1669) from nuns of Port-Royal des Champs to Archbishop Péréfixe, BN, ms. fr. 17750, ff. 9–12; and Kostroun, "Port-Royal Nuns," 291, 296.

164 *Mère* Agnès to Mme. de Foix, 8 June 1669, in *Lettres*, 2:306–307; Weaver, *Joncoux*, 103; and Kostroun, "Port-Royal Nuns," 308–9.

165 "Explication de quelques chapitres des Constitutions de la Veneration du Saint Sacrement" (c. 1679), BHPF, ms. 105.

166 BN, ms. fr. 17776, f. 299.

167 Kostroun, "Port-Royal Nuns," 303; Besoigne, *Port-Royal*, 2:411.

168 Besoigne, ibid., 411–12; Frencken, *Agnès Arnauld*, 178–79.

169 Port-Royal des Champs assembly, 28 June 1669, BN, ms. fr. 17776, ff. 299–300.

170 Louis XIV to Cardinal d'Est, 16 August 1669, BN, ms. fr. 17778; Lowndes, *Nuns*, 391–92.

171 Antoine Arnauld, *Oeuvres*, 1:624; Doyle, *Jansenism*, 34–35.

172 Louis XIV to *Père* Annat, 1668, quoted in Arnauld, *Oeuvres*, 24:155.

173 Richardt, *Jansénisme*, 115.

174 Ibid., 116; BN, ms. fr. 15806, ff. 62–71, 76–79.

175 Maire, *Cause de Dieu*, 38.

176 Robert Arnauld d'Andilly, *Mémoires*, 1:218.

177 Mme. de Sévigné to Mme. de Grignon, 26 January 1674, quoted in Weaver, *Fontpertuis*, 124.

178 Newton, *Port-Royal*, 116; Knox, *Enthusiasm*, 181; and Tregelles, *Jansenists*, 33.

179 Commission for Robert Arnauld d'Andilly de Pomponne, 18 October 1671, BA ms. 6037, ff. 188, 402; Bluche, *Journal*, 79, 88, 121; Sedgwick, *Travails*, 202–208, 215–17; and Angélique de St.-Jean Arnauld to unknown friend, quoted in Crichton, *Jansenisers*, 234.

180 Escholier, *Port-Royal*, 322; Sedgwick, ibid., 223; and Richardt, *Jansénisme*, 119.

181 Conley, *Suspicion*, 29–33. To read 81 examples of Sablé's famous maxims, see Conley, 167–74.

182 Antoine Arnauld to Prince Ernest of Hesse Rhinefils, 19 April 1683, in *Oeuvres*, 2:240–41; idem, *Apologie pour les Catholiques* (1681), in *Oeuvres*, 14:778; idem, "Fragments de la remonstrance au Roi" (1682), in *Oeuvres*, 24:646–48; idem, "duchesse de Longueville," index to *Oeuvres*, 43:162; and Bluche, *Journal*, 118.

183 Préclin and Jarry, *Luttes*, 1:208.

184 Maire, *Cause de Dieu*, 38.

185 Angélique de Saint-Jean Arnauld, 1680, quoted in Sedgwick, *Travails*, 221.

186 Chaunu et al., *Basculement*, 95–96; Neveu, *Erudition*, 259, 263, 393, 402; and Roger Mettam, *Power and Faction in Louis XIV's France* (New York: Basil Blackwell, 1988), 252–54.

187 Antoine Arnauld to Cardinal d'Estrées, October 1676, in *Oeuvres*, 1:768.

188 Parlement of Paris, *arrêt* of 1679, quoted in Antoine Arnauld, *Considerations sur les affaires de l'église* (1681), in *Oeuvres*, 37:663.

189 Antoine Arnauld, *Apologie pour les Catholiques* (1681), in *Oeuvres*, 14:406.

190 Introduction to Antoine Arnauld, *Oeuvres*, 5:LV.

191 Antoine Arnauld to Innocent XI, January 1680 and Innocent XI to Arnauld, 9 April 1680, in *Oeuvres*, 2:80–88; see also the introduction to *Oeuvres*, 5:IV.

192 M. de Pontchâteau to *duchesse* d'Epernon, 1677, quoted in de Pontis, *Mémoires*, 72.
193 Harlay de Champvallon, quoted in ibid., 72.
194 Weaver, *Fontpertuis*, 79, 83, 127–28, 156–57, 236, 242, 257–61, 269, 274, 297, 375, 381.
195 Kostroun, "Port-Royal Nuns," 312–23.
196 "Dictionnaire contenu verité" (c. 1670), BN, ms. fr. 17758, ff. 170–202.
197 Many of the nuns' writings for 1669–1679 have been collected in folio volumes and can be found at the BN, ms. fr. 17778, 17779, and 17782. Weaver, in *Fontpertuis*, 125, states that Angélique de St.-Jean's 800 letters are preserved in archives in Utrecht and Troyes. Her devotional talks or "Reflections de La Mère Angélique de St.-Jean sur les avis précedens qu'elle a faittes dans les entretiens qu'elle faisoit aux Soeurs dans le chap" (March–July 1680) are contained at the BHPF, ms. 126, ff. 4–175.
198 Crichton, *Jansenisers*, 185–87.
199 Angélique de St.-Jean Arnauld to Innocent XI, 22 December 1679, BA, ms. 6038, ff. 324–25.
200 Knox, *Enthusiasm*, 186.
201 Louis XIV to Bishop Vialart of Châlons, 1673, quoted in Richardt, *Jansénisme*, 117.
202 Richardt, ibid., 116.
203 Ibid., 117; Van Kley, *French Revolution*, 63; and Nigel Abercrombie, *The Origins of Jansenism* (Oxford: The Clarendon Press, 1936), 283–84. The archbishop's name appears in the sources as both "Chanvallon" and "Champvallon." I have chosen to use the latter spelling.
204 Abercrombie, ibid., 284–85; BN, ms. fr. 17778, f. 235; BN, ms. fr. 17779, ff. 1, 4, 43–44; and Besoigne, *Port-Royal*, 2:531, 534–35.
205 Richardt, *Jansénisme*, 117–18; Bluche, *Journal*, 119; and Bishop of Châlons to Port-Royal des Champs nuns, 26 May 1679, BN, ms. fr. 19734, ff. 77–78.
206 Antoine Arnauld, "Préface Historique et Critique" (1693), in *Oeuvres*, 24:581; Antoine Arnauld to Harlay de Champvallon, 1679, in *Lettres*, 3:1–4.
207 Emile Jacques, *Les années d'exil d'Antoine Arnauld, 1679–1694* (Louvain: Publications Universitaires de Louvain, 1976), 34.
208 Antoine Arnauld to Louis XIV, 8 May 1679, in *Lettres*, 3:125–31.
209 Sedgwick, *Travails*, 216, 224; Crichton, *Jansenisers*, 173–74.
210 Doyle, *Jansenism*, 41.
211 Archbishop Harlay de Champvallon to President de Guedreville, 1679, cited by Romanes, *Port-Royal*, 436.
212 Louis XIV to Innocent XI, 1680, quoted in Kostroun, "Port-Royal Nuns," 327–28.
213 F. Ellen Weaver, "Angélique de Saint-Jean: Abbesse et 'Mythographe' de Port-Royal," *Chroniques de Port-Royal* 34 (1985):100.
214 Maire, *Cause de Dieu*, 57–58.
215 Venard and Bonzon, *Religion*, 108–9.
216 Slightly different versions of these "Four Gallican Articles" can be found in Doyle, *Jansenism*, 40; Levi, *Louis XIV*, 286; Chaunu et al., *Basculement*, 100–101; and Forrestal, *Visions of Episcopacy*, 131–32.
217 Levi, ibid., 288.
218 Chédozeau, "Port-Royal," 533.
219 Antoine Arnauld, *Considerations sur les affaires de l'Eglise* (1681), cited by Chédozeau, ibid., 535–41.
220 Marie-Florine Bruneau, *Racine, le jansénisme et la modernité* (Paris: José Corti, 1986), 74–75; Goubert, *Louis XIV*, 150; and Phillips, *Church and Culture*, 264.
221 Isaac-Louis Le Maistre de Sacy, *Lettres chréstiennes et spirituelles de messire Isaac Louis Le Maistre de Sacy* (Paris: Guillaume Desprez, 1690), 2 volumes; Delassault, *Sacy*, 260; and Angélique de St.-Jean Arnauld, *Captivité*, 19–22. Although Delassault gives de Sacy's death as January 1682, his cousin Angélique de St.-Jean Arnauld states that he died on 4 January 1684, only fifteen days before her own demise. Because the nuns at Port-Royal had good reasons to keep accurate necrologies, I believe the 1684 date to be the more accurate one.
222 Antoine Arnauld to Mme. de Fontpertuis, 12 February 1684, in *Lettres*, 4:53–55.
223 Antoine Arnauld to M. Dodart, 26 April 1682, in *Oeuvres*, 2:135–37.
224 Antoine Arnauld to Mme. de Fontpertuis, 22 October 1685, quoted in C. Bergeal and A. Durrleman, *Eloge et condemnation de la Révocation de l'Edit de Nantes* (Carrières-sous-Poissey: "La Cause," 1985), 30.

225 Antoine Arnauld to Prince Ernest, Landgrave of Hesse, 17 December 1685, BN, ms. fr. 19727, f. 36.
226 Antoine Arnauld to M. du Vaucel, 13 and 28 December 1685, in Bergeal and Durrleman, *Eloge*, 30–31.
227 Antoine Arnauld to Prince Ernest, Landgrave of Hesse, 14 August 1686, BN, ms. fr. 19727, ff. 72–74; idem to Bishop of Trèves, 14 August 1686, BN, ms. fr. 19723, f. 209.
228 Antoine Arnauld to Paolo Walloni, 9 January 1687, BN, ms. fr. 19724, f. 2.
229 Jacques, *Arnauld*, 491.
230 Bernard Chédozeau, "Huit lettres de Pierre Nicole fort importantes pour le temps des grandes contestations," *Chroniques de Port-Royal* 30 (1981):6, 9–16, 25, 29.
231 Antoine Arnauld to Angélique de St.-Jean Arnauld, 23 April 1680, in *Oeuvres*, 2:88–89.
232 Antoine Arnauld to Angélique de St.-Jean Arnauld, 22 May 1682, in *Oeuvres*, 2:143; Antoine Arnauld to Angélique de St.-Jean Arnauld, 22 May 1682, in *Lettres*, 3:251–53.
233 Antoine Arnauld to Bishop of Castorie, December 1682, in *Lettres*, 3:292–93.
234 Antoine Arnauld, "Remonstrance au Roy," in a letter to the Bishop of Castrie, December 1682, in *Lettres*, 3:291–92; Antoine Arnauld to M. du Vaucel, 29 January 1683, in *Lettres*, 3:308–13.
235 Antoine Arnauld to M. de Fontpertuis, July 1683, in *Lettres*, 3:362–65.
236 Antoine Arnauld to Prince Ernest of Hesse-Rhinfels, 29 January 1683, in *Oeuvres*, 2:198.
237 Antoine Arnauld to the Archbishop of Reims, 17 and 29 January 1683, in *Oeuvres*, 2:189, 193.
238 Antoine Arnauld to M. du Vaucel, 29 January 1683, in *Oeuvres*, 2:194–95.
239 Antoine Arnauld to Prince Ernest of Hesse-Rhinfels, 19 April 1683, in *Oeuvres*, 2:238.
240 Antoine Arnauld, *Jésuites*, 401–2.
241 Antoine Arnauld to M. du Vaucel, 24 August 1685, in *Oeuvres*, 2:553–54.
242 Antoine Arnauld, *Phantosme du Jansenisme ou justification des pretendus Jansenistes par le livre mesme* (Cologne: Nicolas Schouten, 1686), *passim.*
243 Antoine Arnauld to M. du Vaucel, 6 October 1689, in *Lettres*, 6:53.
244 Antoine Arnauld to M. du Vaucel, 17 March 1689, in *Oeuvres*, 3:179; idem, *Innocence opprimée* (1688), 662–63.
245 Antoine Arnauld to Cardinal Paolo Walloni, 20 February 1687, BN, ms. fr. 19724, ff. 13, 31.
246 Ferguson, "Jansenism," 34–35.
247 Ceyssens, "Jansénisme et anti-Jansénisme," 125–26.
248 Chaunu, *Basculement*, 104–105; Maire, *Cause de Dieu*, 41; and Judge, "Church and State," 229–30.
249 Antoine Arnauld to M. du Vaucel, 9 January 1693, in *Lettres*, 7:29.
250 Neveu, *Erudition*, 429–31.
251 Antoine Arnauld to M. du Vaucel, 26 March 1694, in *Oeuvres*, 3:763.
252 Bluche, *Journal*, 216–17; Richardt, *Janénisme*, 118.
253 Quesnel, *Instructions Chrétiennes,* Preface.
254 Richardt, *Jansénisme*, 124; Lucien Ceyssens and Joseph A. G. Tans, *Autour de l'Unigenitus: Recherches sur la genèse de la constitution* (Leuven: Leuven University Press, 1987), 688–89.
255 Obituary for Henri Arnauld, Bishop of Angers, 8 June 1692, quoted in Cochin, *Arnauld*, 405.
256 Maire, *Cause de Dieu*, 40; Cognet, *Lancelot*, 216; and Bluche, *Journal*, 221.
257 Antoine Arnauld to Prince Ernest, Landgrave of Hesse-Rhinfels, 5 October 1691, BN, ms. fr. 19727, f. 123.
258 Antoine Arnauld to Isaac Arnauld d'Andilly de Pomponne, 20 December 1693, in *Oeuvres*, 3:707.
259 Antoine Arnauld to Prince Ernest, 26 October and 2 November 1691, BN, ms. fr. 19727, ff. 129–31.
260 Antoine Arnauld letters to unknown recipients, 5 March, 19 April, 21 May, 29 August 1692; 19 February, 18 March, 8 April 1694, BN, ms. fr. 19726, ff. 8, 16, 73, 108, 132, 141, 151.
261 Antoine Arnauld, "Réflexions sur le Décret du S. Office du 28 janvier 1694," in *Oeuvres*, 24:614–15.
262 Antoine Arnauld to M. du Vaucel, 8 August 1692, in *Lettres*, 6:399.
263 Antoine Arnauld's last will (1690), BN, ms. fr. 15595, ff. 22–32.
264 "Necrologe de Port-Royal" (1694), BHPF, Fonds Ste.-Beuve, ms. 120, ff. 51, 309, 319; speech given by M. Guelphe, 9 November 1694, BHPF, ms. 124; poems, elegies, epitaphs, sonnets, epigrams, and letters honoring Antoine Arnauld, August 1694, Arnauld d'Andilly de Pomponne Papiers, BA, ms. 6039, ff. 280–318.

265 Agnès de St. Theele to Archbishop Noailles, 1697, BN, ms. fr. 17782, ff. 37–38.

266 Marc Venard and Anne Bonzon, in *La religion dans la France moderne, XVIe–XVIIIe siècle*, 180, state that "A case of conscience exists when it is difficult for someone to decide what his moral duty is; how to apply the general law in a particular case."

267 Richardt, *Jansénisme*, 126; Blet, *Clergé*, 167.

268 Richardt, ibid., 127; Tuilier, *Sorbonne*, 2:89.

269 Richardt, ibid.; Tuilier, ibid., 90; Lesaulnier, *Images*, 159; Chaunu et al., *Basculement*, 112; Maire, *Cause de Dieu*, 43, 78–80; Jacques Grès-Gayer, *Théologie et pouvoir en Sorbonne: La Faculté de théologie de Paris et la bulle Unigenitus, 1714–1721* (Paris: Klincksieck, 1991), 21–22; and Pierre Nicole, *Apologie de la Resolution du fameux Cas-de-Conscience, contenue Dans les Ecrits suivants, I. Les Imaginaires, II. Les Visionaires, III. De la foi humaine, IV. Jugement equitable, V. Lettre de Messire Nicolas Pavillon, Evêque d'Alet, à Messire Hardouin de Péréfixe, Archêveque de Paris* (Cologne: Pierre Marteau, 1704), 485–696.

270 Clement XI's "Memoir" of 29 August 1703, quoted in Blet, *Clergé*, 170, 184, 193; Richardt, ibid., 128; Tuilier, ibid., 90; Chaunu et al., ibid., 113; and Grès-Gayer, ibid., 22–23.

271 Letters from Chamillart and La Vrillière, February 1703, quoted in Blet, ibid., 181.

272 Louis XIV to Clement XI, 12 March 1703, quoted in Richardt, *Jansénisme*, 128.

273 Papal nuncio Gualterio to Cardinal Paolucci, 14 May 1703, quoted in Blet, *Clergé*, 183.

274 Mme. de Maintenon to Cardinal Noailles, 19 February 1703, quoted in Richardt, *Jansénisme*, 128; Bournet, *Querelle*, 291–92; and Maire, *Cause de Dieu*, 73.

275 *Arrêt* of the Conseil d'Etat, 5 March 1703, cited by Blet, *Clergé*, 169.

276 Sedgwick, *Travails*, 236.

277 Richardt, *Jansénisme*, 125.

278 Louis XIV to Cardinal Janson, 27 June 1703, quoted in Blet, *Clergé*, 192.

279 Louis XIV to Cardinal Janson, July and August 1703, cited by Richardt, *Jansénisme*, 131–33.

280 Kostroun, "Port-Royal Nuns," 340–41.

281 Louis XIV to Clement XI, 27 January 1705, cited by Richardt, *Jansénisme*, 133; York, "Religious Aspiration"; and Blet, *Clergé*, 212–13.

282 Louis XIV to Cardinal Forbin-Janson, 3 August 1705, quoted in Blet, ibid., 226; Louis XIV to papal nuncio Gualterio, 27 July 1705, quoted in Blet, ibid., 224–25.

283 Ibid., 230–32, 235–37; Bluche, *Journal*, 275.

284 Neveu, *Erudition*, 424; Taveneaux, *Catholicisme*, 2:325; and La Brière, "Jansénisme," 275.

285 Richardt, *Jansénisme*, 134; Préclin and Jarry, *Luttes politiques*, 19:216–17.

286 Richardt, ibid.

287 Richardt, in *Jansénisme*, 138, states that 20 women lived at the convent in 1705; P. Deslandres, in *Histoire de l'église catholique en France* (Paris: Bloud et Gay, 1913), 175, puts the number at 25; and BN, ms. fr. 15806 lists 26 nuns for that year. Because of deaths, the number probably fluctuated during the year.

288 Richardt, *Jansénisme*, 135–39; "Journal de Port-Royal," 22 March 1706, BN, ms. fr. 17781, ff. 1–8, 40.

289 Sedgwick, *Travails*, 236–37; Weaver, *Port-Royal*, 156–57; and Grégoire, *Ruines de Port-Royal des Champs*, 144–45.

290 Sedgwick, ibid., 237; Gastelier, *Angélique*, 400; and Levi, *Louis XIV*, 290.

291 Pasquier Quesnel to M. Schort, 6 November 1706, cited by Le Roy, *Quesnel*, 2:273.

292 Cadet, *Education*, 70–77.

293 Mme. de Maintenon to Cardinal de Noailles, 18 June 1706, cited by Guitton, *La Chaize*, 2:250.

294 Gastelier, *Angélique*, 13; Richardt, *Jansénisme*, 140; and Préclin and Jarry, *Luttes*, 1:218.

295 Taveneaux, *Vie*, 99; Escholier, *Port-Royal*, 281; and Tuilier, *Sorbonne*, 2:94–95.

296 Madame de Maintenon, October 1708, quoted in McManners, *Church and Society*, 2:365; Marcel Langlois, *Madame de Maintenon* (Paris: Plon, 1932), 244–49; and Léon Séché, *Les derniers Jansénistes depuis la ruine de Port-Royal jusqu'à nos jours, 1710–1870* (Paris: Perrin et Cie, 1891), 1:8.

297 Cardinal Noailles, 1709, quoted in Finot, *Port-Royal*, 141.

298 Cardinal Noailles to the *duc* de Noailles and to Louis XIV, 1708, quoted in Edouard de Barthélemy, *Le cardinal de Noailles, evêque de Châlons, archêveque de Paris d'après sa correspondance inédite, 1651–1728* (Paris: Léon Tenchener, 1886), 14.

299 Cardinal Noailles to the *duc* de Noailles, 1708, ibid.; Kostroun, "Port-Royal Nuns," 381.
300 "Extrait du Conseil d'Etat," 7 April 1706, BN, ms. fr. 15809, f. 4.
301 Escholier, *Port-Royal*, 272.
302 Letter of protest by seventeen nuns at Port-Royal des Champs, 14 September 1706, BN, ms. fr. 15809, ff. 11–13.
303 Anonymous letter written from Rome, 15 February 1707, quoted in Gazier, *Port-Royal*, 411 (see also 412, 414, 418, 427).
304 *Arrêt* of the Conseil d'Etat, 3 January 1707, cited by Rogelet, *Port-Royal des Champs*, 17.
305 *Mère* Du Mesnil, 1707, quoted in Gazier, *Port-Royal*, 417.
306 Kostroun, "Port-Royal Nuns," 332–33, 400.
307 "Requêt au Roi," 30 January 1707, BN, ms. fr. 15809, ff. 46–47.
308 Kostroun, "Port-Royal Nuns," 358; Saint-Beuve, *Port-Royal*, 6:191; and Edmond Frédéric Fuzet, *Les Jansénistes du XVIIe siècle; leur histoire et leur dernier historien, M. Sainte-Beuve* (Paris: Bray et Retaux, 1876), 435.
309 Most of the documents relating to Port-Royal des Champs' legal battles can be found in BN, ms. fr. 15809 and 17781; see also Kostroun, ibid., 359, 362, 377, and Richardt, *Jansénisme*, 139.
310 Cardinal de Noailles, *Mandement* of 22 November 1707, BN, ms. fr. 15809, ff. 305–308; letter from nuns at Port-Royal des Champs to Cardinal Sacriponti, 18 March 1708, BN, ms. fr. 15809, ff. 333–75.
311 Gastelier, *Angélique*, 13–14.
312 Pasquier Quesnel to M. Schort, 6 April 1708, quoted in Le Roy, *Quesnel*, 2:296.
313 Nuns of Port-Royal des Champs to Louis XIV, 14 December 1708, BN, ms. fr. 15809, ff. 382–83.
314 Nuns of Port-Royal des Champs to Louis XIV, Cardinal de Noailles, and Cardinal d'Estrées, 14 December 1708, cited by Besoigne, *Port-Royal*, 3:177–80.
315 "Supplement au Nécrologie de Port-Royal," 15 December 1708, BN, ms. fr. 23482, f. 89.
316 Simone Bertière, *Les Reines de France au temps des Bourbons: Les Femmes du Roi-Soleil* (Paris: Editions de Fallois, 1998), 504–5.
317 Cardinal de Noailles' decree of 11 July 1709, quoted in Richardt, *Jansénisme*, 140–41.
318 *Arrêt* of the Conseil d'Etat, 9 September 1709, BN, ms. fr. 17781, ff. 443–46.
319 Escholier, *Port-Royal*, 284–86; Richardt, *Jansénisme*, 141–42.
320 Michel Tronchay, *Histoire abrégé de l'abbaye de Port-Royal depuis sa fondation en 1204 jusqu'à 1709* (N.p, 1710), 68–72; Gastelier, *Angélique,* 15–17; and Gazier, *Port-Royal*, 427–31.
321 *Nécrologie de Port-Royal*, BHPF, Fonds Sainte-Beuve, ms. 120, f. 155.
322 *Lettre de cachet*, 26 October 1709, quoted in Jacques Fouillou, *Mémoires sur la destruction de l'Abbaye de Port-Royal des Champs* (N.p., 1711), 158–59.
323 Bournet, *Querelle*, 294–95.
324 Weaver, *Joncoux*, 241–43, 256.
325 Fouillou, *Mémoires*, 159–62; Olivier Pinault, *Histoire Abrégée de la Dernière Persécution de Port-Royal* (N.p.: Edition Royale, 1750), 229.
326 Besoigne, *Port-Royal*, 3:275–78. While Pinault, in *Histoire Abrégée* (1750), 229, stated that only eight Port-Royal des Champs nuns were still living in 1716, Besoigne (1752) listed twelve.
327 Hallays, *Pélerinage*, 127.
328 Escholier, *Port-Royal*, 290; Cécile Gazier, *Histoire de la Société et de la Bibliothèque de Port-Royal* (Paris: Presses Universitaires de France, 1966), 17; and Mary Anne Schimmelpenninck, *Narrative of the Demolition of the Monastery of Port-Royal des Champs, Including Biographical Memoirs of Its Latter Inhabitants* (London: J. and A. Arch, 1816), 52–53.
329 The list of Port-Royal's benefactors and treasures can be found in BN, ms. fr. 17782, ff. 189–96; Sainte-Beuve, *Port-Royal*, 6:228.
330 Gastelier, *Angélique*, 18–19; Richardt, *Jansénisme*, 142; and Hallays, *Pélérinage*, 128.
331 This estimate of 3000 bodies, widely accepted by writers and historians, is probably greatly exaggerated. It is based on *abbé* Grégoire's calculation in *Les Ruines de Port-Royal des Champs en 1809* (Paris: Levacher, 1809), page 155, that since 1204, there had been about six deaths a year. Thus, 505 years x 6 deaths/year = 3030 bodies. But BHPF, ms. 124, an eleven-page list of former Port-Royal des Champs nuns, postulants, and domestics who died between 1612 and 1736, gives only 298 deaths for

124 years, or about 2.5 per year. Extrapolating that figure over 505 years would yield only about 1263 deaths.

332 Phillips, *Church and Culture*, 204; Richardt, *Jansénisme*, 142; Gastelier, *Angélique*, 19–20; and Monthéard, *Guide*, 124.

333 Schimmelpenninck, *Narrative*, 64–68; Prince Michael, *Louis XIV*, 359.

334 Kostroun, "Port-Royal Nuns," 395.

335 Knox, *Enthusiasm*, 228; Catherine Maire, "Port-Royal: The Jansenist Schism," in *Realms of Memory: Rethinking the French Past*, vol. 1: *Conflicts and Divisions*, ed. Pierre Nora (NY: Columbia Unviersity Press, 1966), 324.

336 "Necrologe de Port-Royal," BHPF, ms. 120.

337 Choudhury, *Convents*, 44–45.

338 Fouillou, *Mémoires*, 124, 143–45.

339 Ibid., 171.

340 These stirring verses can be read in BA, ms. 5346 (vol. 2), ff. 253–54.

341 Tronchay, *Histoire abrégée* (1710), foreword, 81, 88; Quesnel, *Relation de la captivité d'Angélique de St.-Jean Arnauld d'Andilly* (1711) and *Mémoires sur la destruction de Port-Royal des Champs* (1711). See Weaver, *Joncoux*, 258–59.

342 Saint-Simon, *Mémoires*, 9:163, quoted in Lucien Ceyssens, *Le sort de la bulle Unigenitus: recueil d'études offert à Lucien Ceyssens à l'occasion de son 90e anniversaire* (Leuven, Belgium: Leuven University Press, Uitgeverij Peeters, 1992), 501.

343 Maire, *Cause de Dieu*, 47–48; idem, "Agonie religieuse et transfiguration politique du jansénisme," *Chroniques de Port-Royal* 39 (1990):113.

344 See Laporte, *St.-Cyran*, 14 (note 48).

345 Nicolas Fontaine, *Mémoires pour servir à l'histoire de Port-Royal* (Utrecht: Aux dépens de la Compagnie, 1736), 1:iv–v.

346 Pinault, *Port-Royal*, 2:404–7; Clémencet, *Port-Roïal*, 10:36–43. Both M. A. Schimmelpenninck's *Select Memoirs of Port-Royal* (1835) and Marc Escholier's more recent *Port-Royal* (1968), 294–303, echo this jeremiad approach.

347 Leclerc, *Vies*, vols. 1–4; Clemencet's research notes can be found in BHPF, ms. 115; and Cerveau, *Nécrologie*, vols. 1–3, which includes 1,250 names.

348 Rogelet, *Port-Royal des Champs*, 7–20.

349 *Les Nouvelles Ecclésiastiques*, 1 May 1787, p. 72 [Hereafter cited as NE].

350 Grégoire, *Ruins de Port-Royal*, 86, 89–90; Monthéard, *Guide*, 84.

351 J. P. Charpentier, *Tableau historique de la littéraire française*, 328–29, cited by Bremond, *Ecole*, 4:23 (note 2).

352 Bremond, *Ecole*, 4:24–25.

353 Louis Cognet, "Etat présent des études Port-Royalistes," *Critique* 8 (1952):689.

354 Hallays, *Pélerinage*, 46–48; Maire, "Port-Royal," 301–2; Dorival, *Musée*, 9, 35; Monthéard, *Guide*, 84; and Hildesheimer, *Jansénisme*, 173.

5 Jansenism Enters the Political Arena, 1713–1750

1 *Procureur-général* Henri-François d'Aguesseau, 1714, quoted in Maire, *Cause de Dieu*, 9.

2 See Brian E. Strayer, *Huguenots and Camisards as Aliens in France, 1598–1789* (Lewiston, NY: Edwin Mellen Press, 2001), 204–5.

3 Dale Van Kley, *French Revolution*, 6.

4 Maire, *Cause de Dieu*, 9.

5 Godart, *Jansénisme*, 29–30.

6 Maire, *Cause de Dieu*, 83; Lurien Ceyssens, "Autour de la bulle 'Unigenitus': Son acceptation par l'Assemblée du Clergé," *Revue d'histoire ecclésiastique* 80 (1985):369–70. Technically, Church councils came in three forms: An Ecumenical or Universal Council (such as the Council of Trent) brought together all the bishops of the Catholic world; a Gallican or National Council (such as the General

Assembly of the Clergy in France) convened French bishops and clergy; and Provincial Councils, which summoned bishops and local clergy to meet triennially. Because of expense and papal and episcopal distrust, the first and third examples seldom met, but the General Assembly of the Clergy of France met every five years. Cabourdin and Viard, *Lexique historique*, 75.

7 Ceyssens, ibid., 371–76.

8 Ceyssens and Tans, *Unigenitus*, 764, 778.

9 Richardt, *Jansénisme*, 155–60. Although this papal committee at first condemned 155 propositions and Le Tellier found "more than 100 erroneous" statements, the French bishops in 1710 could find only 33 "damnable propositions." The decision to condemn 101 points, therefore, represented a compromise. See Jacques Grès-Gayer, "The Unigenitus of Clement XI: A Fresh Look at the Issues," *Theological Studies* 49 (1988):265–68.

10 Louis XIV to La Trémoille, 5 June and 4 August 1713, quoted in Blet, *Clergé*, 398, 402, 407.

11 Richardt, *Jansénisme*, 100. Because of the large number and importance of the theses it contained, *Unigenitus* was called a "pontifical constitution par excellence" rather than simply a bull. See Tuilier, *Sorbonne*, 2:96.

12 [Anonymous], *L'Esprit de Persécution de la Cour de Rome sous le Pontificat de Clement XI et de la Cour de France sous le Règne de Louis Le Grand, contre les Reformez & les Jansénistes* (Pampelune: Chez les Successeurs de S. Ignace, 1714), 1–36; "Déliberations de l'Assemblée des Cardinaux, Archevêques & Evêques tenue à Paris en 1713 et 1714," BHPF, ms. 739, ff. 7–12; David L. Smith, ed., *Louis XIV* (Cambridge: Cambridge University Press, 1992); and Maire, *Convulsionnaires*, 36.

13 Maire, ibid, 36; Phillips, *Church and Culture*, 109; "Jansénisme et anti-jansénisme," 127; McManners, *Church and Society*, 2:373; and David Parker, *The Making of French Absolutism* (NY: St. Martin's Press, 1983), 137.

14 Van Kley, *Damiens*, 105.

15 Michel, *Paris*, 199–200; Nancy Mitford, *The Sun King* (NY: Harper & Row, 1966), 234.

16 Clement XI's Preamble to the Constitution *Unigenitus*, 8 September 1713, quoted in Smith, *Louis XIV*, 70.

17 Cardinal Noailles, quoted in Richardt, *Jansénius*, 161–62.

18 Louis XIV, "Lettres Patentes," 14 February 1714, BHPF, ms. 739, ff. 33–36.

19 Maire, *Cause de Dieu*, 46; Gres-Gayer, "Unigenitus," 260–62.

20 Blet, *Clergé*, 437–38, 481–85.

21 General Assembly of the Clergy, letters to Clement XI and Louis XIV, 8 September 1713, BHPF, ms. 739, ff. 6, 79–85; Ceyssens, "Unigenitus," 385–92, 397–99, 407, 413; "Mandement of Monsieur le Grand Vicaire" (Charles de Rosset de La Martellière), BHPF, ms. 739, ff. 1–6; "Pastoral Instruction," 23 January 1714, BHPF, ms. 739, ff. 43–78; and McManners, *Church and Society*, 2:378.

22 Richardt, *Jansénisme*, 169; I. Bourlon, *Les Assemblées du Clergé et le Jansénisme* (Paris: Bloud, 1909), 156–58.

23 Chaunu et al., *Basculement*, 156.

24 Blet, *Clergé*, 455; Nelson-Martin Dawson, *Crise d'autorité et clientélisme: Mgr. Jean Joseph Languet de Gergy et la Bulle Unigenitus* (Sherbrooke, Quebec: Editions Les Fous du roi, 1997), 4.

25 Gaston de Noailles to Cardinal de Noailles, 1714, quoted in Richardt, *Jansénisme*, 169.

26 *Lettres de cachet*, 8 February 1714, BN, ms. fr. 17748, f. 71.

27 Blet, *Clergé*, 483, 503, 505, 507–509, 514–16, 522, 524, 526–27; Richardt, *Jansénisme*, 173, 179–80, 186.

28 Cardinal de Noailles to M. de Mirepoix, June 1714, quoted in Richardt, *Jansénisme*, 186.

29 Clement XI, 1714, quoted in Richardt, ibid., 188.

30 Cardinal Fabroni to Louis XIV, 1715, quoted in Richardt, ibid., 190.

31 Clement XI, briefs of 26 February 1715, cited by Richardt, ibid., 189.

32 Cardinal de Noailles to Chancellor Voysin, 15 March 1715, quoted in Richardt, ibid., 189.

33 "Corps de doctrine" and Declaration du Roi, 4 August 1715, cited by Maire, *Cause de Dieu*, 102, 109.

34 Bishop Broglie, quoted in Richardt, *Jansénisme*, 171.

35 Weaver, *Joncoux*, 272.

36 Richardt, *Jansénisme*, 165–66.

37 David A. Bell, *Lawyers and Citizens: The Making of a Political Elite in Old Regime France* (NY: Oxford University Press, 1994), 72; Melton, *Rise of the Public*, 51.
38 These powers of Parlement are discussed in the index to Antoine Arnauld, *Oeuvres*, 43:199–200.
39 Melton, *Rise of the Public*, 53.
40 Henri-François d'Aguesseau to Louis XIV, quoted in Doyle, *Jansenism*, 46.
41 Henri-François d'Aguesseau, Journal, quoted in Richardt, *Jansénisme*, 162.
42 Louis XIV to De Mesmes and Joly de Fleury, 8 February 1714, quoted in Richardt, ibid., 174.
43 Ibid., 176–77.
44 Joly de Fleury to Parlement, 15 February 1714, BHPF, ms. 739, ff. 37–39.
45 Parlement's registration of *Unigenitus*, 15 February 1714, ibid., ff. 39–41; Chaunu et al., *Basculement*, 134.
46 Louis XIV to De Mesmes and Joly de Fleury, 28 July 1715, and their reply to him on 11 August 1715, quoted in Richardt, *Jansénisme,* 191, 193, 195.
47 Hudson, "Regent," 136.
48 Grès-Gayer, *Théologie*, 26–29; Tuilier, *Sorbonne*, 2:96–98.
49 Grès-Gayer, ibid., 34–35; Richardt, *Jansénisme*, 179–82.
50 Cardinal de Trémoille to Torcy, July 1714, quoted in Richardt, ibid., 185–86.
51 Ysoré d'Hervault, Archbishop of Tours, quoted in Grès-Gayer, "Unigenitus," 281.
52 Ibid., 273–81.
53 Merrick, *Desacralization*, 49–50.
54 Bell, *Lawyers*, 68–71.
55 Chaunu et al., *Basculement*, 131.
56 Mettam, *Power and Faction*, 256; Van Kley, *Damiens*, 58; Sedgwick, *Travails*, 248; and Tuilier, *Sorbonne*, 2:117.
57 Tuilier, ibid.; Loupès, *Vie religieuse*, 43; and Peter Campbell, "Les crises parlementaires et les jansénistes, 1727–1740," in *Chroniques de Port-Royal* 39 (1990):149–50.
58 Goubert, *Louis XIV*, 275; McManners, *Church and Society*, 2:394; and Dale Van Kley, "The Jansenist Constitutional Legacy in the French Prerevolution," in Keith Michael Baker, ed., *The French Revolution and the Creation of Modern Political Culture* (Oxford: Pergamon Press, 1987), 1:174–75.
59 Loupès, *Vie religiieuse*, 39; Maire, *Cause de Dieu*, 96; and Daniel Carroll Joynes, "Jansenists & Ideologues: Opposition Theory in the Parlement of Paris, 1750–1775" (Ph.D. diss., University of Chicago, 1981), 24.
60 Selected from 200 letters of eight French bishops to Cardinal de Noailles, 1715, BN, ms. fr. 23216, ff. 5–276.
61 Muchembled et al., *Dictionnaire*, 16–17; Mettam, *Power and Faction*, 168 (note 25); and Cottret, *Lumières*, 280–81.
62 Joynes, "Ideologues," 101; Choudhury, *Convents*, 21; and Hamscher, *Fronde*, 111–12.
63 Doyle, *Jansenism,* 46; Blet, *Clergé*, 606, 609; and Lucien Ceyssens, "Autour de la bulle Unigenitus: La Déclaration, dernière illusion et ultime désillusion de Louis XIV," *Revue d'histoire ecclésiastique* 84 (1989):5–29.
64 Louis XIV to Cardinal de Rohan and Cardinal de Bissy, 1 September 1715, quoted in Maire, *Cause de Dieu*, 85.
65 Louis XIV, quoted in Richardt, *Jansénisme*, 198.
66 Louis XIV, quoted in ibid., 200.
67 *Necrologie de Port-Royal*, f. 78.
68 Vidal, *Miracles*, 15 (note 16); Orcibal, *Louis XIV*, 82.
69 Phillips, *Church and Culture*, 13–14.
70 Hildesheimer, *Jansénisme*, 124; Dominique, "Catholicisme," in Le Goff and Rémond, *French Religion*, 12–13.
71 Weaver, *Joncoux*, 8–9, 15.
72 Anonymous cleric to unnamed archbishop, 1714, BA, ms. 10191.
73 Le Roy, *Quesnel*, 2:328; McManners, "Jansenists," 259; and Pasquier Quesnel, quoted in Jean-Louis Quantin, *Le Catholicisme classique et les Pères de l'Eglise: Un retour aux sources, 1669–1713* (Paris: Institut d'Etudes Augustiniennes, 1999), 132.

74 *Ordonnance et instruction pastorale de Messeigneurs les evesques de Luçon et de La Rochelle, au clergé et au peuple de leurs diocéses, portant condamnation d'un Livre Intitulé Le Nouveau Testament en François, avec des Réflexions Morales sur chaque verset* (Paris: Gregoire Dufuis, 1710), *passim*.
75 "Mandement de Mgr. L'Evêque de Bethléem sur les affaires du tems," undated, BHPF, ms. 114, 729–30.
76 "In Innocentum XI Papum," undated, BA, ms. 12727, ff. 506–9.
77 Catherine Laurence Maire, "L'Eglise et la Nation: Du dépôt de la verité au dépôt des lois: La trajectoire janséniste au XVIIIe siècle," *Annales, Economies, Sociétés, Civilisations* 5 (1991):1178–79; Hudson, "Conciliarism," 402–4.
78 *Duc* de Saint-Simon, March 1711, quoted in Richardt, *Jansénisme*, 145.
79 *Duc* de Saint-Simon, 1714, quoted in Prince Michael, *Louis XIV*, 386.
80 *Princesse* Palatine to unknown, 27 December 1713, quoted in Hildesheimer, *Jansénisme*, 116.
81 Van Kley, *French Revolution*, 76–77; Brongniart, *Saint-Médard*, 68; and Dominique, "Catholicisme,"20.
82 Marie-José Michel, "Clergé et pastorale jansénistes à Paris (1669–1730)," *Revue d'histoire moderne et contemporaine* 26 (April–June 1979):190–94; Bernard Plongeron, "Une Image de l'Eglise d'après les Nouvelles Ecclésiastiques (1728–1790)," *Revue d'Histoire de l'Eglise de France* 53 (1967):242; and Loupès, *Vie religieuse*, 205.
83 Loupès, ibid., 39; Richardt, *Jansénisme*, 201; Christine Pevitt, *The Man Who Would Be King: The Life of Philippe d'Orléans, Regent of France, 1674–1723* (London: Weidenfeld and Nicolson, 1997), 317; and "Mémoire au Conseil de Conscience," undated, BA, ms. 10191.
84 Richardt, ibid., 202; Escholier, *Port-Royal*, 299–301; Fargues, *Nantes*, 266; and Gazier, *Port-Royal*, 440–41.
85 Gazier, *Histoire générale*, 1:252–54; Chaunu et al., *Basculement*, 147.
86 Dorival, *Musée*, 150; Barthélemy, *Noailles*, 27; Chaunu et al., ibid., 147; and *arrêt* of Parlement, 16 December 1716, BA, ms. 10191.
87 Chaunu et al., ibid.; Carreyre, *Régence*, 2:7.
88 Richardt, *Jansénisme*, 202; Cottret, *Lumières*, 281; and McManners, *Church and Society*, 2:393.
89 Pasquier Quesnel, *Deux Actes de l'Appel interjetté de la Constitution Unigenitus Dei Filius au Concile générale* (Amsterdam: Jean Potgieter, 1717), iv–xv, 359, 375–76.
90 Ceyssens, "Penser," 128–29; idem, "Jansénisme et anti-jansénisme," 128–29; and Woodbridge, *Revolt*, 37.
91 Maire, *Cause de Dieu*, 197–200; Bishop Languet de Gergy, *Avertissement de Monseigneur l'Evêque de Soissons à ceux qui dans son diocese se sont declarez appellans de la Constitution Unigenitus* (Reims: B. Multeau le jeune, 1718), 3 volumes (see 3:211).
92 Minutes of the debates in the Parlements of Dijon, Paris, Besançon, Pontoise, and Aix from 1714 to 1727, BN, NAF 3334, ff. 1–10, 46–49, 55–57; minutes for the Parlement of Provence, in *La Faillibilité des papes dans les Decisions dogmatiques demontrée par toute la tradition* (N.p., 1720), 2:704–26.
93 Cardinal de Noailles, "Lettre pastorale," 14 January 1719, quoted in Richardt, *Jansénisme*, 203.
94 Declaration of 5 June 1719 and *lettre de cachet* for 28 June 1720, cited by Carreyre, *Régence*, 2:184–85, 356–57.
95 Declaration of 4 August 1720, BN, Collection Joly de Fleury, ms. 1476, ff. 38–41, 134–60; Jean Egret, *Louis XV et l'opposition parlementaire, 1715–1774* (Paris: Armand Colin, 1970), 25; Thomas, *Unigenitus*, 64–65, 144; and Gilbert Rech, "D'Aguesseau et le jansénisme," in *Le Chancelier Henri-François D'Aguesseau, 1668–1751* (Limoges: Librairie Desvilles, 1953), 119–22.
96 Pevitt, *Orléans*, 261, 273–76; Richardt, *Jansénisme*, 203.
97 Dawson, ed., *Crise d'autorité*, 7; Chaunu et al., *Basculement*, 174, 178–79; and McManners, *Church and Society*, 2:407.
98 Chaunu et al., ibid., 180–83, 186.
99 Marie-Elisabeth-Edmond Maxime de Sars, *Le Cardinal de Fleury: Apôtre de la Paix* (Paris: Hachette, 1942), 128–32; Arlette Farge, *Subversive Words: Public Opinion in Eighteenth-Century France*, trans. Rosemary Morris (University Park, PA: Pennsylvania State University Press, 1994), 22.
100 Farge, ibid., 73.

101 Monsieur Barbier, October 1728, quoted in Maire, *Convulsionnaires*, 49.
102 Xavier Azéma, *Un prélat janséniste, Louis Foucquet, évêque et comte d'Agde, 1656–1702* (Paris: Librairie Philosophique J. Vrin, 1963), 36–37, 47, 51, 53, 140, 187, 229–30.
103 Ibid., 129, 188–95, 202. For copies of Bishop Foucquet's handwritten *Nouvelles Ecclésiastiques*, see BN, ms. fr. 23498–23510.
104 Ibid., 129–38.
105 *Nouvelles Ecclésiastiques* (1675–1696), BN, ms. fr. 23506 and 23498.
106 Azema, *Foucquet*, 215–17, 221.
107 Cottret, *Lumières*, 210; Hudson, "Regent," 135.
108 "*Histoire Ecclésiastique depuis 1708 jusqu'en 1721*," BHPF, ms. 110, 465 *feuilles*.
109 Cottret, *Lumières*, 14; McManners, *Church and Society*, 2:415–16.
110 Chaunu et al., *Basculement*, 86; *Le Figaro* (Paris), 19 juin 2003, p. 1.
111 Choudhury, *Convents*, 42–43; Preclin and Jarry, *Luttes politiques*, 1:252; Palmer, *Unbelievers*, 27; and D. A. Coward, "The Fortunes of a Newspaper: the *Nouvelles Ecclésiastiques*, 1728–1803," *British Journal for Eighteenth-Century Studies* 4 (1981):3–6, 15–16.
112 Coward, ibid., 10; Loupès, *Vie religieuse*, 42; Sars, *Fleury*, 134; and Françoise Bontoux, "Paris janséniste au XVIIIe siècle: Les Nouvelles Ecclésiastiques," *Mémoires de la Fédération des Sociétés historiques et archéologique de Paris et de l'Ile-de-France* 7 (1955):205–207.
113 Fr. Michal Albaric, "Une page d'histoire de la presse clandestine: Les Nouvelles Ecclésiastiques, 1728–1803," *Revue française d'histoire du Livre* 26–27 (1980):321, 324.
114 "Idée de l'ordre observé pour la distribution des Nouvelles eclesiastique [*sic*]," BHPF, Fonds Sainte-Beuve, ms. 121, f. 3.
115 Maire, *Cause de Dieu*, 159–60; Coward, "Newspaper," 5; Chaunu et al., *Basculement*, 266; and Farge, *Subversive Words*, 38.
116 Coward, ibid., 6, 16, 22.
117 Ibid., 23.
118 "Liste de ceux qui recoivent les nouvelles ecclesiastiques," c. 1728–1730, BA, ms. 10195; Chaunu et al., *Basculement*, 203; and Prince Michael, *Louis XIV*, 396.
119 Maire, *Cause de Dieu*, 160; Van Kley, *French Revolution*, 96; and Coward, "Newspaper," 27 (note 68).
120 *Les Nouvelles Ecclésiastiques*, 1728, BHPF, ms. 522 [hereafter cited as *NE*].
121 *NE*, indexes for 1767, 1790, and 1803, cited by Albaric, "Page d'histoire," 328.
122 Ibid., 328–30; Azema, *Foucquet*, 138; Maire, *Cause de Dieu*, 391; and Farge, *Subversive Words*, 38.
123 Farge, ibid., 36–41; Maire, ibid., 221, 225.
124 Farge, ibid., 38–44, 50; see *NE* for 1728, BHPF, ms. 522.
125 *NE*, January 1728, p. 2.
126 Carreyre, "Doctrine," 520; Coward, "Newspaper," 2–3.
127 Chaunu et al., *Basculement*, 261–63.
128 Cottret, *Lumières*, 288; Azema, *Foucquet*, 141–50.
129 *NE*, 1728–29, BHPF, ms. 522.
130 Chaunu et al., *Basculement*, 265–66; Maire, *Cause de Dieu*, 227; Coward, "Newspaper," 3; Van Kley, *French Revolution*, 373.
131 *Arrêt* of the Conseil d'Etat, 4 September 1728, BN, n.a.f. 3333, f. 79.
132 Bontoux, "Janséniste," 211; Pillorget, *Marville*, 168; and Quétal, *Lettres de cachet*, 70.
133 *Lieutenant-général de police* René Hérault, 1728, quoted in Coward, "Newspaper," 1.
134 Ibid., 6; Bontoux, "Janséniste," 216.
135 "A-J" Index to *NE*, pp. 660–868, BHPF, ms. 522.
136 Chaunu et al., *Basculement*, 359–61.
137 Ernest Boysse, *Le Théâtre des Jésuites* (Paris: n.p., 1880; reprint, Genève: Slatkine Reprints, 1970), 110.
138 Coward, "Newspaper," 24 (note 4); Albaric, "Page d'histoire," 330.
139 Coward, ibid., 4–11; Chaunu et al., *Basculement*, 266–67; and Maire, *Convulsionnaires*, 32.
140 Choudhury, *Convents*, 42; "Instruction en forme de catechisme au sujet de la Bulle Unigenitus," c. 1724, BHPF, ms. O2255, 25.
141 Loupès, *Vie religieuse*, 55; Nicolo Lercori's list, 1739, cited by François de Dainville, "La carte du

jansénisme à Paris en 1739, d'après les papiers de la nonciature," *Bulletin de la Société de l'Histoire de Paris et de l'Isle de France* 96 (1969):113–15.

142 Ibid., 56–57.

143 *Placets* from bishops, priests, canons, and *curés* to Cardinal de Noailles and *Lieutenant-général de Police* Hérault, 1724–1753, BA, ms. 10171; Garrioch, *Revolutionary Paris*, 155.

144 Maire, *Cause de Dieu*, 378–80, 385.

145 "Histoire de la Paix des chiens avec les loups: Poeme heureusement Decouvert par un Mandarin de la Société" (Peking: Avec Permission de Sa Majesté Chinoise, 1721), 1–15.

146 Préclin and Jarry, *Luttes politiques*, 19:247.

147 Council of Embrun's condemnation of Jean Soanen, Bishop of Senez, 20 September 1727, BN, NAF 3333, ff. 52–53, 72; bishops' letters for and against *Unigenitus*, 1722–1765, BN, NAF 3333, ff. 6–85; BHPF, ms. 123, ff. 1–96.

148 Bishops' ordinances, pastoral letters, pastoral instructions, responses, remonstrances, and *mandements*, 1726–1736, in *Recueil {des Pièces} sur la Constitution {Unigenitus}, 1724–1738*, BHPF, ms. 3186; see also BN, ms. fr. 23446 *passim.*

149 *Mandement* of 18 October 1720 signed by the Bishops of Senez, Mirepoix, Montpellier, and Boulogne, BHPF, ms. 2386 (vol. 174); "Lettre de Monseigneur l'Evêque de Senez au Roy" (1729), *Recueil*, ff. 1–28.

150 Antoine Fagon, Bishop of Vannes, *Mandement* of 24 February 1722, BHPF, ms. 2126, ff. 169–70; Charles Joachim, Bishop of Montpellier, "Ordonnance et Instruction Pastorale" (1726), "Lettre Pastorale" (1729), and "Projet d'Ordonnance et Instruction Pastorale" (1738), BHPF, ms. 3186; Languet de Gergy, Bishop of Soissons, was known as "the obsessive anti-Jansenist warrior" for his vigorous support of *Unigenitus*. See Bergin, *Crown*, 307, 339.

151 Letters from the Cardinal de Noailles and the Bishops of Auxerre, Troyes, and Bayeux to Louis XV, 1727, BN, ms. fr. 20972, ff. 15–20.

152 Bishop Jean Colbert of Montpellier to *Secrétaire d'Etat* Maurepas, 25 April 1728, quoted in Valentin Durand, *Le jansénisme au XVIIIe siècle et J. Colbert, évêque de Montpellier, 1696–1738* (Toulouse: Librairie Edouard Privat, 1907), 226.

153 Bishop Caylus of Auxerre to Louis XV, 1729, BN, ms. fr. 20972, ff. 199–202.

154 Bishop Caylus, *Mandement* of 24 July 1729, BN, ms. fr. 20972, ff. 51–52.

155 "Mandement et Instruction pastorale de Monseigneur l'Archeveque duc de Cambray," 6 March 1731, BHPF, ms. 1172 (I), pp. 1–166.

156 See dossiers 10172, 10173, 10179, 10181, 10182, 10183, 10184, 10188, 10189, and 10190 at the Bibliothèque de l'Arsenal.

157 Ibid.; see also letters, mandates, *arrêts*, and other documents in BN, ms. fr. 23441, 23442, 23444, 23448, 25088, in BN, NAF 3334, ff. 80–100, 141–90, 228–36, 447, 547–48, and BN, Collection Joly de Fleury, ms. 1490.

158 "Acte de Retraction," 2 October 1741, BA, ms. 10189.

159 Soeur Marie Margueritte Fleury de Saint-Jean Baptiste, "Appeal," 10 May 1734, BA, ms. 10189.

160 See dossiers in BA, mss. 10172, 10173, 10179, 10181, 10182, 10183, 10184, 10188,10190 and BHPF, mss. 109 and 3186(12); Rapley, *Cloister*, 75–77.

161 Archbishop Languet de Gergy, quoted in Rapley, ibid., 77.

162 *Abbé* de Pomponne to Cardinal de Noailles, 25 January 1725, BN, ms. fr. 23222, ff. 21–22.

163 Cardinal de Noailles, "Secret Instruction" to Clement XI, 19 February 1725, BN, ms. fr. 23222, ff. 28–29.

164 Cardinal de Noailles to Cardinal de Polignac, 11 March 1725, BN, ms. fr. 23222, ff. 34–35.

165 Cardinal de Noailles, "Secret Instructions," 23 and 30 July 1725, BN, ms. fr. 23222, ff. 99, 105–11.

166 Cardinal de Noailles, "Projet de Mandement," 17 September 1725, and "Secret Instructions," 9 October and 26 November 1725, BN, ms. fr. 23222, ff. 162–63, 170, 216.

167 "Mémoire" sent to Cardinal Graveson, 17 December 1725, BN, ms. fr. 23222, ff. 238–44.

168 Cardinal de Noailles, "Declaration," 28 October 1727, BN, NAF 3333, ff. 75–78.

169 Cardinal de Noailles "Mandement" to Benedict XIII, October 1728, quoted in Chaunu et al., *Basculement*, 194–95; Loupès, *Vie religieuse*, 41.

170 Benedict XIII to Cardinal de Noailles, 9 November 1978, quoted in Chaunu et al., ibid., 196.
171 Chaunu et al., ibid., 198.
172 "Plaintes que la Religion addresse à Votre Eminence," BA, ms. 11305, ff. 767–68.
173 BHPF, Fonds Ste.-Beuve, ms. 122, ff. 129–30; Chaunu et al., *Basculement*, 199–200; and Loupès, *Vie religieuse*, 41–42.
174 Chaunu et al., ibid., 201–10; McManners, *Church and Society*, 2:421, 434.
175 Vintimille to Fleury, November 1730, quoted in Chaunu et al., ibid., 214.
176 "Approbation pour les Confessions," BN, ms. fr. 23443, f. 115; Chaunu et al., ibid., 215–19, 387.
177 Archbishop of Paris, "Mandement," 8 February 1735, BHPF, ms. 122, ff. 367–69.
178 "Chanson nouvelle sur l'air Voilà mon cousin," c. 1735, BN, ms. fr. 23446, ff. 102.
179 Cardinal de Noailles, quoted in Hudson, "Regent," 143.
180 Cardinal de Fleury to Bishop de Souillac, 1 October 1734, quoted in Emile Appolis, "Une controverse autour d'un 'miracle' janséniste," *Monspeliensis Hippocrates* 44 (1969):27.
181 Hudson, "Regent," 143–45; Farge, *Subversive Words*, 22–23.
182 Norman Ravitch, *Sword and Mitre: Government and Episcopate in France and England in the Age of Aristocracy* (The Hague: Mouton, 1966), 224.
183 Ibid., 225; Kreiser, *Miracles*, 39–43.
184 Sars, *Fleury*, 134–37; Cottret, *Lumières*, 58.
185 Doyle, *Jansenism*, 59–61; Van Kley, *French Revolution*, 122–28.
186 Police spy to Lieutenant-Général Hérault, 27 October 1728, BA, ms. 10158, f. 245.
187 Police report in BA, ms. 10161, f. 403, cited by Van Kley, *French Revolution*, 130.
188 Declaration of 24 March 1730, BA, ms. 10191; Préclin and Jarry, *Luttes politiques*, 1:247.
189 "Relation de ce qui s'est passé au Parlement au sujet de la Declaration du 24 mars 1730," BA, ms. 10191; Suzanne Pillorget, *Claude-Henri Feydeau de Marville, Lieutenant-général de police, 1740–1747* (Paris: Editions Pedone, 1978), 153; Jules Flammermont, ed., *Remonstrances du Parlement de Paris au XVIIIe siècle,* vol. 1: *1715–1753* (Paris: Imprimerie Nationale, 1888–1898), 617–20; and *Conseil d'Etat*, *arrêt* of 5 September 1731, BA, ms. 10192.
190 Préclin and Jarry, *Luttes politiques*, 1:248; Maire, *Cause de Dieu*, 121–22.
191 General Assembly of the Clergy to Louis XV, 11 September 1730, BN, Joly de Fleury, ms. 1476, ff. 209–18.
192 BN, ms. fr. 23453, ff. 62–63; anonymous black and white ink sketch of 100 doctors of theology being expelled from the Sorbonne, BHPF, ms. 123, f. 20; and Tuilier, *Sorbonne*, 2:128–29.
193 Egret, *Louis XV*, 26–29; Maire, "Eglise," 1188; and idem, *Cause de Dieu*, 390–91.
194 *Arrêt* of 25 November 1730, BN, ms. fr. 23449, ff. 38–42; declarations, *arrêts*, *mandements*, and *appels comme d'abus* for the 1730s, BHPF, Fonds Ste.-Beuve, ms. 121; "Mémoire touchant l'origine de l'autorité du Parlement de France appelé Judicium Francorum," 1652, BHPF, ms. 171, ff. 98–105; Maire, *Cause de Dieu*, 393–94; and Bell, *Cult of the Nation*, 58–59.
195 A list of these 140 exiled magistrates is found in BHPF, Fonds Ste.-Beuve, ms. 121, ff. 129–34; anonymous black and white engraving, September 1732, Fonds Ste.-Beuve, ms. 123, f. 53; Chaunu et al., *Basculement*, 228–29; and Gazier, *Histoire générale,* 1:301–305.
196 Remonstrance to Louis XV, 6 April 1737, BN, ms. fr. 23454, ff. 60–94.
197 Louis XV's "Response" to Parlement's 6 April 1737 remonstrance, BN, ms. fr. 23454, ff. 126–30.
198 Clement XII, Brief of 16 February 1738, BN, ms. fr. 23451, ff. 318–28.
199 Parlement's "Address" to Louis XV, 28 June 1738, BN, ms. fr. 23453, ff. 170–77.
200 Louis XV's response to Parlement's "Address," 24 August 1738, cited by Flammermont, *Remonstrances*, 1:373.
201 Conseil d'Etat, *arrêt* of 5 September 1731, BN, ms. fr. 23443, f. 146.
202 Doyle, *Jansenism*, 50.
203 Cottret, "Polémiques," 2:299.
204 Parlement's *arrêt* of 9 February 1731, BHPF, Fonds Ste.-Beuve, ms. 121, ff. 7–10; BA, ms. 10192; and Chaunu et al., *Basculement*, 226.
205 Archbishop Vintimille's *mandement* of 27 April 1732, BHPF, Fonds Ste.-Beuve, ms. 121, ff. 15–18.
206 Archbishop Vintimille to Cardinal de Fleury, 1732, quoted in Chaunu et al., *Basculement*, 227.

207 Bishop of Marseilles, *mandement* of 6 June 1732, BHPF, Fonds Ste.-Beuve, ms. 121, ff. 50–53.
208 Conseil d'Etat, *arrêts* of 3 May and 16 June 1732, BHPF, Fonds Ste.-Beuve, ms. 121, ff. 19, 66.
209 *NE*, 1732, quoted in Melton, *Rise of Public Opinion*, 52.
210 See *NE* for 1730–1739, BHPF, ms. 522; Chaunu et al., *Basculement*, 221–23.
211 "*Abbé* D.G." to a professor of belles-lettres, 28 January and 9 February 1732, quoted in *Réflexions sur l'Ordonnance du roi en date du 27 janvier 1732* (N.p., 1732), 19–31.
212 For satirical songs, see BHPF, Fonds Ste.-Beuve, ms. 121, ff. 35, 46, 54, 71, 97, 136, 138, 169, 174. For poems, see ms. 121, ff. 83, 85, 162, 185. For prints and engravings, see ms. 121, ff. 3, 11, 16, 21, 47, 69, 92, 112, 125, 128, 143, 158 and ms. 122, f. 318.
213 Anonymous black and white engraving (c. 1732), Fonds Ste.-Beuve, ms. 122, f. 318.
214 Louis XV's circular letter to Gallican bishops, 22 July 1731, BN, NAF 3333, ff. 117–18.
215 BN, Collection Joly de Fleury, ms. 1477, ff. 95, 214–16.
216 BN, NAF 3334, ff. 71–72, 194–200, 217–25, 269–313, 438–42.
217 Bishop of Carcassone to Cardinal de Fleury, c. 1730, BN, NAF 3334, ff. 201–202.
218 Archbishop of Aix's "Formulary" of 1733 and Parlement's 23 February 1733 *arrêt* condemning it, BN, ms. fr. 23442, ff. 130–36.
219 *Abbé* J. Languet, "Lettre de L'Abbé des ** à Monseigneur l'Archevesque de Sens sur son Instruction Pastorale" (Paris: n.p., 25 November 1734), 8.
220 "Systeme des tolerans de ce tems," 4 November 1734, BN, ms. fr. 23445, ff. 54–67.
221 Jean Charles de Segur, Bishop of St. Papaul, "Mandement" of 26 February 1735, BN, ms. fr. 23443, ff. 315–65.
222 Conseil d'Etat, *arrêt* of 24 April 1735, ibid., f. 366.
223 François Ilharat de la Chambre, *Traité du Formulaire, ou l'on examine à fond l'affaire du Jansénisme quant au fait, & quant au droit* (Utrecht: Nicolas Le Fevre, 1736), 1:xiv–xxii; 2: table of contents and 161–69.
224 Chabaille d'Anvigny to unknown "Monsieur," 12 November 1736, BA, ms. 11307, ff. 226–38.
225 Pierre-François Lafiteau, *Histoire de la Constitution Unigenitus* (Liège: Everand Kints, 1738), 1:2–6.
226 Bishop Daubrière of Soissons, "Profession of Faith," 23 December 1738, BN, ms. fr. 23452, f. 330.
227 Escholier, *Port-Royal*, 300.
228 *Abbé* Claude-Pierre Goujet, ed., *Mémoires pour servir à l'histoire de Port-Royal* (Paris: n.p., 1734–1737), 3 volumes.
229 Joseph Dedieu, "Un nouveau Port-Royal au diocèse d'Auxerre," *Le Correspondant* 101 (1929):641–60.
230 Chaunu et al., *Basculement*, 234–35.
231 "Lettres de plusieurs evêques sur l'obligation de priver de l'Oblation du Sacrifice de la Messe & des Suffrages de l'Eglise, ceux qui meurent appellans de la Constitution Unigenitus" (1739), BN, Collection Joly de Fleury, ms. 1490, ff. 11–15.
232 These mandates, pastoral letters, reflections, approbations, observations, discourses, notices, ordinances, and memoirs are found in BN, ms. fr. 23441, 23444, 23450, 23451, 23452, 23456, and 23458.
233 Bishop of Laon to Minister Fleury, 12 October 1732, BN, ms. fr. 23441, f. 1.
234 This dramatic "war of words" between the Bishop of Laon and his many opponents can be found in BN, ms. fr. 23441, ff. 1–3, 39–110, 165–79, 406–36, 453–55; ms. fr. 23444, ff. 1–98; ms. fr. 23450, ff. 1–229; and ms. fr. 23456, ff. 1–246.
235 Bishop of Laon to *Lieutenant-général de police* Hérault, 6 February 1738, BN, ms. fr. 23451, ff. 187–89.
236 "Mémoire sur le refus public des Sacremens au lit de mort," c. 1730s, BHPF, ms. 3186(11), ff.1–24.
237 Marquis d'Argenson, *Journal et mémoires du marquis d'Argenson publiés pour la prémière fois d'après les manuscrits autographes de la Bibliothèque du Louvre*, ed: Edme Jacques Benoit Rathery (Paris: Mme. Ve. Jules Renouard, 1859–1867), 2:205.
238 Ibid., 2:90–92.
239 Ibid., 1:369.
240 Anonymous doctor of theology at the Sorbonne to a bishop in the provinces, June 1733, BN, ms. fr. 23441, ff. 136–38, 146.
241 Marquis d'Argenson, 1745, quoted in Dale K. Van Kley, *The Jansenists and the Expulsion of the Jesuits from France, 1757–1765* (New Haven: Yale University Press, 1975), 27.

242 Barbier, May 1752, quoted in ibid., 27.
243 Richard M. Andrews, *Law, Magistracy, and Crime in Old Regime Paris, 1735–1789*. Vol. 1: *The System of Criminal Justice* (Cambridge: Cambridge University Press, 1994), 245, 273.
244 McManners, "Jansenists," 266–69; Maire, *Cause de Dieu*, 396.
245 D'Argenson, *Journal*, 3:49.
246 Oath taken by the Theology Faculty at the Sorbonne in 1741, BN, ms. fr. 20958, f. 147.
247 McManners, *Church and Society*, 1:213; see, for example, the investigations into the Community of Calvaire in Paris from 1740 to 1749, BA, ms. 10174.
248 *Frère* Jean Le Suer, Declaration of 1 April 1744, BA, ms. 10188.
249 Déclaration of *Soeur* Saint-Basile, 22 April 1747, BA, ms. 10189.
250 Chaunu et al., *Basculement*, 245.
251 *NE*, 16 January 1747, p. 9; BN, NAF 3334, ff. 471–81; Loupès, *Vie religieuse*, 55–56; Farge, *Subversive Words*, 155; and Henry Legier Desgranges, *Du Jansénisme à la Révolution, Mme de Moysan et l'extravagante affaire de l'Hôpital Général* (Paris: Hachette, 1954), 257.
252 McManners, *Angers*, 174.
253 Tuilier, *Sorbonne*, 2:142.
254 Farge, *Subversive Words*, 48; Garrioch, *Revolutionary Paris*, 106; and Hildesheimer, *Jansénisme*, 146.
255 Farge, ibid., 48–49; Hildesheimer, ibid., 146–48; Chaunu et al., *Basculement*, 274–77; and Choudhury, *Convents*, 59.
256 Marquis d'Argenson, 1749, quoted in Choudhury, ibid., 59.
257 Arouet de Voltaire, quoted in Hildesheimer, ibid., 146.
258 *NE* for 1740–1749, BHPF, ms. 522. Annual editions varied, however, between 196 and 208 pages.
259 *NE* for 15 December 1742, p. 199; 14 February 1743, p. 21; 14 August 1743, p. 117; 6 March 1745, p. 37; 8 May 1745, p. 73; 6 November 1745, p. 177; 11 December 1745, p. 199; 4 September 1746, p. 142; 4 December 1746, p. 193; 12 June 1747, p. 93; and 13 February 1749, p. 27.
260 *NE*, 5 December 1740, pp. 30–33, 39; for the ongoing battle between the Bishop of Laon and Parlement during the 1740s, see documents contained in BN, ms. fr. 23456, f. 336; ms. fr. 23457, ff. 365–71; and ms. fr. 23458, ff. 1–341.
261 Coward, "Newspaper," 12–13.
262. Choudhury, *Convents*, 53.
263 *NE*, 13 February 1749, p. 27.
264 Charles Arnauld de Pomponne's appeal to Parlement, March 1748, BN, ms. fr. 20972, ff. 380–98.

6 Jansenism Loses Its *Raison d'être*, 1751–1799

1 Marquis d'Argenson, *Journal*, 7:129–30.
2 Ibid., 270.
3 *Père* de Colonia, *Dictionnaire des livres jansénistes* (1752), cited by Garrioch, *Revolutionary Paris*, 41.
4 Julian Swann, "'Fauteurs de toutes les maximes qui sont contraires à la monarchie': le gouvernement face aux magistrats jansénistes sous Louis XV," *Chroniques de Port-Royal* 39(1990):164–68; Emile Régnault, *Christophe de Beaumont, archevêque de Paris, 1703–1781* (Paris: Librairie Victor Lecoffre, 1882), 1:166.
5 Antoine-Louis Rouillé to Joly de Fleury, 19 July 1752, quoted in Dale K. Van Kley, "The Refusal of Sacraments Controversy and the Political Crisis of 1756–57," in *Church, State and Society Under the Bourbon Kings of France*, ed. Richard M. Golden (Lawrence, KS: Coronado Press, 1982), 292–93.
6 Chaunu et al., *Basculement*, 244–50.
7 Cardinal de Bernis, 1758, quoted in Van Kley, "Refusal," 300.
8 Régnault, *Beaumont*, 2:244.
9 Julian Swann, *Politics and the Parlement of Paris under Louis XV, 1754–1774* (Cambridge: Cambridge University Press, 1995), 90.
10 Chaunu et al., *Basculement*, 292–93.

11 Van Kley, *Damiens*, 116.

12 Marquis d'Argenson to the *Président à mortier* of the Paris Parlement, 1 July 1749, in *Journal*, 6:1, 26.

13 Muchembled et al., *Dictionnaire*, 36–37; *billet de confession*, 11 January 1755, BN, Collection Joly de Fleury, ms. 1569, f. 295; Garrioch, *Revolutionary Paris*, 157; and Chaunu et al., *Basculement*, 279, 284.

14 Jeffrey Merrick, "Conscience and Citizenship in Eighteenth-Century France," *Eighteenth Century Studies* 21 (1987):57–58, 62; Strayer, *Huguenots and Camisards*, 408–22; McManners, *Church and Society*, 2:490.

15 Cottret, *Lumières*, 16.

16 Unnamed priest of Boulogne, November 1754, quoted in D'Argenson, *Journal*, 8:373.

17 Chaunu et al., *Basculement*, 288, 291.

18 Régnault, *Beaumont*, 1:159–64; Loupès, *Vie religieuse*, 47; and John Rogister, *Louis XV and the Parlement of Paris, 1737–1755* (Cambridge: Cambridge University Press, 1995), 102.

19 Briefs of the Parlement of Paris, 24 March 1751–30 December 1752, BA, ms. 2453; D'Argenson, *Journal*, 6:322–23; Chaunu et al., *Basculement*, 269–71; Maire, *Cause de Dieu*, 401; and Rogister, *Louis XV*, 103.

20 Rogister, ibid., 104–5; Régnault, *Beaumont*, 1:214–16; and Garrioch, *Revolutionary Paris*, 157.

21 Maire, *Cause de Dieu*, 397.

22 Flammermont, *Remonstrances*, 1:414, 422–23, 436, 439, 442.

23 Doyle, *Jansenism*, 63; Loupès, *Vie religieuse*, 47.

24 *Avocat* Barbier, May 1752, quoted in Loupès, ibid., 48.

25 BA, ms. 2453, ff. 159–61, 169–70; Christophe de Beaumont letters to "Monsieur," 17 December 1752 and 18 January 1753, BN, Collection Joly de Fleury, ms. 1569, ff. 7, 27, 52; and Régnault, *Beaumont*, 1:274.

26 Archbishop Beaumont, 1753, quoted in Flammermont, *Remonstrances*, 1:506–7.

27 Ibid., 507.

28 Louis XV to the First President of Parlement, 21 February 1753, quoted in Régnault, *Beaumont*, 1:288.

29 Ibid., 294.

30 *Lettres de cachet*, 11 March and 28 November 1754, BN, NAF 3335, ff. 159–62, 180; Chaunu et al., *Basculement*, 268–69, 298.

31 For example, the BN, Collection Joly de Fleury, ms. 1568 is full of letters from unnamed sources informing Beaumont of the events in and around Paris in 1755.

32 Christophe de Beaumont to Lamoignon de Malesherbes, 7 September 1754, 30 August 1756, 25 February 1757, BN, ms. fr. 22143, ff. 150, 156 and ms. 22144, f. 104.

33 *Lieutenant-général* Berryer to Lamoignon de Malesherbes, 7 September 1754, BN, ms. fr. 22151, f. 6.

34 Coward, "Newspaper," 13.

35 Egret, *Louis XV*, 70.

36 Marquis d'Argenson, *Journal*, 9:248, 328, 331, 334, 344.

37 See Rogister, *Louis XV*, 103–19.

38 For a cross-section of these documents at the Bibliothèque Nationale, see ms. fr. 23459, ff. 1–258; 23460, ff. 1–86; NAF 3335, ff. 2–8, 13–31, 69–70, 94–99, 118–360; Collection Joly de Fleury, ms. 1490, ff. 68–87; ms. 1567, ff. 1–393; ms. 1568, ff. 1–374; ms. 1569, ff. 1–435; ms. 1571, ff. 1–274; ms. 1572, ff. 1–291. At the Bibliothèque de l'Arsenal, see mss. 2455 and 2456. F. Rocquain, in "Les Refus de sacrements," *Revue Historique* 15 (1877):244–64, also analyzes several of these primary documents.

39 Louis XV, Response to Parlement's Remonstrance, 17 April 1752, BA, ms. 2453 and BN, NAF 3334, f. 535.

40 Louis XV's reply to Parlement, 7 September 1752, quoted in Van Kley, *Damiens*, 133.

41 Louis XV, Declaration of 2 September 1754, quoted in Régnault, *Beaumont*, 1:269–71.

42 Egret, *Louis XV*, 64; Merrick, *Desacralization*, 87–88.

43 Louis XV, Declaration of 8 October 1754, BA, ms. 2454.

44 Marquis d'Argenson, *Journal*, 9:171–72.

45 Louis XV, "Réponse du Roi," 27 February 1756, BA, ms. 2456.

46 *Lit de justice* of 21 August 1756, cited by Chaunu et al., *Basculement*, 295–97.

47 *Declaration du Roi* of 10 December 1756 and *Edit du Roi* of December 1756, BHPF, ms. 1173, ff. 141–48.
48 Van Kley, "Refusal," 294–97.
49 Maire, *Cause de Dieu*, 402–11; Melton, *Rise of the Public*, 54. For a list of those who belonged to the "parti janséniste" and the "parti dévot," see Julian Swann, "Parlement, Politics and the *parti janséniste*: The Grand Conseil Affair, 1755–56," *French History* 6 (1992):435–61 and François Bluche, *Les Magistrats du parlement de Paris au XVIIIe siècle (1715–1771)* in Annales Littéraires de l'Université de Besançon, vol. 35 (Paris: Les Belles Lettres, 1960), 251–52.
50 Chaunu et al., *Basculement*, 283. Of those 65 cases, 20 occupied 30 percent of the magistrates' time.
51 Remonstrance of 15 April 1752, BA, ms. 2453 and BN, NAF 3334, ff. 521–34.
52 *Declaration du Roi*, 11 May 1753, BA, ms. 2453; Rocquain, "Refus," 253–59; and Egret, *Louis XV*, 59–64.
53 Marquis d'Argenson, *Journal*, 8:11.
54 Ibid., 61, 65, 164, 411.
55 BA, ms. 2454, ff. 1–11.
56 *Arrêt* of 18 March 1755, cited by D'Argenson, *Journal*, 8:452, 455–57.
57 "Extrait des Registres de Parlement" for 6 May 1755, BN, Collection Joly de Fleury, ms. 1572, ff. 106–7.
58 Marquis d'Argenson, *Journal*, 8:476.
59 Parlement's letter to Louis XV, 13 December 1756, and Louis XV's response, 21 December 1756, BN, NAF 3335, ff. 233, 236.
60 See, for example, Bell, *Lawyers*, 106, and Hudson, "Regent," 147.
61 Van Kley, "Refusal," 289–91.
62 Christophe de Beaumont to the secretary of the Court at Parlement, 1754, quoted in Régnault, *Beaumont*, 1:273.
63 Marquis d'Argenson, *Journal*, 8:12.
64 Ibid., 330–31.
65 Chaunu et al., *Basculement*, 278.
66 Marquis d'Argenson, *Journal*, 8:429, 437–38; 9:41–42, 45, 334.
67 May 1756 rumors, cited by D'Argenson, *Journal*, 9:267.
68 Renée Haynes, *Philosopher King: The Humanist Pope Benedict XIV* (London: Weidenfeld and Nicolson, 1970), 152; Van Kley, *Damiens*, 141.
69 Benedict XIV's Brief of 16 October 1756, BHPF, ms. 1173, ff. 135–40; Chaunu et al., *Basculement*, 308; and McManners, *Church and Society*, 2:504.
70 Van Kley, *Damiens*, 142; Merrick, *Desacralization*, 90–91.
71 BN, NAF 3335, ff. 9–12, 264–352.
72 Chaunu et al., *Basculement*, 349–54.
73 Ibid., 350–52.
74 *Nouvelles Ecclésiastiques*, 1757, quoted in ibid., 355; David Ogg, *Europe of the Ancien Regime, 1715–1783* (NY: Harper Torchbooks, 1965), 260.
75 Van Kley, *Damiens*, 81–89; Chaunu et al., *Basculement*, 357. While Diderot blamed the Jesuits, Voltaire held both the Jesuits and the Jansenists responsible for inspiring Damiens' crime. "These are the abominable effects of the Bull *Unigenitus* and of the grave impertinences of Quesnel and the insolence of Le Tellier. I have always thought the Jansenists and the Molinists ridiculous, but now they are bloody parricides," he said.
76 Gazier, *Histoire générale*, 2:80.
77 Muchembled et al., *Dictionnaire*, 210.
78 For examples of these printed public sources, see *Recueil des pièces contre Jansénisme*, BHPF, mss. 1172 and 1173, and BA, ms. 2454.
79 St. Augustine, cited by Antoine Arnauld, *Première Lettre de M. Arnauld Docteur de Sorbonne à une personne de condition* (1657), in *Oeuvres*, 19:311–13.
80 Pasquier Quesnel, quoted in Régnault, *Beaumont*, 1:158.
81 Marquis d'Argenson, *Journal*, 7:208, 235.

82 Ibid., 8:289–91.
83 *Abbé* Bon, *Lettres d'un homme du monde au sujet des billets de confession et de la bulle Unigenitus* (1753), cited by Merrick, *Desacralization*, 83.
84 Pierre Guilbert, *Mémoires historiques et chronologiques sur l'Abbaye de Port-Royal des Champs* (Utrecht: n.p., 1755–56), 1:iii, viii–xvii, xxi–xxxi.
85 *NE*, 1750–1759, BHPF, ms. 522; BN, ms. fr. 3335, ff. 248–52, 265, 359–61.
86 *NE*, 20 November 1752, p. 208; 6 March 1758, p. 44; 9 January 1759, p. 9; 16 January 1759, p. 13; 13 February 1759, p. 24.
87 *NE*, 24 April, 1750, p. 65; 1 May 1750, p. 72; 26 June 1754, p. 101; 17 April 1758, pp. 65–68; 8 January 1757, p. 9; 16 January 1759, p. 13; 13 February 1759, p. 24.
88 *NE*, 18 September 1750, p. 201; 16 July 1756; 13 November 1757, p. 188; 12 June 1759, p. 98.
89 *NE*, 18 December 1750, p. 201.
90 *NE*, 13 February 1754, p. 25; 4 December 1754, p. 196.
91 *NE*, 16 October 1755, p. 165.
92 *NE*, 2 January 1757, p. 8.
93 *NE*, 16 January 1757, p. 15.
94 *NE*, 13 December 1759, p. 197.
95 Colonia, *Dictionnaire*, 3:155–74.
96 Rocquain, "Refus," 261–64.
97 Van Kley, *Damiens*, 164.
98 Maire, *Cause de Dieu*, 459; Loupès, *Vie religieuse*, 58; and Cottret, *Lumières*, 87.
99 Palmer, *Unbelievers*, 26.
100 Régnault, *Beaumont*, 1:168.
101 Cottret, *Lumières*, 117; Maire, *Cause de Dieu*, 495, 499; Chaunu et al., *Basculement*, 364; McManners, *Church and Society*, 2:509, 519; and Dale Van Kley, "The Jansenist Constitutional Legacy in the French Prerevolution," in *The French Revolution and the Creation of Modern Political Culture*, ed. Keith Michael Baker (Oxford: Pergamon Press, 1987), 1:179.
102 Maire, ibid., 468–69; McManners, *Church and Society*, 2:533–36.
103 Cottret, *Lumières*, 117–19; McManners, *Church and Society*, 2:546–47.
104 Ibid., 119–29; "Réponse aux questions proposés à l'auteur de l'appel à la Raison," c. 1765, BHPF, ms. 125, ff. 1–88; Maire, *Cause de Dieu*, 501–507; Van Kley, *Jansenists*, 32–33; and Chaunu et al., *Basculement*, 348.
105 BA, ms. 2458 contains 303 pages of documents showing the magistrates' views of the Jesuits.
106 Bell, *Lawyers*, 129.
107 *Arrêt* of Parlement, 6 August 1761, quoted in Chaunu et al., *Basculement*, 363.
108 Louis XV to Choiseul, 1764, quoted in Chaunu, ibid., 363.
109 Cottret, *Lumières*, 119; Maire, *Cause de Dieu*, 518; and McManners, *Church and Society*, 2:558.
110 Dorival, *Musée*, 163–64; Doyle, *Jansenism*, 74.
111 Maire, *Cause de Dieu*, 459.
112 Chaunu et al., *Basculement*, 307.
113 Christophe de Beaumont, *Instruction pastorale sur les atteintes données à l'autorité de l'Eglise par les jugements des tribunaux séculières dans l'affaire des Jésuites* (1763), cited by Chaunu et al., ibid., 309–10.
114 General Assembly of the Clergy, "Declaration of 1765," BN, NAF, ms. 3333, ff. 199–200; Merrick, *Desacralizaiton*, 105, 109.
115 See the documents found in BN, Collection Joly de Fleury, ms. 1569, ff. 277–78; ms. 1570, ff. 1–340; ms. 1490, ff. 48–67; and NAF, ms. 3333, ff. 206–15.
116 General Assembly of the Clergy's "Appeal" to Louis XV, 1760, quoted in Coward, "Newspaper," 14.
117 *NE*, 1760–1769, BHPF, ms. 522.
118 *NE*, 16 May 1763, pp. 81, 84; 25 July 1763, p. 124; 26 August 1767, p. 140.
119 *NE*, 4 August 1760, p. 141; 10 April 1762, p. 57; 8 August 1763, p. 131.
120 *NE*, 9 October 1761, p. 161.
121 *NE*, 9 November 1762, p. 179.
122 *NE*, 17 October 1763, p. 172.

123 *NE*, 18 October 1768, p. 165.

124 See Voltaire and D'Alembert's collaborative work *Sur la destruction des Jesuites en France* and articles on the "Jesuites" and "Jansénistes" in the *Encyclopédie*; Cottret, *Lumières*, 138–41.

125 *NE*, 24 September 1764, p. 61.

126 *NE*, 27 June 1768, p. 101.

127 Brian E. Strayer, Statistical analysis, April 1993. The Bastille has been chosen for analysis because complete records on Jansenists at other prisons are not available.

128 Augustin Gazier, *Histoire générale du mouvement janséniste depuis ses origines jusqu'à nos jours* (Paris: Librairie Ancienne Honoré Champion, 1924), 1:176–77.

129 St.-Cyran's trial transcripts, 14–31 May 1639, BN, ms. fr. 15610, ff. 62–63 and ms. 17804, ff. 1–38; Adam, *Jansénistes*, 138–40; Richardt, *Jansénisme*, 55–58; Gastelier, *Angélique*, 226–27, 232–34, 237; Sedgwick, *Travails*, 107–108; and Richelieu to prince de Condé, 1638, quoted in Kostroun, "Port-Royal Nuns," 181.

130 Jaccard, *St.-Cyran*, 128, 198; Sedgwick, ibid., 129.

131 St.-Cyran, quoted in Jaccard, ibid., 128.

132 Sedgwick, *Travails*, 129; Bremond, *Ecole*, 57, 63; Adam, *Jansénistes*, 141–45; and Gastelier, *Angélique*, 238–40, 254.

133 Chaunu et al., *Basculement*, 82; Mazarin to M. de Fabert, 17 May 1653, in Mazarin, *Lettres*, 5:614–15.

134 BA, ms. 11304.

135 Farge, *Subversive Words*, 23; Maire, *Cause de Dieu*, 138, 143–44.

136 Maire, ibid., 137, 141, 148–50.

137 Ibid., 153.

138 Sainte-Beuve, *Port-Royal*, 3:629–30.

139 Gazier, *Histoire Général*, 1:176–77.

140 Gerberon, *Jansénisme*, 128; Weaver, "Bible and Port-Royal," 75–76; Delassault, *Lettres*, 123–28, 134–37,143–45, 149, 165, 193–94, 203, 206, 298; and Sainte-Beuve, *Port-Royal*, 2:343–54.

141 Du Fossé, *Port-Royal*, 274–89, 316–18; Besoigne, *Port-Royal*, 308–14.

142 Romanes, *Port-Royal*, 469–70; Escholier, *Port-Royal*, 274; and Weaver, *Joncoux*, 298.

143 BA, ms. 11031; Alcime Bachelier, *Le Jansénisme à Nantes* (Paris: Librairie Nizet et Bastard, 1934), 157–58; and Paul Denis, "Quelques lettres de dom Louvard, prisonnier à la Bastille," *Revue Mabillon* 4 (1908–1909): 498–525.

144 BA, ms. 11307, f. 130.

145 BA, ms. 11313, f. 155.

146 BA, ms. 11313, f. 2; ms. 11308, f. 29; ms. 11312, f. 41.

147 BA, ms. 11312, f. 222.

148 Description of Roquette's detention, 1742, in *Nouvelles Ecclésiastiques*, cited by Cottret, *Lumières*, 297; Augustin Gazier, "La Bastille en 1743," *Mémoires de la Société de l'histoire de Paris et de l'Ile de France* 7 (1880):13–36.

149 BA, ms. 11627.

150 BA, ms. 12498; see also Bachelier, *Nantes*, 204.

151 See Strayer, *Huguenots and Camisards*, 238–48.

152 D'Argenson, *Journal*, 9:16–18.

153 *NE*, 6 May 1738, p. 69; 20 November 1743, p. 173; 24 September 1744, p. 153, BHPF, ms. 522.

154 *NE*, poem (undated), quoted in Cottret, *Lumières*, 296, 298.

155 For a comprehensive analysis of long-standing myths concerning conditions at the Bastille and the use of *lettres de cachet*, see Brian E. Strayer, *Lettres de cachet and Social Control in the Ancien Régime, 1659–1789* (NY: Peter Lang, 1992), xi–xxiv, 159–70.

156 The life of Claude Brousson, a Huguenot pastor executed in 1698, is one example of the Huguenots' extreme suffering. See Walter C. Utt and Brian E. Strayer, *Bellicose Dove: Claude Brousson and Protestant Resistance to Louis XIV, 1647–1698* (Brighton & Portland: Sussex Academic Press, 2003).

157 William H. Williams, "The Significance of Jansenism in the History of the French Catholic Clergy in the Pre-Revolutionary Era," *Studies in Eighteenth-Century Culture* 7 (1978):299; Van Kley, "Legacy," 182; and Joynes, "Idealogues," 351–52.

158 Joynes, ibid., 352–53; Garrioch, *Revolutionary Paris*, 294.

159 *Journal Historique de la révolution opérée dans la constitution de la monarchie française* (1772), quoted in Marcel Marion, *Dictionnaire des Institutions de la France aux XVIIe et XVIIIe siècles* (Paris: n.p., 1923; reprint, Editions A. & J. Picard, 1972), 304.

160 Doyle, *Jansenism*, 81; Loupès, *Vie religieuse*, 51.

161 Chaunu et al., *Basculement*, 358.

162 Louis XVI to Archbishop Beaumont, 18 December 1774, quoted in Chaunu et al., ibid., 375.

163 McManners, *Church and* Society, 1:290; Gazette *de France*, 1781, quoted in Chaunu et al., ibid., 377, 381.

164 Maire, *Cause de Dieu*, 531–34; Echeverria, *Maupeou*, 45–46; Doyle, *Jansenism*, 81–82; and Cottret, *Lumières*, 148–50, 153, 172–73, 177.

165 Shanti-Marie Singham, "Vox populi vox Dei: les jansénistes pendant la révolution Maupeou," *Chroniques de Port-Royal* 39(1990): 183–91.

166 Charles H. O'Brien, "The Jansenist Campaign for Toleration of Protestants in Late Eighteenth Century France: Sacred or Secular?" *Journal of the History of Ideas* 46 (1985):523–25; idem, "Jansenists and the Civil Toleration of Protestants in France, 1775–1778: Lepaige, Guidi, and Robert de Saint-Vincent," in *La tolérance civile*, ed. Roland Crahay (Bruxelles: Université de Bruxelles, 1982), 191–92.

167 *Abbé* Clément du Tremblai to Adrien Le Paige, 24 March 1775, quoted in O'Brien, "Jansenists," 183–84.

168 Lamoignon de Malesherbes, *Mémoire* (1776) to Louis XVI, cited by Pierre Grosclaude, *Malesherbes, Témoin et interprète de son temps* (Paris: Librairie Fischbacher, 1961), 416–17.

169 Antoine Arnauld, *De la necessité de la foi* (1641), in *Oeuvres*, 10:179.

170 Antoine Arnauld, *De la Veritable religion* (1656), in *Oeuvres*, 11:673.

171 Index to the writings of Antoine Arnauld, in *Oeuvres*, 43:214.

172 Maire, *Cause de Dieu*, 521; Alexander Sedgwick, "Seventeenth-Century French Jansenism and the Enlightenment," in *Church, State and Society under the Bourbon Kings*, ed. Richard M. Golden (Lawrence, KS: Coronado Press, 1982), 127–30.

173 D'Argenson, *Journal*, 8:333–34.

174 Cottret, *Lumières*, 115; Garrioch, *Revolutionary Paris*, 196.

175 Cottret, ibid., 299–304; Charles H. O'Brien, "Jansenists and Enlightenment: The Attitude of 'Nouvelles Ecclésiastiques' Toward Josephinist Religious Toleration," T*heologische Zeitschrift* 33 (1977):393–407.

176 Cottret, *Lumières*, 28–31, 47–50.

177 Arouet de Voltaire, quoted in Muchembled et al., *Dictionnaire*, 282.

178 Cottret, *Lumières*, 9; Sedgwick, "Jansenism," 125–26.

179 D'Argenson, *Journal*, 2:281.

180 Voltaire, quoted in Cottret, *Lumière*, 23, 25–26, and in Levi, *Louis XIV*, 232.

181 Voltaire, *Poème sur la grâce* (1720), quoted in Cottret, ibid., 24.

182 Voltaire, *Traité sur la tolérance* (1763), quoted in ibid., 37–38.

183 Voltaire, *Ingénu* (1767), quoted in ibid., 39.

184 Voltaire, quoted in ibid., 40–42; Gazier, *Histoire générale*, 2:54–56.

185 Voltaire, *Siècle de Louis XIV* (1751), 488–91.

186 *Nouvelles Ecclésiastiques*, cited by Cottret, *Lumières*, 60, 63, 71.

187 Baron de Montesquieu, quoted in Cottret, ibid., 52–59, 67, 70–71; Shackleton, "Jansenism," 1391.

188 Cottret, ibid., 84–86.

189 Ibid., 76–81; Choudhury, *Convents*, 190 (n. 46).

190 Cottret, ibid., 86; Coward, "Newspaper," 14–15.

191 Marion, *Dictionnaire*, 308; Pierre Dominique, "Port-Royal et les Jésuites, ou les desseins politiques de deux siècles," *Ecrits de Paris* (February 1966):32.

192 D'Alembert, quoted in O'Brien, "Enlightenment," 393.

193 Jean-Jacques Rousseau, *La Nouvelle Héloise* (1763), quoted in Chaunu et al., *Basculement*, 316.

194 Cottret, *Lumières*, 102, 106, 109.

195 Monique Cottret, "Les jansénistes juges de Jean-Jacques," *Chroniques de Port-Royal* 39 (1990):82–83.

196 Cottret, *Lumières*, 89–94; idem, "Jean-Jacques," 81.
197 Cottret, "Jean-Jacques," 84–90.
198 Louis-Adrien Le Paige, quoted in Doyle, *Jansenism*, 73.
199 *NE*, 1770–1779, BHPF, ms. 522.
200 *NE*, 18 January 1770, pp. 10–12; 28 August 1778, p. 137.
201 Doyle, *Jansenism*, 80.
202 *NE*, 1770–1775, 1777. The terms most often used were *ci-devant jésuites* and *exjésuites*.
203 *NE*, 9 January 1774, p. 1.
204 *NE*, 13 June 1770, p. 93; 16 July 1772, p. 113; 13 June 1773, p. 95; 18 July 1773, p. 115; 8 August 1774, p. 125; 16 October 1776, p. 168; 5 June 1777, p. 92; 6 March 1778, p. 19; 22 May 1778, p. 81.
205 *NE*, 1776, 1777, 1778, 1779 (For Arnauld, volumes I–XXVI had appeared by 1779; for Pascal, volumes I–V).
206 *NE*, 5 December 1774, p. 193.
207 *NE*, 1774, 1776, 1778. See especially 19 October 1774, p. 201.
208 Condorcet, *Eloge de Pascal*, quoted in Cottret, *Lumières*, 44.
209 Chaunu et al., *Basculement*, 265; Sedgwick, "Enlightenment," 125–26.
210 Maire, *Cause de Dieu*, 397–98; Van Kley, "Legacy," 182–84, 187, 192; and Nigel Aston, *The End of An Elite: The French Bishops and the Coming of the Revolution, 1786–1790* (Oxford: Clarendon Press, 1992), 26–28.
211 Pius IX, quoted in Loupès, *Vie religieuse*, 224–26.
212 Chaunu et al., *Basculement*, 382, 517.
213 Cottret, *Lumières*, 179–81, 184, 195–97; Doyle, *Jansenism*, 80.
214 Robert de Saint-Vincent, speech to Parlement of Paris, 1787, quoted in Francis G. W. Adams, "The Struggle of the French Protestants for Civil Rights, 1750–1787" (Ph.D. diss., University of Chicago, 1954), 296.
215 Charles H. O'Brien, "Jansénisme et tolérance civile à la veille de la Révolution," *Chroniques de Port-Royal* 39 (1990): 137–39.
216 *NE*, 28 May 1788, pp. 85–86, BHPF, ms. 522.
217 Ruth F. Necheles, *The Abbé Grégoire, 1787–1831: The Odyssey of An Egalitarian* (Westport, CT: Greenwood Publishing, 1971), 10–13, 21 (n. 18).
218 *NE*, 1780–1789, *BHPF*, ms. 522; for the German editions, see *NE*, 27 October 1784, p. 180 and 28 July 1785, p. 124; Michel Albaric, "Regard des jansénistes sur l'Eglise de France de 1780 à 1789 d'après les *Nouvelles Ecclésiastiques*," *Chroniques de Port-Royal* 39 (1990): 65.
219 *NE*, 1780–1789; Albaric, ibid., 65–66.
220 *NE*, 24 April 1780, p. 65; 10 July 1783, p. 122; 20 August 1784, p. 134; 10 July 1786, p. 109.
221 *NE*, 3 July 1781, p. 105; 30 October 1781, p. 173; 6 February 1782, p. 21; 3 April 1782, p. 53; 5 June 1782, p. 90; 10 April 1787, p. 59; 12 March 1788, p. 42.
222 *NE*, 8 August 1780, p. 125; 17 July 1781, p. 116; 10 October 1783, p. 161.
223 Albaric, "*Nouvelles Ecclésiastiques*," 68–69.
224 *NE*, 27 November 1786, p. 189.
225 Meyer, *Controverses*, VII–IX.
226 *Abbé* Grégoire, *Ruines de Port-Royal*, 96–97.
227 Jules Michelet and Jean Jaurès, cited by Woodbridge, *Revolt*, 215 (n. 50).
228 Joseph Dedieu, "Désarroi," 524.
229 René Taveneaux, *Jansénisme et politique*, cited by Woodbridge, *Revolt*, 215 (n. 50).
230 Necheles, *Abbé Grégoire*, xiii.
231 Hildesheimer, *Héritage*, 96.
232 Maire, *Cause de Dieu*, 374–76, 583–85.
233 Doyle, *Jansenism*, 83.
234 Bell, *Cult of the Nation*, 17.
235 Garrioch, *Revolutionary Paris*, 160.
236 Jotham Parsons, *The Church in the Republic: Gallicanism and Political Ideology in Renaissance France* (Washington, DC: Catholic University of America Press, 2004), 10.

237 Maire, *Cause de Dieu*, 562.
238 Van Kley, *French Revolution*, 335; idem, "Legacy," 172–73.
239 Timothy Tackett, *Becoming a Revolutionary: The Deputies of the French National Assembly and the Emergence of a Revolutionary Culture, 1789–1790* (Princeton, NJ: Princeton University Press, 1996), 66–67, 290.
240 McManners, *Church and Society*, 1:519.
241 Doyle, *Jansenism*, 83–84; Tulier, *Sorbonne*, 2:144; and Maire, *Cause de Dieu*, 580.
242 Rabaut de Saint-Etienne, speech before the Constituent Assembly, 1790, quoted in Cottret, *Lumières*, 200.
243 *Nouvelles Ecclésiastiques*, 1790, quoted in ibid., 199.
244 Grégoire, *Ruines de Port-Royal*, 126; Cécile Gazier, *Port-Royal*, 442.
245 Antoine Ricard, *Les premiers Jansénistes et Port-Royal* (Paris: E. Plon, 1883), 470–72.
246 Doyle, *Jansenism*, 85.
247 *NE*, 1790–1799, BHPF, ms 522.
248 *NE*, 1791 and 1794.
249 *NE*, 13 March 1790, p. 41; 15 January 1794, p. 11.
250 *NE*, 2 January 1790, pp. 1–4; see also 4 September 1790, p. 141.
251 *NE*, 10 April 1791, p. 61.
252 *NE*, 9 January 1792, pp. 86–87.
253 *NE*, 14 August-25 December 1793; 24 October 1798; Maire, "Eglise," 1200.
254 *NE*, December 1794, p. 208; 24 October 1798; 21 May 1798, p. 41; 31 July 1799, p. 61.
255 *NE*, 27 February 1799, p. 17.
256 Coward, "Newspaper," 16.

7 The Shaking of Jansenism: Miracle Cures and the *Convulsionnaires*, 1727–1740

1 Minister of State Fleury to *lieutenant-général* Hérault, 23 April 1733, quoted in Farge, *Subversive Words*, 47.
2 Loupès, *Vie religieuse*, 206.
3 For the sake of textual variety, I shall use the terms *convulsionnaires*, *convulsionistes*, convulsionaries, and convulsionists interchangeably.
4 Sedgwick, *Jansenism*, 65.
5 Michel, "Pastoral janséniste," 177–80.
6 Maire, "Agonie," 111; Pillorget, *Marville*, 161.
7 Dainville, "Jansénisme," 113–16, 123.
8 Ibid., 181–91.
9 Maire, *Cause de Dieu*, 273–74, 297.
10 Louis Sébastien Mercier, *Tableau de Paris* (1781), quoted in Alfred Mousset, "Un vent de folie au 'siècle des lumières': Les 'miracles' du cimetière Saint-Médard," *Historia* 127 (1957):567.
11 Kreiser, *Miracles*, 82–83; Maire, *Cause de Dieu*, 243–48; Garrioch, *Revolutionary Paris*, 145; Jean Louis Barbeau de La Bruyère and Claude-Pierre Goujet, *Mémoires pour servir à l'Histoire de Port-Royal ou Supplément aux Mémoires de MM. Fontaine, Lancelot et du Fossé* (Utrecht: Aux dépens de la Compagnie, 1742), 1–14; Pierre-François Mathieu, *Histoire des miraculés et des convulsionnaires de Saint-Médard* (Paris: Didier, 1864), 52–61; Brongniart, 70–71; Albert Mousset, *L'étrange histoire des convulsionnaires de Saint-Médard* (Paris: Editions de Minuit, 1953), 568; and Charles-Henri Manneville, "Une vieille église de Paris: Saint-Médard," *Bulletin de la Montagne Sainte-Geneviève et ses abords* 4 (1903–1904):196–98.
12 Kreiser, *Miracles*, 84–87; Mathieu, *Convulsionnaires*, 62; and A. Borel, "Les convulsionnaires et le diacre Pâris," *L'évolution psychiatrique* 4 (1935):5–7.
13 Kreiser, ibid., 88–90; Barbeau de La Bruyère, *Mémoires*, 15–17; Mathieu, ibid., 63–83; Brongniart, *Saint-Médard*, 71–72; Mousset, "Folie," 568; Loupès, *Vie religieuse*, 44; and Manneville, "Saint-Médard," 200–1.
14 Barbeau de La Bruyère, ibid., 25–30; Mathieu, ibid., 81–85; and Pierre Boyer, *La Vie de Monsieur de*

Pâris, diacre (Bruxelles: Foppens, 1731), 213–17.
15 Manneville, "Saint-Médard," 202; Brongniart, *Saint-Médard*, 72–73; and Maire, *Cause de Dieu*, 249.
16 Unknown Jansenist at Pâris' funeral, quoted in Boyer, *Pâris*, 212.
17 Kreiser, *Miracles*, 90, 407; Bishop of Chartres' request for a *lettre de cachet* against *Sieur* Guisainville, *curé* of Yermenonville, cited by Minister Maurepas to police chief Hérault, 4 June 1736, BA, ms. 11285, ff. 164–75.
18 Brongniart, *Saint-Mêdard*, 73; Kreiser, ibid., 93.
19 Inscription on François Pâris' tombstone, March 1728, quoted in Manneville, "Saint-Médard," 202, 204; Kreiser, ibid., 93; and Paul Valet, "Le diacre Pâris et les convulsionnaires de Saint-Médard," *Bulletin de la Montagne Sainte-Geneviève et ses abords* 2 (1896):365–66.
20 Voltaire, quoted in Bernard Mercier de Lacombe, *La résistance janséniste et parlementaire au temps de Louis XV: L'abbé Nigon de Berty, 1702–1772* (Paris: Société du Grand Armorial de France, 1948), 50–51.
21 Deacon Pâris' "Profession of Faith," BHPF, ms. 108, ff. 3–9; see also Séché, *Jansénistes*, 1:42–43.
22 François Pâris, *Compendium Theologiae Dogmaticae et Moralis* (1714), cited by Alphonse Adhémar d'Alès, "La Théologie du diacre Pâris," *Recherches de science religieuse* 10 (1920):374–76.
23 Prayers attributed to Deacon Pâris, BA, ms. 5346 (vol. 2), ff. 168–69.
24 Songs and prayers to Deacon Pâris, 1728–1733, in "Tombeau," BA, ms. 2056.
25 "Prière du bienheureux François Pâris," BN, NAF 4264, f. 157.
26 Prayer to Deacon Pâris, quoted in Jean-Louis Barbeau de La Bruyère, *La Vie de M. François de Pâris, diacre* (N.p., 1731), 36–48.
27 "Tombeau," BA, ms. 2056, f. 343; Patouillet and Colonia, *Dictionnaire*, 2:116; and Manneville, "Saint-Médard," 222–25.
28 La Bruyère, *Vie*, 49–50, 79; Maire, *Convulsionnaires*, 78–79; and idem, *Cause de Dieu*, 243, 258.
29 Barthélemy Doyen, *Vie de Monsieur de Pâris, diacre du diocès de Paris* (En France: n.p., 1732), "Avertissement," 93–105.
30 Muchembled et al., *Dictionnaire*, 194.
31 Cottret, "Polémiques," 1:43–45.
32 Maire, *Convulsionnaires*, 58.
33 Antoine Arnauld, *De l'autorité des Miracles*, cited by Jean-Louis Quantin, "Port-Royal entre l'histoire et le miracle, de *l'Augustinus* à la *Perpétuité*," *Chroniques de Port-Royal* 46 (1998):123, 127.
34 Index to the writings of Antoine Arnauld, in *Oeuvres*, 43:177–78.
35 Antoine Arnauld, *Frequent Communion*, 783.
36 "Relation de Quelques miracles opérés par l'intercession du Bf. François Charinnes Curé de la Paroisse de La Tourette," BN, NAF., ms. 4262, f. 2; Maire, *Convulsionnaires*, 56–58.
37 Knox, *Enthusiasm*, 227.
38 Ibid., 227–28.
39 Louis-Florentin Calmeil, *De la Folie considerée sous le point de vue pathologique, philosophique, historique et judiciaire* (Paris: J.-B. Ballière, 1845), 503–8.
40 Venard and Bonzon, *Religion*, 186.
41 Vidal, *Miracles*, 12.
42 Ibid., 13.
43 Ibid., 15.
44 Maire, *Convulsionnaires*, 25.
45 Gazier, *Histoire générale*, 1:276.
46 Kreiser, *Miracles*, 78–79.
47 Durand, *Jansénisme*, 315; Maire, *Cause de Dieu*, 241; and [Claude Hohl], *Le Jansénisme dans l'Yonne* (Auxerre, France: Archives départmentales de l'Yonne, 1986), 26.
48 Police Inspector Guillotte to *lieutenant-général* Hérault, 5 June 1726, and *lettres de cachet* for 11 June 1726, BA, ms. 10196.
49 Taveneaux, *Vie*, 193–94.
50 Auguste Marie, "Les Convulsionnaires de Saint-Médard," *Aesculape* 14 (1924):31.
51 Hildesheimer, in *Jansénisme*, 137, lists eight miracles for 1727, ten for 1728, three for 1727, three for 1730, and fifteen for 1731. However, Kreiser, in *Miracles*, 149, counts only 24 miracles between May

1727 and the spring of 1731, while Doyen, *Miracles*, 1–153, cites only the thirteen miracle cures that 24 *curés* reported to Archbishop Vintimille on 4 October 1731.

52 Valet, "Pâris," 367–77, gives the names of these fourteen as Madeleine Beigney (62), Pierre Lero (35), Marie-Jeanne Orget (57), Elisabeth de la Loe (25), Marie-Madeleine Massaron (27), Dom Alphonse de Palacious (a Spaniard), Demoiselle Thibault (61), Marie-Anne Couronneau (68), Marguerite-Françoise du Chêre, Philippe Sergent, Pierre Gautier, Demoiselle Coirin, Marie Carteri, and Demoiselle Hardouin.

53 Mathieu, *Convulsionnaires*, 115–77; Anne Le Franc, "To the Most Great Glory of God" (1730) and 129 testimonies of physicians, surgeons, neighbors, and relatives regarding her incurable disease, quoted in *Dissertation sur les Miracles*, 33–48; Kreiser, *Miracles*, 120–29; Georges Gilles de la Tourette, "Le miracle opéré sur Marie-Anne Couronneau le 13 juin 1731," *Nouvelle iconographie de la Salpêtrière* 2 (1889):241–47; Maire, *Convulsionnaires*, 65–72; and idem, *Cause de Dieu*, 251, 254–55, 282.

54 Kreiser, ibid., ix; Maire, *Convulsionnaires*, 90–95.

55 Maire, *Convulsionnaires* (1985), 90–95; idem, *Cause de Dieu* (1998), 269–71, 275, 280. In addition, Daniel Vidal's *Miracles et convulsions jansénistes au XVIIIe siècle* (1987), which examines a wider range of healing miracles and convulsions in seventeenth and eighteenth-century France, provides a broader context for Maire's statistical analysis. See tables in Vidal, *Miracles*, 177–81.

56 "Extrait des Informationne" for 16 and 21 June 1728, BA, ms. 10191; Kreiser, ibid., ix; and Vidal, *Miracles*, 37. Vidal lists these physicians as Elie Col de Vilors, L.-P. Lehoc, Charles Dorlet, H. Le Dran, F.-B. Dalton, B. Pibrac, Chirac, Winslow, and Vernage.

57 Police reports on St.-Médard visitors, BA, ms. 10196; Hildesheimer, *Heritage*, 77, 79; Kreiser, *Miracles*, 147–48, 153–54, 395–96; Maire, *Cause de Dieu*, 261–64; and Mousset, "Folie," 573.

58 Maire, ibid., 271–72.

59 Hildesheimer, *Héritage*, 79. Again, for a broader comparative context in seventeenth and eighteenth-century France, see the tables in Vidal, *Miracles*, 173–76.

60 Kreiser, *Miracles*, 395–96.

61 Kreiser, *Miracles*, 154–56; Mousset, "Folie," 572; Brongniart, *Saint-Médard*, 74; Maire, *Cause de Dieu*, 257; Vidal, *Miracles*, 329; and Augustin Noyon, "Un miracle du diacre Pâris: La guérison de l'abbé de Bécherand (1731–1732)," *Etudes* 156 (1918):412.

62 McManners, "Jansenism," 264; Maire, *Convulsionnaires*, 17, 251 For a comparison with the Camisard phenomenon, see Strayer, *Huguenots and Camisards*, 294–316.

63 Documents presented to Archbishop Noailles, BA, ms. 5346 (vol. 2) and BHPF, ms. 2386; Maire, *Cause de Dieu*, 253; Chaunu et al., *Basculement*, 193–94; Kreiser, *Miracles*, 94–96; Doyen, *Miracles*, 1–127; and Minister Fleury to Cardinal de Noailles, c. 1728, quoted in Kreiser, *Miracles*, 94–95.

64 Archbishop Vintimille, "Mandement," 15 July 1731, cited by Kreiser, *Miracles*, 149; Doyen, *Miracles*, 1–140.

65 Maire, *Cause de Dieu*, 253, 257; Vidal, *Miracles*, 15 (n. 16).

66 Maire, *Convulsionnaires*, 25; Kreiser, *Miracles*, x; and Georges Hardy, *Le Cardinal de Fleury et le mouvement janséniste* (Paris: Honoré Champion, 1925), 256–61.

67 *NE*, July 1728, BHPF, ms. 522; Maire, *Convulsionnaires*, 68.

68 *NE*, 17 December 1733, p. 205.

69 Kreiser, *Miracles*, 166–74; Marie, "Saint-Médard," 54.

70 Marie, ibid., 54; Kreiser, ibid., 173–75.

71 Maire, *Convulsionnaires*, 72; Escholier, *Port-Royal*, 301.

72 Haynes, *Benedict XIV*, 78; Borel, "Convulsionnaires," 10–12.

73 Séché, *Jansénistes*, 1:56–58; Maire, *Convulsionnaires*, 17–18, 103; and idem, *Cause de Dieu*, 243, 254.

74 Maire, *Cause de Dieu*, 260; Neveu, *Erudition*, 280–83.

75 Neveu, ibid., 284–88; Maire, ibid., 116, 119. The eight "Figurist" parishes included St.-Jacques-du-Haut-Pas, St.-Etienne-du-Mont, St.-Benoît, St.-Séverin, St.-André-des Arts, St.-Germain-l'Auxerrois, St.-Gervais, and St.-Marguerite.

76 *Abbé* d'Etemare, quoted in Neveu, ibid., 287.

77 Ibid.; Knox, *Enthusiasm*, 375–79.

78 Maire, *Convulsionnaires*, 17–18.

79 Marguerite de Roux-Sigy, c. 1650s, quoted in Vidal, *Miracles*, 11.
80 Undated police report on Pierre Lalair, quoted in Maire, *Cause de Dieu*, 287.
81 Maire, *Convulsionnaires*, 103–105.
82 Vidal, *Miracles*, 233.
83 Monsieur Duguet, December 1732, BA, ms. 5784, ff. 9, 24–25.
84 Jean Vinehon, in "Les convulsionnaires de Saint-Médard, ont-ils dépassé les limites des pouvoirs humains?" *Etudes carmélitaines* 32 (1953):45, posits between 400 and 500 *convulsionnaires*, while Hans-Jurgen Lusebrink and Rolf Reichardt, in *The Bastille: A History of a Symbol of Despotism and Freedom*, trans. Norbert Schurer (Durham, NC: Duke University Press, 1997), 16, estimate closer to 600. Valentin Durand, in *Jansénisme* (1907), 338, puts the total number at 800.
85 Mme. Duguet-Mol, *Journal historique des Convulsions du tems* (N.p., 1743), 56.
86 Bournet, *Querelle*, 324–25.
87 These titles are found in BN, NAF 4262, ff. 107, 110–12, 115, 171.
88 Séché, *Jansénistes*, 1:61.
89 B. Robert Kreiser, "Religious Enthusiasm in Early Eighteenth-Century Paris—Convulsionaries of Saint-Médard," *Catholic Historical Review* 61, no. 3 (1975):364–65.
90 Dominique Julia, "Le catholicisme, religion du royaume (1715–1789)," in Jacques Le Goff and René Rémond, *Histoire de la France religieuse*, vol. 3: *Du roi Très Chrétien à la laicité républicaine, XVIIIe–XIXe siècle* (Paris: Editions du Seuil, 1991), 32.
91 Cottret, *Lumières*, 291.
92 Vidal, *Miracles*, 195.
93 Ibid., 197.
94 Maire, *Cause de Dieu*, 283.
95 Knox, *Enthusiasm*, 376–77.
96 *Abbé* Marc-Antoine Reynaud, cited by Maire, *Cause de Dieu*, 305; idem, *Convulsionnaires*, 198–201.
97 Maire, *Cause de Dieu*, 306; Cottret, "Polemiques," 1:64, 77.
98 Maire, *Convulsionnaires*, 184–201, 211–19; Kreiser, "Convulsionaries," 359–61; Joseph Dedieu, "L'Agonie du jansénisme (1715–1790): Essai de Bio-Bibliographie," *Revue d'histoire de l'Eglise de France* 14 (1928):186–87; and a "New Song" of twelve stanzas, 7 August 1731, quoted in the "Tombeau," BA, ms. 2056.
99 *Convulsionnaire* prayers, BA, ms. 10203; Cottret, "Polémiques," 1:287–88.
100 "Explication de l'Apocalypse," BHPF, ms. 112; Maire, *Convulsionnaires*, 16, 137; idem, *Cause de Dieu*, 311, 314; Neveu, *Erudition*, 307–308; and Taveneaux, *Vie*, 195–96.
101 Daniel Vidal, *La Morte-Raison: Isaac la juive, convulsionnaire janséniste de Lyon, 1791–1841* (Grenoble: Editions Jérôme Millon, 1994), 64–72; André de Maricourt and Georges Firmin-Didot, "Les Convulsionnaires," *La Nouvelle revue* 54, 3d series (1908):359, 362–63.
102 Maire, *Cause de Dieu*, 86, 203; idem, "Eglise," 1180; Loupès, *Vie religieuse*, 47; and Choudhury, *Convents*, 35.
103 Catherine-Laurence Maire, "Le figurisme: de l'abbé d'Etemare à l'abbé Grégoire," *Politica hermetica* 10 (1996):28–34, 42–43; Doyle, *Jansenism*, 49–50.
104 Maire, *Cause de Dieu*, 237.
105 *Abbé* d'Etemare, *Essai d'un parallèle du tempts de Jésus-Christ et des nôtres* (undated), cited by Cottret, *Lumières*, 233, 236, 239; idem, "Polémiques," 1:79–80.
106 Neveu, *Erudition*, 303.
107 Ibid., 14, 305–6; Maire, *Cause de Dieu*, 308.
108 Maire, ibid., 238.
109 Vidal, *Miracles*, 33–41, 49–67, 75–76, 91–105, 111–17, 122, 128, 133–35, 146–47, 151–53, 160–62.
110 Collection of letters, testimonies, and reports regarding alleged miracles at Pâris' tomb, 1727–1734, BN, ms. fr. 22245, ff. 3–40, 99–53, 206–12; Maire, *Convulsionnaires*, 13; and idem, *Cause de Dieu*, 242–43.
111 "*Arrêt* du Grand Conseil du Roi," 14 June 1731, cited by "Tombeau," BA, ms. 2056.
112 Kreiser, *Miracles*, 175–76; Manneville, "St.-Médard," 218–19.

113 Police report for 6 August 1731, BA, ms. 10196.

114 Kreiser, *Miracles*, 151–52.

115 "Requeste presentée à Monseigneur l'Archevêque par les curés de Paris," August and October 1731, in "Tombeau," BA, ms. 2056, ff. 106–10 and in BN, ms. fr. 22245, ff. 1–2.

116 "*Mandement* de Monseigneur l'Archevêque de Paris" (1731) and "Requeste Presentée au Parlement," cited by "Tombeau," BA, ms. 2056, ff. 1–34, 129–32; Archbishop Vintimille, *Mandement* of 18 October 1731, BN, ms. fr. 22245, ff. 43–46; Maire, *Cause de Dieu*, 255; and Chaunu et al., *Basculement*, 222–23, 232.

117 Police chief Hérault to Chancellor D'Aguesseau, 6 August 1731, BA, ms. 10196.

118 Police report for 24 September 1731, BA, ms. 10196.

119 Police reports on Louis Sabinet, Monsieur Pinault, the chevalier de Blaru, the marquis d'Arbois, Monsieur de Fontaine, Monsieur Auffroi, and Alexandre Ottin can be found in BN, NAF 4262, ff. 25–32, 75–107, 118–31.

120 Marion, *Histoire de l'église*, 3:392–94.

121 Police reports and gazettes for 1732, BA, ms. 10161, ff. 41–48, 53–62, 67, 125, 173, and ms. 5784, ff. 19–25.

122 Knox, *Enthusiasm*, 377, 380–81; Kreiser, "Convulsionnaires," 376–79; and Hippolyte Blanc, *Le Merveilleux dans le Jansénisme, le magnetisme, le Methodisme, et le Baptisme americains, l'épidémie de Morzine, le spiritisme* (Paris: Henri Plon, 1865), 12.

123 See, for example, BHPF, ms. 2386, which concerns the alleged healing of 20 individuals, giving their former illnesses, how Deacon Pâris intervened to answer their prayers, their subsequent healing, and testimonies of its genuineness; Palmer, *Unbelievers*, 94–95; Maire, *Convulsionnaires*, 154–55; idem, *Cause de Dieu*, 352–53; and Henri Pensa, *Sorcellerie et religion: Du désordre dans les esprits et dans les moeurs aux XVIIe et XVIIIe siècles* (Paris: Librairie Felix Alcan, 1933), 291.

124 Doyle, *Jansenism*, 56.

125 Crichton, *Jansenisers*, 247, 263; Durand, *Jansénisme*, 343.

126 "Hypocrisy Demasquée ou l'Hérésie confoundue dans ses faux miracles," 1731, BN, NAF, ms. 3333, ff. 122–33; see also ms. 3333, ff. 135–50.

127 P. Bougeant, "Le Saint déniché" (1732), quoted in Armogathe, "Miracles," 160.

128 Maire, *Cause de Dieu*, 286.

129 Maricourt and Firmin-Didot, "Convulsionnaires," 368; Kreiser, *Miracles*, 179.

130 Kreiser, "Convulsionaries," 384; Van Kley, *French Revolution*, 99; and Williams, "Jansenism," 294.

131 Farge, *Subversive Words*, 24–25, 33, 69; Maire, *Convulsionnaires*, 161–63; Cottret, "Polémiques," 2:389; and a *Decret* of the Holy Congregation of the Inquisition, 22 August 1731, BN, NAF, ms. 3333, f. 121.

132 Kreiser, *Miracles*, 158–60; Maire, *Convulsionnaires*, 106, 109–10; and Mousset, *Convulsionnaires*, 52, 55, 58–59.

133 Kreiser, ibid., 282; Cottret, "Polémiques," 2:392–401; and *Père* Gagnol, *Le Jansénisme convulsionnaire et l'Affaire de la Planchette (1747) d'après les Archives de la Bastille* (Paris: Libraire générale catholique, 1911), 131.

134 Archbishop Vintimille to Joly de Fleury, 21 January 1732, quoted in Sars, *Fleury*, 143.

135 *Ordonnance* of 27 January 1732, cited by Manneville, "St.-Médard," 234–36; Merrick, *Desacralization*, 68; Cognet, *Jansénisme*, 114–15; Maire, *Convulsionnaires*, 110–11; and Borel, "Convulsionnaires," 3.

136 Sign posted at St.-Médard Cemetery, quoted in Mousset, *Convulsionnaires*, 73–74; in *Subversive Words*, 70, Arlette Farge gives a more poetic version of this message: "From King to God, a message clear: Miracles are forbidden here."

137 Mousset, *Convulsionnaires*, 76–77; Van Kley, "Sacraments," 301–2.

138 Blanc, *Jansénisme*, 14.

139 The subsequent history of the cemetery proved no more peaceful than its troubled past. From 1753 to 1773, it became the theatre for "the war of the Marguillers," a battle over whether Jansenist curates should be allowed to celebrate Mass there. During the French Revolution, rivalry between Constitutional and Refractory clergy over who should control its affairs once again led to the chapel being closed in 1793, only to be reopened two years later. In 1798 a third faction, the Cult of the

Theophilanthropiques, transformed the chapel into a "Temple of Work," but soon sold it to the locksmith Citizen Hanriot. In 1807, after the *abbé* Berthier had removed the funerary enclosure around Pâris' tomb and "purified" the grounds, burials were resumed there. The Deacon's body was exhumed and moved, but one woman retrieved Pâris'skull and buried it near her church door. Profaned once again during the Revolution of 1871, St.-Médard found relative tranquility only after 1901 when a new *Salle des Catéchismes* was built on its grounds. See Marie, 56–57; Mousset, "Folie," 574; Farge, *Subversive Words*, 23; and Marc Thibout, *Saint-Médard: Nefs et clochers* (Paris: Musées nationaux, 1947), 6.

140 Mousset, ibid., 574; Gagnol, *Jansénisme*, 16–17.

141 Cabourdin and Viard, eds., *Lexique historique*, s.v. "Convulsionnaires," 84; Mousset, *Convulsionnaires*, 175–81; G. Arnaud d'Agnel, "Les convulsionnaires de Pignans," *Annales du Midi* 19 (1907):206–11; Preclin and Jarry, *Luttes*, 1:251; and Emile Appolis, "Les 'miracles' jansénistes dans le Bas-Languedoc (1732–1745)," *Annales du Midi* 67 (1955):269–79.

142 Appolis, "Controverse," 20, 27. This broader history of the spread of convulsionism throughout France after 1732 still needs to be written.

143 Maire, *Convulsionnaires*, 125–26, 130; idem, *Cause de Dieu*, 291–92; and Roxane Kural, "Contribution à l'Histoire des mentalités de l'Occident pré-industriel: Etude de deux manuscrits de Convulsionnaires Jansénistes du milieu du XVIIIème siècle," TMs (photocopy), 1970–71, BHPF, ms. 2824, pp. 28–29.

144 Maire, *Cause de Dieu*, 293–94. The social backgrounds for 27 men (8%) and 37 women (40.5%) are unknown.

145 Ibid., 295.

146 Ibid.; records of attendees and participants at seances in 1732–34, 1739, 1741–43, BHPF, Fonds Ste.-Beuve, ms. 127; and Maire, *Convulsionnaires*, 119–20.

147 Maire, ibid., 121–23.

148 Ibid., 296.

149 Knox, *Enthusiasm*, 374.

150 The *abbé* Grégoire estimated, probably with some exaggeration, that by the end of the 1730s, the *convulsionnaires* were holding about 800 seances in Paris and the provinces. Knox, *Enthusiasm*, 382.

151 Preclin and Jarry, *Luttes*, 1:250; Vidal, *Miracles*, 375, 390.

152 Kural, "Contribution," 24–26; records of convulsionist meetings in the 1730s and 1740s, BHPF, Fonds Ste.-Beuve, ms. 127, ff. 1–238 and ms. 197, ff. 1–739; and Vidal, *Miracles*, 396.

153 Records of convulsionist seances in 1732–34, 1739, and 1741–43, BHPF, Fonds Ste.-Beuve, ms. 127, ff. 1–238.

154 Vidal, *Miracles*, 390.

155 Kreiser, *Miracles*, 309–15; Léon Cahen, *Les Querelles religieuses et parlementaires sous Louis XV* (Paris: Hachette, 1913), 49.

156 Cahen, ibid., 50; Loupès, *Vie religieuse*, 45; Kreiser, *Miracles*, 306–8; Vidal, *Miracles*, 278–79; Arnaud d'Agnel, "Pignons," 214; and BA, ms. 11032.

157 BA, mss. 11032 and 11033.

158 Kural, "Contribution," 42; Maire, *Convulsionnaires*, 113–16; Taveneaux, *Vie*, 197; Borel, "Convulsionnaires," 15–18; and Kreiser, "Convulsionaries," 119–25.

159 Maire, ibid., 119–25.

160 Records of convulsionist seances for 1732–1737, 1739, 1741–1743, BHPF, Fonds Ste.-Beuve, mss. 118 (I and II), 127, and 197; Kural, "Contribution," 75–77, 81.

161 BHPF, Fonds Ste.-Beuve, mss. 118 (I) and 127, ff. 1–238; BA, ms. 11283, ff. 115–53; and Mousset, *Convulsionnaires*, 167–70.

162 Knox, *Enthusiasm*, 372; police reports on the five sisters arrested on 6 March 1734, BA, ms. 11283, ff. 115–53.

163 BHPF, Fonds Ste.-Beuve, mss. 117, 118 (III), and 127; *Deux siècles de jansénisme: à travers les documents du fonds Port-Royal d'Utrecht* (Paris: Archives Nationales, 1974), 75–76; Blanc, *Jansénisme*, 24–26; and Knox, *Enthusiasm*, 372, 382–84.

164 Maire, *Convulsionnaires*, 16; Maricourt and Firmin-Didot, "Convulsionnaires," 360–61.

165 Kreiser, "Convulsionaries," 373; Vidal, *Miracles*, 324–25.

166 *Dom* Samson to Hérault, 16 May 1736, BA, ms. 10193; Vidal, ibid., 326.
167 Kreiser, "Convulsionaries," 374–76; Valet, "Pâris," 383; and Daniel Vidal, *Le Malheur et son prophète: inspirés et sectaires en Languedoc calviniste, 1685–1725* (Paris: Payot, 1983), 281–83.
168 Gertrude Rachel, 1771, quoted in Vidal, *Miracles*, 386.
169 Vidal, ibid., 277.
170 Ibid., 230–31, 309–13, 335, 338–39.
171 Ibid., 359–61, 366.
172 Ibid., 382–83.
173 Bournet, *Querelle*, 328; Kreiser, *Miracles*, xi; and Maire, *Convulsionnaires*, 11–13, 17.
174 "List of Works composed for and against the miracles and the convulsions from 1656 to 1785," BHPF, Fonds Ste.-Beuve, ms. 119, ff. 1–24; see also Kural, "Contribution," BHPF, mss. 196 and 197.
175 The above precis of *convulsionnaire* beliefs is drawn from many sources, including BHPF, Fonds Ste.-Beuve, mss. 118 (II, III), 127, and 197; BN, NAF 4264, ff. 111–24; BA, mss. 11033 and 11034; and Kural, "Contribution," 82–87.
176 Undated anonymous exhortation, quoted in Kural, "Contribution," Fonds Ste.-Beuve, ms. 197, ff. 650–51.
177 Vidal, *Miracles*, 367–68.
178 Bishop Colbert's "Instruction pastorale," 1 February 1733 and Clement XII's Brief of 3 October 1733, cited by Durand, *Jansénisme*, 317, 326.
179 *Abbé* Languet, "Lettre," 2–10.
180 Maire, "Eglise," 1185.
181 Dr. Le Thieullier to Archbishop Vintimille, 27 December 1735, BN, ms. fr. 22245, ff. 97–98.
182 Maire, *Cause de Dieu*, 412.
183 Kreiser, *Miracles*, 391–93.
184 Ibid., xi; Maire, *Convulsionnaires*, 11–13.
185 "Requête" of 19 Paris *curés*, 22 January 1738, BN, ms. fr. 23455, ff. 161–63; Bournet, *Querelle*, 328; and Knox, *Enthusiasm*, 387.
186 Archbishop of Sens, "Instruction pastorale," undated, quoted in Dawson, ed., *Crise d'autorité*, 81–85.
187 *Abbé* B. Fourgon, *Jugement équitable sur les convulsions* (Paris: n.p., June 1733), 2–22.
188 Archbishop of Embrun, "Instruction Pastorale," 1735, BN, ms. fr. 23447, ff. 76–99.
189 Charles Gaspard Guillaume de Vintimille du Luc, "Ordonnance . . . Rendue sur la Requête du Promoteur-général de l'Archevêché de Paris, au sujet des prétendus miracles attribuéz à l'intercession du sieur Pâris, Diacre, inhumé dans le Cimetière de la Paroisse de Saint-Médard," 8 November 1735, BN, Collection Clairambault, ms. 525, ff. 652–746.
190 Statement by 30 Paris physicians, 7 January 1735, cited by Durand, *Jansénisme*, 341–42.
191 BA, ms. 12727, ff. 262–65.
192 *NE*, 30 March 1737, p. 49, BHPF, ms. 522. Catherine Maire, in *Cause de Dieu*, 148, 153, mentions the locations of ten secret presses.
193 *NE*, 4 May 1737, p. 69.
194 Police reports, 1731–1734, BA, ms. 10192; inspector Duval to Hérault, March (?) 1732, cited by François Ravaisson-Mollien, *Archives de la Bastille* (Paris: n.p., 1866–1884; reprint, Genève: Slatkine-Megariotis Reprints, 1975), 14:299.
195 *Ordonnance* of 17 February 1733, BA, ms. 11218.
196 Maire, *Convulsionnaires*, 126; Kreiser, *Miracles*, 282–83, 297; and Borel, "Convulsionnaires," 16.
197 Kreiser, ibid., 279–81; Monsieur Duguet to Monsieur Fauillous, 30 September 1733, BA, ms. 5784, f. 16. Duguet may have been a police spy, but he was also a sympathetic observer who provided detailed and mostly accurate accounts of convulsionary activity. From first-hand observation, interviews of eye witnesses, and careful verification of the facts, he concluded that 20 cures had been genuine while most of the rest were "condemnable" as frauds and impostures. Jean Le Bel told police chief Hérault, in a letter of 18 September 1740, that he could be "useful" by exposing the convulsionists' "scandalous assemblies all around Paris." See BA, ms. 11327, ff. 83–96.
198 Fleury to Hérault, 23 April 1733, quoted in Ravaisson, *Archives*, 14:340.

199 Fleury to Hérault, 30 August 1734, BA, ms. 11257 (a slightly different version is quoted in Ravaisson, ibid., 14:373); McManners, *Church and Society*, 2:451.
200 Maire, *Convulsionnaires*, 125–27, 130; Séché, *Jansénistes*, 1:57–58.
201 Police reports regarding a 25 May 1736 plot against Louis XV, BA, ms. 11310, ff. 153–66; Kreiser, *Miracles*, 300, 304–305, 320–26; Maire, ibid., 129–36; and idem, *Cause de Dieu*, 299–300, 638.
202 Anonymous *convulsionnaire* tract, 1734, quoted in Kreiser, *Miracles*, 317.
203 Police dossier for Adam Antoine Royer, 1735, BA, ms. 11285, ff. 72–75.
204 "Mémoire concernant les convulsionnaires augustinian," 27 January 1736, BA, mss. 10193 and 11422; Port-Royal des Champs arrests, 12 and 15 January 1736, BA, ms. 11314, ff. 322–26 and ms. 11315, ff. 79–134. It appears as though the police used the term *convulsionnaire* primarily to refer to men and *convulsioniste* mainly to refer to women. See BA, ms. 11306, ff. 102–103.
205 Police dossier for Anne Catherine de Montfreuve, 27 May 1736 to 21 October 1742, BA, ms. 11327, ff. 332–47.
206 *Ordonnance* of 17 February 1737, cited by Maire, *Cause de Dieu*, 300.
207 Kreiser, *Miracles*, 375–76; for Hérault's undated letter regarding Montgeron, see BA, ms. 11366.
208 Kreiser, ibid., 375–82; Patouillet and Colonia, *Dictionnaire*, 4:186–87; and McManners, *Church and Society*, 2:453–54.
209 Armogathe, "Miracles," 136; Kreiser, *Miracles*, 383–88; Cottret, *Lumières*, 57; and Maire, *Convulsionnaires*, 173.
210 Louis-Basile Carré de Montgeron, *Le verité des miracles opérés par l'intercession de M. de Pâris et autres appellans démontrée contre M. l'Archêveque de Sens* (Utrecht: Libraires de la Compagnie, 1737), title page and "Lettre au Roi," 1–58.
211 Dossier for Sieur de Montgeron, 1736–1754, BA, ms. 11366, ff. 311–28; Maire, ibid., 173–74.

8 Crucifying Jansenism: *Grands Secours* and the Death of Convulsionism, 1741–1799

1 François Arouet de Voltaire, quoted in Augustin Gazier, "Le frère de Voltaire (1685–1745)," *Revue des deux mondes* 32 (1906):623.
2 Borel, "Convulsionnaires," 19.
3 Duguet-Mol, *Journal*, 1–13, 20, 24, 36, 41–46, 67, 95.
4 *NE*, 30 September 1742, pp. 153–56; Maire, *Cause de Dieu*, 301–2, 347; idem, *Convulsionnaires*, 142–44; and Cottret, *Lumières*, 234–36.
5 Maire, *Cause de Dieu*, 334, 339, 343–45, 348–49.
6 Police dossiers for Jansenists and convulsionists during the 1740s, BA, ms. 10194 and 11606, ff. 27, 183, 200; and Vidal, *Miracles*, 20.
7 Records of various convulsionist group seances, BHPF, Fonds Ste.-Beuve, mss. 117, 128, and 129; John Hearsey, *Voltaire* (New York: Barnes & Noble, 1976), 7, 30, 46.
8 M. Le Blanc to Bishop of Auxerre, 24 November 1745, BN, ms. fr. 20972, ff. 247–48.
9 Police report, c. 1744, BA, ms. 10194.
10 Gagnol, *Jansénisme*, 58, 87–95.
11 Maire, *Convulsionnaires*, 132–34.
12 Dossier for Lioutaud Ebeniste, February 1751, BA, ms. 10195.
13 Maire, *Cause de Dieu*, 302.
14 Vidal, *Morte-Raison*, 24.
15 BHPF, Fonds Ste.-Beuve, ms. 117, ff. 451–70.
16 Vidal, *Miracles*, 353–54.
17 BHPF, Fonds Ste.-Beuve, ms. 117, ff. 361–63.
18 Ibid., ff. 359–429.
19 Ibid., ff. 223–81, 299–356; BHPF, ms. 197, ff. 303–18; and BA, ms. 11635, ff. 535–46.
20 BHPF, Fonds Ste.-Beuve, ms. 118 (III), f. 295; Vidal, *Miracles*, 273–76.
21 These and many other Figurist symbols can be found in the manuscripts contained in the BN, NAF 4262, f. 100+; BA, ms. 11600, ff. 304–305; BHPF, Fonds Ste.-Beuve, ms. 128, ff. 1–160 and ms. 129; see also Vidal, ibid., 280–81, 290–96, 301, 305.

22 BA, ms. 11606, f. 337. In this rather simplistic code, the letters of the alphabet are assigned numbers (i.e., a = 2, b = 3, c = 4, etc.) or alternate letters (i.e., a = b, b = c, c = d, etc.).
23 Séance of 20 December 1743, BHPF, Fonds Ste.-Beuve, ms. 117, ff. 439–44.
24 Vidal, *Miracles*, 399.
25 Police reports, BA, ms. 11525, ff. 180–84; ms. 11577, f. 128; ms. 11630, ff. 65–66.
26 Kural, "Contribution," f. 13.
27 BA, ms. 10195; Vidal, *Miracles*, 19.
28 Maire, "Port-Royal," in Nora, ed., *Realms*, 1:328–30; Bell, *Lawyers*, 18, 98, 107–8.
29 Kural, "Contribution," ff. 12, 20, 26, 29, 32, 36; Vidal, *Miracles*, 19. This estimate of about 800 convulsionaries for all of France is based on numbers provided by the *abbé* Le Sesne and the *abbé* d'Etemare.
30 "Confession of Faith," 11 January 1752, cited by Mathieu, *Convulsionnaires*, 393–95.
31 BHPF, Fonds Ste.-Beuve, ms. 196, ff.1–300, and ms. 197, ff. 439–42, 551–55, 681–91; Kural, "Contribution," ff. 36–45, 51–77, 85, 89, 130, 141–45.
32 Maire, *Convulsionnaires*, 224; idem, *Cause de Dieu*, 303–4; and Vidal, *Miracles*, 346.
33 Van Kley, "Refusal," 301–3; BN, Collection Joly de Fleury, ms. 1569, ff. 112, 122, 193.
34 Kural, "Contribution," ff. 106–7, 132–40, 164–65.
35 Vidal, *Miracles*, 391–94.
36 Maire, *Cause de Dieu*, 320–23.
37 Sister Dorothée, 1750, quoted in Vidal, *Miracles*, 396–97.
38 Sister Alexis' dream, c. 1754, BHPF, Fonds Ste.-Beuve, ms. 196, cited by Kural, "Contribution," ff. 171–72.
39 Ibid., ff. 97.
40 Ibid., f. 99.
41 Ibid., ff. 99–104.
42 Préclin and Jarry, *Luttes politiques*, 19:251.
43 BN, NAF 4262, ff. 144–71.
44 Knox, *Enthusiasm*, 388.
45 For police-actions, from 1735 to 1760, see the BA, Archives de la Bastille, dossiers 1193–94, 5784, 10183–84, 10194–96, 10203–10206, 1134, 11349, 11366, 11375, 11525, 11628, 11630.
46 Farge, *Subversive Words*, 23; Blanc, *Jansénisme*, 45; and Cottret, "Polemiques," 1:65–67.
47 BA, ms. 11349; Quétel, *Lettres de cachet*, 72; Maricourt and Firmin-Didot, "Convulsionnaires," 368; Maire, *Convulsionnaires*, 108; and idem., *Cause de Dieu*, 260.
48 BA, ms. 11314, ff. 322–26 and ms. 11315, ff. 79–134; Vidal, *Miracles*, 239–40; Maire, *Convulsionnaires*, 108; and Mathieu, *Convulsionnaires*, 411–14.
49 BA, ms. 11268.
50 BA, ms. 11253.
51 Strayer, *Lettres de cachet*, 44–45.
52 BA, ms. 11201.
53 BA, ms. 11310, ff. 153–66.
54 Maricourt and Firmin-Didot, "Convulsionnaires," 368.
55 Strayer, *Lettres de cachet*, 133–34.
56 Police dossier for Margueritte Dousson, 1731, BA, ms. 11141 and 11151.
57 Police dossier for Jeanne and Gabrielle Moulère, 1737–1748, BA, ms. 11375; Maire, *Convulsionnaires*, 132–34.
58 Police dossier for Jeanne Coutelier, 1742–1761, BA, ms. 11509.
59 Mousset, "Folie," 574.
60 Strayer, *Lettres de cachet*, 46–47.
61 Police dossiers for Jean Le Roux, Duval, Jacques Guillebert, Le Maistre, Verdive, and Hamelin, 1731, BA, ms. 11154.
62 Police dossier for Prior Brayer, 1739, BA, ms. 11416.
63 Strayer, *Lettres de cachet*, 47–49.
64 Police dossier for the *comte* d'Avernes, 1737, BA, ms. 11422.

65 Strayer, *Lettres de cachet*, 59–60.
66 Police dossier for Paul François Langlade, 1734, BA, ms. 11258.
67 Police dossier for the son of Adam Antoine Royer, 1735, BA, ms. 11285.
68 Police dossier for Jacques Pierre Guillani Fleur de Rouvroy, 1735, BA, ms. 11305.
69 Mathieu, *Convulsionnaires*, 414–15.
70 Strayer, statistical analysis of 176 *convulsionnaires* at the Bastille, June 2004.
71 Gazier, *Histoire générale*, 1:176–77.
72 Police dossier for Thérèse Langlois, 1731, BA, ms. 11154.
73 Police dossier for Marguerite Giroux, 1732, BA, ms. 11097.
74 *Anecdotes aussi sûre que curieuses touchant la conduite tyrannique & barbare qu'on a exercée sur Denyse Régné à la Bastille* (N.p., 1760), 1–160; Maire, *Convulsionnaires*, 158–60; and Strayer, *Lettres de cachet*, 159–70, which analyzes this genre of popular propaganda against the Bastille.
75 Police dossier for Antoinette and Galois Prudhomme, 1734, BA, ms. 11253.
76 Police dossier for Milord Edward Donald Drummond, 1739–1755, BA, mss. 11422 and 11440.
77 Police dossier for Alexandre Fleury, 1741, BA, ms. 11487.
78 Police dossier for the Charles Hébert family, 1746–47, BA, ms. 11606.
79 Police dossiers for Pelagie Rousseau, 1747–48, BA, ms. 11624 and 11630.
80 Police dossiers for Claude De S____ and *Sieur* Baudin, 1747–49, BA, ms. 11630.
81 Police dossier for the *abbé* Vaillant, 1740–1761, BA, ms. 11032; Ravaisson, *Archives*, 14:384, 396.
82 Susanne Raubeau Duchenne, "Confession," 15 March 1748, BA, ms. 11630, f. 146.
83 BHPF, Fonds Ste.-Beuve, ms. 121, ff. 12–13.
84 Police dossier for *Sieur* Earotanacq, 1733, BA, ms. 11241.
85 Police dossier for Jeanne Desbarbert, 1734, BA, ms. 11249.
86 Police dossier for Pierre de La Barre, 1760, BA, ms. 12077.
87 Merrick, *Desacralization*, 125.
88 Maire, *Cause de Dieu*, 328–29.
89 Vidal, *Miracles*, 217.
90 Pensa, *Sorcellerie*, 285, 290–94; Dedieu, "Désarroi," 586–87.
91 BHPF, Fonds Ste.-Beuve, ms. 130, ff. 1–182.
92 Ibid., ff. 1, 5, 7, 20, 23–25, 28, 33, 38, 56, 71, 87, 148, 159.
93 Cottret, *Lumières*, 111.
94 Shackleton, "Jansenism," 1394–95; Kreiser, *Miracles*, 398–99.
95 David Hume, *An Inquiry Concerning Human Understanding*, cited by Kreiser, ibid., 399.
96 Cottret, *Lumières*, 56.
97 Vidal, *Miracles*, 369–70; Blanc, *Jansénisme*, 22
98 Voltaire, *Dictionnaire philosophique*, s.v. "Convulsions" and "Fanatisme," cited by Maire, *Convulsionnaires*, 19.
99 Voltaire, *Le Siècle de Louis XIV*, 494.
100 Voltaire, *Discours en verse sur l'homme, septième discours: sur la vraie vertu* (1734), quoted in Cottret, *Lumière*, 24–25.
101 Voltaire, "Treatise sur la Tolérance," 506.
102 Gazier, "Frère de Voltaire," 617–33; Hearsey, *Voltaire*, 7, 30, 46, 168.
103 Father of François and Armand Voltaire, quoted in Cottret, *Lumières*, 23.
104 D'Alembert, quoted in Maire, *Convulsionnaires*, 21–22.
105 Denis Diderot, quoted in Cottret, *Lumières*, 79, 81.
106 Diderot and D'Alembert, *Encyclopédie*, cited by Kay S. Wilkins, "The Treatment of the Supernatural in the *Encyclopédie*," *Studies on Voltaire and the Eighteenth Century* 90 (1972):1762.
107 Vidal, *Morte-Raison*, 26–27; Nicolas Restif de la Bretonne, Les *Nuits de Paris* (London: n.p, 1788), 142.
108 Pensa, *Sorcellerie*, 317–20, 325–26; Vidal, ibid., 29.
109 Vidal, ibid., 32.
110 Vidal, ibid., 24–25; idem, *Miracles*, 397–98.
111 Mousset, *Convulsionnaires*, 173.

112 Cottret, "Polémiques," 1:164–65.

113 Maire, *Convulsionnaires*, 238–40; Georges Desdevises du Dézert, *L'Eglise & l'Etat en France, depuis l'Edit de Nantes jusqu'au concordat*, 2 vols. (Paris: Société française imprimerie et de librairie, 1907–1908), 1:187–88.

114 Vidal, *Miracles*, 239, 365; Pensa, *Sorcellerie*, 309.

115 Maire, *Convulsionnaires*, 229; idem, *Cause de Dieu*, 325.

116 Knox, *Enthusiasm*, 373; Maire, ibid., 229; and Rita Herman-Belot, "L'abbé Grégoire et le 'retour des Juifs,'" *Chroniques de Port-Royal* 39 (1990): 211–17.

117 Vidal, *Morte-Raison*, 27–29.

118 Ibid., 29.

119 Maire, *Cause de Dieu*, 595.

120 Vidal, *Morte-Raison*, 26.

121 Ibid., 36–37.

9 Jansenism and Convulsionism, 1650–2000: An Historiographic Essay

1 Jean-François Chomel to Armand Wallon, 12 December 1731, quoted in Mousset, *Convulsionnaires*, 60–61.

2 Antoine Arnauld, *Oeuvres*, 23:54, quoted in Sedgwick, *Jansenism*, 102.

3 Blaise Pascal, *Pensées* (1662), quoted in *Great Books of the Western World*, vol. 33: *Pascal: The Provincial Letters, Pensées, Scientific Treatises*, ed. Robert M. Hutchins (Chicago: Encyclopaedia Britannica, 1952), 328–38, 341.

4 Edward Donald James, *Pierre Nicole, Jansenist and Humanist: A Study of His Thought* (The Hague: Martinius Nijhoff, 1972), 1–2, 68–71.

5 Haynes, *Benedict XIV*, 78–79.

6 [Anonymous], *Dissertation sur les miracles* (N.p., 1731), 3–5, 9–10, 13, 23.

7 Boyer, *Pâris*, i–xxxv.

8 Jean-François Chomel to Armand Wallon, 12 December 1731, quoted in Mousset, *Convulsionnaires*, 60–61.

9 Inspector Duguet's report, December 1732, BA, ms. 5784, f. 24.

10 *Frère* Augustin, speech before Parlement, January 1736, quoted in Maricourt and Firmin-Didot, "Convulsionnaires," 363–65, 368.

11 Paquier, *Jansénisme*, 476; Joseph Dedieu, *L'Agonie du Jansénisme, 1715–1790* (Paris: Société d'histoire ecclésiastique de la France, 1928), 45–48; idem, "Port-Royal," 656–57; Augustin Gazier, "Jean Restout et les miracles du diacre Pâris (1737)," *Revue de l'art chrétien* 62 (1912):118–21; and idem, *Histoire générale*, 1:280–82.

12 Maire, *Convulsionnaires*, 170; Armogathe, "Miracles," 137–47, 156–57.

13 Carré de Montgeron, *Le verité des miracles opérés par l'intercession de M. de Pâris et autres appellans démontrée contre M. l'archêveque de Sens*, 2 vols. (Utrecht: Libraires de la Compagnie, 1737), 1:i–xxxvi.

14 Ibid., xxvii–xxviii, 1–18.

15 Calmeil, *Folie*, 360–61, 367, 371, 376, 380.

16 Maire, *Convulsionnaires*, 98–99; Mousset, "Folie," 570–71.

17 Armogathe, "Miracles," 150.

18 Archbishop Vintimille, *Ordonnance* (1735), 2–3, 8, 20–25. Benedict XIV's criteria for genuine miracles in the 1740s stated that the disease must be serious, its existence objectively proved by medical science, its symptoms incurable by natural means, and its miraculous cure must be rapid and permanent. See Greg Burke, "Modern Miracles Have Strict Rules," *Time Magazine*, 10 April 1995, p. 72.

19 Maire, *Convulsionnaires*, 153–54; Kreiser, *Miracles*, xii–xiii, 176–79, 277.

20 *Règle infaillible pour discerner les vrais des faux miracles* (N.p., c. 1730s), 3–7, 12–13, 23.

21 Debate between Archbishop Jean-Joseph Languet de Gergy and Bishop Colbert de Croissy, 1733–1734, cited by Mousset, *Convulsionnaires*, 113; Bishop Charles-Daniel-Gabriel de Thubières-Grimoard de Pestels de Le Caylus, "Lettres . . . au sujet du second Tome de M. de Montgeron, 24 août

1742–25 janvier 1746" (N.p., 1746), 1–12.

22 Philippe Hecquet, *Le Naturalisme des Convulsions dans les Maladies de l'Epidémie Convulsionnaire* (Soleure: Andreas Gymnicus, 1733), 1–4, 7, 10–12, 16, 141–42, 147, 165, 189–90; Vinehon, "Convulsionnaires," 39–43; Maire, *Convulsionnaires*, 155, 167–69; and idem, *Cause de Dieu*, 278–29.

23 Dom La Taste, "Theological Letter XIXe" (1737), quoted in Maire, *Convulsionnaires*, 155–56, 174–76.

24 Louis de Bonnaire, *Traités polémiques sur la fin du monde* (1738), quoted in Maire, ibid., 178.

25 *Abbé* Jacques Vincent Bidal d'Asfeld, *Vains efforts des mélangistes ou discernans dans l'oeuvre des convulsions* (Paris: n.p., 1738), 3–6, 13–15, 43–44, 136–37; Maire, ibid., 176–77.

26 Lafiteau, *Unigenitus*, 2:327–35.

27 Antoine Vinchon Des Voeux, *Critique générale du livre de Mr. de Montgeron sur les Miracles de Mr. l'abbé* [sic] de *Pâris ou Nouvelles Lettres sur les Miracles* (Amsterdam: Henri Dusauzet, 1740), 1:iv–vi, x–xii, 1–46, 78–164; 2:217–506.

28 Denis Diderot, *Encyclopédie*, s.v. "Miracles," 10:560–62.

29 Ibid., s.v. "Convulsionnaire," 4:171.

30 Louis-Sébastien Mercier, *Tableau de Paris* (Neufchâtel: Samuel Fauche, 1781; reprint, Amsterdam: n.p., 1782–1788), 1:19–21, 174–76.

31 Bishop Grégoire, *Histoire des sectes religieuses*, 2d ed. (Paris: Baudouin Frères, 1828), 128–40.

32 Dr. L. F. Calmeil, *De la Folie* (1845), cited by Maire, *Convulsionnaires*, 241.

33 Dr. J. M. Charcot, *De la contracture hystérique permanente* (1872). For terminology employed by Drs. Bourneville, Regnard, Richer, and Pitres from 1877 to 1891, see Maire, ibid., 242–44.

34 Léon Séché, *Les derniers Jansénistes depuis la ruine de Port-Royal jusqu'à nos jours, 1710–1870*, 3 vols. (Paris: Perrin, 1891), 1:66–67.

35 Ibid., 58–61.

36 Maricourt and Firmin-Didot, "Convulsionnaires," 356–58.

37 Julien Noir, "La foi qui guérit à Saint-Médard. A propos d'un portrait du diacre Pâris," *Bulletin de la Montagne Saint-Geneviève et ses abords* 6 (1909–1912):71–79, 81.

38 Paquier, *Jansénisme*, 497, 500–16, 522–23.

39 L. Loevenbruck, "Convulsionnaires," in *Dictionnaire de théologie catholique,* ed. A. Vacant and E. Mangenot (Paris: Letouzey et Ané, 1923), 3: cols. 1757–62.

40 Marie, "Convulsionnaires," 88.

41 *Abbé* Léon Bournet, *La querelle janséniste* (Paris: Pierre Téqui, 1924), 329–36.

42 G.-J. Waffelaert, "Convulsionnaires," in *Dictionnaire apologétique de la foi catholique*, ed. Alphonse Adhemar d'Alès (Paris: Gabriel Beauchesne, 1925), 1: cols. 705–13.

43 Knox, *Enthusiasm*, 386.

44 Vinehon, "Convulsionnaires," 43–46.

45 Preclin and Jarry, *Luttes politiques*, 1:251.

46 Mousset, *Convulsionnaires*, 21–23.

47 Haynes, *Benedict XIV*, 78.

48 McManners, "Jansenism," 253–54.

49 Kreiser, *Miracles*, 383.

50 Ibid., 120–21.

51 Ibid., see footnote 77.

52 Vidal, *Miracles*, 186–98.

53 Maire, *Convulsionnaires*, 156, 246–50; idem, *Cause de Dieu*, 266–67, 347.

Conclusion: The Impact of Jansenism in France

1 Jacques Alfred Galland, *Essai sur l'histoire du protestantisme à Caen et en Basse-Normandie de l'Edit de Nantes à la Révolution* (Paris: Société d'Histoire du Protestantisme en Normandie, 1898), 471.

2 Valet, "Paris," 406.

3 Bournet, *Querelle*, 366–72.

4 Ibid., 372–73.

5 Ferguson, "Jansenism," 38.

6 Godart, *Jansénisme*, 5–6.
7 Knox, *Enthusiasm*, 228–30.
8 Weaver, *Port-Royal*, 154.
9 Dominique Dinet, "Le jansénisme et les origines de la déchristianisation au XVIIIe siècle, l'exemple des pays de l'Yonne," in *Du jansénisme à la laicité: Le jansénisme et les origines de la déchristianisation*, ed. Léo Hamon (Paris: Editions de la Maison des Sciences de l'Homme, 1983), 1–10, 18, 21–26. Dinet's dechristianization thesis had earlier been expressed by the *abbé* Charrier (1920), Pierre Ordioni (1932), and Edmond Préclin (1936).
10 Sedgwick, "Jansenists," 42.
11 Cardinal Jean-Marie Lustiger, "Homélie de S. Em. Le Cardinal Jean-Marie Lustiger, 8 septembre 1991," quoted in *La Mère Angélique Arnauld (1591–1661): Relation Colloque* (Paris: Bibliothèque Mazarine, 1992), 97–102.
12 Hildesheimer, *Jansénisme* (1991), 205–8; idem, *Héritage* (1992), 96–101.
13 Leszek Kolakowski, *God Owes Us Nothing: A Brief Remark on Pascal's Religion and on the Spirit of Jansenism* (Chicago and London: University of Chicago Press, 1995), 64–65.
14 Van Kley, *French Revolution*, 7, 372.

Bibliography

Unpublished Primary Sources

Bibliothèque de l'Arsenal (Paris)

Archives de la Bastille: 1193, 1194, 10161, 10191, 10203, 11031, 11032, 11033, 11034, 11097, 11141, 11151, 11154, 11218, 11249, 11253, 11257, 11258, 11283, 11285, 11304, 11305, 11306, 11307, 11308, 11309, 11310, 11312, 11313, 11314, 11315, 11327, 11329, 11336, 11366, 11628, 11630, 11635, 12077, 12498, 12727

Dossiers divers: 2056, 2453, 2454, 2455, 2456, 2457, 2458, 5180, 5181, 5182, 5346, 5784, 6034, 6035, 6036, 6937, 6038, 6039, 6040, 10158, 10171, 10172, 10173, 10174, 10179, 10181, 10182, 10183, 10184, 10188, 10189, 10190,10192, 10193, 10194, 10195, 10196, 10197, 10198, 10199, 10200, 10201, 10202, 10204, 10205, 10206, 11344, 11349, 11375, 11416, 11422, 11440, 11487, 11489, 11509, 11525, 11577, 11600, 11606, 11624, 11627

Bibliothèque de l'Histoire du Protestantisme Français (Paris)

Fonds Sainte-Beuve: 101, 102, 103, 104, 105, 106, 107, 108, 109, 110, 111, 112, 113, 114, 115, 116, 117, 118, 119, 120, 121, 122, 123, 124, 125, 126, 127, 128, 129, 130, 196, 197

Bibliothèque Nationale (Paris)

Collection Clairambault: 525

Collection Joly de Fleury: 1476, 1477, 1490, 1567, 1568, 1569, 1570, 1571, 1572

Collection Manuscrits Français: 10587, 12886, 12887, 13894, 15271, 15595, 15610, 15611, 15805, 15806, 15809, 17589, 17748, 17750, 17758, 17775, 17776, 17778, 17779, 17781, 17782, 17790, 17791, 17792, 17793, 17794, 17795, 17804, 19723, 19724, 19725, 19726, 19727, 19734, 20958, 20972, 22143, 22144, 22151, 22245, 23216, 23222, 23441, 23442, 23443, 23444, 23445, 23446, 23447, 23448, 23449, 23450, 23451, 23452, 23453, 23454, 23455, 23456, 23457, 23458, 23459, 23460, 23481, 23482, 23498, 23499, 23500, 23501, 23502, 23503, 23504, 23505, 23506, 23507, 23508, 23509, 23510, 25088

Collection Nouveaux Acquisitions Français: 1525, 3333, 3334, 3335, 4262, 4264

Theses and Dissertations

Adams, Francis G. W. "The Struggle of the French Protestants for Civil Rights, 1750–1787." Ph.D. diss., University of Chicago, 1954.

Chill, Emanuel S. "The Company of the Holy Sacrament, 1630–1666: Social Aspects of the French Counter-Reformation." Ph.D. diss., Columbia University, 1960.

Cottret, Monique. "Les Représentations mythiques de l'Eglise primitive dans les polémiques entre les jansénistes et les jésuites (1713–1760)." Thèse de 3e cycle, University of Paris, 1979.

Joynes, Daniel Carroll. "Jansenists & Idealogues: Opposition Theory in the Parlement of Paris, 1750–1775." Ph.D. diss., University of Chicago, 1981.

Kostroun, Daniella J. "Undermining Obedience in Absolutist France: The Case of the Port-Royal Nuns, 1690–1709." Ph.D. diss., Duke University, 2000.

Newton, William Ritchey. "Port-Royal and Jansenism: Social Experience, Group Formation and Religious Attitudes in Seventeenth-Century France." Ph.D. diss., University of Michigan, 1974.

Perrier, Henry Charles. "Quelques Remarques sur les écoles de Port-Royal." Thèse de la Faculté libre de théologie protestante de Paris, 1911.

Published Primary Sources

Abra de Raconis, Charles François. *Examen et jugement du livre de la Fréquente Communion, fait contre La Frequente Communion & publié sous le nom du Sieur Arnauld, Docteur de Sorbonne.* Paris: Sébastien Cramoisy, 1644.

Anecdotes aussi sûre que curieuses touchant la conduite tyrannique & barbare qu'on a exercisée sur Denyse Régné à la Bastille. N.p., 1760.

Annat, François. *La conduitte de l'Eglise et du Roy justifiée dans la condamnation des jansénistes.* Paris: Sébastien Cramoisy, 1664.

——. *Reflexions de la Mère Angélique de S. Jean Arnauld Pendant sa captivité au Monastère des Religieuses Annonciades de Paris en l'année 1664 sur la conformité de l'état, où etoient alors les Religieuses de Port-Royal, avec celui de Jesus-Christ dans l'Eucharistе.* N.p., 1710.

Arnauld, Antoine. *Apologie de Monsieur Jansénius, evesque d'Ipres & de la Doctrine de S. Augustin, expliquée dans son Livre, intitulé AUGUSTINUS.* Paris: n.p., 1644.

——. *Considerations sur les affaires de l'Eglise qui doivent estre proposées dans la prochaine Assemblée Générale du Clergé de France.* N.p., 1681.

——. *De la fréquente communion, où les sentimens des pères, des papes, et des conciles, touchant l'usage des Sacramens de Pénitence, & d'Eucharistie, sont fidélement exposez.* Paris: n.p., 1643. Reprint, Lyon: C. Plaignard, 1739.

——. *Oeuvres de Messire Antoine Arnauld, docteur de la maison et société de Sorbonne.* 44 vols. Paris and Lausanne: Sigismond d'Arnay, 1775–1783; reprint, Bruxelles: Culture et Civilisation, 1964–1967.

——. *Phantosme du Jansenisme ou justification des pretendus Jansenistes par le livre mesme.* Cologne: Nicolas Schouten, 1686.

——. *Morale Pratique des Jésuites.* 8 vols. N.p., 1683. Reprint, Nancy: Joseph Nicolai, 1716–1735.

——. *Seconde lettre de M. Arnauld, docteur de la maison et société de Sorbonne à un duc et pair de France.* In *Lettres de Monsieur Antoine Arnuald, Docteur de Sorbonne.* 9 vols. Paris: n.p., 1655. Reprint, Nancy: Joseph Nicolai, 1727.

——. *Theologie Morale des Jesuites extraitte fidellement de leurs livres contre la Morale Chrestienne en général.* Paris: n.p., 1643.

Arnauld, Antoine, Pierre Nicole, and Claude de Sainte-Marthe. *Apologie pour les religieuses de Port-Royal du Saint Sacrement, contre les injustices & les violences du procédé dont on a usé envers ce Monastère.* N.p., 1665.

Arnauld, Isaac. *Le Mépris du monde; résolution vertueuse de l'obéissance deu au roy; Meditations sur la Veillesse.* N.p., 1618. Reprint, Genève: Pour Jean Ant. & Samuel De Tournes, 1618.

Arnauld, Jacqueline Marie Angélique. *Lettres de la Reverende Mère Marie Angélique Arnauld, abbesse et réformatrice de Port-Royal, 1620–1661.* Utrecht: Aux Depens de la Compagnie, 1742.

——. *Mémoires et relations sur ce qui s'est passé à Port-Royal des Champs, depuis le commencement de la réforme de cette abbaye.* N.p., 1716.

——. *Relation écrite par la Mère Angélique Arnauld sur Port-Royal.* Edited and annotated by Jean Lesaulnier. Paris: Bibliothèque Mazarine, 1992.

Arnauld, Jeanne Catherine Agnès. *Lettres de la Mère Agnès Arnauld, abbesse de Port-Royal.* 2 vols. Edited by M.P. Faugère. N.p., 1626–1671. Reprint, Paris: Ernest Thorin, 1866.

Arnauld d'Andilly, Angélique de Saint-Jean. *Relation de captivité d'Angélique de Saint-Jean Arnauld d'Andilly*, 3d ed. Paris: Gallimard, 1954.

Arnauld d'Andilly, Robert. *Mémoires. Collection des Mémoires relatifs à l'histoire de France*, ed. M. Petitot, vols. 33–34. Paris: Foucault, Libraire, 1824.

Barbeau de La Bruyère, Jean Louis. *La Vie de M. François de Pâris, diacre.* N.p., 1731.

Barbeau de La Bruyère, Jean Louis and Claude-Pierre Goujet. *Mémoires pour servir à l'Histoire de Port-Royal ou Supplément aux Mémoires de MM. Fontaine, Lancelot et du Fossé.* Utrecht: Aux dépens de la Compagnie, 1742.

Barnes, Annie, ed. *Lettres inédites de Jean Duvergier de Hauranne, abbé de Saint-Cyran.* Paris: Librairie Philosophique J. Vrin, 1962.

Besoigne, Jérome. *Histoire de l'Abbaye de Port-Royal.* Cologne: Aux dépens de la Compagnie, 1752–1753.

Bibliothèque Janséniste. Bruxelles: Chez Simon T'Sertetevens, 1740.

Boyer, Pierre. *La Vie de Monsieur de Pâris, diacre.* Bruxelles: Foppens, 1731.

Carré de Montgeron, Louis-Basile. *La verité des miracles opérés par l'intercession de M. de Pâris et autres appellans, démontrée contre M. l'archêveque de Sens.* 2 vols. Utrecht: Libraires de la Compagnie, 1737.

[Cerveau, René]. *L'Esprit de M. Nicole, ou Instructions sur les Verités de la Religion tirées des Ouvrages de ce Grand Théologien tant sur les Dogmes de la Foi et les Mystères, que sur la Morale.* Paris: G. Desprez, 1765.

——. *Nécrologie des plus célèbres défenseurs et confesseurs de la vérité des XVIIe et XVIIIe siècles.* 2 vols. Paris: n.p., 1760.

Cléméncet, Charles. *Histoire générale de Port-Roïal, depuis la réforme de l'abbaïe jusqu'à son entière destruction.* 10 vols. Amsterdam: Jean Vanduren, 1755–1757.

D'Argenson, marquis. *Journal et mémoires du marquis d'Argenson publiés pour la première fois d'après les manuscrits autographes de la Bibliothèque du Louvre.* 9 vols. Edited by Edme Jacques Benoit Rathery. Paris: Mme. Ve. Jules Renouard, 1859–1867.

D'Asfeld, Jacques Vincent Bidal. *Vains efforts des mélangistes ou discernans dans l'oeuvre des convulsions.* Paris: n.p., 1738.

de Brisacier, Jean. *Les Jansénistes reconnus Calvinistes.* Paris: Sébastien Cramoisy et Gabriel Cramoisy, 1652.

de Colonia, Dominique. *Dictionnaire des livres jansénistes, ou qui favorisent le jansénisme.* 5 vols. Antwerp: Chez Jean-Baptiste Verdussen aux deux Cicognes, 1752.

Defense des Religieuses de Port-Royal et de leurs directeurs, sur tous les faits alleguez par M. Chamillard Docteur de Sorbonne dans ses deux libelles contre ces Religieuses. N.p., 1667.

de Marandé, Léonard. *Inconvénients d'estat procedans du Jansénisme, adressez à Mr. Arnauld.* Paris: Sébastien et Gabriel Cramoisy, 1653.

de Pontis, Louis. *Mémoires du Sieur de Pontis officier des armées du Roi contenant plusieurs circonstances des guerres et du gouvernement sous les règnes des rois Henri IV, Louis XIII et Louis XIV.* N.p., 1676. Reprint, Paris: Honoré Champion, 2000.

de Retz, Jean François Paul de Gondi, Cardinal. *Mémoirs of Cardinal de Retz.* Ed. David Ogg. London: J. M. Dent, 1917. Reprint, Paris: Pléiade, 1956.

de Saint-Amour, Louis Gorin. *The Journal of Mons. De Saint Amour, Doctor of the Sorbonne, containing a full Account of all the Transactions both in France and at Rome concerning the Five Famous Propositions controverted between the Jansenists and the Molinists from the beginning of the Affair till the Popes {sic} Decision, 1646–1653.* London: T. Ratcliff, 1664.

de Saint-Cyran, Jean Du Vergier de Hauranne, *abbé. Considerations chrétiennes sur la Mort.* 3d ed. Paris: Veuve de Guillaume Desprez, 1710.

——. *Oeuvres chrétiennes et spirituelles de Messire Jean Du Vergier de Hauranne, abbé de Saint-Cyran.* 4 vols. N.p., 1645. Reprint, Lyon: Thomas Amaulry, 1679.

de Sainte-Marthe, Claude. *Déffense des religieuses de Port-Royal et de leurs directeurs sur tous les faits alleguez par M. Chamillard, Docteur de Sorbonne, dans ses deux libelles contre ces Religieuses.* N.p., 1667.

Des Voeux, Antoine Vinchon. *Critique générale du livre de Mr. de Montgeron sur les Miracles de Mr. l'abbé {sic} de Pâris ou Nouvelles Lettres sur les Miracles.* Amsterdam: Henri Dusauzet, 1740.

de Vintimille du Luc, Charles Gaspard Guillaume. *Ordonnance . . . Rendue sur la Requête du Promoteur-général de l'Archevêché de Paris, au sujet des prétendus miracles attribuéz à l'intercession du sieur Pâris, Diacre, inhumé dans le cimetière de la Paroisse de Saint Médard.* Paris: Pierre Simon, 1735.

Dissertation Dans laquelle on démontre que la Bulle Unigenitus n'est ni Loi de l'Eglise Ni Loi de l'Etat. N.p., 1752.

Dissertation sur les miracles. N.p., 1731.

Doyen, Barthélemy. *Recueil des Miracles operés au tombeau de M. de Pâris Diacre.* N.p., 1732.

——. *Vie de Monsieur de Pâris, diacre du diocese de Paris.* En France: n.p., 1732.

Du Fossé, Pierre Thomas. *Mémoires pour servir à l'histoire de Port-Royal.* Cologne and Utrecht:Aux Depens de la Compagnie, 1739.

Duguet-Mol, Mme. *Journal historique des Convulsions du tems.* N.p., 1743.

L'Esprit de Persécution de la Cour de Rome sous le Pontificat de Clement XI et de la Cour de France sous le Règne de

Louis Le Grand, contre les Reformez & les Jansénistes. Pampelune: Chez les successeurs de S. Ignace, 1714.

La Faillibilité des papes dans les Decisions dogmatiques démontrée par toute la tradition. 2 vols. N.p., 1720.

Fontaine, Nicolas. *Mémoires pour sevir à l'histoire de Port-Royal.* 2 vols. Utrecht: Aux dépens de la Compagnie, 1736.

Fouillou, Jacques. *Chimère du Jansénisme ou Dissertation sur le sens dans lequel les cinq Propositions ont été condamnées.* N.p., 1708.

——. *Histoire abrégée du Jansénisme, et Remarques sur l'Ordonnance de M. L'Archevêque de Paris.* Cologne: Jean Druckerus, 1698.

——. *Mémoires sur la destruction de l'Abbaye de Port-Royal des Champs.* N.p., 1711.

Fourgon, B. *Jugement équitable sur les convulsions.* Paris: n.p., 1733.

Gerberon, Gabriel. *Histoire générale du Jansénisme, contenant ce qui s'est passé en France, en Espagne, en Italie, dans les pais bas.* 5 vols. Amsterdam: Chez J. Louis De Lorme, 1701.

Goujet, Claude-Pierre. *Mémoires pour servir à l'histoire de Port-Royal.* 3 vols. Paris: N.p., 1734–1737.

Grégoire, Henri. *Oeuvres de l'abbé Grégoire.* Vol. 12, *Les Ruines de Port-Royal en*Paris: Imprimerie-Librairie chrétienne, 1801.

Guilbert, Pierre. *Mémoires historiques et chronologiques sur l'Abbaye de Port-Royal des Champs.* 7 vols. Utrecht: n.p., 1755–1756.

Hecquet, Philippe. *Le Naturalisme des Convulsions dans les Maladies de l'Epidémie Convulsionnaire.* Soleure: Andreas Gymnicus, 1733.

Hermant, Godefroi. *Mémoires de Godefroi Hermant sur l'histoire ecclésiastique du XVIIe siècle (1630–1663).* 6 vols. Edited by A. Gazier. Paris: Plon-Nourrit, 1905–1910.

"Histoire de la Paix des chiens avec les loups: Poeme heureusement Decouvert par un Mandarin de la Société." Peking: Avec Permission de Sa Majesté Chinoise, 1721.

Ilharat de la Chambre, Françoise. *Traité du Formulaire, ou l'on examine à fond l'affaire du Jansénisme quant au fait, & quant au droit.* 4 vols. Utrecht: Nicolas Le Fevre, 1736.

"Instruction en forme de catechisme au sujet de la Bulle Unigenitus." N.p., c. 1724.

Jansénius, Cornelius. *Augustinus; Réforme de l'homme intérieur.* Translated by Robert Arnauld d'Andilly. N.p.: Joannis Berthelin, 1643.

Jurieu, Pierre. *L'Esprit de MR. Arnauld: Tiré de sa conduite & des Ecrits tant de lui que de ses Disciples, particulièrement de l'Apologie pour les Catholiques.* 2 vols. Deventer: Jean Colombius, 1684.

Kural, Roxane. "Contribution à l'Histoire des mentalités de l'Occident pré-industriel: Etude de deux mansucrits de Convulsionnaires Jansénistes du milieu du XVIIIème siècle." TMs (photocopy, 1970–1971). Special Collections, Bibliothèque de l'Histoire du Protestantisme Français, Paris.

Lafitau, Pierre-François. *Histoire de la Constitution Unigenitus.* 2 vols. Liège: Everand Kints, 1738.

Lallemant, Jacques-Philippes. *Jansénius condamné par l'église, par luy-mesme et ses défenseurs, et par S. Augustin.* Bruxelles: François Van den Abbeelen, 1705.

Lancelot, Claude. *Mémoires touchant la vie de Monsieur de Saint-Cyran par M. Lancelot pour servir l'éclaircissement à l'histoire de Port-Royal.* 2 vols. Cologne: Aux dépens de la Compagnie, 1738.

Languet de Gergy, Bishop of Soissons. *Avertissement de Monseigneur l'Evêque de Soissons à ceux qui dans son diocese se sont declarez appellans de la Constitution Unigenitus.* 3 vols. Reims: B. Multeau le jeune, 1718.

Languet, J. "Lettre de L'Abbé des ** à Monseigneur l'Archevesque de Sens sur son Instruction Pastorale." Paris: n.p., 1734.

Leclerc, Pierre, ed. *Histoire des persécutions des Religieuses de Port-Royal, écrites par elles-mêmes.* Villefranche: n.p., 1753.

Le Maistre de Sacy, Isaac-Louis. *Lettres chréstiennes et spirituelles de messire Isaac Louis Le Maistre de Sacy.* 2 vols. Paris: Guillaume Desprez, 1690.

Le Paige, Louis-Adrien and J.B.F. Du Rey de Meinières. *Histoire de la détention du Cardinal de Rets, Archevesque de Paris, et de ses suites.* Vincennes: n.p., 1755.

Mazarin, Jules. *Lettres du cardinal Mazarin pendant son ministère.* 9 vols. Paris: Imprimerie Nationale, 1872–1906.

Mercier, Louis-Sébastien. *Tableau de Paris.* Neufchâtel: Samuel Fauche, 1781. Reprint, Amsterdam: n.p., 1782–1788.

Nicole, Pierre. *Apologie de la Resolution du fameux Cas-de-Conscience, contenue Dans les Ecrits suivants, I. Les*

Imaginaires, II. Les Visionaires, III. De la foi humaine, IV. Jugement equitable, V. Lettre de Messire Nicolas Pavillon, Evêque d'Alet, à Messire Hardouin de Péréfixe, Archêveque de Paris. Cologne: Pierre Marteau, 1704.

——. *Traité de la Prière Divisé en sept Livres.* 2 vols. Paris: Louis Josse et Charles Robustel, 1714.

——. *Traitté de l'éducation d'un prince.* Paris: Chez la veuve Chas. Sarreux, 1671.

Nivelle, Gabriel-Nicolas. *Les Hexaples, ou, Les six colomnes sur la constitution Unigenitus.* 6 vols. Amsterdam: Nicolas Potgieter, 1721.

Nouvelles ecclésiastiques ou Mémoires pour servir à l'histoire ecclésiastique de la Constitution Unigenitus. 24 vols. Paris and Utrecht: n.p., 1728–1803.

Orcibal, Jean, ed. *Correspondance de Jansénius.* Louvain: Bureaux de la Revue, 1947.

Ordonnance et instruction pastorale de Messeigneurs les evesques de Luçon et de La Rochelle, au clergé et au peuple de leurs diocéses, portant condamnation d'un Livre Intitulé Le Nouveau Testament en françois, avec des Réflexions Morales sur chaque verset. Paris: Gregoire Dufuis, 1710.

Pascal, Blaise. *The Provincial Letters, Pensées, Scientific Treatises.* Great Books of the Western World, ed. Robert M. Hutchins, vol. 33. Chicago: Encyclopaedia Britannica, 1952.

Pascal, Jacqueline. *A Rule for Children and Other Writings* [1665]. Edited and translated by John J. Conley. N.p., 1665. Reprint, Chicago and London: University of Chicago Press, 2003.

Patouillet, L. and D. Colonia. *Dictionnaire des Livres jansénistes ou qui favorisent le Jansénisme.* 4 vols. Anvers: Jean-Baptiste Verdussen, 1754.

Pinault, Olivier. *Histoire Abrégée de la Dernière Persecution de Port-Royal.* 3 vols. N.p.: Edition Royale, 1750.

Pirot, Georges. "Extraict de quelques propositions tirées d'un livre intitulé, Apologie pour casuistes contre les calomnies des Jansénistes." Paris: n.p., 1657.

Quesnel, Pasquier. *Deux Actes de l'Appel interjetté de la Constitution Unigenitus Dei Filius au Concile générale.* Amsterdam: Jean Potgieter, 1717.

——. *Histoire abrégée de la vie et des ouvrages de MR. Arnauld.* Cologne: n.p., 1695.

——. *Instructions chrétiennes et élévations à Dieu sur la passion avec les octaves de Pasque, de la Pentecoste, du S. Sacrement de Noel.* Paris: André Pralard, 1702.

——. *Le Nouveau Testament en François avec des Réflexions morales sur chaque verset, pour en rendre la lecture plus utile, & la Meditation plus aisée.* Paris: André Pralard, 1698.

Racine, Jean-Baptiste. *Abrégé de l'histoire de Port-Royal* [written in 1695, first published in 1742]. N.p.: Editions d'aujourdhui, 1981.

Recueil des pièces contre Jansénisme. 2 vols. N.p., 1731–1759. Bibliothèque de l'Histoire du Protestantisme Français.

Recueil des pièces sur la Constitution {Unigenitus}. N.p., 1724–1738. Bibliothèque de l'Histoire du Protestantisme Français.

Recueil des pièces sur l'Affaire de l'Archevêque de Paris. N.p., 1750–1759.

Réflexions sur l'Ordonnance du roi en date du 27 janvier 1732. N.p., 1732.

Règle infaillible pour discerner les vrais des faux miracles. N.p., c. 1730.

Restif de la Bretonne, Nicolas Edme. *Les Nuits de Paris.* London: n.p., 1788.

Tronchay, Michel. *Histoire abrégé de l'abbaye de Port-Royal depuis sa fondation en 1204 jusqu'à 1709.* N.p., 1710.

Secondary Sources

Articles

Adhémar d'Alès, Alphonse. "La théologie du diacre Pâris." *Recherches de science religieuse* 10 (1920):373–87.

Albaric, Fr. Michel. "Une page d'histoire de la presse clandestine: Les Nouvelles Ecclésiastiques, 1728–1803." *Revue française d'histoire du Livre* 26–27 (1980): 319–330.

——. "Regard des jansénistes sur l'Eglise de France de 1780 à 1789 d'après les *Nouvelles Ecclésiastiques*." *Chroniques de Port-Royal* 39 (1990):65–79.

Appolis, Emile. "Une controverse autour d'un 'miracle' janséniste." *Monspeliensis Hippocrates* 44 (1969):20–28.

——. "Les 'miracles' jansénistes dans le Bas-Languedoc (1732–1745)." *Annales du Midi* 67 (1955):269–79.

Armogathe, Jean-Robert. "A propos des miracles de Saint-Médard: Les preuves de Carré de Montgeron et le positivisme des Lumières." *Revue de l'histoire des religions* 180 (1971):135–60.

——. "Le 'Phantôme du Jansénisme' ou la rhétorique de la déviance." In *Vie ecclésiale, communauté et communautés*, 95–106. Paris: Didier-Erudition, 1989.

Arnaud d'Agnel, G. "Les convulsionnaires de Pignans." *Annales du Midi* 19 (1907):206–20.

Basset, Guy. "Eclats de vie d'Henri Arnauld: Rencontres, accords et affrontements." *Chroniques de Port-Royal* 32 (1983):80–100.

Blet, Pierre. "Louis XIV et les Papes aux prises avec le Jansénisme." *Archivum Historiae Pontificiae* 31 (1993):109–92 and 32 (1994):65–148.

——. "Le nonce Nicolo di Bagno et le Jansénisme, 1651–1656." In *La vie, la mort, la foi, le temps.* Edited by Jean-Pierre Barde and Madeleine Foisil. Paris: Presses Universitaires de France, 1993.

Bontoux, Françoise. "Paris janséniste au XVIIIe siècle: Les Nouvelles Ecclésiastiques." *Mémoires de la Fédération des Sociétés historiques et archéologique de Paris et de l'Ile-de-France* 7 (1955):205–20.

Borel, A. "Les convulsionnaires et le diacre Pâris." *L'évolution psychiatrique* 4 (1935): 3–24.

Briggs, Robin. "The Catholic Puritans: Jansenists and Rigorists in France." In *Communities of Belief: Cultural and Social Tension in Early Modern France*, 339–63. Oxford: Clarendon Press, 1989.

Bugnion-Secretan, Perle. "La Mère Angélique Arnauld à Travers ses écrits." *Chroniques de Port-Royal* 37 (1987):75–87.

Burke, Greg. "Modern Miracles Have Strict Rules." *Time Magazine*, 10 April 1995, p. 72.

Campbell, Peter. "Les crises parlementaires et les jansénistes,1727–1740." *Chroniques de Port-Royal* 39 (1990):147–61.

Carreyre, Jean. "La Doctrine janséniste." In *Introduction aux études d'histoire Ecclésiastique locale.* Edited by Victor Carrière, vol. 3:513–39. Paris: Libraire Letouzey et Ané, 1934.

——. "Le quesnellisme." In *Introduction aux études d'histoire cclésiastique locale.* Edited by Victor Carrière, vol. 3:541–89. Paris: Libraire Letouzey et Ané, 1934.

Carrier, Hurbert. "Port-Royal et la Fronde: Deux Mazarinades inconnues d'Arnauld d'Andilly." *Revue d'histoire littéraire de la France* 75 (1975):3–29.

Ceyssens, Lucien. "Autour de la bulle Unigenitus: La Déclaration, dernière illusion et ultime désillusion de Louis XIV." *Revue d'histoire ecclastique* 84 (1989):5–29.

——. "Autour de la bulle Unigenitus: Louis XIV." *Bulletin de l'Institut historique belge de Rome* 55–56 (1985–1986):123–66.

——. "Autour de la bulle 'Unigenitus': Son acceptation par l'Assemblée du Clergé." *Revue d'histoire ecclesiastique* 80 (1985):369–414.

——. "Les Cinq propositions de Jansénius à Rome." *Revue d'histoire ecclésiastique* 66 (1971):449–501, 821–86.

——. "Le jansénisme: Considérations historiques préliminaires à sa notion." *Analecta gregoriana* 71 (1952):3–32.

——. "La lettre circulaire du Port-Royal: un faux indestructible." *Bulletin de l'Institut historique belge de Rome* 43 (1973):509–44.

——. "Que penser finalement de l'histoire du jansénisme et de l'antijansénisme?" *Revue d'Histoire ecclésiastique* 88 (1993):108–30.

Chaunu, Pierre. "Jansénisme et frontière de Catholicité (XVIIe et XVIIIe siècles)." *Revue historique* 227 (1962):115–38.

Chédozeau, Bernard. "Les années de jeunesse de Pierre Nicole et son entrée à Port-Royal, 1625–1654." *XVIIe siècle* 101 (1973):51–69.

——. "Huit lettres de Pierre Nicole fort importantes pour le temps des grandes contestations." *Chroniques de Port-Royal* 30 (1981):3–37.

——. "Idéal intellectuel et vie monastique à Port-Royal." *Chroniques de Port-Royal* 37 (1987):57–74.

——. "Port-Royal et le jansénisme: la revendication d'une autre forme du tridentinisme?" *XVIIe siècle* 171 (1991):119–25.

——. "Port-Royal, les Gallicans et les Politiques à la veille de la *Déclaration des Quatres Articles* (1679–1681)." *Revue des sciences philosophiques et théologiques* 77 (1993):533–46.

Cognet, Louis. "La direction de conscience à Port-Royal." *Supplément de la vie spirituelle* 8 (1955):289–305.

——. "Etat présent des études Port-Royalistes." *Critique* 8 (1952):689–702.

——. "Le mépris du monde à Port-Royal et dans le jansénisme." *Revue d'ascétique et de mystique* 41 (1965):387–402.

"Convulsionnaires à la Bastille (1732)." *Revue retrospective* 10 (1889):140–41.

Cottret, Monique. "Aux origines du républicanisme janséniste: le mythe de l'église primitive et le primitivisme des lumières." *Revue d'histoire moderne et contemporaine* 31 (1984):99–115.

——. "Les jansénistes juges de Jean-Jacques." *Chroniques de Port-Royal* 39 (1990):81–102.

Coward, D. A. "The Fortunes of a Newspaper: the *Nouvelles Ecclésiastiques*, 1728–1803." *British Journal for Eighteenth Century Studies* 4 (1981):1–27.

Dedieu, Joseph. "Le désarroi janséniste pendant la période du quesnellisme." In *Introduction aux études d'histoire ecclésiastique locale*, edited by Victor Carrière, Volume 3: 513–635. Paris: Librairie Letouzey et Ané, 1936.

Daniel, Charles. "Les méthodes de Port-Royal et les jésuites." *Etudes religieuses, philosophiaues, historiques et littéraires* 42 (1880):117–37.

de Dainville, François. "La carte du jansénisme à Paris en 1739, d'après les papiers de la nonciature." *Bulletin de la Société de l'Histoire de Paris et de l'Isle de France* 96 (1969):113–24.

Dedieu, Joseph. "L'agonie du jansénisme (1715–1790): Essai de Bio-Bibliographie." *Revue d'histoire de l'Eglise de France* 14 (1928):161–214.

——. "Un nouveau Port-Royal au diocèse d'Auxerre." *Le Correspondant* 101 (1929):641–61.

de Falguerolles, G. E. "La Tour de Constance dans la lutte pour le rétablissement des libertés de pensée et de réunion." *Bulletin de la société de l'histoire du protestantisme français* 114 (1968):173–291.

de La Brière, Yves. "Le Jansénisme de Jansénius. Etude critique des Cinq Propositions." *Recherches de science religieuse* 6 (1916):270–301.

——. "Les premiers contradicteurs de l'*Augustinus*." *Recherches de science religieuse* 1 (1910):497–99.

de la Tourette, Georges Gilles. "Le miracle opéré sur Marie-Anne Couronneau le 13 juin 1731." *Nouvelle iconographie de la Salpêtrière* 2 (1889):241–50.

de Maricourt, André and Georges Firmin-Didot. "Les Convulsionnaires." *La Nouvelle revue*, 3d series, 54 (1908):356–68.

Denis, Paul. "Quelques lettres de dom Louvard, prisonnier à la Bastille." *Revue Mabillon* 4 (1908–1909):498–525.

Deyon, Pierre. "Perspectives et limites d'une 'sociologie' du jansénisme." *Annales: Economies, Sociétés, Civilisations* 21 (1966):428–34.

Dinet, Dominique. "Le jansénisme et les origines de la déchristianisation au XVIIIe siècle, l'exemple des pays de l'Yonne." In *Du jansénisme à la laicité: Le jansénisme et les origines de la déchristianisation*, edited by Léo Hamon. Paris: Editions de la Maison des Sciences de l'Homme, 1983.

Dominique, Pierre. "Port-Royal et les Jésuites, ou les desseins politiques de deux siècles." *Ecrits de Paris* (February 1966):26–33.

Dubois, Elfrieda T. "A Jesuit History of Jansenism." *The Modern Language Review* 64 (1969):764–73.

Ferguson, Wallace K. "The Place of Jansenism in French History." *Journal of Religion* 7 (1927):16–42.

Ferreyrolles, Gérard. "Jansénius politique: le *Mars Gallicus*." *Actes du colloque de Clermont-Ferrand* (September 1990):95–108.

Gazier, Augustin. "La Bastille en 1743." *Mémoires de la Société de l'histoire de Paris et de l'Ile de France* 7 (1880):11–36.

——. "Les Christs prétendus Jansénistes." *Revue de l'art chrétien* 60 (1910):77–94.

——. "Claude Lancelot d'après sa correspondance inédite (1664–1665)." *Revue hebdomadaire*, 8 August 1908, pp. 193–227.

——. "Le frère de Voltaire (1685–1745)." *Revue des deux mondes* 32 (1906):615–46.

——. "Jean Restout et les miracles du diacre Pâris (1737)." *Revue de l'art chrétien* 62 (1912):117–30.

Golden, Richard M. "The Mentality of Opposition: The Jansenism of the Parisian *Curés* during the Religious Fronde." *The Catholic Historical Review* 64 (1978):565–80.

Grès-Gayer, Jacques. "The Unigenitus of Clement XI: A Fresh Look at the Issues." *Theological Studies* 49 (1988):259–82.

Guitton, Georges. "Le Père François de la Chaize au milieu des intrigues jansénistes." *Nouvelle revue théologique* 74 (1952):160–80.

Haillant, M. "Jansénius et ses défenseurs dans l'*Instruction pastorale* de Fénelon, Archevêque de Cambrai, portant condamnation du *Cas de conscience*, le 10 février de l'an 1701." In *L'Image de C. Jansénius jusqu'à la fin du XVIIIe siècle*. Edited by Edmond J. M. Van Eijl. Leuven: University Press, 1987.

Hamscher, Albert N. "The Parlement of Paris and the Social Interpretation of Early French Jansenism." *The Catholic Historical Review* 63 (July 1977):392–410.

Herman-Belot, Rita. "L'abbé Grégoire et le 'retour des Juifs.'" *Chroniques de Port-Royal* 39 (1990):211–18.

Hudson, David C. "The *Nouvelles ecclésiastiques*: Jansenism and Conciliarism, 1717–1735." *Catholic Historical Review* 70 (1984):389–406.

——. "The Regent, Fleury, Jansenism and the Sorbonne." *French History* 8 (1994):135–48.

Jansen, Paule. "L'Assemblée générale du Clergé de 1655 et l'Affaire janséniste." *Chroniques de Port-Royal* 32 (1983):161–77.

——. "Les Travaux et les jours." *Chroniques de Port-Royal* 37 (1987):45–56.

Janssen, A. "Un Polémiste anti-janséniste. Le Père Fr. Annat, S.J.: Son role dans la condamnation des cinq propositions de l'Augustinus." In *Mélanges d'histoire offerts à Charles Moeller*, 349–58. Louvain and Paris: Van Linthout, 1914.

Judge, H.G. "Church and State under Louis XIV." *History* (UK) 45 (1960):217–33.

——. "Louis XIV and the Church." In *Louis XIV and the Craft of Kingship*. Edited by John C. Rule, 240–64. N.p.: Ohio State University Press, 1969.

Julia, Dominique. "Le catholicisme, religion du royaume (1715–1789)." In *Histoire de la France religieuse*. 4 vols. Edited by Jacques Le Goff and René Rémond. Volume 3: d*u roi Très Chrétien à la laicité républicaine, XVIIIe–XIX siècle,* 11–50. Paris: Editions du Seuil, 1991.

Kostroun, Daniella. "A Formula for Disobedience: Jansenism, Gender and the Feminist Paradox." *Journal of Modern History* 75 (September 2003):483–522.

Kreiser, B. Robert. "Religious Enthusiasm in Early 18th Century Paris—Convulsionaries of Saint-Médard." *Catholic Historical Review* 61, no. 3 (1975):353–85.

Kurland, N. D. "Antoine Arnauld's First Controversy: *De la Fréquente Communion.*" In *The Dawn of Modern Civilization.* Edited by Kenneth A. Strand, 239–51. Ann Arbor: University of Michigan Press, 1962.

Laporte, Jean. "Le Jansénisme." In *Etudes d'histoire de la philosophie française au XVII siècle,* 88–105. Paris: Librairie philosophique J. Vrin, 1951.

Latreille, André. "Innocent XI, Pape 'Janséniste': Directeur de Conscience de Louis XIV." *Cahiers d'Histoire: Publiées par les Universités Clermont-Lyon-Grenoble* 1 (1956):9–39.

Lesaulnier, Jean. "Petite galerie des personnalités familières de Port-Royal." *Chroniques de Port-Royal* 40 (1991):137–83.

Lustiger, Jean-Marie. "Homélie de S. Em. Le Cardinal Jean-Marie Lustiger, 8 septembre 1991." In *La Mère Angélique Arnauld (1591–1661): Relation-Colloque.* Paris: Bibliothèque Mazarine, 1992.

Magnard, Pierre. "Angelique de Saint-Jean ou l'Esprit de resistance." *Chroniques de Port-Royal* 34 (1985):13–32.

——. "De l'obéissance en temps de persecution." *Chroniques de Port-Royal* 37 (1987):89–106.

Maire, Catherine-Laurence. "Agonie religieuse et transfiguration politique du jansénisme." *Chroniques de Port-Royal* 39 (1990):103–14.

——. "L'Eglise et la Nation: Du dépôt de la verité au dépôt des lois—La trajectoire janséniste au XVIIIe siècle." *Annales, Economies, Sociétés, Civilisations* 5 (1991):1177–1205.

——. "Le figurisme: de l'abbé d'Etemare à l'abbé Grégoire." *Politica hermetica* 10 (1996):28–47.

Manneville, Charles-Henri. "Une vieille église de Paris: Saint-Médard." *Bulletin de la Montagne Sainte-Geneviève et ses abords* 4 (1903–1904):3–298.

Marie, Auguste. "Les convulsionnaires de Saint-Médard." *Aesculape* 14 (1924):29–33, 54–58, 86–88.

McGuire, Martin R. P. "Louis-Sébastien Le Nain de Tillemont." *The Catholic Historical Review* 52 (July 1966):186–200.

McKenna, Antony. "Les petites écoles de Port-Royal." *Chroniques de Port-Royal* (1975):13–40.

McManners, John. "Jansenism and Politics in the Eighteenth Century." *Studies in Church History* 12 (1975):253–73.

Merrick, Jeffrey. "Conscience and citizenship in Eighteenth-Century France." *Eighteenth-Century Studies* 21 (1987):48–70.

Mesnard, Jean. "Fideles de Port-Royal en France et en Hollande du XVIIe au XIXe siècle." *Chroniques de Port-Royal* 35 (1986):17–28.

——. "Les séjours de Pascal à Port-Royal des Champs." *Chroniques de Port-Royal* 1 (1951):15–28.

Michel, Marie-José. "Clergé et pastorale jansénistes à Paris (1669–1730)." *Revue d'histoire moderne et contemporaine* 26 (1979):177–97.

Mousset, Alfred. "Un vent de folie au 'siècle des lumières': Les 'miracles' du cimetière Saint-Médard." *Historia* 127 (1957):567–74.

Neveu, Bruno. "Un ami de Port-Royal: Guillaume Du Gué de Bagnols (1616–1657)." *Chroniques de Port-Royal* 15–16 (1966):45–92.

——. "Augustinisme janséniste et magistère romain." *XVIIe siècle* 135 (1982):191–209.

——. "Un Parlementaire parisien érudit et janséniste: Jean Le Nain (1609–1698)." *Paris et Ile-de-France. Mémoires* 16–17 (1965–1966):191–230.

Noir, Julien. "La foi qui guérit à Saint-Médard. A propos d'un portrait du diacre Pâris." *Bulletin de la Montagne Saint-Geneviève et ses abords* 6 (1909–1912):69–82.

Noyon, Augustin. "Un miracle du diacre Pâris: La guérison de l'abbé de Bécherand (1731–1732)." *Etudes* 156 (1918):412–32.

O'Brien, Charles H. "Jansenists and Enlightenment: The Attitude of 'Nouvelles Ecclésiastiques' toward Josephinist Religious Toleration." *Theologische Zeitschrift* 33 (1977):393–407.

——. "Jansénisme et tolérance civile à la veille de la Révolution." *Chroniques de Port-Royal* 39 (1990):131–45.

——. "The Jansenist campaign for Toleration of Protestants in Late Eighteenth Century France: Sacred or Secular?" *Journal of the History of Ideas* 46 (1985):523–38.

Orcibal, Jean. "L'enfance de Racine." *Revue d'histoire littéraire de la France* 51 (1951): 1–16.

——. "Jansénius et Rome." *Actes du colloque sur le jansénisme organisé par l'Academia belgica, Rome, 1973*: Louvain: Editions Nauwelaerts, 1973.

——. "Le premier Port-Royal, réforme ou contre-réforme." *Nouvelle Clio* (1950): 238–80.

Pascal, Pierre. "L'Abbé de Saint-Cyran, les Chartreux et les Solitaires de Port-Royal." *Revue historique* 191 (1941):232–48.

Plainmaison, Jacques. "Pourquoi 'les Provinciales' ou une guerre perdue d'avance." *Revue historique* 287 (1992):61–88.

Plongeron, Bernard. "Une Image de l'Eglise d'après les Nouvelles Ecclésiastiques (1728–1790)." *Revue d'Histoire de l'Eglise de France* 53 (1967):241–68.

Pommier, Jean. "Port-Royal et la Sainte-Epine." *Mercure de France,* 1 March 1956, pp. 437–57.

Préclin, Edmond. "Les conséquences sociales du jansénisme." *Revue d'Histoire de l'Eglise de France* 21 (1935):355–91.

——. "Les conséquences sociales du jansénisme." *Introduction aux études d'histoire ecclésiastique locale* 3 (1936):592–635.

——. "Edmond Richer." *Revue d'histoire moderne* 5 (1930):241–69, 321–36.

Quantin, Jean-Louis. "Port-Royal entre l'histoire et le miracle, de *L'Augustinus* à *la Perpétuité.*" *Chroniques de Port-Royal* 46 (1998):119–36.

Raymond, Marcel. "Du jansénisme à la morale de l'intérêt." *Mercure de France* 330 (June 1957):238–55.Rébelliau, Alfred. "Deux ennemis de la Compagnie du Saint-Sacrement, Molière et Port-Royal." *Revue des Deux-Mondes*, 2d series, 15 octobre 1909, pp. 892–923.

Rech, Gilbert. "D'Aguesseau et le jansénisme." In *Le Chancelier Henri-François D'Aguesseau, 1668–1751*, 119–30. Limoges: Librairie Desvilles, 1953.

Rivaud, Albert. "Claude Lancelot, éducateur janséniste." *Revue des Deux-Mondes,* July 1951, pp. 305–12.

Rocquain, F. "Les Refus de sacrements." *Revue Historique* 15 (1877):241–64.

Sabatier, Auguste. "Port-Royal et le protestantisme." *Révue Chrétienne* 2 (1897):81–95.

Sedgwick, Alexander. "Jansen and the Jansenists: Grace and the Free Will Controversy in 17th Century France." *History Today* 40 (July 1990):36–42.

——. "Seventeenth-Century French Jansenism and the Enlightenment." In *Church, State and Society under the Bourbon Kings*. Edited by Richard M. Golden, 125–47. Lawrence, KS: Coronado Press, 1982.

Sellier, Philippe. "Port-Royal: Un emblème de la Réforme Catholique." *Chroniques de Port-Royal* 37 (1987):15–26.

Shackleton, Robert. "Jansenism and the Enlighenment." *Studies on Voltaire and the Eighteenth Century* 57 (1967):1387–97.

Singham, Shanti-Marie. "Vox populi vox Dei: les jansénistes pendant la révolution Maupeou." *Chroniques de Port-Royal* 39 (1990):183–93.

Swann, Julian. "'Fauteurs de toutes les maximes qui sont contraires à la monarchie': le gouvernement face aux magistrats jansénistes sous Louis XV." *Chroniques de Port-Royal* 39 (1990):163–72.

——. "Parlement, Politics and the *parti janséniste*: the Grand Conseil Affair, 1755–56." *French History* 6 (1992):435–61.

Tallon, Alain. "Prière et charité dans la Compagnie du Saint-Sacrement (1629–1667)." *Histoire économie et société* 10 (1991):331–44.

Tans, J.A.G. "Les Idées politiques des jansénistes." *Neophilologus* 40 (January 1956):1–18.

Taveneaux, René. "Jansénisme et vie sociale en France au XVIIe siècle." *Revue d'Histoire de l'Eglise de France* 54 (1968):27–46.

Tinayre, Marcelle. "Une journée à Port-Royal-des-Champs (1654)." *Revue de Paris* 2 (1902):809–34.

Valet, Paul. "Le diacre Pâris et les convulsionnaires de Saint-Médard." *Bulletin de la Montagne Sainte-Geneviève et ses abords* 2 (1896):343–420.

Van Kley, Dale K. "The Refusal of Sacraments Controversy and the Political Crisis of 1756–57." In *Church, State and Society Under the Bourbon Kings of France.* Edited by Richard M. Golden, 284–326. Lawrence, KS: Coronado Press, 1982.

——. "The Jansenist Constitutional Legacy in the French Prerevolution." In *The French Revolution and the Creation of Modern Political Culture*. Edited by Keith Michael Baker, 169–201. Oxford: Pergamon Press, 1987.

Vinehon, Jean. "Les convulsionnaires de Saint-Médard ont-ils dépassé les limites des pouvoirs humains?" *Etudes carmélitaines* 32 (1953):39–47.

Walgrave, J. "*L'Augustinus* de Jansénius." In *Jansénius et le Jansénisme dans les Pays-Bas*. Edited by J. Van Bavel and M. Schrama, 27–38. Leuven: University Press, 1982.

Weaver, F. Ellen. "Angélique de Saint-Jean: Abbesse et 'Mythographe' de Port-Royal." *Chroniques de Port-Royal* 34 (1985):93–108.

——. "The Bible and Port-Royal." *Cîteaux* 41 (1990):66–100.

——. "Jansenist Bishops and Liturgical-Social Reform." In *Church, State and Society under the Bourbon Kings.* Edited by Richard M. Golden, 24–82. Lawrence, KS: Coronado Press, 1982.

Wilkins, Kay S. "The Treatment of the Supernatural in the *Encyclopédie*." *Studies on Voltaire and the Eighteenth Century* 90 (1972):1757–71.

Williams, William H. "The Significance of Jansenism in the History of the French Catholic Clergy in the Pre-Revolutionary Era." *Studies in Eighteenth-Century Culture* 7 (1978):289–306.

York, Anne. "Religious Aspiration and Janséniste Confrontation." Paper given at the Western Society for French History, Orcas Island, Washington, 15 October 1992.

Books

Abercrombie, Nigel. *The Origins of Jansenism.* Oxford: The Clarendon Press, 1936.

Adam, Antoine. *Du mysticisme à la révolte. Les jansénistes du XVIIe siècle.* Paris: M. Fayard, 1968.

Adams, Geoffrey. *The Huguenots & French Opinion.* Atlantic Highlands, NJ: Humanities Press International, 1991.

Allier, Raoul. *La cabale des dévôts, 1627–1666.* Paris: n.p., 1902. Reprint, Geneva: Slatkine Reprints, 1970.

André, Louis. *Michel Le Tellier et Louvois*, 2d ed. Paris: Armand Colin, 1943.

Andrews, Richard M. *Law, Magistracy, and Crime in Old Regime Paris, 1735–1789.* Volume 1, *The System of Criminal Justice.* Cambridge: Cambridge University Press, 1994.

Aston, Nigel. *The End of An Elite: The French Bishops and the Coming of the Revolution, 1786–1790.* Oxford: Clarendon Press, 1992.

Azéma, Xavier. *Un prélat janséniste, Louis Foucquet, évêque et comte d'Agde, 1656–1702.* Paris: Librairie Philosophique J. Vrin, 1963.
Bachelier, Alcime. *Le Jansénisme à Nantes.* Paris: Librairie Nizet et Bastard, 1934.
Barbiche, Bernard, ed. *Les institution de la monarchie française à l'époque moderne.* Paris: Presses Universitaires de France, 1999.
Barnard, Howard Clive. *The Little Schools of Port-Royal.* Cambridge: Cambridge University Press, 1913.
——. *The Port-Royalists on Education: Extracts from the Educational Writings of the Port-Royalists.* Cambridge: Cambridge University Press, 1918.
Batiffol, Louis. *Biographie du Cardinal de Retz.* Paris: Librairie Hachette, 1929.
Bayrou, François. *Ils portaient l'écharpe blanche: L'aventure des prémiers réformés, des guerres de religion à l'Edit de Nantes, de la Révocation à la Révolution.* Paris: Editions Grasset & Fasquelle, 1998.
Bell, David. *The Cult of the Nation in France: Inventing Nationalism, 1680–1800.* Cambridge, MA: Harvard University Press, 2001.
——. *Lawyers and Citizens: The Making of a Political Elite in Old Regime France.* New York: Oxford University Press, 1994.
Berenguier, Raoul. *Port-Royal et la vallée de Chevreuse.* Paris: Nouvelles Editions Latines, [c. 1962].
Bergeal, C. and A. Durrleman. *Eloge et condemnation de la Révocation de l'Edit de Nantes.* Carrières-sous-Poissey: "La Cause," 1985.
Bergin, Joseph. *Crown, Church and Episcopate under Louis XIV.* New Haven and London: Yale University Press, 2004.
Bertière, Simone. *Les Reines de France au temps des Bourbons: Les Femmes du Roi-Soleil.* Paris: Editions de Fallois, 1998.
Blanc, Hippolyte. *Le Merveilleux dans le Jansénisme, le magnetisme, le Methodisme, et le Baptisme americains, l'épidémie de Morzine, le spiritisme.* Paris: Henri Plon, 1865.
Blet, Pierre. *Le Clergé de France: Louis XIV et le Saint-Siège de 1695 à 1715.* Vatican: Archivio Vaticano, 1989.
Bluche, François. *Les Magistrats du parlement de Paris au XVIIIe siècle (1715–1771).* Annales Littéraires de l'Université de Besançon, volume 35. Paris: Les Belles Lettres, 1960.
——. *Le Journal secret de Louis XIV.* Paris: Editions du Rocher, 1998.
Bonnot, Isabelle. *Hérétique ou saint? Henry Arnauld, évêque janséniste d'Angers au XVIIe siècle.* Paris: Nouvelles Editions Latines, 1984.
Bordonove, Georges. *Les Rois qui ont fait la France: Les Bourbons.* Volume 3, *Louis XIV.* Paris: Pygmalion, 1982.
Borella, Luisa. *Plaidoyer pour Arnauld. Lecture des trois premières 'Provinciales' de Pascal.* Parme: Edizioni Universitaire, 1988.
Bourlon, I. *Les Assemblées du Clergé et le Jansénisme.* Paris: Bloud, 1909.
Bournet, Léon. *La querelle janséniste.* Paris: Pierre Téqui, 1924.
Boysse, Ernest. *Le Théâtre des Jésuites.* Paris: n.p., 1880. Reprint, Geneva: Slatkine Reprints, 1970.
Bremond, H. *Histoire littéraire du sentiment religieux en France.* Volume 4, *L'école de Port-Royal.* Paris: Bloud, 1923.
Brongniart, Marcel. *La Paroisse Saint-Médard au faubourg Saint-Marceau.* Paris: A. et J. Picard, 1951.
Browning, William Shipton. *History of the Huguenots, from 1598 to 1838.* London: W. Pickering, 1839.
Bruggeman, J. and A. J. Van de ven. *Inventaire des pièces d'archives françaises se rapportant à l'abbaye de Port-Royal-des-Champs et son cercle et à la résistance contre la bulle Unigenitus et à l'appel.* La Haye: Martinus Nijhoff, 1972.
Bruneau, Marie-Florine. *Racine, le jansénisme et la modernité.* Paris: José Corti, 1986.
Bugnion-Secretan, Perle. *La Mère Angélique Arnauld (1591–1661), d'après ses écrits: Abbesse et réformatrice de Port-Royal.* Paris: Les éditions du Cerf, 1991.
Cabourdin, Guy and Georges Viard, eds. *Lexique historique de la France d'Ancien Régime*, 2d ed. Paris: Armand Colin, 1990.
Cadet, Felix. *L'éducation à Port-Royal.* Paris: Librairie Hachette, 1887.
Cahen, Léon. *Les Querelles religieuses et parlementaires sous Louis XV.* Paris: Hachette, 1913.
Calmeil, Louis-Florentin. *De la Folie considerée sous le point de vue pathologique, philosophique, historique et judiciaire.* Paris: J.-B. Baillière, 1845.

Calot, François and Louis-Marie Michon. *Port-Royal et le Jansénisme.* Paris: Albert Morancé, 1928.

Carr, Thomas M. *Voix des Abbesses du Grand Siècle: La Prédication au féminin à Port-Royal, Contexte rhétorique et Dossier.* Tubingen: Gunter Narr Verlag, 2006.

Carreyre, Jean. *Le Jansénisme durant la Régence.* 3 volumes. Louvain: Bureau de la Revue, 1929–1933.

Carrière, Victor, ed. *Introduction aux études d'histoire ecclésiastique locale.* Vol. 3, *Questions d'histoire générale à développer dans le cadre régional au diocèseain.* Paris: Libraire Letouzey et Ané, 1936.

Ceyssens, Lucien. *Le sort de la bulle Unigenitus: recueil d'études offert à Lucien Ceyssens à l'occasion de son 90e anniversaire.* Leuven, Belgium: Leuven University Press, Uitgeverij Peeters, 1992.

Ceyssens, Lucien and Tans, Joseph A. G. *Autour de l'Unigenitus: Recherches sur la genèse de la constitution.* Leuven, Belgium: Leuven University Press, 1987.

Chaunu, Pierre, Madeleine Foisil, and Françoise de Noirfontaine. *Le basculement religieux de Paris au XVIIIe siècle.* Paris: Fayard, 1998.

Choudhury, Mita. *Convents and Nuns in Eighteenth-Century French Politics and Culture.* Ithaca, NY: Cornell University Press, 2004.

Clark, Ruth. *Strangers & Sojourners at Port-Royal.* Cambridge: University Press, 1932.

Cochin, Claude. *Henry Arnauld, evêque d'Angers, 1597–1692.* Paris: Auguste Picard, 1921.

Cognet, Louis. *Claude Lancelot, Solitaire de Port-Royal.* Paris: Editions Sulliver, 1950.

——. *Le Jansénisme.* Paris: Presses Universitaires de France, 1961.

——. *La Mère Angélique et Saint François de Sales, 1618–1626.* Paris: Editions Sulliver, 1951.

——. *La Réforme de Port-Royal, 1591–1618.* Paris: Editions Sulliver, 1950.

Conley, John J. *The Suspicion of Virtue: Women Philosophers in Neoclassical France.* Ithaca and London: Cornell University Press, 2002.

Coquerel, Athanase. *Les forçats pour la foi. Etude historique (1684–1775).* Paris: Michel Lévy Frères, 1866.

Corvisier, André. *Louvois.* Paris: Fayard, 1983.

Cottret, Monique. *Jansénismes et Lumières: Pour un autre XVIIIe siècle.* Paris: Editions Albin Michel, 1998.

Crahay, Roland, ed. *La tolérance civile.* Bruxelles: Université de Bruxelles, 1982.

Crichton, J.D. *Saints or Sinners? Jansenism and Jansenisers in Seventeenth Century France.* Dublin: Veritas Publications, Criterion Press, 1996.

Cristiani, Chanoine. *L'hérésie de Port-Royal.* Paris: Arthème Fayard, 1955.

Dall, Guillaume. *La Mère Angélique, abbesse de Port-Royal, d'après sa correspondance.* Paris: Librairie Académique Didier, 1893.

Dawson, Nelson-Martin. *Crise d'autorité et clientélisme: Mgr. Jean Joseph Languet de Gergy et la Bulle Unigenitus.* Sherbrooke, Quebec: Editions Les Fous du roi, 1997.

de Barthélemy, Edouard. *Le cardinal de Noailles, evêque de Châlons, archevêque de Paris, d'après sa correspondance inédite, 1651–1728.* Paris: Léon Techener, 1886.

de Courcelles, Dominique. *Le Sang de Port-Royal.* Edited by de l'Herne. Paris: l'Herne, 1994.de Lacombe, Bernard Mercier. *La résistance janséniste et parlementaire au temps de Louis XV: l'abbé Nigon de Berty, 1702–1772.* Paris: Société du Grand Armorial de France, 1948.

de Montherlant, Henry. *Port-Royal.* Edited by Robert Hagspiel. Paris: n.p., 1954. Reprint, Engelwood Cliffs, NJ: Prentice-Hall, 1967.

Dedieu, Joseph. *L'Agonie du Jansénisme, 1715–1790.* Paris: Société d'histoire ecclésiastique de la France, 1928.

Delassault, Geneviève, ed. *Choix des lettres inédites de Louis-Isaac Le Maistre de Sacy, 1650–1683.* Paris: Librairie Nizet, 1959.

——. *Le Maistre de Sacy et son temps.* Paris: Librairie Nizet, 1957.

Delforge, Frédéric. *Les petites écoles de Port-Royal, 1637–1660.* Paris: Les Editions du Cerf, 1985.

Delmont, Théodore. *Bossuet et le Jansénisme d'après les plus récentes publications.* Arras: Sueur-Charruey, 1899.

de Meyer, Albert. *Les Premières Controverses jansénistes en France, 1640–1649.* Louvain: Imprimerie Veuve Joseph Van Linthout, 1917.

de Sars, Marie-Elisabeth-Edmond Maxime. *Le Cardinal de Fleury: Apôtre de la Paix.* Paris: Hachette, 1942.

Desdevises du Dézert, Georges. *L'Eglise & l'Etat en France, depuis l'Edit de Nantes jusqu'au concordat.* 2 vols. Paris: Société française imprimerie et de librairie, 1907–1908.

Deslandres, P. *Histoire de l'église catholique en France.* Paris: Bloud et Gay, 1913.

Deux siècles de jansénisme: à travers les documents du fonds Port-Royal d'Utrecht. Paris: Archives Nationales, 1974.

Diefendorf, Barbara. *From Penitence to Charity: Pious Women and the Catholic Reformation in Paris.* New York: Oxford University Press, 2004.

Dorival, Bernard. *Pascal et les Provinciales. Catalogue de l'exposition du Musée national des Granges de Port-Royal.* Paris: Editions des Musées nationaux, 1963.

Doyle, William. *Jansenism: Catholic Resistance to Authority from the Reformation to the French Revolution.* New York: St. Martin's Press, 2000.

Duinker, Anna Catharina Marie. *Claude de Sainte-Marthe, prêtre et confesseur de Port-Royal.* Haarlem, Netherlands: N/V H.D. TjeenkWillink, 1932.

Dunn, Marilynn. *The Emergence of Monasticism: From the Desert Fathers to the Early Middle Ages.* Melden, MA: Blackwell Publishers, 2000.

Durand, Valentin. *Le jansénisme au XVIIIe siècle et J. Colbert, évêque de Montpellier,* Toulouse: Librairie Edouard Privat, 1907.

Echeverria, Durand. *The Maupeou Revolution: A Study in the History of Libertarianism, France, 1770–1774.* Baton Rouge: Louisiana State University Press, 1985.

Egret, Jean. *Louis XV et l'opposition parlementaire, 1715–1774.* Paris: Armand Colin, 1970.

Escholier, Marc. *Port-Royal: The Drama of the Jansenists.* New York: Hawthorn Books, 1968.

Farge, Arlette. *Subversive Words: Public Opinion in Eighteenth-Century France.* Translated by Rosemary Morris. University Park, PA: Pennsylvania State University Press, 1994.

Fargues, Paul. *Histoire du Christianisme.* Volume 5, *De l'Edit de Nantes à la Révolution.* Paris: Librairie Fischbacher, 1938.

Finot, Ed. *Port-Royal et Magny.* Paris: Georges Chamerot, 1888.

Flammermont, Jules, ed. *Remonstrances du Parlement de Paris au XVIII siècle.* Volume 1, *1715–1753.* Paris: Imprimerie Nationale, 1888–1898.

Forrestal, Alison. *Fathers, Pastors and Kings: Visions of Episcopacy in Seventeenth-Century France.* Manchester and New York: Manchester University Press, 2004.

Fouqueray, Henry. *Histoire de la Compagnie de Jésus en France des origines à la suppression, 1528–1762.* 5 vols. Paris: Bureaux des Etudes, 1910–1925.

Fraigneau, André. *Port-Royal des Champs.* Paris: Editions Sun, 1949.

Frencken, J. L. A. A. *Agnès Arnauld.* Nimègue-Utrecht: N. V. Dekker en Van de Vigt en J.. van Leeuwen, 1932.

Fuzet, Edmond Frédéric. *Les Jansénistes du XVIIe siècle; leur histoire et leur dernier historien, M. Sainte-Beuve.* Paris: Bray et Retaux, 1876.

Gagnol, Père. *Le Jansénisme convulsionnaire et l'affaire de la Planchette (1747) d'après les Archives de la Bastille.* Paris: Libraire générale catholique, 1911.

Galland, Jacques Alfred. *Essai sur l'histoire du protestantisme à Caen et en Basse-Normandie, de l'Edit de Nantes à la Révolution.* Paris: Société d'Histoire du Protestantisme en Normandie, 1898.

Garrioch, David. *The Making of Revolutionary Paris.* Los Angeles: University of California Press, 2002.

Gastelier, Fabian. *Angélique Arnauld.* Paris: Librairie Arthème Fayard, 1998.

Gazier, Augustin. *Les Dernières années du cardinal de Retz (1655–1679): Etude historique et littéraire.* Paris: Ernest Thorin, éditeur, 1875.

——. *Histoire générale du mouvement janséniste depuis ses origines jusqu'à nos jours.* 2 vols. Paris: Librairie Ancienne Honoré Champion, 1924.

——. *Jeanne de Chantal et Angélique Arnauld d'après leur correspondance, 1620–1641.* Paris: Librairie Ancienne Honoré Champion, 1915.

Gazier, Cécile. *Les Belles amies de Port-Royal.* Paris: Perrin et Cie, 1930.

——. *Histoire de la Société et de la Bibliothèque de Port-Royal.* Paris: Presses Universitaires de France, 1966.

——. *Histoire du monastère de Port-Royal.* Paris: Perrin, 1929.

——. *Ces Messieurs de Port-Royal.* Paris: Perrin, 1932.

Godard, Philippe. *La querelle des refus des sacrements (1730–1765).* Paris: Domat-Montchrestien, 1937.

Godart, Justin. *Le jansénisme à Lyon; Benôit Fourgon, 1687–1773.* Paris: Félix Alcan, 1934.

Golden, Richard M. *The Godly Rebellion. Parisian Curés and the Religious Fronde.* Chapel Hill, NC: University of North Carolina Press, 1981.

Goldmann, Lucien, ed. *Correspondance de Martin de Barcos, abbé de Saint-Cyran, avec les abbesses de Port-Royal et les principaux personnages du groupe janséniste.* Paris: Presses Universitaires de France, 1956.

——. *Le Dieu caché* [*The Hidden God*]. Translanted by Philip Thody. Paris: Gallimard, 1955. Reprint, New York: The Humanities Press, 1964.

Goubert, Pierre. *Louis XIV and Twenty Million Frenchmen.* New York: Vintage Books, 1966.

——. *Mazarin.* Paris: Fayard, 1990.

Grégoire, Bishop. *Histoire des sectes religieuses,* 2d ed. Paris: Baudouin Frères, 1828.

Grès-Gayer, Jacques M. *Le Gallicanisme de Sorbonne: Chroniques de la Faculté de Théologie de Paris, 1657–1688.* Paris: Honoré Champion, 2002.

——*Le Jansénisme en Sorbonne, 1643–1656.* Paris: Klincksieck, 1996.

——. *Théologie et pouvoir en Sorbonne. La Faculté de théologie de Paris et la bulle Unigenitus, 1714–1721.* Paris: Klincksieck, 1991.

Grosclaude, Pierre. *Malesherbes. Témoin et interprète de son temps.* Paris: Librairie Fischbacher, 1961.

Guitton, Georges. *Le Père de la Chaize, confesseur de Louis XIV.* 2 vols. Paris: Beauchesne et ses fils, 1959.

Hallays, André. *Le pélerinage de Port-Royal.* Paris: Libraire Academique Perrin, 1914.

——. *Les solitaires de Port-Royal.* Paris: Plon, 1927.

Hamscher, Albert N. *The Parlement of Paris After the Fronde, 1653–1673.* Pittsburgh, PA: University of Pittsburgh Press, 1976.

Hardy, Georges. *Le cardinal de Fleury et le mouvement janséniste.* Paris: Honoré Champion, 1925.

Haynes, Renée. *Philosopher King: The Humanist Pope Benedict XIV.* London: Weidenfeld and Nicolson, 1970.

Hearsey, John. *Voltaire.* New York: Barnes & Noble, 1976.

Hildesheimer, Françoise. *Le Jansénisme en France au XVII et XVIIIe siècles.* Paris: Publisud, 1991.

——. *Le Jansénisme: l'histoire et l'héritage.* Paris: Desclée de Brouzer, 1992.

[Hohl, Claude]. *Le Jansénisme dans l'Yonne.* Auxerre, France: Archives départmentales de l'Yonne, 1986.

Jaccard, L.-Frédéric. *Saint-Cyran, précurseur de Pascal.* Lausanne: Editions La Concorde, 1945.

Jacques, Emile. *Les années d'exil d'Antoine Arnauld, 1679–1694.* Louvain: Publications universitaires de Louvain, 1976.

James, Edward Donald. *Pierre Nicole, Jansenist and Humanist: A Study of His Thought.* The Hague: Martinus Nijhoff, 1972.

Jansen, Paule. *Arnauld d'Andilly, défenseur de Port-Royal (1654–1659): Sa correspondance inédite avec la Cour conservée dans les Archives du Ministère des Affaires Etrangères.* Paris: Libraire philosophique J. Vrin, 1973.

——. *Le Cardinal Mazarin et le mouvement janséniste français, 1653–1659.* Paris: Libraire philosophique J. Vrin, 1967.

Knox, R. A. *Enthusiasm: A Chapter in the History of Religion with Special Reference to the XVII and XVIII Centuries.* Oxford: n.p., 1950. Reprint, Westminster, MD: Christian Classics, 1983.

Kolakowski, Leszek. *God Owes Us Nothing: A Brief Remark on Pascal's Religion and on the Spirit of Jansenism.* Chicago and London: University of Chicago Press, 1995.

Kreiser, B. Robert. *Miracles, Convulsions, and Ecclesiastical Politics in Early Eighteenth Century Paris.* Princeton: Princeton University Press, 1978.

Langlois, Marcel. *Madame de Maintenon.* Paris: Plon, 1932.

Laporte, Jean-Pierre. *La Doctrine de Port-Royal: Essai sur la formation et le développement de la doctrine: Saint-Cyran.* 2 vols. Paris: Presses Universitaires de France, 1923.

——. *La Doctrine de Port-Royal: La morale, d'après Arnauld.* 2 vols. Paris: Libraire Philosophique J. Vrin, 1951–1952.

——. *Saint-Cyran.* Paris: Presses Universitaires de France, 1922.

Lefebvre, Henri. *Pascal.* 2 vols. Paris: Les éditions Nagel, 1949.

Legier Desgranges, Henry. *Du Jansénisme à la Révolution, Mme. de Moysan et l'extravagante affaire de l'Hôpital Général.* Paris: Hachette, 1954.

Le Goff, Jacques and René Rémond. *Histoire de la France religieuse.* Ed. François Lebrun. Volume 2, *Du Christianisme flamboyant à l'aube des Lumières (XIVe–XVIIIe siècle).* Paris: Editions du Seuil, 1988.

Le Roy, Albert. *Un Janséniste en exil: Correspondance de Pasquier Quesnel, prêtre de l'Oratoire, sur les affaires politiques et religieuses de son temps.* 2 vols. Paris: Librairie Academique Perrin, 1900.

Lesaulnier, Jean. *Images de Port-Royal.* Paris: Nolin, 2002.

Levi, Anthony. *Cardinal Richelieu and the Making of France.* New York: Carroll and Graf, 2000.

——. *Louis XIV.* New York: Carroll & Graf, 2004.

Lewis, W. H. *The Splendid Century: Life in the France of Louis XIV.* N.p.: William Morrow, 1954.

Lhermitte, Jean. *Le problème des miracles*, 7th ed. Paris: Gallimard, 1956.

Lossky, Andrew. *Louis XIV and the French Monarchy.* New Brunswick, NJ: Rutgers University Press, 1994.

Loupès, Philippe. *La vie religieuse en France au XVIIIe siècle.* Paris: SEDES, 1993.

Lowndes, M.E. *The Nuns of Port-Royal as Seen in Their Own Narratives.* Oxford: Oxford University Press, 1909.

Lusebrink, Hans-Jurgen and Rolf Reichardt. *The Bastille: A History of a Symbol of Despotism and Freedom.* Translated by Norbert Schurer. Durham, NC: Duke University Press, 1997.

Maire, Catherine-Laurence. *De la cause de Dieu à la cause de la Nation: Le jansénisme au XVIIIe siècle.* Paris: Editions Gallimard, 1998.

——. *Les convulsionnaires de Saint-Médard: Miracles, Convulsions et prophéties à Paris au XVIIIe siècle.* Paris: Gallimard, Julliard, 1985.

Marion, Marcel. *Dictionnaire des Institutions de la France aux XVIIe et XVIIIe siècles.* Paris: n.p., 1923. Reprint, Paris: Editions A. & J. Picard, 1972.

Martin, Henri-Jean. *The French Book: Religion, Absolutism, and Readership, 1585.* Translated by Paul Saenger and Nadine Saenger. Geneva: n.p., 1969. Reprint, Baltimore and London: The Johns Hopkins University Press, 1996.

Mathieu, Pierre-François. *Histoire des miraculés et des convulsionnaires de Saint-Médard.* Paris: Didier, 1864.

Maulvault, Achille. *Répertoire alphabétique des personnes et des choses de Port-Royale.* Paris: Honoré Champion, 1902.

McManners, John. *Church and Society in Eighteenth Century France.* Vol. 1, *The Clerical Establishment and Its Social Ramifications*; Vol. 2, *The Religion of the People and the Politics of Religion.* Oxford: Clarendon Press, 1998.

——. *French Ecclesiastical Society under the Ancien Régime. A Study of Angers in the Eighteenth Century.* Manchester: Manchester University Press, 1960.

Melton, James Van Horn. *The Rise of the Public in Enlightenment Europe.* Cambridge and New York: Cambridge University Press, 2001.

Merrick, Jeffrey W. *The Desacralization of the French Monarchy in the Eighteenth Century.* Baton Rouge, LA: Louisiana State University, 1990.

Mesnard, Jean. *Pascal et les Roannez.* 2 vols. Paris: Desçlée de Brouwer, 1965.

——. *Pascal, His Life and Works.* New York: Philosophical Library, 1952.

Mettam, Roger. *Power and Faction in Louis XIV's France.* New York: Basil Blackwell, 1988.

Michel, Jacqueline. *"L'aventure janséniste" dans l'oeuvre de Henry de Montherlant.* Paris: A. G. Nizet, 1976.

Michel, Marie-José. *Jansénisme et Paris, 1640–1730.* N.p.: Klincksieck, 2000.

Minois, Georges. *Le confesseur du roi: Les directeurs de conscience sous la monarchie français.* Paris: Fayard, 1988.

Mitford, Nancy. *The Sun King.* New York: Harper & Row, 1966.

Monthéard, Thérèse. *Le Guide de la vallée de Chevreuse et de Port-Royal.* Besançon: Editions de la Manufacture, 1992.

Mousnier, Roland et al., eds. *Le Conseil du roi, de Louis XII à la Révolution.* Paris: Presses Universitaires de France, 1970.

Mousset, Albert. *L'étrange histoire des convulsionnaires de Saint-Médard.* Paris: Editions de Minuit, 1953.

Muchembled, Robert, Anne Conchon, Bruno Maes, and Isabelle Paresys, eds. *Dictionnaire de l'Ancien Régime.* Paris: Armand Colin, 2004.

Namer, Gérard. *L'Abbé Leroy et ses amis: Essai sur le Jansénisme extrémiste intramondain.* Paris: SEVPEN, 1964.

Necheles, Ruth F. *The Abbé Grégoire, 1787–1831: The Odyssey of An Egalitarian.* Westport, CT: Greenwood Publishing, 1971.

Neveu, Bruno. *Erudition et religion aux XVIIe et XVIIIe siècles.* Paris: Editions Albin Michel, 1994.

——. *Un historien à l'école de Port-Royal: Sébastien LeNain de Tillemont, 1637.* La Haye: Martinus Nijhoff, 1966.

Newton, William Ritchey. *Sociologie de la communauté de Port-Royal, Histoire, économie.* Paris: Klincksieck, Collection "Port-Royal," 1999.

Nora, Pierre, ed. *Realms of Memory: Rethinking the French Past.* Volume 1, *Conflicts and Divisions.* New York: Columbia University Press, 1966.

O'Connell, Marvin R. *Blaise Pascal: Reasons of the Heart.* Library of Religious Biography. Edited by Mark A. Noll, Nathan O. Hatch, Allen C. Guelzo. Grand Rapids, MI: William B. Eerdmans, 1997.

Ogg, David. *Europe of the Ancien Regime, 1715–1783.* New York: Harper Torchbooks, 1965.

Orcibal, Jean. *Jansénius d'Ypres (1585–1638).* Paris: Etudes Augustiniennes, 1989.

——. *Louis XIV contre Innocent XI. Les appels au futur concile de 1688 et l'opinion française.* Paris: Librairie Philosophique J. Vrin, 1949.

——. *Les Origines de Jansénisme.* Volume 3, *Jean Duvergier de Hauranne, abbé de Saint-Cyran et son temps, 1581–1638.* Paris: Librairie Philosophique J. Vrin, 1948.

——. *Port-Royal entre le miracle et l'obéissance: Flavie Passart et Angélique de Saint-Jean Arnauld d'Andilly.* Paris: Desclée de Brouwer, 1957.

______. *Saint-Cyran et le jansénisme.* Paris: Editions du Seuil, 1961.

Palmer, Robert R. *Catholics and Unbelievers in Eighteenth-Century France.* Princeton, NJ: n.p., 1939. Reprint, New York: Cooper Square Publishers, 1961.

Paquier, Jules. *Le Jansénisme.* Paris: Librairie Bloud, 1909.

Paradis, Edouard. *La Pédagogie janséniste comparée à la pédagogie catholique.* Lyon and Paris: Librairie Catholique Emmanuel Vitte, 1910.

Parguez, Jacques. *La bulle Unigenitus et le Jansénisme politique: Avant-coureur de la Révolution Française.* Paris: Librairie Maurice Glomeau, 1936.

Parker, David. *The Making of French Absolutism.* New York: St. Martin's Press, 1983.

Parsons, Jotham. *The Church in the Republic: Gallicanism and Political Ideology in Renaissance France.* Washington, DC: Catholic University of America Press, 2004.

Pensa, Henri. *Sorcellerie et religion: Du désordre dans les esprits et dans les moeurs aux XVIIe et XVIIIe siècles.* Paris: Librairie Felix Alcan, 1933.

Perruchot, Henri. *Port-Royal.* Paris: Livre de Paris, 1947.

Pevitt, Christine. *The Man Who Would Be King: The Life of Philippe d'Orléans, Regent of France, 1674–1723.* London: Weidenfeld and Nicolson, 1997.

Phillips, Henry. *Church and Culture in Seventeenth-Century France.* Cambridge: Cambridge University Press, 1997.

Pillorget, Suzanne. *Claude-Henri Feydeau de Marville, Lieutenant-général de police.* Paris: Editions Pedone, 1978.

Poulet, Charles. *Histoire de l'église de France.* 3 vols. Paris: Beauchesne, 1946–1949.

Préclin, Edmond. *Sébastien Zamet, sa vie et ses oeuvres: Les origines du Jansénisme.* Paris: Librairie Alphonse Picard et Fils, 1912.

Préclin, Edmond and Eugène Jarry. *Les luttes politiques et doctrinales aux XVII et XVIIIe siècle,* vol. 19. In *Histoire de l'Eglise depuis les origines jusqu'à nos jours.* Edited by Augustin Fliche and Victor Martin. Paris: Bloud & Gay, 1955–1956.

Prince Michael of Greece. *Louis XIV: The Other Side of the Sun.* Translated by Alan Sheridan. New York: Harper & Row, 1983.

Prunel, Louis. *Sébastien Zamet, évêque, duc de Langres, pair de France (1588–1655). Sa vie et ses oeuvres.* Paris: Thèse, Librairie Alphonse Picard, 1912.

Quantin, Jean-Louis. *Le Catholicisme classique et les Pères de l'Eglise: Un retour aux sources, 1669–1713.* Paris: Institut d'Etudes Augustiniennes, 1999.

Quétal, Claude. *De Par Le Roy: Essai sur les lettres de cachet.* Toulouse: Privat Editeur, 1981.

Rapley, Elizabeth. *The Dévotes: Women and Church in Seventeenth-Century France.* Montreal and Kingston: McGill–Queen's University Press, 1990.

——. *A Social History of the Cloister: Daily Life in the Teaching Monasteries of the Old Regime.* Montreal and Kingston: McGill–Queen's University Press, 2001.

Ravaisson-Mollien, François. *Archives de la Bastille.* Volume 14, *Règne de Louis XV (1726 à 1737).* Paris: n.p., 1866–1884. Reprint, Genève: Slatkine-Megariotis Reprints, 1975.

Ravitch, Norman. *Sword and Mitre: Government and Episcopate in France and England in the Age of Aristocracy.* The Hague: Mouton, 1966.

Rea, Lilian. *The Enthusiasts of Port-Royal.* New York: Scribners, 1912.

Rébelliau, Alfred. *Bossuet.* Paris: Hacette, 1900.

Régnault, Emile. *Christophe de Beaumont, archevêque de Paris, 1703–1781.* 2 vols. Paris: Librairie Victor Lecoffre, 1882.

Remsberg, Robert. *Wisdom and Science at Port-Royal and the Oratory: A Study of Contrasting Augustinianisms.* Yellow Springs, OH: Antioch Press, 1940.

Ricard, Antoine. *Les premiers Jansénistes et Port-Royal.* Paris: E. Plon, 1883.

Richardt, Aimé. *Le Jansénisme de Jansénius à la mort de Louis XIV.* Paris: François-Xavier de Guibert, 2002.

Rogelet, Christine. *Port-Royal des Champs en notre temps.* Paris: Eiditions du Temps, 1969.

Rogister, John. *Louis XV and the Parlement of Paris, 1737–1755.* Cambridge: Cambridge University Press, 1995.

Romanes, Ethel. *The Story of Port-Royal.* London: John Murray, 1907.

Sainte-Beuve, Charles. *Port-Royal.* 7 vols. 3d ed. Paris: Hachette, 1867.

Salmon, J. H. M. *Cardinal de Retz: The Anatomy of a Conspirator.* New York: The Macmillan Company, 1969.

Schimmelpenninck, Mary Anne. *Narrative of the Demolition of the Monastery of Port-Royal des Champs, Including Biographical Memoirs of Its Latter Inhabitants.* London: J. and A. Arch, 1816.

——. *Select Memoirs of Port-Royal.* 2 vols. 5th ed. Philadelphia: Henry Longstretch, 1853.

Séché, Léon. *Les derniers Jansénistes depuis la ruine de Port-Royal jusqu'à nos jours, 1710–1870.* 3 vols. Paris: Perrin et Cie, 1891.

Sedgwick, Alexander. *Jansenism in Seventeenth-Century France: Voices from the Wilderness.* Charlottesville: University Press of Virginia, 1977.

——. *The Travails of Conscience: The Arnauld Family and the Ancien Régime.* Cambridge, MA: Harvard University Press, 1998.

Shennon, J. H. *Louis XIV.* London: Routledge, 1986.

Shiokawa, Tetsuya. *Pascal et les miracles.* Paris: Librairie A.-G. Nizet, 1977.

Smith, David L., ed. *Louis XIV.* Cambridge: Cambridge University Press, 1992.

Sonnino, Paul. *Louis XIV's View of the Papacy (1661–1667).* Berkeley: University of California Press, 1966.

——, ed. and trans. *Louis XIV: Mémoires for the Instruction of the Dauphin.* New York: Free Press, 1970.

Speake, Jennifer and Thomas G. Bergin, eds. *Encyclopedia of the Renaissance and the Reformation.* Aylesbury, United Kingdom: Market House Books Ltd., 2004.

Strayer, Brian E. *Huguenots and Camisards as Aliens in France, 1598–1789.* Lewiston, NY: Edwin Mellen Press, 2001.

——. *Lettres de cachet and Social Control in the Ancien Régime, 1659–1789.* New York: Peter Lang, 1992.

Swann, Julian. *Politics and the Parlement of Paris under Louis XV, 1754–1774.* Cambridge: Cambridge University Press, 1995.

Tackett, Timothy. *Becoming a Revolutionary: The Deputies of the French National Assembly and the Emergence of a Revolutionary Culture, 1789–1790.* Princeton, NJ: Princeton University Press, 1996.

Tans, J.A.G., ed. *Pasquier Quesnel et les Pays-Bas: Correspondance publiée avec introduction et annotations.* Paris: Librairie Vrin, 1960.

Tans, J.A.G. and H. Schmitz du Moulin, eds. *La Correspondance de Pasquier Quesnel, inventaire et index analytique.* 2 vols. Bruxelles: Editions Nauwelaerts, 1989.

Tans, J.A.G. and H. Schmitz du Moulin. *Pasquier Quesnel devant la Congregation de l'Index.* La Haye: Martinus Nijhoff, 1974.

Tapié, Victor-L. *France in the Age of Louis XIII and Richelieu.* Translated and edited by D. McN. Lockie. New York: Praeger Publishers, 1975.

Taveneaux, René. *Le Catholicisme dans la France classique, 1610–1715.* 2 vols. Paris: Société d'Edition d'Enseignement Superieur, 1994.

——. *Jansénisme et politique.* Paris: Armand Colin, 1965.

——. *Jansénisme et Réforme catholique.* Nancy: Presses Universitaires de Nancy, 1992.

——. *La Vie quotidienne des jansénistes aux XVIIe et XVIIIe siècles.* Paris: Hachette, 1973.

Thibout, Marc. *Saint-Médard: Nefs et clochers.* Paris: Musée nationaux, 1947.

Thomas, Jacques-François. *La Querelle de l'Unigenitus.* Paris: Presses Universitaires de France, 1950.

Tollemache, Marguerite. *French Jansenists.* London: Kegan Paul, Trench, Trubner, 1893.

Treasure, G.R.R. *Cardinal Richelieu and the Development of Absolutism.* New York: St. Martin's Press, 1972.

Tregelles, Samuel P. *The Jansenists: Their Rise, Persecutions by the Jesuits, and Existing Remnant: A Chapter in Church History.* London: Samuel Bagster, 1851.

Tuilier, André. *Histoire de l'Université de Paris et de la Sorbonne.* 2 vols. Paris: Nouvelle Librairie de France, 1995.

Utt, Walter C. and Brian E. Strayer. *The Bellicose Dove: Claude Brousson and Protestant Resistance to Louis XIV, 1647–1698.* Brighton & Portland: Sussex Academic Press, 2003.

Van Kley, Dale K. *The Damiens Affair and the Unraveling of the Ancien Régime, 1750.* Princeton: Princeton University Press, 1984.

——. *The Jansenists and the Expulsion of the Jesuits from France, 1757–1765.* New Haven: Yale University Press, 1975.

——. *The Religious Origins of the French Revolution: From Calvin to the Civil Constitution, 1560–1791.* New Haven, CT: Yale University Press, 1996.

Venard, Marc and Anne Bonzon. *La religion dans la France moderne XVIe–XVIIIe siècle.* Paris: Hachette, 1998.

Vidal, Daniel. *Le Malheur et son prophète: inspirés et sectaires en Languedoc calviniste, 1685–1725.* Paris: Payot, 1983.

——. *La Morte-Raison: Isaac la juive, convulsionnaire janséniste de Lyon, 1791–1841.* Grenoble: Editions Jérôme Millon, 1994.

——. *Miracles et convulsions jansénistes au XVIIIe siècle. Le mal et sa connaissance.* Paris: Presses Universitaires de France, 1987.

Weaver, F. Ellen. *The Evolution of the Reform of Port-Royal from the Rule of Cîteaux to Jansenism.* Paris: Editions Beauchesne, 1978.

——. *Madame de Fontpertuis: une dévote janséniste, amie et gérante d'Antoine Arnauld et de Port-Royal.* Paris: Klincksieck, 1998.

——. *Mademoiselle de Joncoux: polémique janséniste à la veille de la bulle Unigenitus.* Paris: Les Editions du Cerf, 2002.

Wilhelm, Jacques. *La Vie Quotidienne: Des Parisiens au temps du Roi-Soleil, 1660–1715.* Paris: Hachette, 1977.

Willaert, Léopold. *Les Origines du jansénisme dans les Pays-Bas catholiques.* Volume 1, *Le Milieu: Le Jansénisme avant la lettre.* Gembloux: Editions J. Duculot, 1948.

Wolf, John B. *Louis XIV.* New York: The Norton Library, 1968.

Woodbridge, John D. *Revolt in Prerevolutionary France: The Prince de Conti's Conspiracy against Louis XV, 1755–1757.* Baltimore, MD: Johns Hopkins University Press, 1995.

Wright, Jonathan. *God's Soldiers: Adventure, Politics, Intrigue and Power—A History of the Jesuits.* New York: Doubleday, 2004.

Index

www.ingramcontent.com/pod-product-compliance
Lightning Source LLC
LaVergne TN
LVHW081935200926
848484LV00009B/2442
* 9 7 8 1 8 4 5 1 9 2 4 5 7 *